Thieme

Shoulder Surgery

Tricks of the Trade

Joshua S. Dines, MD
Orthopaedic Surgeon
Hospital for Special Surgery
Uniondale, New York
Associate Professor
Department of Orthopaedic Surgery
Weill Cornell Medical College
New York, New York

David M. Dines, MD
Orthopaedic Surgeon
Hospital for Special Surgery
Uniondale, New York
Professor
Weill Cornell Medical College
New York, New York

Lawrence V. Gulotta, MD
Associate Attending Orthopaedic Surgeon
Hospital for Special Surgery
Uniondale, New York
Associate Professor
Department of Orthopaedic Surgery
Weill Cornell Medical College
New York, New York

476 illustrations

Thieme
New York • Stuttgart • Delhi • Rio de Janeiro

Executive Editor: William Lamsback
Managing Editor: Nikole Y. Connors
Director, Editorial Services: Mary Jo Casey
Production Editor: Torsten Scheihagen
International Production Director: Andreas Schabert
Editorial Director: Sue Hodgson
International Marketing Director: Fiona Henderson
International Sales Director: Louisa Turrell
Director of Institutional Sales: Adam Bernacki
Senior Vice President and Chief Operating Officer: Sarah Vanderbilt
President: Brian D. Scanlan
Printer: King Printing Co., Inc.
Medical illustrator: Andrea Hines
Cover design by Rebecca Symonds

Library of Congress Cataloging-in-Publication Data

Names: Dines, Joshua S., author. | Dines, David M., author. | Gulotta, Lawrence V., author.
Title: Shoulder surgery : tricks of the trade / Joshua S. Dines, MD, Orthopaedic Surgeon, Hospital for Special Surgery, Uniondale, New York, Associate Professor, Orthopaedic Surgery, Weill Cornell Medical College, New York, New York, USA, David M. Dines, MD, Orthopaedic Surgeon Hospital for Special Surgery, Uniondale, New York, Professor, Weill Cornell Medical College, New York, New York, USA, Lawrence V. Gulotta, MD, Associate Attending Orthopedic Surgeon, Hospital for Special Surgery, Uniondale, New York, Associate Professor, Orthopaedic Surgery, Weill Cornell Medical College, New York, New York, USA.
Description: First edition. | New York : Thieme, 2019. |
Identifiers: LCCN 2018054049 (print) | LCCN 2018054896 (ebook) | ISBN 9781626238077 (e-book) | ISBN 9781626235168 (print)
Subjects: LCSH: Shoulders surgery.
Classification: LCC RD557.5 (ebook) | LCC RD557.5 .D55 2019 (print) | DDC 617.5/72059--dc23
LC record available at https://lccn.loc.gov/2018054049

Thieme Publishers New York
333 Seventh Avenue, New York, NY 10001 USA
+1 800 782 3488, customerservice@thieme.com

Thieme Publishers Stuttgart
Rüdigerstrasse 14, 70469 Stuttgart, Germany
+49 [0]711 8931 421, customerservice@thieme.de

Thieme Publishers Delhi
A-12, Second Floor, Sector-2, Noida-201301
Uttar Pradesh, India
+91 120 45 566 00, customerservice@thieme.in

Thieme Publishers Rio de Janeiro, Thieme Publicações Ltda.
Edifício Rodolpho de Paoli, 25º andar
Av. Nilo Peçanha, 50 – Sala 2508
Rio de Janeiro 20020-906 Brasil
+55 21 3172-2297 / +55 21 3172-1896

Cover design: Thieme Publishing Group
Typesetting by DiTech Process Solutions

Printed in the United States of America by King Printing Co., Inc.

5 4 3 2 1

ISBN 978-1-62623-516-8

Also available as an e-book:
eISBN 978-1-62623-515-1

To Kathryn, Poppy, and my parents: Thank you for your unwavering love, support, and encouragement. And to the residents, fellows, and colleagues with whom I work: Thank you for inspiring me to always continue learning and teaching.

-Joshua S. Dines

I dedicate this text to my family for their loving support over these many years which has made it possible for me to produce this book and be successful in all other aspects of my professional career.

I also dedicate this book to my students, residents, and fellows, who by their thirst for knowledge stimulate me every day to be the best orthopedic educator and surgeon that I can be.

-David M. Dines

For my residents, fellows, and patients, who are a constant source of inspiration and education.

-Lawrence V. Gulotta

Contents

Video Legends

Video 7.1 Arthroscopic subscapularis repair.

Video 9.1 Arthroscopic rotator cuff repair with knotted and knotless margin convergence techniques.

Video 10.1 Revision RCR with patch augmentation.

Video 13.1 Shoulder arthroscopy and suprapectoral space visualization. LHB preparation. Proximal humeral intraosseous tunnel drilling and Cobra guide positioning. Two lateral bone tunnels drilling to enable two shuttle sutures passing and shuttling the holding sutures of LHB through the lateral cortex. Final placement of LHB into the bone socket and suture bridge fixation at the lateral humeral cortex.

Video 15.1 Open subpectoral biceps tenodesis.

Video 16.1 Arthroscopic biceps transfer.

Video 17.1 SLAP repair.

Video 22.1 Arthroscopic Remplissage and Bankart Repair.

Video 23.1 Arthroscopic double-row anterior stabilization, labral repair of shoulder.

Video 27.1 The Guided All-Arthroscopic Latarjet Procedure Using Cortical Button Fixation. A step by step demonstration of the surgical technique on a live patient.

Video 29.1 Revision of a failed Latarjet procedure with distal tibia allograft augmentation to the anterior glenoid.

Video 31.1 Arthroscopic Posterior Instability/Labrum Repair.

Video 34.1 Arthroscopic Modified McLaughlin Procedure Utilizing the MGHL.

Video 36.1 Arthroscopic-assisted lower trapezius tendon transfer for massive irreparable posterior-superior rotator cuff tears.

Video 38.1 Comprehensive arthroscopic management procedure for the treatment of glenohumeral osteoarthritis.

Video 41.1 Subscapularis takedown and repair during a total shoulder arthroplasty by means of a peel technique.

Video 41.2 Subscapularis tenotomy and repair during a total shoulder arthroplasty.

Video 41.3 Takedown of the subscapularis during a total shoulder arthroplasty by means of a lesser tuberosity osteotomy.

Foreword

It is an honor and privilege to write the foreword for this magnificent textbook edited by Drs. David Dines, Joshua Dines, and Lawrence Gulotta. The three editors, with their tremendous experience and the help of world renowned subject matter experts, have created an essential resource for all surgeons in training or practice to improve their knowledge of shoulder surgery.

This comprehensive textbook excels in providing clear and practical tips and techniques to effectively address a wide spectrum of shoulder pathology from rotator cuff disease and instability to arthritis and trauma. The organization of the book's content provides a logical approach to the management of shoulder disorders. The consistent layout of each of the chapters facilitates learning essential steps in pre-operative evaluation and surgical treatment. The figures have been carefully chosen to highlight the most critical steps in the surgical procedure.

One of the unique aspects of the book is the focus on the most important aspects of the operating room setup, relevant operative anatomy, awareness of potential pitfalls, and a dedicated list of pearls. There is no doubt that this book will serve as an extremely useful reference and will be used repeatedly by surgeons to expand their knowledge with essential technical information.

The editors are to be congratulated for this tremendous book and a wonderful contribution that will greatly benefit patient care worldwide.

John W. Sperling, MD, MBA
Professor and Vice-Chair
Department of Orthopedic Surgery
Mayo Clinic
Rochester, Minnesota

Preface

Shoulder surgery is a rapidly advancing field. At one end of the spectrum, more pathologies are being treated in a minimally invasive or arthroscopic fashion, and at the other end, more difficult clinical situations are being addressed with advanced arthroplasty techniques. The authors of *Shoulder Surgery: Tricks of the Trade* wrote this book with the goal of reinforcing basic principles of arthroscopy and shoulder surgery while highlighting more contemporary procedures currently being done by shoulder surgeons. To do this, an international team of expert shoulder surgeons was assembled to provide step-by-step instructions on how to perform both common and not-so-common procedures.

There are 73 chapters divided into four sections. With the goal of making this an easy-to-use resource for medical students, residents, fellows, and surgeons specializing in shoulder surgery or sports medicine, each chapter follows the same format. Indications and contraindications are discussed, details of the surgical approach and steps required to complete the procedure effectively are described, and postoperative management is outlined. Tips and pearls of each procedure are highlighted. The goal was to make each chapter high-yield in the sense that it provides the physician with the knowledge necessary to treat the patient appropriately in a concise but comprehensive format.

Contributors

Joseph A. Abboud, MD
Professor of Shoulder and Elbow Surgery
Senior Vice President Rothman Institute
The Sidney Kimmel Medical College
Thomas Jefferson University
Philadelphia, Pennsylvania

Jeffrey S. Abrams, MD
Clinical Professor, Seton Hall University
Orange, New Jersey
Senior Attending, Princeton Medical Center
Princeton, New Jersey
Clinical Association Orthopaedics, University of Pennsylvania
Philadelphia, Pennsylvania

Jens D. Agneskirchner, MD, PhD
Specialist in Orthopedics and Traumatology
Gelenkchirurgie Orthopädie
Hannover, Germany

William R. Aibinder, MD
Resident
Department of Orthopedic Surgery
Mayo Clinic
Rochester, Minnesota

Answorth A. Allen, MD
Professor Clinical Orthopedic Surgery
Weill Cornell Medical College
Attending Physician Hospital for Special Surgery
New York, New York

David W. Altchek, MD
Attending Orthopedic Surgeon
Co-Chief Emeritus, Sports Medicine Hospital for Special Surgery
Professor of Clinical Orthopedic Surgery
Weill Cornell Medical College
New York, New York

Michael Angeline, MD
Department of Orthopaedic Surgery
Mercy Health
Janesville, Wisconsin

George S. Athwal, MD, FRCSC
Associate Professor of Surgery
Clinician-Scientist
University of Western Ontario
London, Ontario, Canada

George C. Balazs, MD
Sports Medicine Service
Hospital for Special Surgery
New York, New York

Jonathan D. Barlow, MD
Shoulder and Elbow/Trauma Surgeon
Mayo Clinic
Columbus, Ohio

Jessica Bear, MD
Clinical Assistant Professor
Department of Orthopedic Surgery
University of Nevada, Las Vegas
OptumCare Orthopaedics and Spine
Las Vegas, Nevada

Asheesh Bedi, MD
Professor and Chief
Shoulder and Sports Medicine Service
University of Michigan
Ann Arbor, Michigan

Jonathan Berkowitz, MD
Attending Orthopedic Surgeon
Department of Sports Medicine
Lose Angeles Orthopedic Institute
Los Angeles, California

Pascal Boileau, MD
Head of Orthopaedic and Trauma Surgery
Nice Shoulder Institute
Nice, France

James P. Bradley, MD
Clinical Professor Orthopedics
Head Team Physician Pittsburgh Steelers
UPMC
Pittsburgh, Pennsylvania

Stephen F. Brockmeier, MD
Sports Medicine & Shoulder Surgery
Associate Professor
Department of Orthopaedic Surgery
University of Virginia
Team Physician, UVA Athletics
Director, UVA Sports Medicine Fellowship
Charlottesville Virginia

Tyler J. Brolin, MD
Clinical Instructor
Department of Orthopaedic Surgery
Campbell Clinic-University of Tennessee Health Science Center
Collierville, Tennessee

Aydin Budeyri, MD, FEBOT
Postdoctoral Research Fellow
The Shoulder Center
Baylor University Medical Center at Dallas
Dallas, Texas
Assistant Professor
Department of Orthopedics and Traumatology
SANKO University, Faculty of Medicine
Gaziantep, Turkey

Stephen S. Burkhart, MD
President, The San Antonio Orthopaedic Group
Chairman of BRIO (Burkhart Research Institute for Orthopedics)
San Antonio, Texas

Curtis A. Bush, MD
Department of Orthopaedic Surgery
Texas Health Physicians Group/ Orthopedic Specialty Associates
Fort Worth, Texas

Brandon C. Cabarcas, BS
Research Coordinator
Midwest Orthopaedics at Rush
Chicago, Illinois

Paul J. Cagle Jr., MD
Shoulder and Elbow Surgery
Assistant Professor
Associate Residence Program Director
Leni & Peter May Department of Orthopedics
Icahn School of Medicine at Mount Sinai
New York, New York

Jacob G. Calcei, MD
Orthopaedic Surgery Resident
Department of Sports Medicine and Shoulder
Hospital for Special Surgery
New York, New York

Christopher L. Camp, MD
Senior Associate Consultant
Assistant Professor of Orthopaedics
Department of Orthopedic Surgery and Sports Medicine
Mayo Clinic
Rochester, Minnesota

Lauren Casnovsky, MD
Resident
Department of Orthopaedic Surgery
University of Minnesota
Minneapolis, Minnesota

Michelle J. Chang, MD
Resident
Department of Internal Medicine
Columbia University
New York, New York

Neal C. Chen, MD
Assistant Professor
Department of Orthopaedic Surgery
Harvard Medical School
Boston, Massachusetts

John E. Conway, MD
Department of Orthopaedic Surgery
Texas Health Physicians Group/ Orthopedic Specialty Associates
Fort Worth, Texas

Frank A. Cordasco, MD, MS
Professor of Orthopaedic Surgery, Weill Cornell Medical College
Attending Surgeon, Sports Medicine and Shoulder Service
Senior Scientist, Research Division
Hospital for Special Surgery
New York, New York

Edward Craig, MD
Professor
Department of Orthopaedic Surgery
University of Minnesota
Minneapolis, Minnesota

Kathryn Crum, MD
Central Florida Bone & Joint Institute
Orange City, Florida

Derek Cuff, MD
Suncoast Orthopaedic Surgery and Sports Medicine
Venice, Florida

William E. Daner III, MD
Department of Orthopaedic Surgery
Virginia Commonwealth University Health System
Richmond, Virginia

David M. Dare
Orthopaedic Surgeon, Sports Medicine and Shoulder Surgery
Raleigh Orthopaedic Clinic
Raleigh, North Carolina

Daniel E. Davis, MD, MS
Assistant Professor
Department of Orthopaedic Surgery
Shoulder and Elbow Division
The Rothman Institute
Sidney Kimmel Medical College at Thomas Jefferson University
Philadelphia, Pennsylvania

Bradley K. Deafenbaugh, MD
Orthopaedic Trauma Surgeon
Naval Medical Center San Diego
San Diego, California

Ryan M. Degen, MSc, MD, FRCSC
Assistant Professor
Department of Surgery
Western University
London, Ontario, Canada

Patrick J. Denard, MD
Southern Oregon Orthopedics
Medford, Oregon, USA
Clinical Instructor
Department of Orthopedics and Rehabilitation
Oregon Health and Science University
Portland, Oregon

David M. Dines, MD
Orthopaedic Surgeon
Hospital for Special Surgery
Uniondale, New York
Professor
Weill Cornell Medical College
New York, New York

Joshua S. Dines, MD
Orthopaedic Surgeon
Hospital for Special Surgery
Uniondale, New York
Associate Professor
Department of Orthopaedic Surgery
Weill Cornell Medical College
New York, New York

Christopher C. Dodson, MD
Associate Professor
Department of Orthopaedic Surgery
Sidney Kimmel Medical College of Thomas Jefferson University
Philadelphia, Pennsylvania

Johanna C. E. Donders, MD
Department of Orthopedic Trauma Surgery
Hospital for Special Surgery
New York, New York

T. Bradley Edwards, MD
Attending Shoulder Surgeon
Fondren Orthopedic Group
Texas Orthopedic Hospital
Houston, Texas

Bassem T. Elhassan, MD
Professor
Department of Orthopedics
Mayo Clinic
Rochester, Minnesota

Brandon J. Erickson, MD
Sports Medicine Orthopaedic Surgeon
Department of Orthopaedic Surgery
Rothman Orthopaedics
New York, New York

Zachary J. Finley, MD
Resident
Department of Orthopaedic Surgery
Tulane University
New Orleans, Louisiana

Evan L. Flatow, MD
Lasker Professor of Orthopaedic Surgery
Icahn School of Medicine at Mount Sinai
President, Mount Sinai West
New York, New York

Salvatore J. Frangiamore, MD, MS
Orthopaedic Sports Medicine Surgeon
Summa Health
Cleveland, Ohio

Rachel M. Frank, MD
Assistant Professor
Department of Orthopaedic Surgery
University of Colorado
Boulder, Colorado

Erik M. Fritz, MD
Department of Orthopaedic Surgery
University of Minnesota
Minneapolis, Minnesota

Leesa M. Galatz, MD
Mount Sinai Professor and System Chair
Department of Orthopedic Surgery
Icahn School of Medicine, Mount Sinai Health System
New York, New York

Seth Gamradt, MD
Director of Orthopaedic Athletic Medicine
Associate Professor of Clinical Orthopaedic Surgery
Department of Orthopaedic Surgery
Keck Medical Center of the University of Southern California
Los Angeles, California

Raffaele Garofalo, MD
Director of Upper Limb Unit
F Miulli Hospital
Acquaviva delle fonti-Ba Italy

Joseph M. Gentile, MD
Novant Health Orthopedics & Sports Medicine
Huntersville, North Carolina

Anirudh K. Gowd, BS
Research Coordinator
Midwest Orthopaedics at Rush
Chicago, Illinois

Lawrence V. Gulotta, MD
Associate Attending Orthopaedic Surgeon
Hospital for Special Surgery
Uniondale, New York
Associate Professor
Department of Orthopaedic Surgery
Weill Cornell Medical College
New York, New York

Philippe Hardy, MD, PhD, Pr
Hôpital Ambroise Paré-APHP
CHU Paris Ile de France Ouest
Boulogne Billancourt, France

Samuel M. Harmsen, MD
Clinical Faculty, Shoulder and Elbow
The University of Arizona - Phoenix Orthopedic Residency
Shoulder and Elbow Specialist
The Orthopedic Clinic Association
Phoenix, Arizona

Alicia K. Harrison, MD
Assistant Professor
Department of Orthopaedic Surgery
University of Minnesota
Minneapolis, Minnesota

Robert U. Hartzler, MD, MS
Clinical Assistant Professor
Department of Orthopaedic Surgery
Baylor College of Medicine and BRIO (Burkhart Research Institute for Orthopedics)
San Antonio, Texas

Eiko Hashimoto, MD
Department of Orthopaedic Surgery
Chiba University Graduate School of Medicine
Chiba, Japan

David L. Helfet, MD
Professor
Department of Orthopaedic Surgery
Weill Cornell Medicine
Hospital for Special Surgery
New York, New York

Jessica H. Heyer, MD
Resident
Department of Orthopaedic Surgery
George Washington School of Medicine & Health Sciences
Washington, D.C.

Laurence D. Higgins, MD, MBA
Vice President of Strategic Development
Arthrex
Naples, Florida

Jason C. Ho, MD
Orthopedics Sports Medicine
Walnut Creek Medical Center
Walnut Creek, California

Malte Holschen, MD
Department for Shoulder and Elbow Surgery
Orthopedic Practice Clinic
Münster, Germany

Brandon Horn, DO
Orthopedic Surgeon
Witham Health Services
Lebanon/Zionsville, Indiana

Joseph P. Iannotti, MD, PhD
Chairman, Orthopaedic and Rheumatologic Institute
Department of Orthopaedic Surgery
Cleveland Clinic
Cleveland, Ohio

Bradley Jaquith, MD
Department of Orthopaedic Surgery
University of Tennessee-Campbell Clinic
Memphis, Tennessee

Jay D. Keener, MD
Professor
Department of Orthopedic Surgery
Washington University
St. Louis, Missouri

Jacob M. Kirsch, MD
Resident
Department of Orthopedic Surgery
University of Michigan
Ann Arbor, Michigan

Sumant G. Krishnan, MD
Director
The Shoulder Center
Baylor University Medical Center at Dallas
Dallas, Texas

Neil S. Kumar, MD, MBA
Department of Orthopaedic Surgery
UConn Health
Farmington, Connecticut

Laurent Lafosse, MD
Chairman
Alps Surgery Institute
Clinique Générale d'Annecy
Annecy, France

Philippe Landreau, MD
Assistant Professor of Clinical Orthopaedic Surgery
Chief of Surgery
Aspetar (Qatar Orthopaedic and Sports Medicine Hospital)
Doha, Qatar

Lionel E. Lazaro, MD
Fellow
Department of Orthopaedic Surgery-Sports Medicine
Kerlan-Jobe Orthopedic Institute
Los Angeles, California

Mark D. Lazarus, MD
Professor
The Rothman Institute
Department of Orthopaedic Surgery
Sidney Kimmel Medical College
Thomas Jefferson University
Philadelphia, Pennsylvania

Evan S. Lederman, MD
The Orthopedic Association, PC
Phoenix, Arizona

William N. Levine, MD
Frank E. Stinchfield Professor and Chair
NYP/Columbia University Irving Medical Center
New York, New York

Jonathan C. Levy, MD
Shoulder & Elbow Surgery
Chief of Orthopedics, Holy Cross Orthopedic Institute
Program Director, Holy Cross Shoulder & Elbow Fellowship
Medical Director, Holy Cross Orthopedic Research Institute
Holy Cross Orthopedic Institute
Fort Lauderdale, Florida

Xinning (Tiger) Li, MD
Associate Professor
Sports Medicine and Shoulder Surgery
Department of Orthopaedic Surgery
Boston University School of Medicine
Boston Medical Center
Boston, Massachusetts

Orr Limpisvasti, MD
Orthopaedic Surgeon
Kerlan-Jobe Orthopaedic Surgeon
Los Angeles, California

Robert B. Litchfield, MD, FRCSC
Medical Director, Fowler Kennedy Sport Medicine Clinic
University of Western Ontario
London, Ontario, Canada

Josh Locker, MD
Resident
Department of Orthopaedic Surgery and Rehabilitation
University of Nebraska Medical Center
Omaha, Nebraska

Dean G. Lorich, MD (deceased)
Associate Director
Department of Orthopaedic Trauma Service
Hospital for Special Surgery, New York Presbyterian Hospital
Weill Cornell Medicine
New York, New York

Jared M. Mahylis, MD
Orthopedic Surgeon
Specialty Physicians of Illinois, LLC
Olympia Fields, Illinois

Devin R. Mangold, MD
Resident Physician
Department of Orthopedic Surgery
Mayo Clinic
Rochester, Minnesota

Sandeep Mannava, MD, PhD
Assistant Professor
Department of Orthopaedics
University of Rochester Medical Center
Rochester, New York

Benjamin Marjanovic, MD
Head of the Department of Arthroscopy and Sports Orthopedic
Orthopedic Hospital Valdoltra
Ankaran, Slovenia

Augustus D. Mazzocca, MS, MD
Professor
Department of Orthopaedic Surgery
UConn Health
Farmington, Connecticut

Lucas S. McDonald, MD, MPHTM, CDR MC USN
Assistant Professor of Surgery USUHS
Department of Orthopaedic Surgery
Naval Medical Center San Diego
San Diego, California

Michael H. McGraw, MD
Assistant Team Physician East Carolina University
Orthopaedics East and Sports Medicine Center
Greenville, North Carolina

Sean McIntire, MD, LCDR MC USN
Department of Orthopaedic Surgery
Naval Medical Center San Diego
San Diego, California

Heather M. Menzer, MD
Department of Orthopedic Surgery & Sports Medicine
Phoenix Children's Medical Group
Phoenix, Arizona

Teruhisa Mihata, MD, PhD
Director, Shoulder and Elbow Surgery, and Sports Medicine
Associate Professor, Department of Orthopedic Surgery
Osaka Medical College
Takatsuki, Osaka, Japan

Peter J. Millett, MD, MSc
Chief Medical Officer
Director of Shoulder Surgery
Shoulder, Knee, Elbow, and Sports Medicine Orthopaedic Surgery
The Steadman Clinic
Vail, Colorado

Kyong S. Min, MD
Assistant Professor
Department of Orthopaedic Surgery
Tripler Army Medical Center
Honolulu, Hawaii

Justin J. Mitchell, MD
Orthopaedics Sports Medicine Surgeon
Gunderson Health System
La Crosse, Wisconsin

Colin P. Murphy, BA
MD Candidate
Georgetown University School of Medicine
Washington, DC

Andrew S. Neviaser, MD
Associate Professor of Orthopaedic Surgery
Shoulder Division
Ohio State University Wexner Medical Center
Columbus, Ohio

Tom Norris, MD
Past President
American Shoulder and Elbow Surgeons
Fellowship Director
San Francisco Shoulder, Elbow, and Hand Clinic
California Pacific Medical Center
San Francisco, California

Alejandro Novoa-Boldo, MD
Shoulder Fellow
Sports Medicine and Shoulder Service
Hospital for Special Surgery
New York, New York

Matthew P. Noyes, MD
Canton Orthopaedic Institute
Canton, Ohio
Clinical Instructor
Northeast Ohio University College of Medicine
Rootstown, Ohio

Michael O'Brien, MD
Physician, Sports Medicine Division Boston Children's Hospital
Director, Sports Concussion Clinic
Assistant Professor of Orthopedic Surgery
Harvard Medical School
Boston, Massachusetts

Stephen J. O'Brien, MD, MS
Attending Orthopaedic Surgeon
Hospital for Special Surgery
Professor of Clinical Orthopaedic Surgery
Department of Orthopedic Surgery
Weill Cornell Medical College
New York, New York

Joo Han Oh, MD, PhD
Professor
Chief, Shoulder Surgery & Sports Medicine Division
Department of Orthopaedic Surgery
Seoul National University College of Medicine
Chairman, Joint Reconstruction Center
Seoul National University Bundang Hospital
Seoul, South Korea

Victor A. Olujimi, MD
Shoulder & Elbow Fellow
Leni & Peter May Department of Orthopedics
Icahn School of Medicine at Mount Sinai
New York, New York

Dean N. Papaliodis, MD
Department of Orthopaedic Surgery
Texas Health Physicians Group/ Orthopedic Specialty Associates
Fort Worth, Texas

Nicholas R. Pagani, MD
Resident Physician
Department of Orthopaedic Surgery
Tufts University School of Medicine
Boston, Massachusetts

Bradford O. Parsons, MD
Surgery/Residency Director
Leni & Peter W. May Department of Orthopaedic Surgery
Icahn School of Medicine at Mount Sinai Medical Center
Mount Sinai Hospital
New York, New York

Nirav K. Patel, MD, FRCS
Assistant Professor
Department of Orthopaedic Surgery
Virginia Commonwealth University
Richmond, Virginia

Brendan M. Patterson, MD
Department Chair
Department of Orthopaedic Surgery
Cleveland Clinic
Cleveland, Ohio

Diana Patterson, MD
Resident
Department of Orthopedic Surgery
Icahn School of Medicine, Mount Sinai Health System
New York, New York

Liam A. Peebles, BA
Research Coordinator
Center for Outcomes-Based Orthopaedic Research
The Steadman Philippon Research Institute
Vail, Colorado

Christos D. Photopoulos, MD
Orthopaedic Surgeon
Kerlan-Jobe Orthopaedic Clinic
Los Angeles, California

Boris Poberaj, MD
Orthopaedic Surgeon
Department of Surgery
Aspetar (Qatar Orthopaedic and Sports Medicine Hospital)
Doha, Qatar

Matthew T. Provencher, MD, MC, USNR
Shoulder, Knee, and Sports Surgeon
The Steadman Clinic
The Steadman Philippon Research Institute
Vail, Colorado

Richard Puzzitiello, BS
Midwest Orthopaedics at Rush
Rush University Medical Center
Chicago, Illinois

Prem N. Ramkumar, MD
Resident
Department of Orthopaedic Surgery
Cleveland Clinic
Cleveland, Ohio

Matthew L. Ramsey, MD
Professor of Orthopaedic Surgery
Sidney Kimmel College of Medicine at Thomas Jefferson University
Chief, Shoulder and Elbow Service
Rothman Institute
Philadelphia, Pennsylvania

Jonathan C. Riboh, MD
Assistant Professor
Department of Orthopaedic Surgery
Duke University School of Medicine
Durham, North Carolina

Eric T. Ricchetti, MD
Associate Professor
Director, Shoulder Center
Director, Shoulder and Elbow Surgery Fellowship Program
Department of Orthopedic Surgery, Cleveland Clinic
Cleveland, Ohio

Kent Rinehart, MD
Resident
Department of Orthopaedic Surgery and Rehabilitation
University of Nebraska Medical Center
Omaha, Nebraska

Anthony A. Romeo, MD
Chief of Orthopaedics
Rothman Orthopaedic Institute- New York
New York, New York

Frank Russo, MD
Resident Physician
Department of Orthopaedic Surgery
Keck Medical Center of USC
Los Angeles, California

Ramin Sadeghpour, MD
Maimonides Bone & Joint Center
Brooklyn, New York

David Saliken, MD, FRCSC
Clinical Instructor
Department of Orthopedic Surgery
University of British Columbia, RebalanceMD
Victoria, BC, Canada

Anthony Sanchez, BS
MD Candidate
School of Medicine, Oregon Health & Science University
Portland, Oregon

George Sanchez, BS
MD Candidate
Geisel School of Medicine at Dartmouth
Hanover, New Hampshire

C. Craig Satterlee, MD
Shoulder and Elbow Surgery
Drisko, Fee and Parkins Orthopaedics
Kansas City, Missouri

Felix H. Savoie, MD
Ray J. Haddad Professor and Chairman
Department of Orthopaedics
Tulane University School of Medicine
New Orleans, Louisiana

Mark A. Schrumpf, MD
Orthopaedic Surgeon
San Francisco Shoulder, Elbow and Hand Clinic
San Francisco, California

Sarav S. Shah, MD
Orthopaedic Shoulder Reconstruction Fellow
Hospital for Special Surgery
New York, New York

Andrew J. Sheean, MD
Department of Orthopaedic Surgery
University of Pittsburgh
Pittsburgh, Pennsylvania

Dave R. Shukla, MD
Shoulder and Elbow Surgery
Newport Orthopedic Institute
Newport Beach, California

Danielle N. Sin
Cardiothoracic Surgery Research Coordinator
NYU Langone Health
New York, New York

John W. Sperling, MD, MBA
Professor and Vice-Chair
Department of Orthopedic Surgery
Mayo Clinic
Rochester, Minnesota

Samuel R.H. Steiner, MD
Sports Orthopedic Surgeon
Orthopaedic Associates of Wisconsin
Pewaukee, Wisconsin

Matthew A. Tao, MD
Assistant Professor
Department of Orthopaedic Surgery
University of Nebraska Medical Center
Omaha, Nebraska

Samuel A. Taylor, MD
Assistant Attending Surgeon
Hospital for Special Surgery
Sports Medicine and Shoulder Service Assistant Professor
Weill Cornell Medical College
New York, New
York

André Thès, MD
Assistant Professor
Department of Orthopedic Surgery
Hôpital Ambroise Paré - APHP
Boulogne Billancourt, France

Matthew M. Thompson, MD
Assistant Professor
Department of Orthopaedic Surgery
University of Maryland School of Medicine
Baltimore, Maryland

Thomas (Quin) Throckmorton, MD
Professor
Shoulder and Elbow Surgery
Residency Program Director
University of Tennessee-Campbell Clinic
Department of Orthopaedic Surgery
Memphis, Tennessee

Camden Tissue, MD
Assistant Professor
Department of Orthopedic Surgery
University of Texas at Houston
Houston, Texas

Fotios P. Tjoumakaris, MD
Associate Professor
Department of Orthopaedic Surgery
Sidney Kimmel College of Medicine, Thomas Jefferson University
Rothman Orthopaedic Institute
Philadelphia, Pennsylvania

Philippe Valenti, MD
Paris Shoulder Unit
Clinique Bizet
Paris, France

Carola F. van Eck, MD, PhD
Team Physician Robert Morris University
Team Physician Pittsburgh Passion Women's Football
Co-Medical Director Orthopaedic Engineering & Sports Medicine Laboratory
Assistant Professor Orthopaedic Surgery, School of Medicine, Department of Orthopaedic Surgery
Assistant Professor of Sports Medicine and Nutrition,
School of Health and Rehabilitation Sciences,
Department of Sports Medicine and Nutrition
University of Pittsburgh Medical Center
Rooney Sports Complex
Pittsburgh Pennsylvania

Danica D. Vance, MD
Resident
New York Presbyterian/ Columbia Orthopedics
New York, New York

Shreya Veera, BS
Research Coordinator
Midwest Orthopaedics at Rush
Chicago, Illinois

Nikhil N. Verma, MD
Professor and Director, Division of Sports Medicine
Fellowship Director, Sports Medicine
Department of Orthopedics
Rush University Medical Center
Midwest Orthopedics at Rush
Team Physician, Chicago White Sox/Chicago Bulls
Chicago, Illinois

Wame N. Waggenspack, Jr., MD
Shoulder, Elbow, and Sports Medicine
Baton Rouge Orthopaedic Clinic
Baton Rouge, Louisana

Tim Wang, MD
Clinical Assistant Professor
Department of Orthopaedic Surgery
Stanford University School of Medicine
Stanford, California

Jon J.P. Warner, MD
Chief, MGH Shoulder Service
Chair Quality and Safety Committee for Orthopedics
Massachusetts General Hospital
Professor of Orthopaedic Surgery
Harvard Medical School
Director, Boston Shoulder Institute
Boston, Massachusetts

Russell Warren, MD
Attending Orthopedic Surgeon
Hospital for Special Surgery
Professor of Orthopedic Surgery
Weill Cornell Medical College
New York, New York

Brian R. Waterman, MD
Associate Professor, Sports Medicine
Team Physician, Wake Forest University Athletics
Team Physician, Winston-Salem Dash / Chicago White Sox
Department of Orthopaedic Surgery
Wake Forest University School of Medicine Medical Center Boulevard
Winston-Salem, North Carolina

David S. Wellman, MD
Assistant Professor
Department of Orthopedic Surgery
Hospital for Special Surgery
Weill Cornell Medical College
New York, New York

Brian C. Werner, MD
Assistant Professor
Department of Orthopaedic Surgery
University of Virginia
Team Physician, James Madison University
Charlottesville, Virginia

Helen S. Zitkovsky, BA
Medical Student
Tufts University School of Medicine
Boston, Massachusetts

Part I

Rotator Cuff/Biceps

1 Subacromial Decompression and Acromioplasty

Jessica H. Heyer and Andrew S. Neviaser

Abstract
Subacromial decompression and acromioplasty are used to treat shoulder impingement symptoms refractory to nonoperative management. This chapter will review the preoperative considerations for determining whether a patient is a candidate for a subacromial decompression and the procedural steps for performing a subacromial decompression and acromioplasty in the beach-chair position. It will conclude with ways to avoid and manage complications.

Keywords: *rotator cuff disease, impingement, acromioplasty, subacromial decompression*

1.1 Goals of Procedure

Subacromial impingement is one of the most common causes of anterior shoulder pain and occurs when the undersurface of the anterior acromion compresses the subacromial bursa, supraspinatus insertion, and biceps tendon during elevation of the arm. This was long considered the primary cause of rotator cuff tearing,[1] but is now thought to be a consequence of rotator cuff dysfunction resulting in loss of effective humeral head depression. Decompression of the acromion's undersurface increases the size of the subacromial space, allowing for unfettered movement of the rotator cuff and bursa as well as diminished pain. An arthroscopic approach to acromioplasty has many advantages over open approaches and is now the most popular method of decompression.

1.2 Advantages

Historically, subacromial decompression and acromioplasty were done through an open approach. An oblique incision was made from the anterolateral corner of the acromion to just lateral to the coracoid, to expose the coracoacromial (CA) ligament and the undersurface of the anterior acromion.[2] This approach required detachment and reattachment of the deltoid, and longer postoperative rehabilitation, and could result in chronic deltoid dehiscence. Arthroscopic treatment is a minimally invasive technique that, when compared to open acromioplasty, allows for earlier return to work, reduced complications, and superior long-term functional results.[3,4] Arthroscopy also allows for visualization of the glenohumeral joint as well as the subacromial space, providing a more comprehensive assessment of the shoulder. Rotator cuff and biceps pathology can be concurrently treated through the same portals used for decompression

1.3 Indications

Subacromial decompression is indicated for patients with symptoms of shoulder impingement that are refractory to nonsurgical treatment. This procedure is often done in conjunction with rotator cuff repair and biceps tenodesis. The diagnosis of shoulder impingement is made based on history and physical examination. Patients typically report pain on the anterior aspect of the shoulder often radiating to the biceps and/or the deltoid insertion. Symptoms are typically exacerbated by elevation of the arm above shoulder level and with internal rotation. Several tests for impingement have been described and found to be sensitive, but not specific.[5] In addition to impingement tests, a comprehensive physical examination should include rotator cuff strength testing, as well as palpation and provocative testing of the biceps.

Radiographs should include a true anteroposterior view of the shoulder (Grashey view), axillary view, and a scapular outlet view. The scapular outlet view allows for assessment of acromial morphology and pathology. Bigliani et al classified the acromion morphologically: type I being flat, type II curved, and type III hooked.[6] Type III morphology has the strongest association with full-thickness rotator cuff tears.

The critical shoulder angle as described by Moor et al is another exciting radiographic assessment of the shoulder.[7] This angle is subtended by a line drawn along the vertical inclination of the glenoid and a tangent to the most lateral extent of the acromion. Larger angles are associated with rotator cuff pathology, whereas smaller angles may correlate with the development of osteoarthritis. Further investigation of this measurement is needed before it can alter the method of routine acromioplasty, however. MRI is useful for defining the severity of other shoulder pathology including the extent of rotator cuff tearing.

The initial treatment of shoulder impingement is nonoperative. Patients can be offered a subacromial cortisone injection and physical therapy, both of which have been shown to be successful in the management of shoulder impingement. When nonsurgical management has failed, a subacromial decompression can be considered. In the absence of full-thickness rotator cuff tearing, physical therapy lasting 6 to 12 weeks and one or two injections are reasonable trials of nonoperative management.

1.4 Contraindications

The main contraindication to a complete subacromial decompression is an unrepairable anterosuperior rotator cuff tear. In the absence of the anterosuperior rotator cuff, the CA arch prevents superior escape of the humeral head. Loss of the arch, typically from resection of the CA ligament, results in complete loss of elevation because the humerus has no stable foundation to act as a fulcrum during elevation (superior escape). In the setting of such a tear, a limited decompression can be done with preservation of the CA ligament and superior escape avoided.

Os acromiale is typically an asymptomatic, incidental finding, but has been implicated in shoulder impingement. This is thought to be due to separate bony components of the acromion moving in opposition and causing compression of the anterior shoulder tendons during elevation.[8] If the os acromiale is stable (i.e., the components move as one unit), subacromial decompression can be utilized, but care should be taken to avoid excessive bony resection leading to a painful mobile os. An unstable os acromiale are those that are tender to palpation and have significant mobility between components. Prior to decompression of an unstable os acromiale, fusion with internal fixation is recommended to avoid persistent pain at the fibrous connection.

1.5 Preoperative Preparation/ Positioning

Imaging, both radiographs and MRI, is essential for preoperative planning, particularly when determining what other procedures may need to be performed.

The authors prefer a beach-chair position with a limb positioner, which can be used for mild traction. The patient is seated sufficiently upright so that the acromion is parallel to the floor. Anatomic landmarks are marked. The clavicle, acromion, scapular spine, and coracoid process are drawn out.

1.6 Operative Technique

The posterior portal is made approximately 1 cm inferior and 1 cm medial to the posterolateral corner of the acromion in the "soft spot" of the glenohumeral joint. By aiming the trocar toward the coracoid, it can be inserted atraumatically into the joint. The anterior portal is made just lateral to the coracoid, and should be placed through the rotator interval, inferior to the biceps tendon and slightly lateral to superior glenohumeral ligament. After the joint is inspected and intra-articular pathology addressed, the camera is inserted into the subacromial space. This is done using the same posterior portal and sliding the trocar along the deep surface of the acromion. It is then pushed to the anterior aspect of the subacromial space until it contacts the insertion of the CA ligament. Once the ligament is reached, firm resistance is felt. The camera is then pulled posteriorly with lens directed superiorly to visualize the ligament and anterolateral acromion.

The lateral portal is the main working portal for subacromial decompression. It is made in line with the posterior border of the clavicle, approximately 2 cm inferior to the lateral acromion. A spinal needle can be used to guide portal placement. The optimal position of the needle is parallel and immediately superior to the rotator cuff (**Fig. 1.1**). This allows for easy manipulation of the burr underneath the acromion.

An arthroscopic electrocautery device is inserted through the lateral portal and the subacromial bursa ablated to visualize the subacromial space, rotator cuff, and inferior aspect of the acromion. Complete resection of the soft tissue off the acromion at this stage aids in the later bony work.

The CA ligament is resected off of the acromion with the electrocautery. A relaxing incision can be made along the lateral border of the ligament to release it from the deltoid. This allows for complete resection of the ligament via a biting tool rather than simply releasing it from the acromion (**Fig. 1.2**).

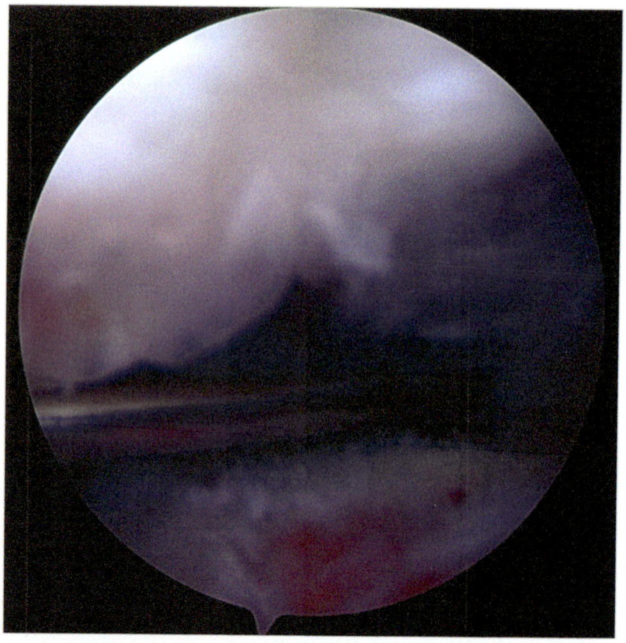

Fig. 1.1 This view from the posterior portal in a left shoulder demonstrates optimal position of the spinal needle to direct positioning of a lateral subacromial portal. The needle sits superior and parallel to the rotator cuff (bottom).

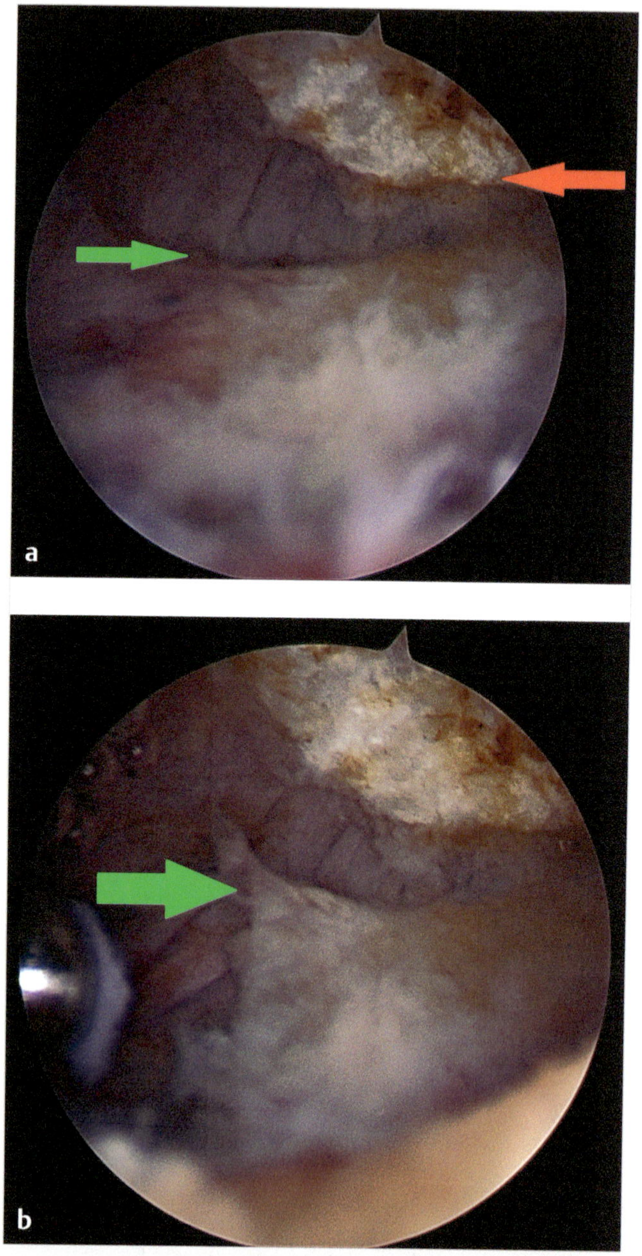

Fig. 1.2 **(a)** Viewing a left shoulder from the posterior portal: the coracoacromial ligament (*green arrow*) has been released from the anterolateral acromion but remains adherent to the deep surface of the deltoid. **(b)** The lateral margin of the ligament has been released with the electrocautery device. This exposes an edge (*green arrow*) that can be used to excise the ligament.

A burr is inserted through the lateral portal and positioned on the anterolateral corner of the acromion. The goal of bone resection is to produce a flat acromial undersurface. The anterolateral corner is resected to the desired level establishing the amount of the resection for the remainder of the bone (**Fig. 1.3**). Care is taken to avoid detachment of the deltoid insertion. Most arthroscopic burrs have a guard that can be used to avoid contacting the proximal tendinous deltoid attachment (**Fig. 1.4**). Once the entire acromion is flattened to the desired level, the arthroscope is moved to the lateral portal to evaluate the transition zone between the resected portion and the unresected portion (**Fig. 1.5**). The transition zone can be smoothed with the burr brought through the posterior portal (**Fig. 1.6**). The acromion should be viewed

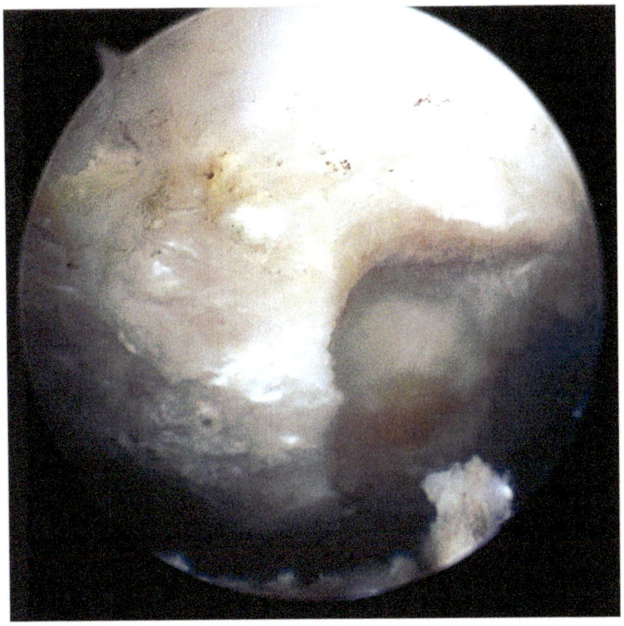

Fig. 1.3 Viewing a right shoulder from the posterior portal: the amount of resection has been established on the lateral side. The remainder of the acromial can now be resected to match this height. Working in a stepwise fashion helps avoid excessive removal of bone and minimizes the risk of fracture.

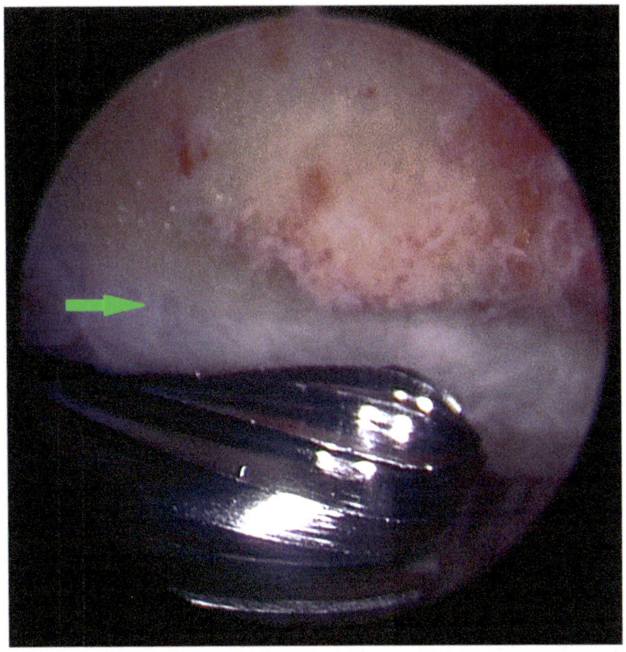

Fig. 1.4 Viewing a left shoulder from the posterior portal: the burr, brought from the lateral portal, is rotated so that the tendinous deltoid insertion (*green arrow*) is protected from the blades. This allows the anterior margin of the acromion to be resected atraumatically.

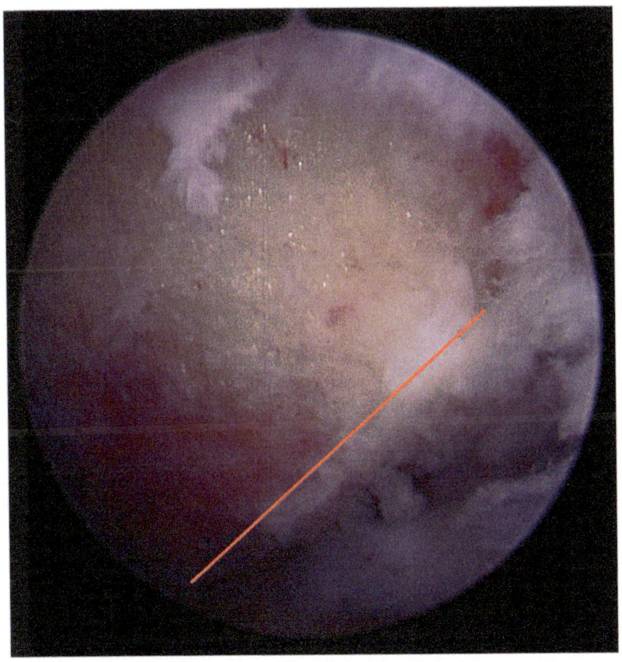

Fig. 1.5 Viewing a left shoulder from the lateral portal: the transition zone (*red line*) often remains prominent after initial resection. The burr can then be inserted through the posterior portal to address this area.

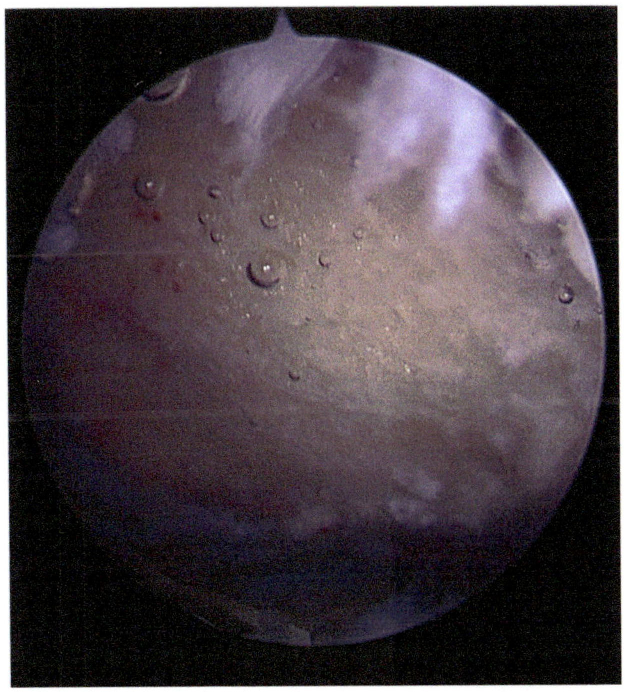

Fig. 1.6 The final results viewed from the lateral portal in a left shoulder is a flat acromion.

from both portals to ensure that the final result is a flat acromion (**Fig. 1.6**).

1.7 Tips and Pearls/Expert Suggestions

- Establishing a lateral portal that permits the burr to be held parallel to the acromion is a critical step and allows for a smooth bony resection. Establishing the portal position with a spinal needle aids in achieving perfect portal placement.
- Spurs on the deep surface of the acromioclavicular joint can also be resected without concern for aggravating previously asymptomatic arthritis of this joint.
- In the setting of a massive rotator cuff tear, limited acromioplasty with preservation of the CA ligament avoids the devastating complication of anterosuperior escape.

1.8 What to Avoid

Care should be taken to avoid releasing the proximal deltoid attachment from the acromion. This has be demonstrated to diminish abduction strength and most commonly occurs during exposure of the lateral and anterior acromial margins.[9] Careful dissection with the electrocautery device and use of the burr guard during resection at the acromial edges minimizes deltoid damage.

Excessive bony resection can lead to a thin acromion that is prone to fracture. There is no singular amount of resection that can be applied to every patient. Creating a flat acromion that opens the subacromial space is the main goal of this procedure and should be the guiding principle for resection. Establishing the desired amount of resection at the lateral acromial edge initially and then completing that amount of resection across the remaining acromion allows for a controlled amount of bone removal.

1.9 Complications/Bailout/Salvage

Fortunately, complications from subacromial decompression are rare. The most devastating is anterosuperior escape. This is only recognized postoperatively and is best treated by prevention. Care should be taken to avoid disruption of the CA arch in the setting of large rotator cuff tears even when they are repairable. Avoiding resection of the CA ligament does not have detrimental effects on outcomes following repair of large tears.[10] If the anterosuperior escape does occur, reverse shoulder arthroplasty provides the most reliable functional outcome. Other, less invasive techniques, such as superior capsular reconstruction, remain unproven at this time but could become an acceptable alternative treatment in younger patients.

1.10 Postoperative Care

Postoperatively the patient is placed into either a sling or an abduction brace. An abduction brace is utilized if there was a concurrent rotator cuff repair performed. Our patients typically receive regional analgesia via a peripheral nerve block preoperatively and are discharged with a pump that allows for continuous infusion for 3 to 5 days. Patients are discharged from the postanesthesia care unit (PACU) to home. They receive a multimodal regime of oral analgesics, including a short-acting narcotic, a long-acting narcotic, and medication addressing neuropathic pain (i.e., gabapentin or pregabalin).

The postoperative regimen is dependent on what other procedures were performed. If a subacromial decompression and acromioplasty were performed in isolation, the patient can start passive range of motion of the shoulder on postoperative day 1. If a patient has a rotator cuff repair, the shoulder is typically immobilized for 6 weeks before range-of-motion exercises are begun.

References

1. Neer CS II. Impingement lesions. Clin Orthop Relat Res 1983(173):70–77
2. Neer CS II. Anterior acromioplasty for the chronic impingement syndrome in the shoulder: a preliminary report. J Bone Joint Surg Am 1972;54(1):41–50
3. Davis AD, Kakar S, Moros C, Kaye EK, Schepsis AA, Voloshin I. Arthroscopic versus open acromioplasty: a meta-analysis. Am J Sports Med 2010;38(3):613–618
4. Odenbring S, Wagner P, Atroshi I. Long-term outcomes of arthroscopic acromioplasty for chronic shoulder impingement syndrome: a prospective cohort study with a minimum of 12 years' follow-up. Arthroscopy 2008; 24(10):1092–1098
5. Park HB, Yokota A, Gill HS, El Rassi G, McFarland EG. Diagnostic accuracy of clinical tests for the different degrees of subacromial impingement syndrome. J Bone Joint Surg Am 2005;87(7):1446–1455
6. Bigliani BU, Morrison ES, April EW. The morphology of the acromion and its relationship to rotator cuff tears. Orthop Trans 1986;10:216
7. Moor BK, Bouaicha S, Rothenfluh DA, Sukthankar A, Gerber C. Is there an association between the individual anatomy of the scapula and the development of rotator cuff tears or osteoarthritis of the glenohumeral joint?: A radiological study of the critical shoulder angle. Bone Joint J 2013;95-B(7):935–941
8. Kurtz CA, Humble BJ, Rodosky MW, Sekiya JK. Symptomatic os acromiale. J Am Acad Orthop Surg 2006; 14(1):12–19
9. Rockwood CA Jr, Williams GR Jr, Burkhead WZ Jr. Débridement of degenerative, irreparable lesions of the rotator cuff. J Bone Joint Surg Am 1995;77(6):857–866
10. Fealy S, April EW, Khazzam M, Armengol-Barallat J, Bigliani LU. The coracoacromial ligament: morphology and study of acromial enthesopathy. J Shoulder Elbow Surg 2005;14(5):542–548

2 Arthroscopic Acromioclavicular Joint Resection

Jeffrey S. Abrams

Abstract

Acromioclavicular joint arthritis is a common shoulder etiology of pain and contributes to bursal compression of the supraspinatus. Isolated resection has previously been performed with an open procedure. An arthroscopic approach can be performed that removes the clavicle facet from the acromion and combines distal clavicle excision, centering the decompression and preserves the joint capsule. The direct method can be performed within the capsule with smaller instruments for painful clavicle osteolysis. The indirect bursal approach can combine a subacromial decompression with distal clavicle excision. This can be applied to a patient with impingement and bursal sided rotator cuff pathology.

Keywords: *acromioclavicular joint arthritis, arthroscopic Mumford procedure, distal clavicle excision*

2.1 Goals of Procedure

The goals of arthroscopic acromioclavicular joint (ACJ) resection are to decompress and create a space between the acromion and arthritic clavicle, and preserve the ACJ capsule. The indirect approach utilizes an arthroscope placed in the subacromial bursa and resects bone, beginning along the inferior margins and progressing to the superior capsule. Capsular boundaries are limited, so resection is partially achieved from the acromion, and the balance of the 1-cm resection is accomplished with distal clavicle resection (**Fig. 2.1**).

2.2 Advantages

The dorsal and posterior capsular stabilizing ligaments are not cut when performing decompression of the ACJ. By centering the decompression, the medial capsular extension of the capsuloligaments and the coracoclavicular (CC) ligaments are preserved. Cosmesis and avoiding a painful scar in the area of a shoulder strap is an advantage of the arthroscopic approach. Also, visualization of the glenohumeral articulation can be achieved using the same portals.

2.3 Indications

- Unresponsive pain to nonoperative treatment for a 6-month period.
- Painful distal clavicle osteolysis in a younger patient with repetitive stresses.
- Treatment of soft-tissue ganglions that extend from the glenohumeral joint via a rotator cuff defect.

2.4 Contraindications

- Traumatic ACJ capsular injury that may exacerbate symptoms with distal clavicle excision.
- Unstable os acromiale can be further destabilized with distal clavicle resection.
- Revision surgery where prior distal clavicle resection has resected the medial ACJ capsule.

2.5 Preoperative Planning/ Positioning

- Clinical examination identifying symptomatic ACJ: direct palpation and cross-chest provocative testing.
- Imaging studies: radiograph (**Fig. 2.2**) and MRI (**Fig. 2.3**).
- Beach-chair or lateral decubitus.

2.6 Operative Technique

- Examination under anesthesia.
- Marking structures, landmarks, and portal placement (**Fig. 2.4**).
- Glenohumeral joint inflation with saline.
- Posterior portal: outside-in technique.
- Anterior portal:
  - Skin inferior to ACJ entering rotator interval.
- Replace viewing portal via the posterior puncture into the subacromial space.

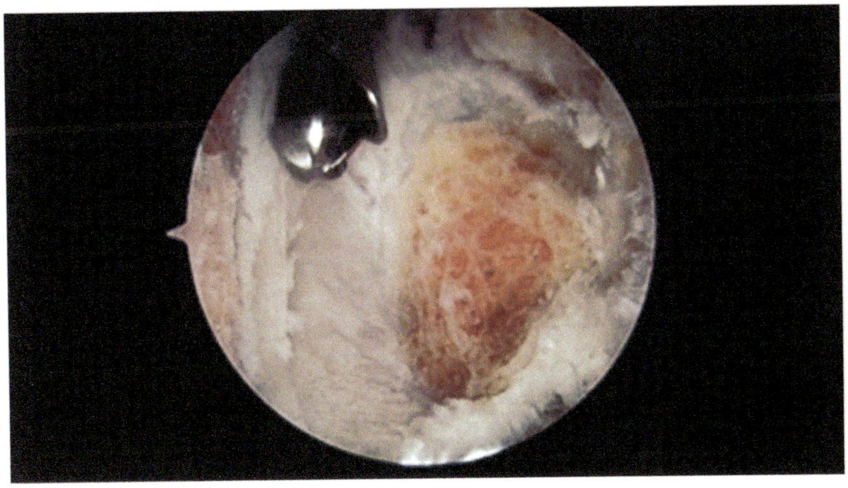

Fig. 2.1 Complete distal clavicle resection with preserved dorsal and posterior capsule.

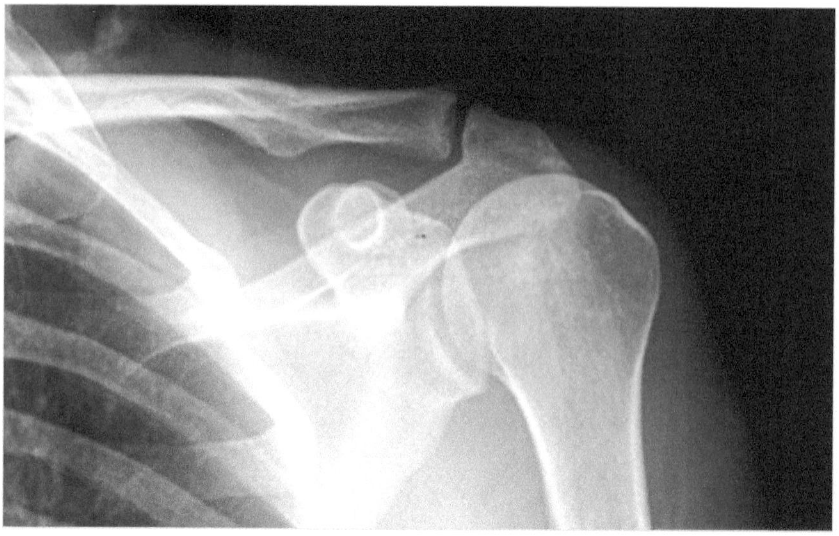

Fig. 2.2 Anteroposterior radiograph of arthritic acromioclavicular joint.

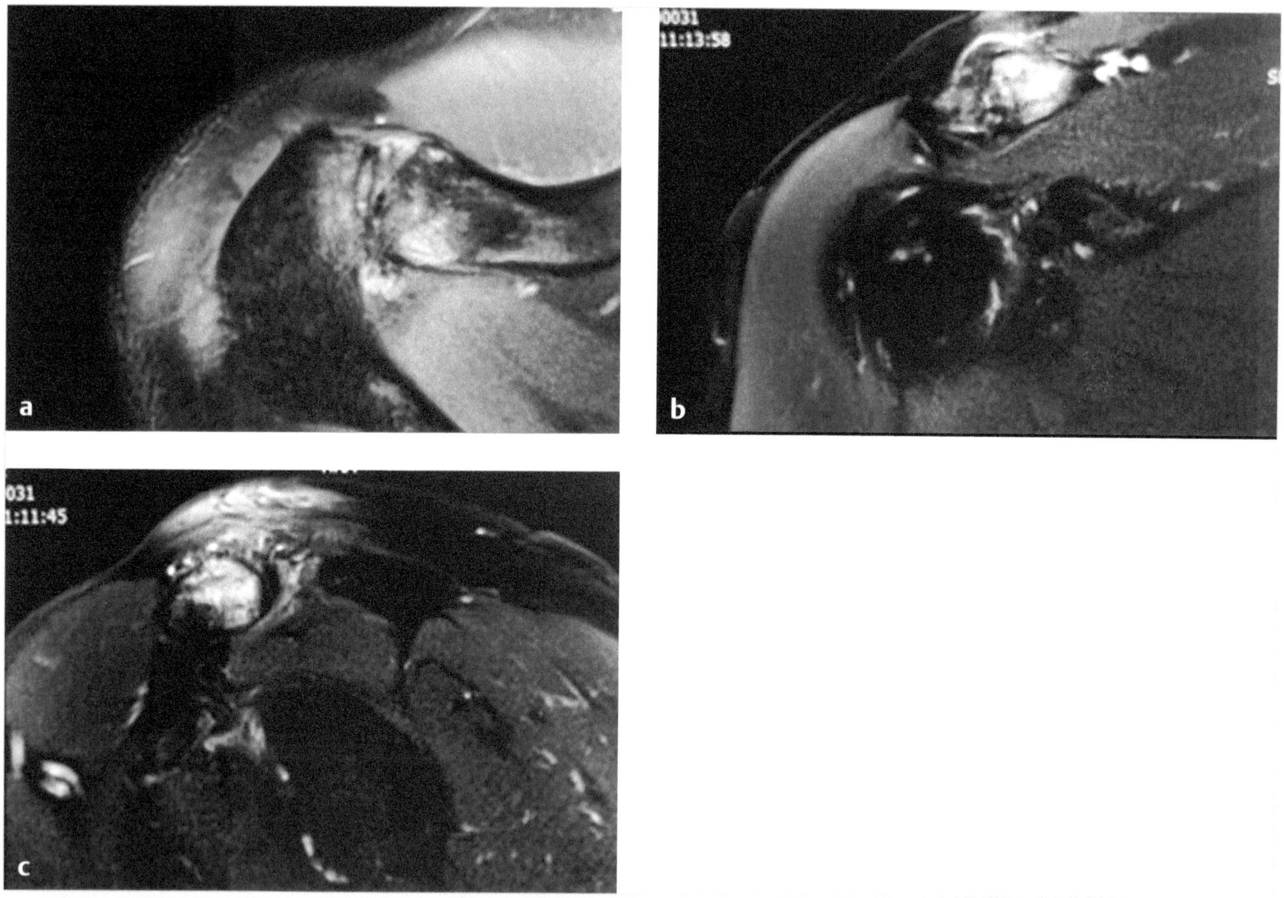

Fig. 2.3 MRI of symptomatic acromioclavicular pain.

- Create a lateral bursal portal in line with midclavicle with the acromion, 3 cm lateral.
- Bursectomy.
- Subacromial resection performed via the posterior and lateral viewing portals (**Fig. 2.5**).
- Place scope in the posterior viewing portal and introduce cannula in the anterior portal (**Fig. 2.6**).
- Use shaver and cautery to debride soft tissue beneath the ACJ.
- Begin decompression by resecting the clavicle facet of the acromion in an anterior-to-posterior direction. Superior visualization of the distal clavicle is achieved (**Fig. 2.7**).
- Anterior clavicle resection is begun through the anterior portal beginning along the inferior surface and progressing to the capsule (**Fig. 2.8**).
- The posterior clavicle resection continues by elevating the posterior capsuloligaments and resecting bone with the capsule (**Fig. 2.9**).
- Symmetric resection is achieved and confirmed from posterior, lateral, and anterior viewing portals (**Fig. 2.10**).

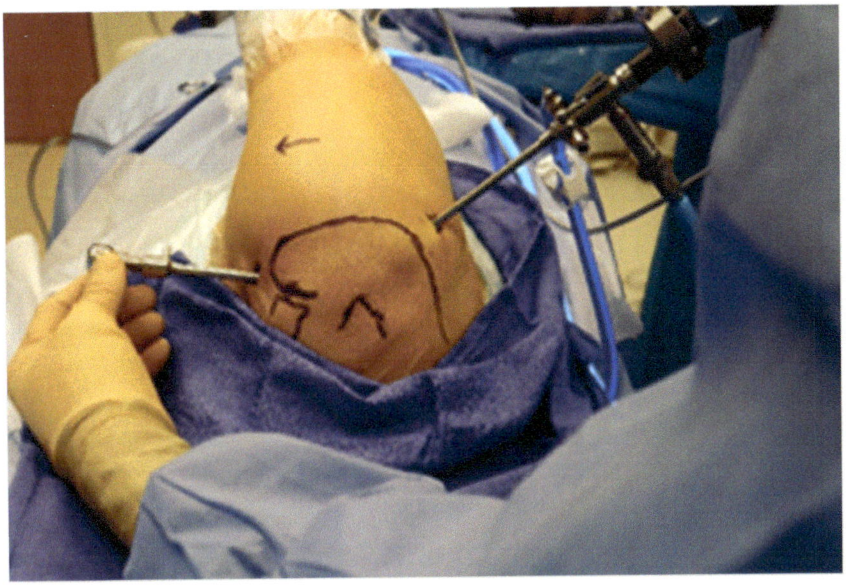

Fig. 2.4 Portal placement for acromioclavicular joint resection.

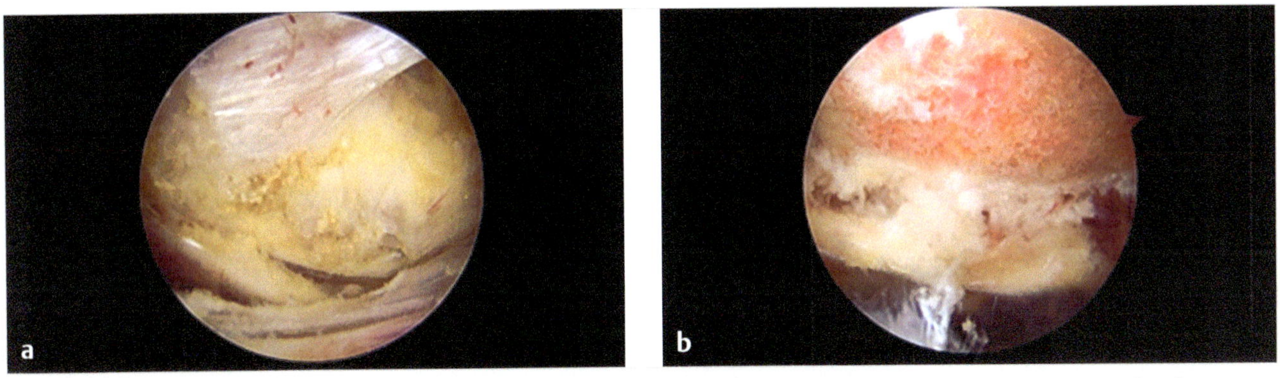

Fig. 2.5 Subacromial decompression. (a) Posterior view of hypertrophic acromioclavicular joint pressing on bursal rotator cuff surface. (b) Posterior view of acromioplasty.

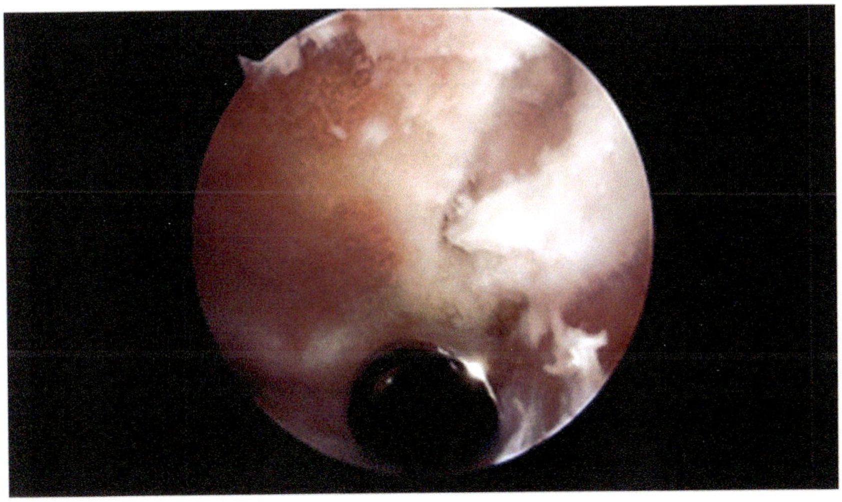

Fig. 2.6 Reposition anterior cannula in line with acromioclavicular joint.

2.7 Tips and Pearls

- Patient selection should identify complex anatomy, that is, os acromiale, superior clavicle positioning due to capsular injury.
- Hemostasis is best achieved with cautery and water ingress and egress.
- Begin the joint decompression on the acromion aspect of the joint to remain intrascapular.
- Resect ACJ meniscus, if present, to avoid painful articulation.
- Bevel clavicle resection to minimize risk of heterotopic bone formation.
- Visualize the posterior capsule and distal clavicle resection to avoid persistent contact with cross-chest positioning.

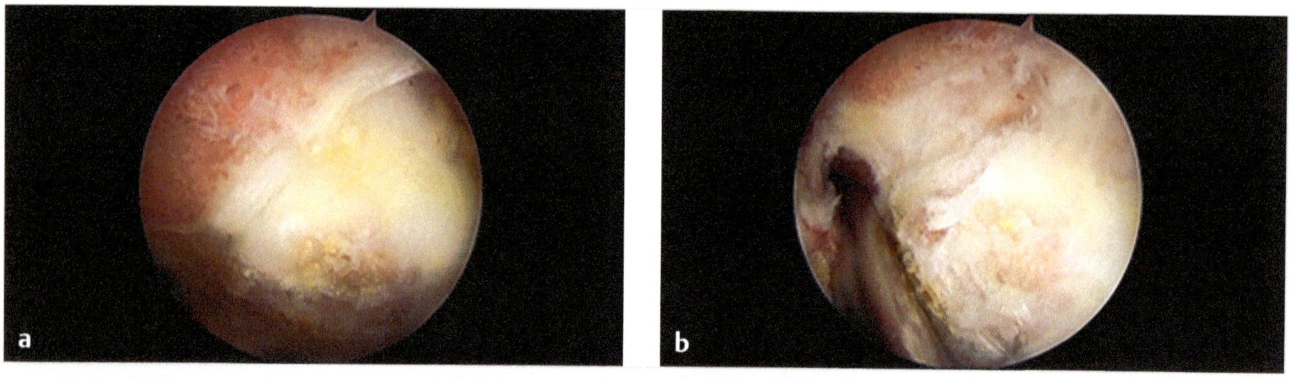

Fig. 2.7 Resection begins with clavicle facet of the acromion. **(a)** View of clavicle is partially hidden by clavicle facet of the acromion. **(b)** Acromial resection to better visualize the clavicle.

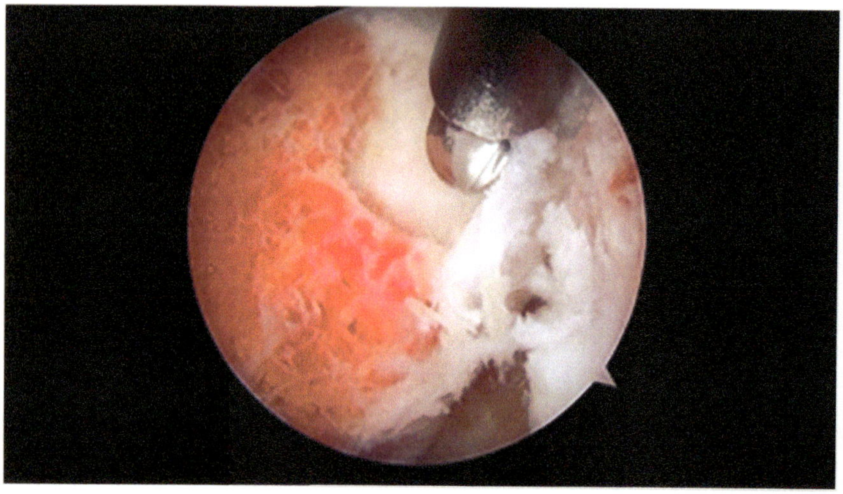

Fig. 2.8 Clavicle resection begins anteriorly and works gently to protect the capsule.

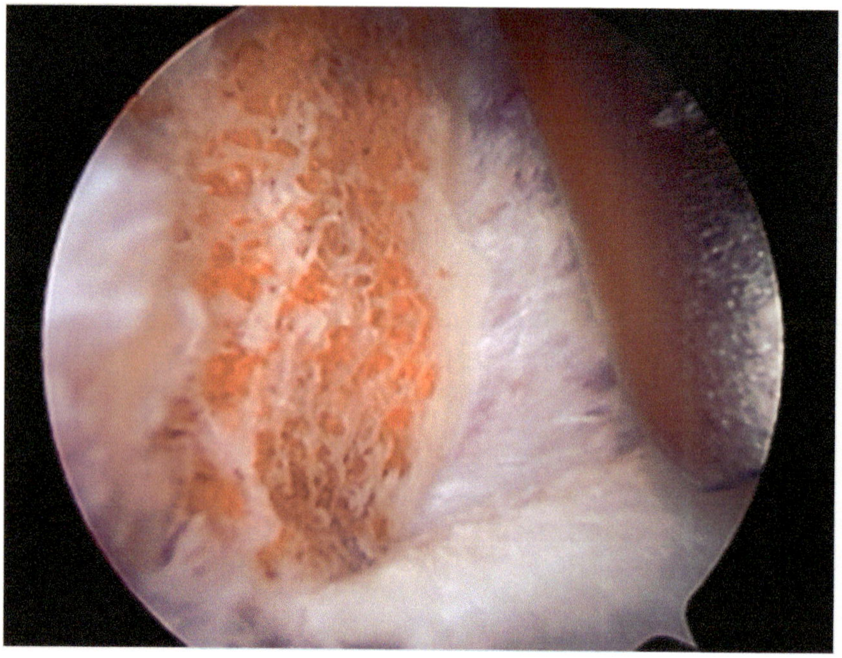

Fig. 2.9 Posterior capsule is elevated off the clavicle prior to completing the resection.

2.8 What to Avoid

- Poor visualization that can lead to CC ligament injury, unresected posterior clavicle, and destabilization due to inadvertent capsular ablation or excision. Confirm landmarks before performing bone resection (**Fig. 2.11**).
- Capsular calcification can occur along the distal clavicle. Bevel the distal clavicle and remove any residual bone (**Fig. 2.12**).

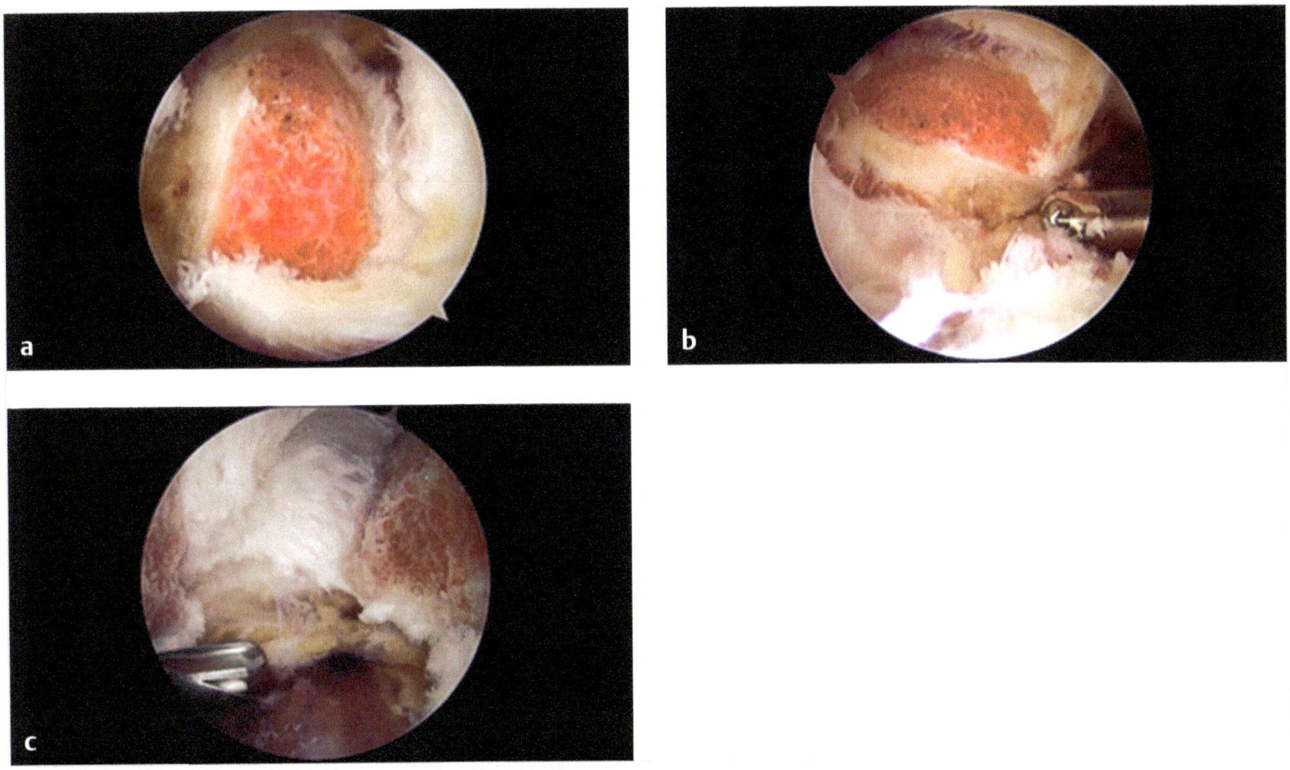

Fig. 2.10 Three views of completed acromioclavicular joint resection. (a) Posterior view. (b) Lateral view. (c) Anterior view.

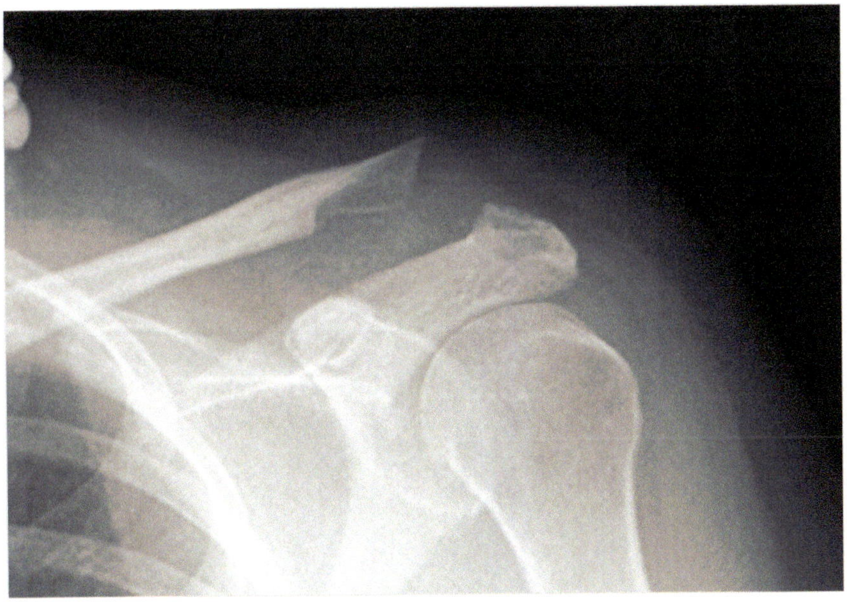

Fig. 2.11 Medial extension of the acromioclavicular joint resection has injured the coracoclavicular ligament resection.

- Os acromiale can be destabilized with distal clavicle resection. Preoperative recognition and intraoperative assessment of fragment mobility may require stabilization or resection (**Fig. 2.13**).

2.9 Complications

Destabilization can occur following prior or intraoperative injury to capsule and CC ligaments. This can be associated with overzealous resection of the clavicle. This can be repaired with CC ligament repair combined with suture anchor placed in the coracoid and sutured into the distal margin of the resected clavicle. Sutures through the CC ligaments can be combined (**Fig. 2.12**).

- With unstable os acromiale, a small posterior clavicle resection can be combined with os excision. Preserve soft-tissue capsular tissue to avoid deltoid injury (**Fig. 2.13**).

2.10 Postoperative Care

- Sling: on for 24 hours, then remove as pain allows.
- Ice: on/off for initial pain relief and for weeks/months during rehabilitation.

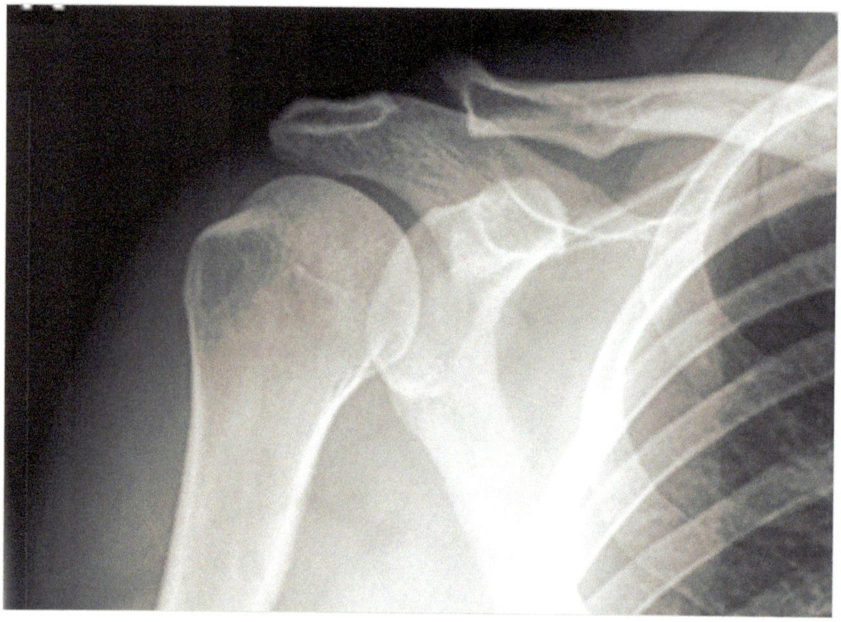

Fig. 2.12 Heterotopic bone can develop along the distal clavicle resection.

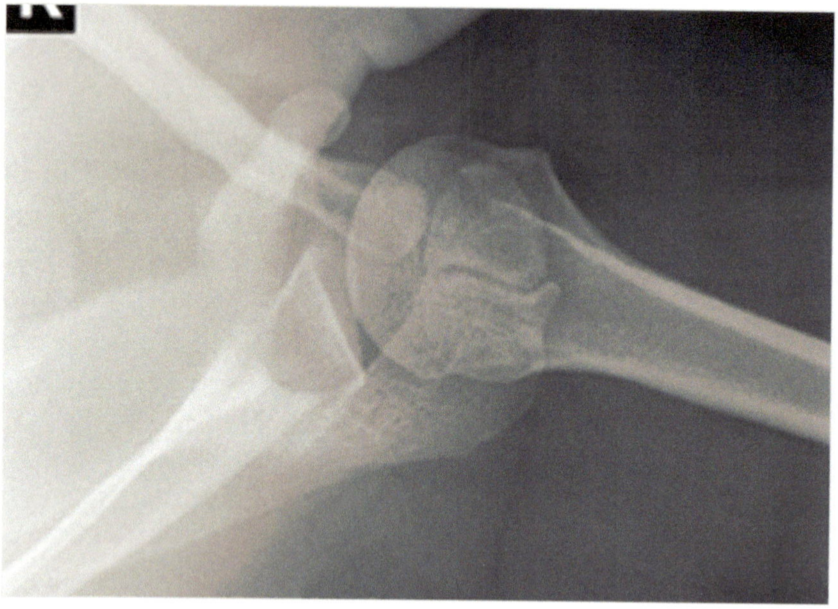

Fig. 2.13 Axillary view of os acromiale.

- Early range of motion, passive and active flexion and rotation.
- Table slides.
- Shoulder shrugs + core strengthening.
- Strengthening and gentle resistive exercise at 4 to 6 weeks.
- More advanced strengthening after 8 weeks.

Suggested Readings

Edwards SL, Wilson NA, Flores SE, Koh JL, Zhang LQ. Arthroscopic distal clavicle resection: a biomechanical analysis of resection length and joint compliance in a cadaveric model. Arthroscopy 2007;23(12):1278–1284

DeFroda SF, Nacca C, Waryasz GR, Owens BD. Diagnosis and management of distal clavicle osteolysis. Orthopedics 2017;40(2):119–124

Martin SD, Baumgarten TE, Andrews JR. Arthroscopic resection of the distal aspect of the clavicle with concomitant subacromial decompression. J Bone Joint Surg Am 2001; 83-A(3):328–335

Pandhi NG, Esquivel AO, Hanna JD, Lemos DW, Staron JS, Lemos SE. The biomechanical stability of distal clavicle excision versus symmetric acromioclavicular joint resection. Am J Sports Med 2013;41(2):291–295

Robertson WJ, Griffith MH, Carroll K, O'Donnell T, Gill TJ. Arthroscopic versus open distal clavicle excision: a comparative assessment at intermediate-term follow-up. Am J Sports Med 2011;39(11):2415–2420

Walton J, Mahajan S, Paxinos A, et al. Diagnostic values of tests for acromioclavicular joint pain. J Bone Joint Surg Am 2004;86-A(4):807–812

3 Arthroscopic Capsular Release

Danica D. Vance and William N. Levine

Abstract

Adhesive capsulitis or "frozen shoulder" is a debilitating condition that results in pain and significant loss of shoulder range of motion. The majority of cases are of idiopathic etiology, although the condition may develop after shoulder trauma or previous shoulder surgery. Initial treatment includes nonoperative management with physical therapy, nonsteroidal anti-inflammatory medications and intraarticular corticosteroid injections. Arthroscopic capsular release should be considered for those patients with refractory shoulder stiffness who fail 6 months of nonoperative management. This minimally invasive procedure involves arthroscopic release of the inflamed and fibrotic shoulder capsule to restore shoulder range of motion. This chapter describes in detail the steps to perform a successful arthroscopic capsular release.

Keywords: *adhesive capsulitis, shoulder arthroscopy, manipulation under anesthesia, frozen shoulder*

3.1 Goals of Procedure

- Restore shoulder range of motion (ROM) in a stiff or frozen shoulder secondary to capsule inflammation and fibrosis, termed adhesive capsulitis.

3.2 Advantages

- Minimally invasive procedure.
- Relatively short recovery time.
- Faster return to full activity.
- Shorter operative time than an open procedure.
- Can be performed under regional anesthesia.

3.3 Indications

- Failure to improve with nonoperative treatment of at least 6 months. Nonoperative treatment can vary but includes the following:
  - Physical therapy to improve ROM.
  - Nonsteroidal anti-inflammatory drug (NSAID) medications.
  - Intra-articular corticosteroid injections for pain relief and to allow release of adhesions with therapy and home stretching.
- Idiopathic adhesive capsulitis is most common in women between the ages of 40 and 60 years:
  - This generally presents with a gradual onset and no predisposing factor.
- Risk factors for adhesive capsulitis include diabetes mellitus, thyroid conditions, cardiac disease, Parkinson's disease, Peyronie's disease, Dupuytren's contracture, cardiac disease, and pulmonary disease:
  - Three to six times higher incidence in diabetic patients.
- Secondary adhesive capsulitis may occur after previous shoulder trauma or surgery.

3.4 Contraindications

- Motion loss with shoulder prosthesis.
- Myositis ossificans.

3.5 Preoperative Preparation/ Positioning

- Clinical evaluation:
  - Important to obtain complete injury history including onset and duration of symptoms and prior shoulder trauma, surgery, or period of immobilization:
    - Three clinical phases of adhesive capsulitis:
      i. Freezing or painful stage:
        a. Pain at night and with shoulder ROM.
        b. Duration of 6 weeks to 9 months.
      ii. Frozen phase:
        a. The loss of global shoulder ROM.
      iii. Thawing phase:
        a. Return of shoulder ROM toward normal.
        b. At least 10% of patients have incomplete recovery without surgical intervention.
    - Equal loss of passive and active ROM.
    - Passive ROM evaluation:
      i. Certain physical examination findings may correlate with contractures in specific areas of the capsule:
        a. Loss of external rotation (ER) in adduction → anterosuperior capsule.
        b. Loss of ER in abduction → anteroinferior capsule.
        c. Loss of internal rotation (IR) → posterior capsule.
        d. Loss of flexion and abduction → inferior capsule.
  - Adhesive capsulitis is a clinical diagnosis. Imaging is obtained to rule out other diagnoses.
    - Routine shoulder radiographs include anteroposterior, scapular Y, and axillary lateral shoulder view. Typical finding may include the following:
      i. Normal shoulder anatomy.
      ii. Calcific tendinitis.
    - MRI:
      i. Coracohumeral ligament and joint capsule thickening at the rotator cuff interval.
      ii. Rule out rotator cuff pathology.
  - If not contraindicated, we prefer regional anesthesia for muscle paralysis and immediate postoperative pain control.

3.6 Positioning

- Arthroscopy can be performed with the patient in either beach-chair or lateral decubitus position. For this procedure, we prefer the patient in the beach-chair position (**Fig. 3.1**).
- A hydraulic arm positioner is used to maintain arm position throughout the procedure (**Fig. 3.1**).
- All bony prominences are well padded.

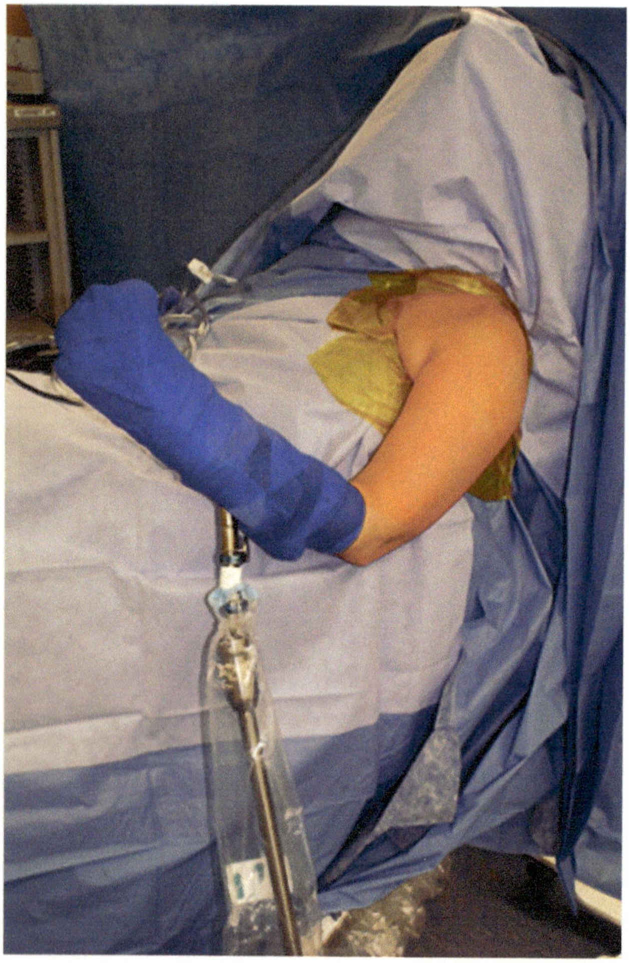

Fig. 3.1 Beach-chair position with hydraulic arm positioner.

- An examination under anesthesia is performed to evaluate shoulder ROM before incision.

3.7 Operative Technique

3.7.1 Shoulder Portals

- The acromion, distal clavicle, acromioclavicular (AC) joint, and coracoid process are drawn on the shoulder with a marking pen.
- Access to the glenohumeral joint is first obtained through the posterior portal.
- The posterior portal is created at the "soft spot" located approximately 1 cm medial and 2 cm inferior to the posterolateral edge of the acromion:
  - An incision is made through skin using a number 11 blade and the arthroscopic trocar is advanced into the glenohumeral joint.
  - Pearl: in shoulders with adhesive capsulitis, you have to be very careful to avoid "transhumeral" placement of the trocar. Aim a little more superior than normal.
- Once inside the glenohumeral joint, a standard anterior portal is created under direct visualization just lateral to the coracoid:
  - An 18-gauge spinal needle is used to achieve the proper location and direction of the anterior portal.

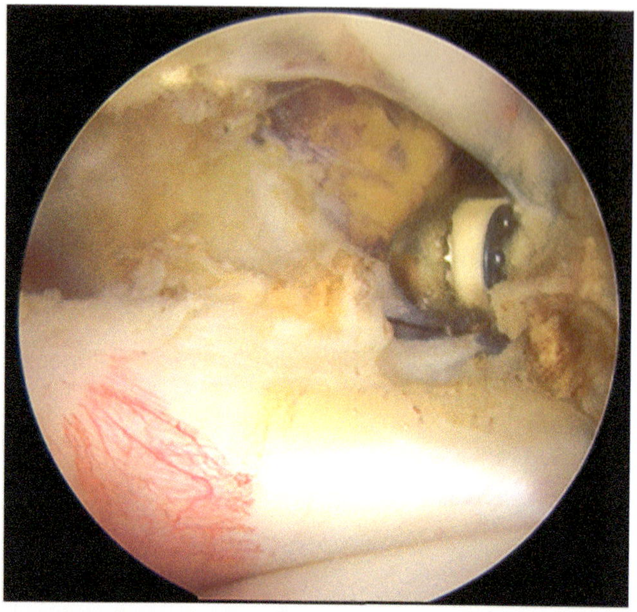

Fig. 3.2 Release of rotator interval.

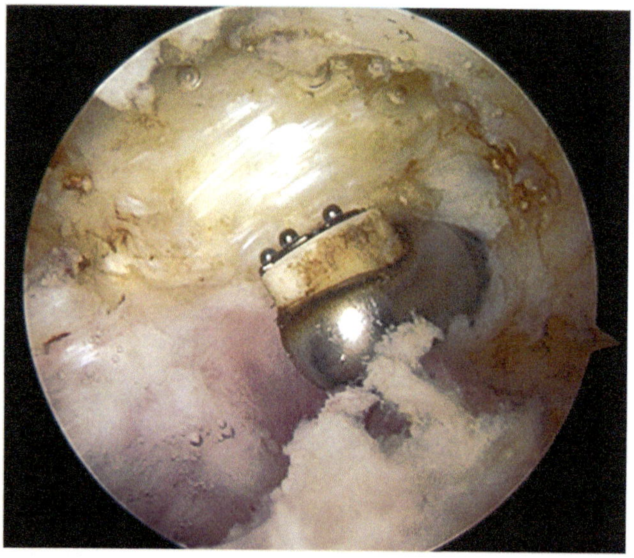

Fig. 3.3 Visualization of the coracoacromial ligament.

  - The portal is created between the long head of the biceps and subscapularis tendons within the rotator interval.
- Additional anterior and lateral portals may be created for full capsular release.

3.8 Procedure

3.8.1 Anterosuperior Capsule Release

- The procedure begins with release of the rotator interval and anterior capsule. This can be achieved using a radiofrequency device, arthroscopic biter, or shaver. We prefer to use a radiofrequency device (**Fig. 3.2**):
  - Release all fibrous tissue superior to subscapularis.
- The interval is released until the coracoid is visualized, sweeping tissue from the coracoacromial ligament (**Fig. 3.3**).

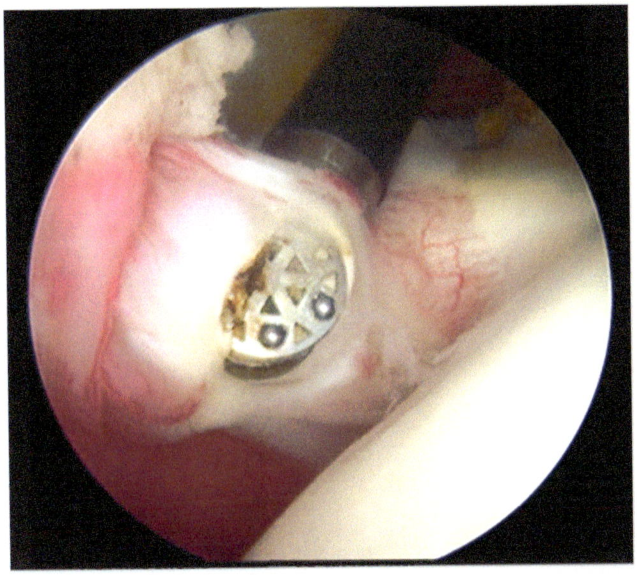

Fig. 3.4 Anteroinferior capsular release.

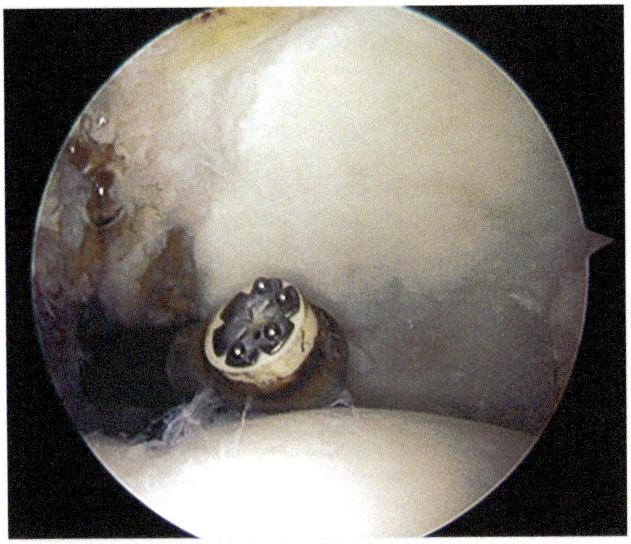

Fig. 3.5 Posterior capsular release.

- The capsule will be thicker than normal.
- Following release of the rotator interval, the remaining anterior capsule is released systematically in the anteroinferior direction to just lateral to the inferior labrum.
- A blunt obturator is used to separate the capsule (middle glenohumeral ligament) and inferior labrum from the subscapularis tendon. This interval is important to ensure there is no iatrogenic injury to the subscapularis or labral tissue.
- Once the interval is created, continue releasing the capsule inferiorly. The capsule can be released safely up to the 5 o'clock position (right shoulder) or 7 o'clock position (left shoulder; **Fig. 3.4**).
- The axillary nerve is located just 2.5 mm inferior to the inferior capsule around the 6 o'clock position. To avoid iatrogenic injury to the nerve, use a duckbill biter to release the capsule when approaching this area.
- A substantial interval of at least 1 cm should be created to avoid reformation of the scarred capsular tissue.

3.8.2 First Manipulation under Anesthesia

- Following complete release of the anterior capsule, a manipulation under anesthesia is performed to release the remaining inferior capsule.
- The humerus is held close to the joint with one hand and the other is used to stabilize the scapula.
- Test forward flexion, and ER at both 0- and 90-degree abductions. This should be performed in a safe, but aggressive manner to release the inferior capsule.
- Following manipulation, place the arthroscope back into the posterior portal to evaluate the release of the anteroinferior capsule.

3.8.3 Posterior Capsule Release

- The arthroscope is now switched to the anterior portal in order to view and release the posterior capsule.

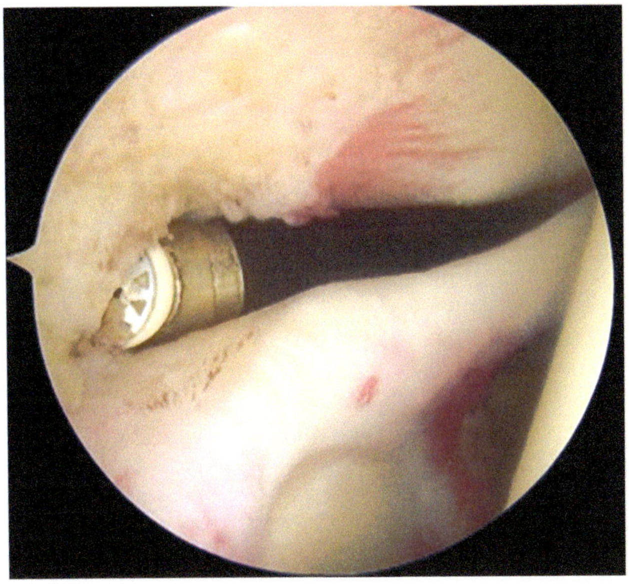

Fig. 3.6 Superior capsule release.

- Using a switching stick, a cannula is placed in the posterior portal.
- The posterior capsule is released using electrocautery (**Fig. 3.5**).
- Release posteriorly until fibers of the infraspinatus muscle are visualized.
- Work in the superior direction, releasing the capsule above the biceps to connect to the anterior release previously performed (**Fig. 3.6**).
- Widen the interval to at least 1 cm.

3.8.4 Second Manipulation under Anesthesia

- After completion of the capsular release, a second round of shoulder ROM is performed.
- Test IR at 0 and 90 degrees of abduction.

3.9 Tips and Pearls/Expert Suggestions

- Entering the glenohumeral joint may be difficult secondary to contraction and thickening of the posterior capsule.
- When releasing the anterior capsule, place the electrocautery anterior to the tissue you wish to release. Work toward yourself, so the tissue released is visualized at all times.
- The posterior portal may be made higher than normal to avoid iatrogenic cartilage injury.
- During the manipulation under anesthesia, hold the humerus close to the joint to avoid creating a long lever arm that may result in a humeral shaft fracture.
- Ensure a balanced capsular release:
  - Always release the rotator interval and evaluate the subacromial space.

3.10 What to Avoid

- Axillary nerve:
  - Potential injury during anteroinferior capsule release.
  - Runs parallel to the inferior border of the subscapularis, approximately 2.5 mm inferior to the inferior capsule.
  - Abduction and ER increase the distance between the axillary nerve and the inferior capsule.

3.11 Complications/Bailout/Salvage

- Axillary nerve injury:
  - Caution must be taken during the anteroinferior capsule release.
- Iatrogenic chondral or rotator cuff injury:
  - Forceful entry into the glenohumeral joint may damage the articular surface of the glenoid or humeral head.
- Humerus fracture during manipulation:
  - When performing gentle shoulder manipulation, hold the proximal humerus to decrease the leverage arm and reduce the risk of humeral shaft fracture.
- Dislocation:
  - With extensive adhesiolysis and gentle manipulation under anesthesia, it is possible to dislocate the shoulder. Check ROM is full and confirm with radiographs in the postanesthesia care unit (PACU).
  - Radiographs are obtained in the postanesthesia care unit (PACU) to confirm there is no fracture.
- Recurrent stiffness:
  - Check ROM in PACU. If there is any apprehension and resistance by the patient, do not hesitate to have anesthesia perform additional regional block.
  - Demonstrate full ROM in PACU so the patient sees their shoulder should move through a full ROM.

3.12 Postoperative Care

- Operative shoulder is placed in simple sling for comfort.
- Patient may use the operative shoulder as tolerated
- Physical therapy is initiated immediately following surgery for shoulder ROM:
  - Both passive and active assisted exercises.
  - Critical to schedule postoperative physical therapy sessions when patient schedules surgery.
  - Patients typically undergo physical therapy for 3 to 6 months postoperatively.
- Evaluate the patient closely to confirm progress in shoulder strength and ROM postoperatively.

Suggested Readings

Bridgman JF. Periarthritis of the shoulder and diabetes mellitus. Ann Rheum Dis 1972;31(1):69–71

Farrell CM, Sperling JW. Cofield RH. Manipulation for frozen shoulder: long-term results. J Shoulder Elbow Surg 2005;14(5):480–484

Grey RG. The natural history of "idiopathic" frozen shoulder. J Bone Joint Surg Am 1978;60(4):564

Kim YS, Lee HJ. Essential surgical technique for arthroscopic capsular release in the treatment of shoulder stiffness. JBJS Essential Surg Tech 2015;5(3):e14

Manske RC, Prohaska D. Diagnosis and management of adhesive capsulitis. Curr Rev Musculoskelet Med 2008; 1(3–4):180–189

Nicholson GP. Arthroscopic capsular release for stiff shoulders: effect of etiology on outcomes. Arthroscopy 2003;19(1):40–49

Pearsall AW IV, Osbahr DC, Speer KP. An arthroscopic technique for treating patients with frozen shoulder. Arthroscopy 1999;15(1):2–11

Price MR, Tillett ED, Acland RD, Nettleton GS. Determining the relationship of the axillary nerve to the shoulder joint capsule from an arthroscopic perspective. J Bone Joint Surg Am 2004;86-A(10):2135–2142

Sedeek S, Chye Andrew TH. Adhesive capsulitis: is arthroscopic capsular release necessary? Current review. OA. Orthopaedics 2013;1(1):8

Snow M, Boutros I, Funk L. Posterior arthroscopic capsular release in frozen shoulder. Arthroscopy 2009;25(1):19–23

Warner JJ, Allen A, Marks PH, Wong P. Arthroscopic release for chronic, refractory adhesive capsulitis of the shoulder. J Bone Joint Surg Am 1996;78(12):1808–1816

Zanotti RM, Kuhn JE. Arthroscopic capsular release for the stiff shoulder. Description of technique and anatomic considerations. Am J Sports Med 1997;25(3):294–298

4 Arthroscopic Treatment of Calcific Tendinitis

Brandon C. Cabarcas, Anirudh K. Gowd, Shreya Veera, Rachel M. Frank, and Nikhil N. Verma

Abstract

This chapter outlines the evaluation, diagnosis, and management of calcific tendinitis of the rotator cuff, with special attention given to surgical technique. The advantages of arthroscopic intervention, clinical pearls and pitfalls, and expert tips and suggestions to help optimize outcomes and limit complications are discussed in detail. By the end of the chapter, the reader will gain a better understanding of the etiology of this condition, as well as the evidence-based treatment options available for clinical use. They will also learn valuable arthroscopic technical skills and strategies that can be immediately utilized in the operative setting.

Keywords: *calcific tendinitis, rotator cuff, tendinitis, arthroscopic treatment, arthroscopy*

4.1 Goals of Procedure

Calcific tendinitis, characterized by the formation of calcium deposits within the rotator cuff tendons, occurs in up to 20% of adults.[1] The disease has been found to occur more frequently in patients between ages 50 and 60 years, with a predilection in sedentary workers and females.[2] While the etiology of this disease process is not entirely understood, the pathogenesis of calcification is cyclical in nature, beginning with cell-mediated fibrocartilaginous metaplasia, progressing to calcification of the tendon, and, finally, resorption. Pain is most severe in the resorptive phase.[3] This is in contrast to insertional calcification at the bone–tendon junction, such as what occurs in other anatomical areas including the Achilles–calcaneus interface.[4] Calcium deposits, consisting of hydroxyapatite crystals, are found in the supraspinatus tendon in 50% of cases and commonly extend into the infraspinatus, but are rarely found in the subscapularis or teres minor tendons of the rotator cuff.[5]

While acute pain is the most common clinical manifestation, calcific tendinitis is also associated with muscle spasms, bursitis, inflammation of the long head of the biceps, and acute or gradual restriction of movement.[6] Twenty percent of cases are found incidentally in asymptomatic patients.[7] Although calcific tendinitis may resolve on its own, repeated episodes may warrant specific treatment to manage pain.

The management of calcific tendinitis may consist of both nonoperative and operative treatments, depending on the patient's age, activity level, and symptoms. Nonoperative options are almost always the first line of treatment. These treatments can include activity modification, physical therapy including range-of-motion exercises, cryotherapy, and nonsteroidal anti-inflammatory drugs (NSAIDs) for pain relief. Other nonoperative treatments, including extracorporeal shock wave therapy (ECSW) and needling with/without steroid injections, have also been described. ECSW has been shown to have some short-term symptomatic improvement in some studies, but is dose dependent and can be accompanied by bone marrow edema and humeral head necrosis.[8] Ultrasound-guided needle lavage is another described minimally invasive technique aimed at decompressing the deposits to reduce pain.[9] The use of a corticosteroid injection following the needling process has been shown to improve results; however, when used alone, it is generally short acting and may be contraindicated in patient populations with medical history of insulin resistance, immunosuppression, and high blood pressure.[10] If nonoperative treatment options fail, surgical intervention in the form of an arthroscopic debridement can be attempted. The overall goal of arthroscopic treatment of calcific tendinitis is to reduce pain and improve function.

4.2 Advantages of Arthroscopic Management

While nonoperative treatments as described earlier may be successful for the majority of patients, in some cases, symptoms persist and surgical intervention is necessary. Arthroscopic debridement has been shown to provide excellent results in unresponsive or worsening cases.[11] In comparison to ECSW and ultrasound-guided needle lavage, surgical management provides direct visualization of the lesion as well as complete breakdown of the deposit. While nonsurgical treatments such as ECSW and ultrasound-guided needle lavage are less invasive, they may not provide complete removal of deposit when compared with surgery. Notably, while open surgery can be performed, this approach is typically unnecessary as complete deposit removal is not essential and can cause iatrogenic damage to the tendon.

Several clinical investigations have highlighted favorable clinical outcome measures associated with arthroscopic surgery for calcific tendonitis. In a cohort of 23 patients who had failed at least 1 year of nonoperative management, Ark et al demonstrated that arthroscopic calcium removal and concomitant subacromial bursectomy produced results graded as good (full motion and complete pain relief) in 50% of patients and satisfactory (full motion and occasional episodes of pain) in 41% of patients at average follow-up of over 2 years.[12] In an investigation by Seil et al, 54 patients with calcific tendinitis of the supraspinatus tendon underwent arthroscopic removal of the calcific deposits. Clinical follow-up at 2 years showed significant improvement in shoulder function according to the Constant score, 32.8 points (±19.8) preoperatively and 90.9 (±13.0) postoperatively ($p < 0.001$), as well as 92% patient satisfaction with the overall outcome.[13] Additionally, Maier et al conducted a therapeutic case series with 99 patients who underwent arthroscopic removal of rotator cuff calcific deposits with preservation of the integrity of the rotator cuff. Good to excellent results were reported in 90% of patients measured by the Constant score (overall mean CS_{abs} = 88.8 points (±10.4); CS_{rel} = 99.0% [±3.7]; $p < 0.05$) at average follow-up of 37 months and avoided iatrogenic tendon defects in all patients. Overall, the literature clearly demonstrates improved short- and long-term postoperative clinical outcome measures after arthroscopic intervention for calcific tendonitis.[11–18]

4.3 Indications

Calcific tendinitis has been well reported in the literature. Indications for surgery are widely dependent on symptom involvement, although there is no clearly defined time period for when surgery should be performed (**Table 4.1**). Patients are best indicated for arthroscopic treatment of calcific tendinitis after failure of nonoperative management. Failure of nonoperative therapy is typically defined by the persistence of symptomatic calcific tendinitis of the shoulder after a minimum of 6 months.[19] Physical examination findings may be variable due to the severity of the disease and any associated pain at the time of the examination. The following radiographic classification system described by Mole et al is commonly used to classify these lesions[20]:

- Type A: sharply delineated, dense, and homogeneous.
- Type B: sharply delineated and dense in appearance, with multiple fragments.
- Type C: heterogeneous in appearance, with a fluffy deposit.
- Type D: dystrophic calcifications at the tendon insertion.

Calcific deposits can be visualized as a single localized deposit, several localized deposits, or one large deposit consisting of several compartments.[11] Each compartment or localized deposit can require separate release during surgery for complete evacuation of symptomatic deposits. Preoperative advanced imaging with MRI can also be helpful as this modality can detect partial- or full-thickness rotator cuff tears as well as other concomitant pathologies. An example of a calcific deposit in the anteroposterior view is shown in **Fig. 4.1**. Notably, in the presence of calcifications, shadows visible on imaging may cause false-positive and false-negative findings.[25]

4.4 Contraindications

Active resorption of calcified deposits is a contraindication to surgery as the tendon is returning to its normal function. During this phase, pain medication is the best mode of management.[3,26] Patients of poor cardiac function, geriatric populations older than 65 years, or those intolerant of anesthesia are not indicated for surgery.

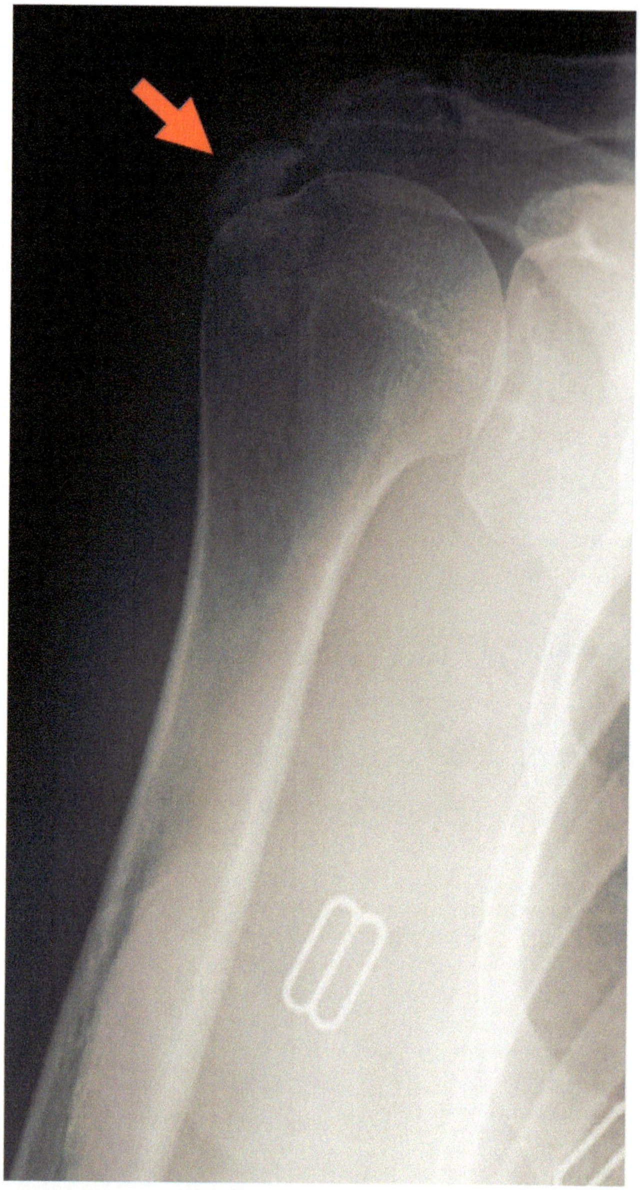

Fig. 4.1 Calcific tendinitis can be easily identified on the anteroposterior view of the shoulder (*red arrow*).

Table 4.1 Indications for operative treatment for calcific tendinitis[13,15,17,21–24]

Study	Year	Average symptom duration (mo)	Surgery performed	Indication for surgery
Rubenthaler et al	2003	17.1	Arthroscopic removal + subacromial decompression	
Porcellini et al	2004	20	Bursal debridement and arthroscopic removal of deposit	Type A and B calcifications refractory to non-op
Seil et al	2006	52	Arthroscopic removal	Type A and B calcifications refractory to non-op
Balke et al	2012	31.2	Bursal debridement + subacromial decompression	Refractory to non-op for at least 6 mo
Maier et al	2013	39.9	Arthroscopic removal of deposit	Refractory to non-op for at least 6 mo
Ranalletta et al	2015	5.5	Arthroscopic removal + tendon defect repair	Refractory to non-op for at least 4 mo and visualization on radiograph
Clement et al	2015		Arthroscopic removal ± subacromial decompression	Refractory calcific tendinitis

4.5 Preoperative Preparation/ Positioning

Our preference is to perform arthroscopic removal under both general and regional anesthesia with the patient in the beach-chair position as seen in **Fig. 4.2**. The shoulder is prepped and draped in standard, sterile fashion. Radiographs should be available at the time of surgery to assist with the localization and assessment of the calcium deposition.[11] In some cases, intraoperative fluoroscopy can be used, though this is rarely required.

4.6 Operative Technique

The arthroscopic procedure is initiated with establishment of the standard posterior and anterior (midglenoid) portals, followed by a diagnostic arthroscopy of the entire glenohumeral joint. After initial inspection, attention should be turned to the subacromial space. A lateral portal can be established once this space is entered. A bursectomy is performed for symptom relief as well as to properly visualize the integrity of the rotator cuff. It is crucial to inspect the entire rotator cuff for the presence of edema, neovascularity, or frank calcium deposits, all of which can be present depending on the particular phase and stage of calcification occurring within the tendon.[11,27]

Attention is then directed to the area of the tendon with the presumed deposit. In most cases, this will be the posterior aspect of the supraspinatus and the leading edge of the infraspinatus.[5] The area is then probed in order to detect any irregularities in tissue consistency and texture. If a calcific lesion is suspected, a 14-gauge needle can be used to puncture the site of interest. This may result in the release of visible calcified deposits, which can resemble a "toothpaste" or "chalk-dust" consistency as seen in **Fig. 4.3**.[11] Using a bladeless shaver barrel, the shaver suction is used to remove the debris in a manner similar to a vacuum cleaner. This technique should be used to remove the maximum possible amount of calcific debris from the subacromial space, as significant residual deposits have been associated with decreased clinical outcome measures.[21]

Examination of remaining tendon defects should always follow any excision of calcified lesions. Arthroscopic excision may inadvertently result in iatrogenic rotator cuff tendon defects. Preoperatively, patients should be counseled on this potential risk, and additional repair of full-thickness and large partial-thickness tears should be strongly considered, as repairs have been associated with positive postoperative outcomes.[15,27,28] Before the scope is removed from the subacromial space, all soft tissue and bony debris are irrigated out thoroughly and the procedure is completed. The wounds are irrigated and closed in standard fashion.

4.7 Tips and Pearls/Expert Suggestions

The cyclic and idiopathic nature of calcific tendinitis pathogenesis can result in highly variable clinical presentations. Patients with symptomatic calcific tendinitis can present very similarly

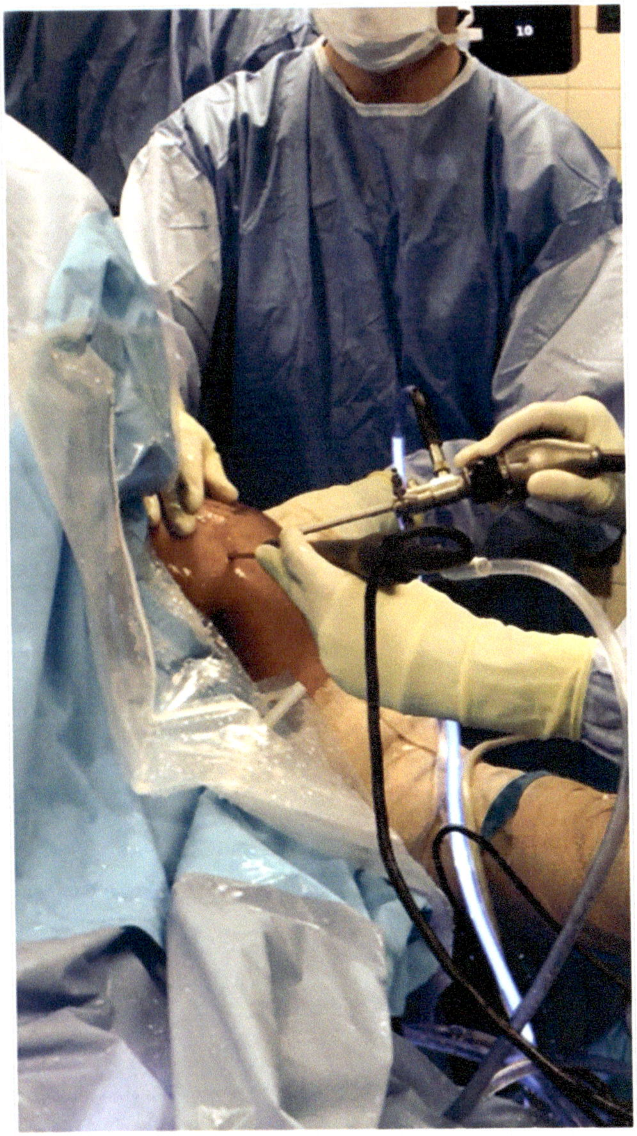

Fig. 4.2 Patient in the preferred beach-chair surgical position.

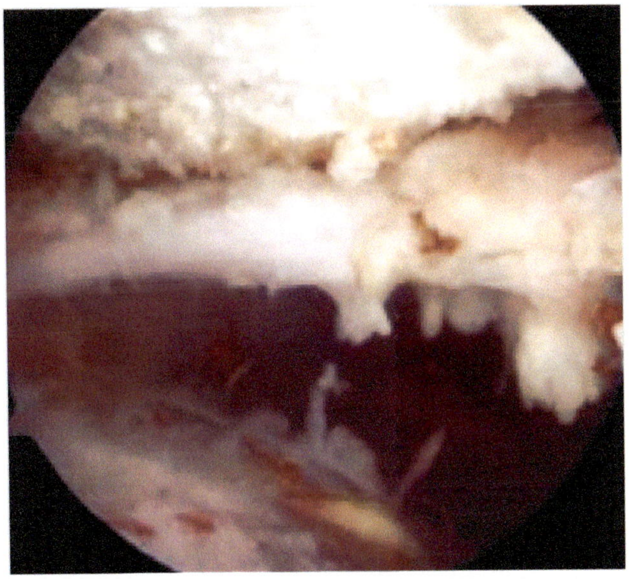

Fig. 4.3 Calcific tendinitis of the supraspinatus tendon.

to patients with other pathological conditions of the shoulder, including acute subacromial bursitis, rotator cuff tendinitis, and impingement syndrome.[11] It is critical to thoroughly examine the radiographs of patients presenting with shoulder pain to assess for both calcific tendinitis and other potential pain-generating pathologies. Diagnosis and follow-up of calcific tendinitis is usually performed with standard anteroposterior, outlet, and axillary view radiographs because it allows for localization and assessment of the texture and morphology of the calcium deposits.[6]

If arthroscopic intervention is necessary, it is important to note that it can be very challenging to determine the location of the calcium deposits upon arthroscopic evaluation of the rotator cuff. The calcium deposits may not be readily noticeable via standard arthroscopic techniques. One technique that may prove useful in such cases is marking areas of increased vascularity with a spinal needle as a reference.[11] These areas of increased vascularity can often be associated with the resorptive phase of calcific tendinitis, where spontaneous resorption of the calcium deposit may occur.[11]

Another issue worthy of attention is the potential for removal of calcium deposits to create significant defects in the rotator cuff. Evidence in the literature suggests that concomitant repair of significant rotator cuff defects found after removal of calcific deposits is associated with favorable clinical outcomes.[15,28] After removal of the calcium deposits has been completed, a detailed inspection of the rotator cuff tendons is warranted in order to identify any potentially significant tears. The decision to perform repair should be made based on evaluation of the size of the tendon defect, as minor rotator cuff tears have not been shown to negatively affect clinical outcomes.[15]

Complete removal of all calcium deposits from the rotator cuff tendons may pose a technical challenge during surgery. Residual calcium deposits sometimes persist despite thorough arthroscopic debridement. There is no clear consensus in the literature regarding the impact of residual calcium deposits on clinical outcomes for rotator cuff calcific tendinitis. Most authors report significant improvements and strong correlations in clinical outcome measures after complete removal or partial reduction of calcium deposits.[11,29,30] Some report that the persistence of residual calcium deposits after arthroscopy are actually associated with decreased Constant scores.[21] However, other studies have demonstrated that minor residual calcium does not significantly affect the Disabilities of the Arm, Shoulder and Hand (DASH) or Constant scores.[15,31] Given that the clinical impact of minor residual calcium deposits has yet to be clearly established, it is recommended that arthroscopic debridement of calcium deposits be as complete and thorough as possible.

4.8 What to Avoid

It is imperative to obtain adequate visualization and localization of the calcific deposits in the preoperative setting in order to create an adequate surgical plan. Performing a complete subacromial bursectomy can help avoid problems with visualization. Large lesions can have multiple areas of calcific deposition, and the goal should be to remove the greatest amount of deposits possible.[11] Although no clear consensus exists regarding residual calcium deposits, there is enough clinical evidence to encourage surgeons to perform a thorough and complete debridement of calcific lesions.[11,29,30] It is advisable to avoid unnecessarily leaving behind accessible and excisable calcium deposits within the tendons of the rotator cuff or subacromial space. Additionally, it is crucial to keep in mind the potential risk for creation of iatrogenic tendon defects in the rotator cuff tendons while excising calcific lesions. Although the risk is essentially unavoidable given the nature of the procedure, care should be taken to perform a thorough arthroscopic examination of the rotator cuff once debridement is complete in order to assure no significant tendon defects go unnoticed. It is recommended to repair full-thickness or significant partial-thickness tears present after arthroscopic excision of calcific tendon deposits to improve clinical postoperative outcomes.[15,28]

4.9 Complications/Bailout/Salvage

Pain is a major complication of calcific tendinitis of the rotator cuff tendons. Pain associated with this condition most often presents as nonradiating "shooting" pain in the shoulder, and is commonly associated with the resorptive phase of the calcific stage in the development of calcific tendinitis.[11,32] Management of patients presenting with acute pain involves periodic visits approximately every 4 months with evaluation of calcium deposits by ultrasound. Standard radiographs should be performed annually to document the morphology of the deposits, and NSAIDs are recommended once the pain reaches a score of 5 on the Visual Analog Scale, in addition to regimented physical therapy and exercise to prevent stiffness.[27] Adhesive capsulitis is also sometimes seen as a complication of rotator cuff calcific tendinitis. In patients with chronic calcific tendinitis, the calcium deposits become hardened and dried, producing limited range of motion, pain, and possibly frozen shoulder.[27] An investigation done by Jacobs et al found that 18% of 57 patients who underwent arthroscopic excision of rotator cuff calcifications developed frozen shoulder within an average follow-up of 15 months.[31] The authors attributed the complication to residual calcium debris irritating the glenohumeral capsule, but they also noted no difference in the final DASH or Constant scores after conservative treatment for all affected patients. In general, physical therapy is highly recommended in order to assist in recovering mobility of the affected shoulder. NSAIDs, articular corticosteroid injections, and long-term regimented rehabilitation may be necessary in refractory adhesive capsulitis cases.[27]

Rotator cuff tear is a potential complication of calcific tendinitis with significant clinical consequences. Evidence in the literature suggests that rotator cuff tears are commonly found in the preoperative setting.[27] A study by Kernwein demonstrated a 90% probability of discovering a rotator cuff tear in patients older than 40 years with chronic calcific tendinitis via arthrography.[33] In a retrospective analysis of 73 patients who underwent rotator cuff repair, Wolfgang documented an incidence of calcific tendinitis of 23%.[34] Arthroscopic removal of calcific deposits can sometimes create rotator cuff tendon defects necessitating repair. A detailed arthroscopic examination of the glenohumeral joint, capsule, and rotator cuff should be performed once excision of the calcium deposits is complete in order to identify any potential tendon defects. Repair of the rotator cuff tendon is generally recommended if there is a full-thickness or large partial-thickness tear, as these additional repairs have been associated with positive clinical postoperative outcomes.[15,27,28]

4.10 Postoperative Care

Most of the evidence in the literature suggests that it generally takes more than 6 months of postoperative recovery time for patients to report significant pain relief.[12,13,17,22] It is highly recommended to educate patients regarding the postoperative protocol and likely slowly progressive nature of symptom improvement. Pharmacotherapy for pain relief and limiting inflammation are mainstays of the postoperative period, along with regular physical therapy sessions to regain shoulder range of motion, strength, and function. An example of an acceptable postoperative care regimen includes prescription pain medications and antiemetics as needed in the immediate postoperative period. Prescription or over-the-counter anti-inflammatory drugs (e.g., NSAIDs) and possibly corticosteroid intra-articular injections are deemed clinically appropriate in the following weeks to months. Physical therapy can begin with a passive range of motion only program for the first 4 weeks, and then a gradual progression to active-assisted and active range of motion as tolerated to improve strength, mobility, and function.

References

1. Speed CA, Hazleman BL. Calcific tendinitis of the shoulder. N Engl J Med 1999;340(20):1582–1584
2. ElShewy MT. Calcific tendinitis of the rotator cuff. World J Orthop 2016;7(1):55–60
3. Suzuki K, Potts A, Anakwenze O, Singh A. Calcific tendinitis of the rotator cuff: management options. J Am Acad Orthop Surg 2014;22(11):707–717
4. Oliva F, Via AG, Maffulli N. Calcific tendinopathy of the rotator cuff tendons. Sports Med Arthrosc Rev 2011;19(3): 237–243
5. Seyahi A, Demirhan M. Arthroscopic removal of intraosseous and intratendinous deposits in calcifying tendinitis of the rotator cuff. Arthroscopy 2009;25(6):590–596
6. Merolla G, Singh S, Paladini P, Porcellini G. Calcific tendinitis of the rotator cuff: state of the art in diagnosis and treatment. J Orthop Traumatol 2016;17(1):7–14
7. Depalma AF, Kruper JS. Long-term study of shoulder joints afflicted with and treated for calcific tendinitis. Clin Orthop 1961;20(20):61–72
8. Bannuru RR, Flavin NE, Vaysbrot E, Harvey W, McAlindon T. High-energy extracorporeal shock-wave therapy for treating chronic calcific tendinitis of the shoulder: a systematic review. Ann Intern Med 2014;160(8):542–549
9. Castillo-González FD, Ramos-Álvarez JJ, Rodríguez-Fabián G, González-Pérez J, Calderón-Montero J. Treatment of the calcific tendinopathy of the rotator cuff by ultrasound-guided percutaneous needle lavage. Two years prospective study. Muscles Ligaments Tendons J 2014;4(2):220–225
10. de Witte PB, Kolk A, Overes F, Nelissen RGHH, Reijnierse M. Rotator cuff calcific tendinitis: ultrasound-guided needling and lavage versus subacromial corticosteroids—five-year outcomes of a randomized controlled trial. Am J Sports Med 2017;45(14):3305–3314
11. Barber FA, Cowden CH III. Arthroscopic treatment of calcific tendonitis. Arthrosc Tech 2014;3(2):e237–e240
12. Ark JW, Flock TJ, Flatow EL, Bigliani LU. Arthroscopic treatment of calcific tendinitis of the shoulder. Arthroscopy 1992;8(2):183–188
13. Seil R, Litzenburger H, Kohn D, Rupp S. Arthroscopic treatment of chronically painful calcifying tendinitis of the supraspinatus tendon. Arthroscopy 2006;22(5): 521–527
14. Lam F, Bhatia D, Van Rooyen K, de Beer J. Modern management of calcifying tendinitis of the shoulder. Curr Orthop 2006;20(6):446–452
15. Maier D, Jaeger M, Izadpanah K, Bornebusch L, Suedkamp NP, Ogon P. Rotator cuff preservation in arthroscopic treatment of calcific tendinitis. Arthroscopy 2013;29(5):824–831
16. Marder RA, Heiden EA, Kim S. Calcific tendonitis of the shoulder: is subacromial decompression in combination with removal of the calcific deposit beneficial? J Shoulder Elbow Surg 2011;20(6):955–960
17. Balke M, Bielefeld R, Schmidt C, Dedy N, Liem D. Calcifying tendinitis of the shoulder: midterm results after arthroscopic treatment. Am J Sports Med 2012;40(3):657–661
18. Castagna A, DE Giorgi S, Garofalo R, Conti M, Tafuri S, Moretti B. Calcifying tendinitis of the shoulder: arthroscopic needling versus complete calcium removal and rotator cuff repair. A prospective comparative study. Joints 2016;3(4):166–172
19. Ogon P, Suedkamp NP, Jaeger M, Izadpanah K, Koestler W, Maier D. Prognostic factors in nonoperative therapy for chronic symptomatic calcific tendinitis of the shoulder. Arthritis Rheum 2009;60(10):2978–2984
20. Mole D, Kempf JF, Gleyze P, Rio B, Bonnomet F, Walch G. Results of endoscopic treatment of non-broken tendinopathies of the rotator cuff. 2. Calcifications of the rotator cuff. Rev Chir Orthop Repar Appar Mot 1993;79(7):532–541
21. Porcellini G, Paladini P, Campi F, Paganelli M. Arthroscopic treatment of calcifying tendinitis of the shoulder: clinical and ultrasonographic follow-up findings at two to five years. J Shoulder Elbow Surg 2004;13(5):503–508
22. Rubenthaler F, Ludwig J, Wiese M, Wittenberg RH. Prospective randomized surgical treatments for calcifying tendinopathy. Clin Orthop Relat Res 2003(410):278–284
23. Clement ND, Watts AC, Phillips C, McBirnie JM. Short-term outcome after arthroscopic bursectomy debridement of rotator cuff calcific tendonopathy with and without subacromial decompression: a prospective randomized controlled trial. Arthroscopy 2015;31(9):1680–1687
24. Ranalletta M, Rossi LA, Bongiovanni SL, Tanoira I, Piuzzi N, Maignon G. Arthroscopic removal and rotator cuff repair without acromioplasty for the treatment of symptomatic calcifying tendinitis of the supraspinatus tendon. Orthop J Sports Med 2015;3(4):2325967115577957
25. Gosens T, Hofstee DJ. Calcifying tendinitis of the shoulder: advances in imaging and management. Curr Rheumatol Rep 2009;11(2):129–134
26. Uhthoff HK, Loehr JW. Calcific tendinopathy of the rotator cuff: pathogenesis, diagnosis, and management. J Am Acad Orthop Surg 1997;5(4):183–191
27. Merolla G, Bhat MG, Paladini P, Porcellini G. Complications of calcific tendinitis of the shoulder: a concise review. J Orthop Traumatol 2015;16(3):175–183
28. Yoo JC, Park WH, Koh KH, Kim SM. Arthroscopic treatment of chronic calcific tendinitis with complete removal and rotator cuff tendon repair. Knee Surg Sports Traumatol Arthrosc 2010;18(12):1694–1699

29. Jerosch J, Strauss JM, Schmiel S. Arthroscopic treatment of calcific tendinitis of the shoulder. J Shoulder Elbow Surg 1998;7(1):30–37
30. Wang C-J, Yang KD, Wang F-S, Chen H-H, Wang J-W. Shock wave therapy for calcific tendinitis of the shoulder: a prospective clinical study with two-year follow-up. Am J Sports Med 2003;31(3):425–430
31. Jacobs R, Debeer P. Calcifying tendinitis of the rotator cuff: functional outcome after arthroscopic treatment. Acta Orthop Belg 2006;72(3):276–281
32. Bayam L, Ahmad MA, Naqui SZ, Chouhan A, Funk L. Pain mapping for common shoulder disorders. Am J Orthop 2011;40(7):353–358
33. Kernwein GA. Roentgenographic diagnosis of shoulder dysfunction. JAMA 1965;194(10):1081–1085
34. Wolfgang GL. Surgical repair of tears of the rotator cuff of the shoulder. Factors influencing the result. J Bone Joint Surg Am 1974;56(1):14–26

5 Arthroscopic Rotator Cuff Repair

Christos D. Photopoulos, Carola F. van Eck, and Orr Limpisvasti

Abstract

Rotator cuff pathology is a common cause of pain and dysfunction in the shoulder, and it is well known that the incidence of rotator cuff disease increases with age. Rotator cuff repair is one of the most commonly performed procedures in the United States, and over the past two decades, the field of orthopaedic surgery has witnessed the evolution of surgical approaches, techniques, and constructs involved in rotator cuff repair. Although commonly performed, arthroscopic rotator cuff repair can be a technically challenging procedure, even for experienced orthopaedic surgeons. The goal of this chapter is to outline a preferred technique for arthroscopic rotator cuff repair and to provide tips for success in preoperative, intraoperative, and postoperative management.

Keywords: *arthroscopy, rotator cuff, tear, repair, technique, transosseous equivalent*

5.1 Goals of Procedure

The clinical goals of arthroscopic rotator cuff repair are to alleviate patient suffering, improve pain, and restore function. Technical goals of the procedure are to restore native anatomy,[1] achieve strong initial fixation, and maintain durable stability at the repair site until biologic healing takes place.[2,3]

5.2 Advantages

There are several advantages to performing an arthroscopic rotator cuff repair. The use of arthroscopy allows for a comprehensive evaluation of the glenohumeral joint. As the cause of shoulder pain and dysfunction is frequently multifactorial, arthroscopy permits the treatment of intra-articular lesions, including those involving the labrum, biceps, or articular cartilage. Other commonly cited advantages include surgeon preference and comfort, the use of smaller incisions with less soft-tissue dissection, and a minimized risk of deltoid injury seen with nonarthroscopic procedures.[2,4–6]

5.3 Indications

Patient symptoms are the primary driving indicators for surgical repair, as the primary function of rotator cuff surgery is to alleviate pain and functional impairment. When deciding which patients are indicated for surgery, the natural history of the disease must be discussed with the patient, and several factors must be taken into account. Generally, surgical intervention is reserved for those who have failed some degree of nonoperative management, including physical therapy, anti-inflammatories, and injection therapy. Patient age and tear chronicity are important considerations, as younger patients with acute tears are more commonly indicated for surgical repair than physiologically older patients with chronic disease. Tear size, morphology, and location are likewise of importance, as larger and full-thickness tears, especially those that involve the anterior cable, are generally more accepted for surgical repair.[7–9]

5.4 Contraindications

There are few relative and absolute contraindications to surgical repair. Important preoperative factors to consider are those precluding patients from anesthesia and elective surgical intervention, including recent infections, recent illnesses, and patient comorbidities that would render necessary anesthesia difficult or dangerous. Factors such as fatty infiltration, marked rotator cuff retraction, and rotator cuff arthropathy with superior humeral head migration must also be recognized preoperatively. Factors that would prevent a successful postoperative rehabilitation program, such as a patient's ability or willingness to comply with postoperative instructions, should also be taken into account. Factors portending a poor outcome must be taken into consideration and discussed with the patient, as alternate treatment options to surgical repair exist.

5.5 Preoperative Preparation/ Positioning

In the preoperative holding area, the surgical site, including the axilla, is shaved and cleansed. Chlorhexidine (2%) is the preferred skin-preparation solution given its efficacy in decreasing the bacterial burden of the skin.[10,11] Regional anesthesia, consisting of an interscalene nerve block, is commonly performed prior to surgery.

The patient is transferred to the operating table and placed atop a well-padded bean bag. After induction, the operative extremity is examined to evaluate shoulder stability and range of motion. **Tip:** Perform this while the patient is supine so that examination can be referenced against the contralateral shoulder. The patient is then placed in the lateral decubitus position and secured in position with bean bag suction. Together, the patient and the bean bag are translated closer to the surgeon to optimize ergonomics during the procedure; the patient is stabilized with two straight posts posteriorly and one curved post anteriorly. A careful assessment of all neurovascular structures and bony prominences must be performed. The hips are slightly abducted and externally rotated with pillows to relieve stress on the spine; the knees are flexed and padded to protect the peroneal nerves; and the upper torso and scapula are tilted toward the surgeon to assist in maintaining parallelism of the glenoid face to the floor. When positioning the patient's head, the cervical spine should not be hyperextended, laterally bent, or rotated. Reverse Trendelenburg facilitates proper scapular positioning under traction and helps create clearance between the shoulder and the head during surgery. The arm holder should be positioned in a manner that when balance suspension is applied, the arm is held in 40 degrees of forward

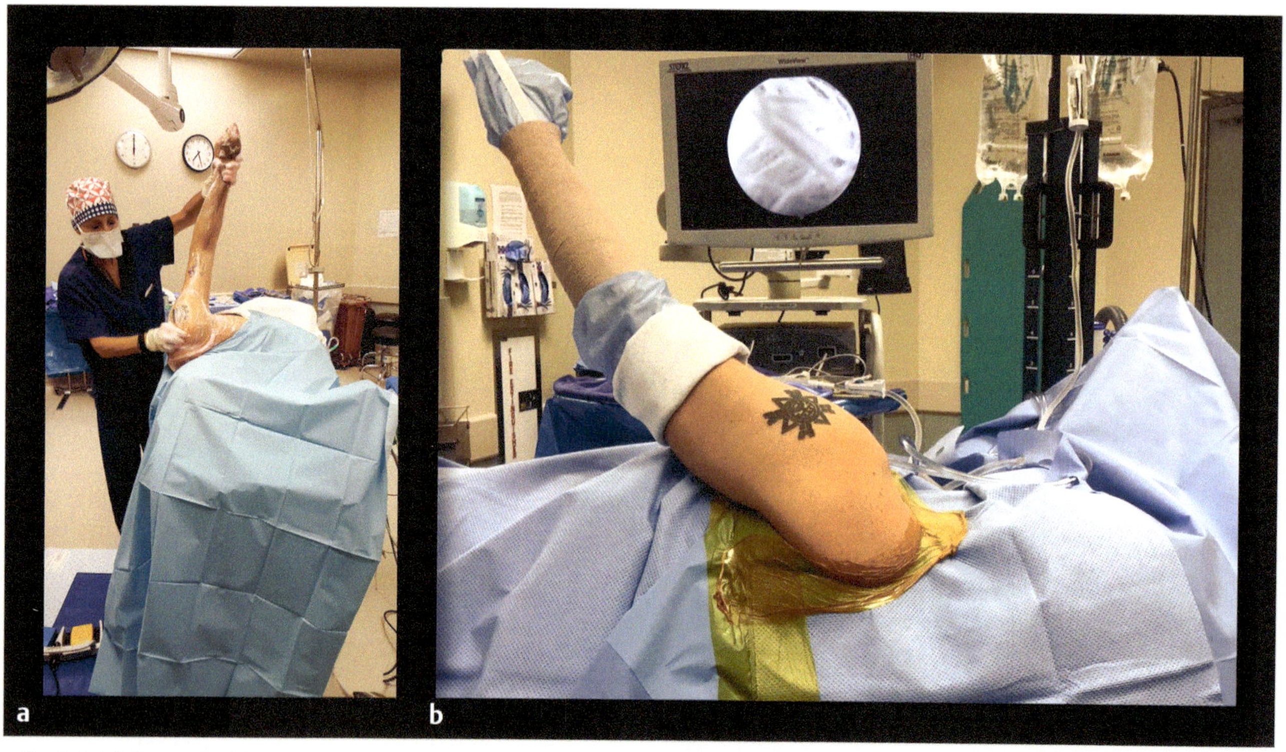

Fig. 5.1 (a) Prepping of the operative extremity with chlorhexidine soap. (b) Surgical setup after prepping and draping are completed.

flexion and 40 degrees of abduction. A belt is placed to secure the patient to the table (**Fig. 5.1**).

Chlorhexidine (2%) solution is again used to clean the extremity. The sequence of draping is as follows: (1) downdrape over the body, (2) four blue towels squared around shoulder, and (3) two impervious U-drapes applied in opposing directions. Any remaining soap is then dried with a sterile towel. The drapes are sealed at the skin interface with antimicrobial adhesive strips (3M Ioban, St. Paul, MN). A sterile impervious stockinet with attachment for the balance suspension is then applied from the hand to just above the elbow. This is secured in place with an elastic compressive bandage (3M Coban), paying careful attention that no bandage is applied over the cubital tunnel and that all bony prominences are free of point compression (**Fig. 5.1**).

Ten to 15 lb of balanced suspension is then applied to the arm. Bony landmarks, portals, and planned incisions can be drawn onto the skin if necessary. The projected portal sites should be infiltrated with local anesthetic to aid in postoperative pain control. **Tip:** Epinephrine may be added to the local anesthetic to reduce portal site bleeding during the surgery.

Operating room setup is important in facilitating surgical ergonomics. The operating room table may be turned to ensure there is enough room for the surgical team, while minimizing the risk of surgical field contamination (**Fig. 5.1**). The Mayo stand (and the surgical instruments) and the arthroscopy tower are positioned on the opposite side of the operating table from the surgeon. If gravity inflow is to be utilized, a Y-connector and very firm tubing must be used to ensure maintenance of adequate pressure. Foot controls for the shaver, burr, and electrocautery should be set up prior to incision.

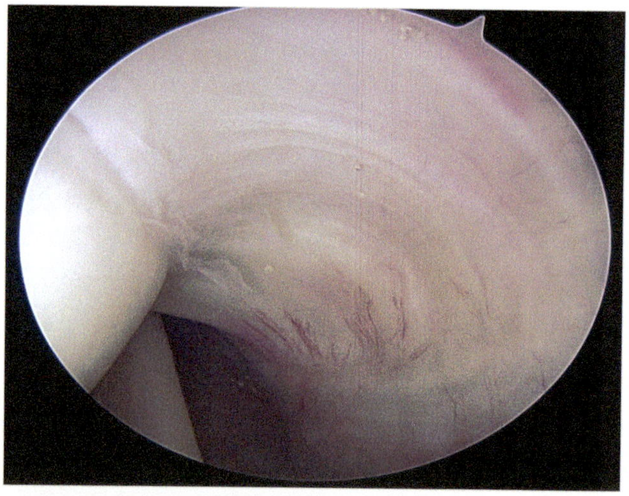

Fig. 5.2 Evaluation of the articular aspect of the rotator cuff through the posterior glenohumeral portal.

5.6 Operative Technique

5.6.1 Portals

To begin with, a standard posterior portal is established and a diagnostic arthroscopy is performed to assess for associated chondral, labral, bicipital, and articular-sided rotator cuff pathology (**Fig. 5.2**). To create a working anterosuperior portal (ASP), a spinal needle is placed in an outside-in fashion through the rotator interval (**Fig. 5.3**). The exact location of the

ASP should be determined based on its function. For instance, if a distal clavicle excision is to be performed, this portal can be moved slightly medially. During the case, 7 × 70 mm threaded cannulas (Arthrex, Naples, FL) are the workhorse cannulas for all working portals. PassPort cannulas (Arthrex), whose low-profile flanges prevent cannula loss during instrument insertion and removal, can also be used.

Intra-articular evaluation of the subscapularis tendon is critical, and if repair is required, this must be done first (**Fig. 5.4**). To better examine the subscapularis enthesis, the humerus can be internally rotated, or a 70-degree scope may be used. During surgical repair, the assistant may be asked to perform a lever-push maneuver in order to deliver the footprint into the field of view. This is done by placing a posteriorly directed force onto the proximal humerus, while providing counter pressure to the posterior elbow.

The subacromial space is entered using the existing posterior portal. A lateral working portal is established two finger breadths lateral to the lateral border of the acromion (in line with the acromioclavicular joint from an anteroposterior standpoint). A posterolateral portal can likewise be added as needed. **Tip:** To avoid turbulence, keep accessory portals in the subacromial space small. In addition, avoid violation of the deltoid fascia, which can lead to fluid extravasation and soft-tissue swelling.

5.6.2 Visualization

Once in the subacromial space, a 4.0 shaver (Dissector, Arthrex) is used to perform a complete bursectomy. This not only will aid in visualization but is also effective in reducing pain, as inflamed bursal tissue has been shown to be rich with afferent nerve fibers and inflammatory mediators.[12,13] **Tip:** This step is essential to facilitate lateral row implant placement and suture management.

Using a shaver and electrocautery (Apollo, Arthrex), the coracoacromial ligament can be dissected off the acromion to further aid in visualization. This may be done completely or partially, depending on the concern for creating instability or superior escape. An acromioplasty is then performed using a 5.5 round burr (Arthrex; **Fig. 5.5**). If a distal clavicle resection is performed,

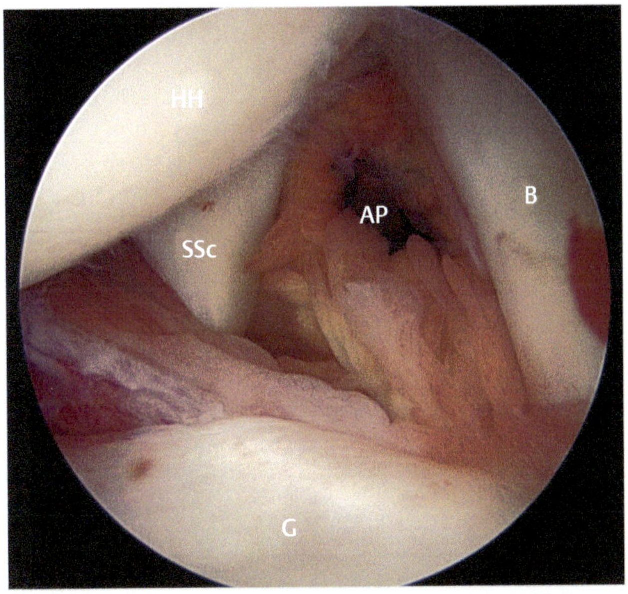

Fig. 5.3 Location of the anterosuperior portal (AP) as viewed from the posterior portal. G, glenoid; HH, humeral head; B, long head of the biceps tendon; SSc, subscapularis tendon.

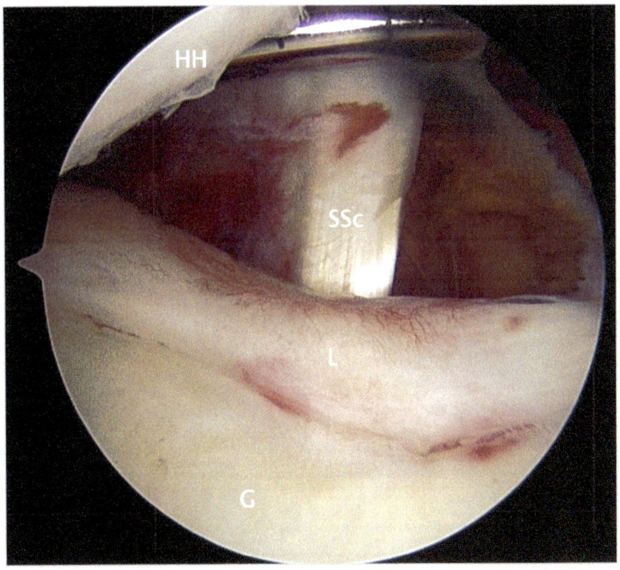

Fig. 5.4 Evaluation of the integrity of the subscapular tendon (SSc) from the posterior portal. G, glenoid; HH, humeral head; L, glenoid labrum.

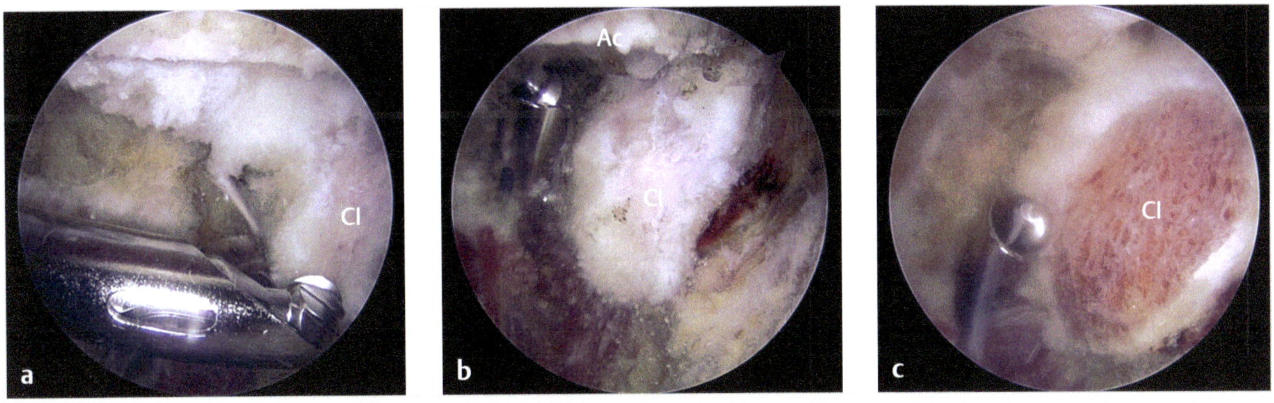

Fig. 5.5 **(a)** A subacromial decompression is performed using a burr through the lateral portal. **(b)** After this is done, the distal clavicle can be visualized. **(c)** A distal clavicle excision is then performed through the anterosuperior portal. Ac, acromion; Cl, distal clavicle.

the coracoclavicular ligaments must be carefully identified and preserved. In addition, the posterosuperior capsule of the acromioclavicular joint must be left intact to preserve stability of the acromioclavicular joint.[14–17] Commonly, more bone is resected anteriorly than it is posteriorly, leading to residual posterior bony contact and continued pain.[18,19] To ensure that this does not occur, the arthroscope can be placed in an anterior portal to evaluate the symmetry of the resection. Similarly, a 70-degree scope can be used from the posterior portal in lieu of placing the arthroscope in the anterior portal. **Tip:** Advance the 7-mm cannula from the anterior portal into the acromioclavicular joint interval to ensure adequate and symmetric resection.

5.6.3 Evaluation and Releases

After thorough visualization is achieved and any acromioclavicular work is performed, the rotator cuff is thoroughly examined. **Tip:** It may be necessary to temporarily release the balanced suspension at this time. This will allow rotation of the humeral head under tension in order to (1) distinguish bursal tissue from rotator cuff tissue and to (2) better determine the sufficiency of the rotator cable. If the rotator cuff tear is not adequately visualized through the posterior portal, a 70-degree scope can be used to get the desired "50-yard line view" (**Fig. 5.6**). Alternatively, an additional, more posterolateral viewing portal can be established.

The edges of the tear are debrided and the native footprint is evaluated. **Tip**: Note that although the supraspinatus inserts directly lateral to the articular cartilage border, there is a bare area between the articular margin and the infraspinatus insertion. Reattachment of the infraspinatus tendon immediately adjacent to the articular cartilage can lead to overtensioning of the rotator cuff. An arthroscopic grasper (KingFisher or Rotator Cuff Grasper, Arthrex) can be used to pull the torn rotator cuff back to the footprint in order evaluate the tension and rotation of the final construct (**Fig. 5.7**). Should tissue mobilization be necessary, an elevator can be used to release the rotator cuff tendon on both the articular and bursal aspects. **Tip**: To avoid injury to the suprascapular nerve, be careful not to go further than 2.5 cm medial to the glenoid with the elevator and electrocautery.

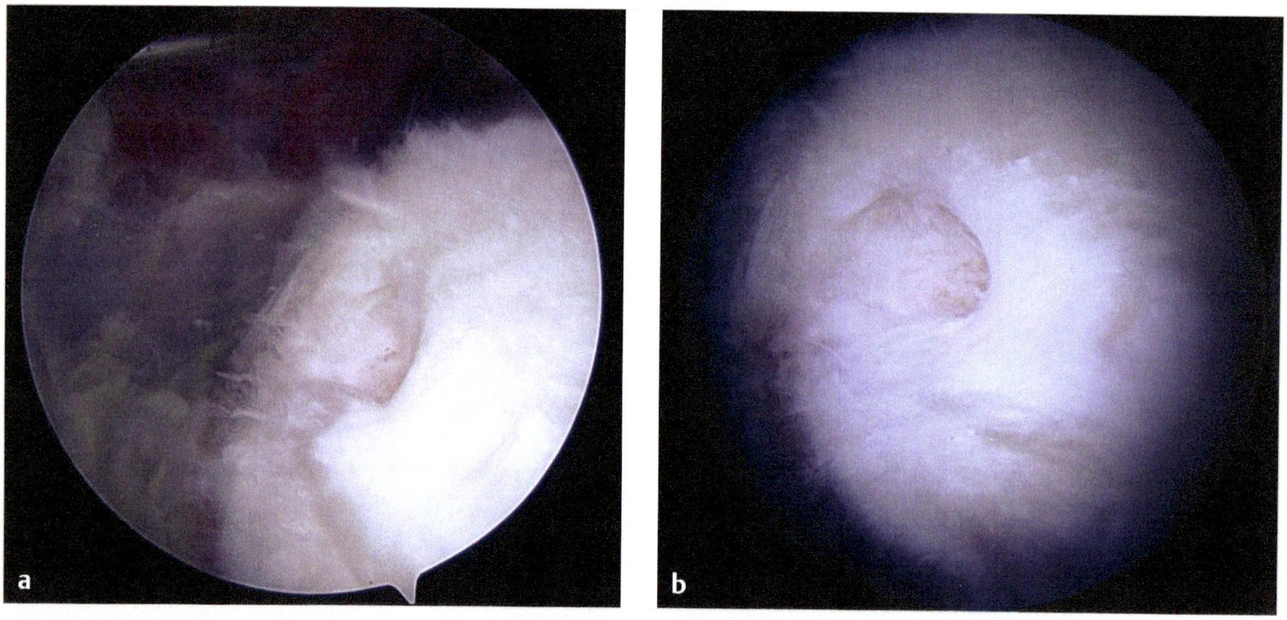

Fig. 5.6 (a) Suboptimal visualization of a smaller size rotator cuff tear through the posterior portal using the 30-degree scope. (b) Improved visualization using a 70-degree scope through the same portal.

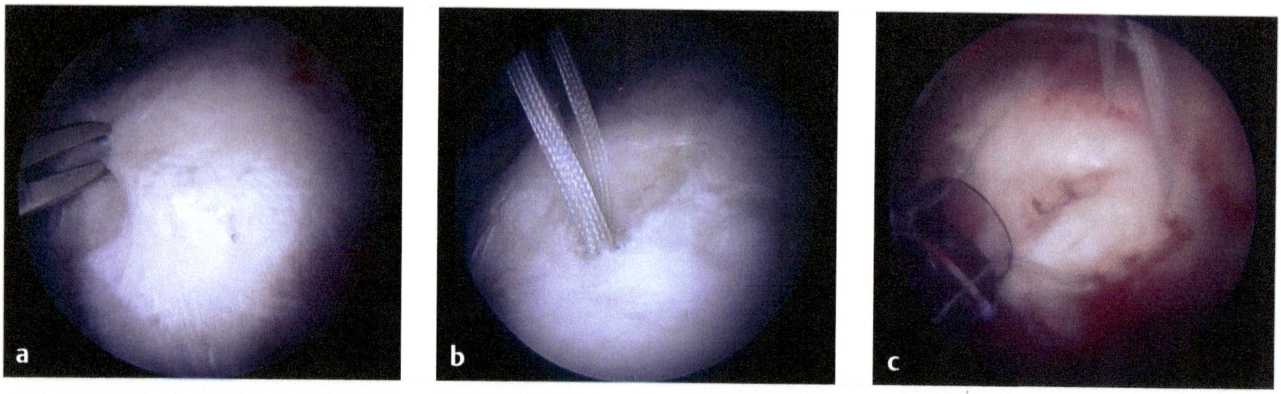

Fig. 5.7 Repair of a smaller rotator cuff tear. (a) A grasper is used to determine the native location of the tendon. (b) This location is then used to place the anchor. (c) Sutures are then passed through the tendon and tied to complete the repair.

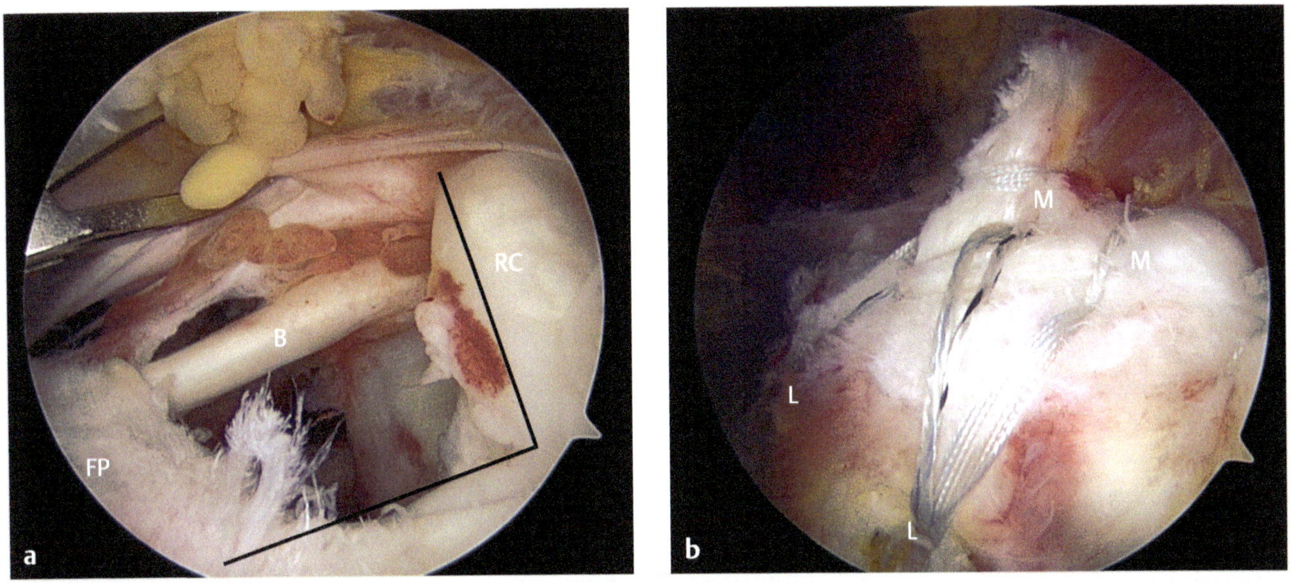

Fig. 5.8 Repair of a larger, retracted rotator cuff tear. **(a)** L-shaped tear (*black line*) involving the entire supraspinatus tendon and the majority of the infraspinatus tendon. **(b)** The tendon is mobilized and repair using a transosseous-equivalent (TOE) construct. FP, footprint; B, long head of biceps tendon; RC, retracted rotator cuff tear; M, medial row anchor; L, lateral row anchor.

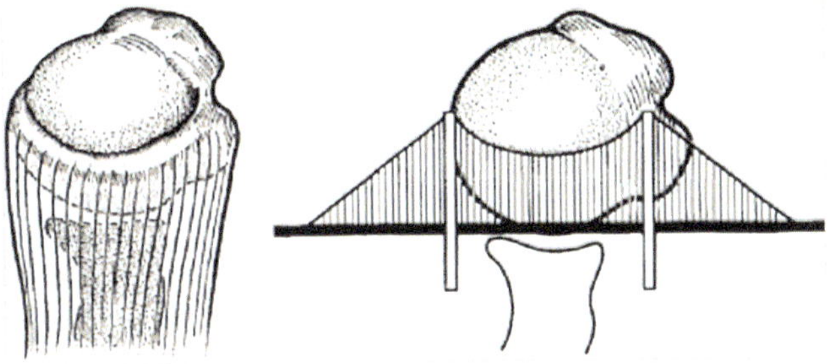

Fig. 5.9 The rotator cable functions like a suspension bridge to confer a balanced force-couple about the glenohumeral joint. (Reprinted with permission: Burkhart, S. S., et al. (1993). "The rotator crescent and rotator cable: an anatomic description of the shoulder's 'suspension bridge.'"Arthroscopy 9 (6):611–616.)

A PoweRasp or PowerPick (1.5-mm depth, 30-degree curve, Arthrex) can be used to create a bleeding bony surface at the site of the native footprint, in accordance with the Grimson-Duvey principle.[20] Preparation of the footprint should be gentle, as excessive decortication can compromise anchor fixation. When it comes to footprint preparation, channeling can offer improved outcomes for healing.[21]

In evaluation of the rotator cuff tear, the final construct should be planned out to determine the need for interval slides.[22] The rotational function of the shoulder must be kept in mind, and restoration of balanced suspension via the anterior and posterior cable insertions should take precedence over full restoration of the mediolateral footprint (**Fig. 5.9**).[23–26] The end result should be a repair that maximizes restoration of this cable, enhances footprint apposition and contact pressure, and maximizes load-sharing and interconnectivity.[3,27]

5.6.4 Repair Technique

Several different types of repair constructs can be utilized in arthroscopic rotator cuff repair, including single-row repair, double-row repair, and transosseous equivalent (TOE).[3] For the purpose of this chapter, the TOE repair technique will be described. The basic premise of this construct relies on the use of medial anchors, lateral anchors, and bridging suture material between the two, which provides compression of the repaired tendon atop the native footprint.[27–29]

A medial row of anchors is first placed along the articular margin of the humeral head. To do this, percutaneous portals along the lateral edge of the acromion can be created with the help of spinal needles for localization. It is important to ensure that a 45-degree angle between the bone and the anchor is achievable in order to maximize anchor pullout strength.[30] The 4.75 SwiveLock anchor (Arthrex) is the workhorse for the medial row anchor(s), as (1) it is versatile with regard to the types and number of sutures/tapes that can be placed, (2) it has a central retention suture that can also be used to tie medial knots and pulley constructs, and (3) it is vented, thus permitting blood flow from the bone to reach the repaired tendon.[20,31] FiberTape (Arthrex) is typically used given its strength and its decreased risk of tissue cut-through (**Figs. 5.7, 5.8**). In addition, FiberTape has been shown to provide the best traction in the lateral SwiveLock for bridge constructs.[32] For anchor insertion, a punch is best used to breach the hard cortical bone, and a tap is then used to compress and preserve bone density. Multiple portals can be created as needed, and multiple medial row anchors may be used depending on the size of the tear.

Suture limbs from these medial anchors are then passed through the rotator cuff. This can be done in an antegrade fashion with a Scorpion suture passer (Arthrex), or in a retrograde fashion with suture lassos. **Tip**: A free FiberLink (Arthrex) is very helpful for passing multiple strands of suture through a single tissue pass. Once all suture limbs from the medial anchors are passed, they should be tied to provide compression of the tendon tissue onto the bone (**Figs. 5.7, 5.8**).[33] **Tip**: If the tissue is friable and there is concern the sutures might rip out during reduction of the rotator cuff tendon to the footprint, an additional FiberLink or SutureTape can be used as a reduction stitch. Alternatively, rip-stop sutures employing Modified Mason–Allen constructs are useful for load-sharing, improving edge apposition in footprint reconstructions, as well as for single-row repairs of small tears (**Fig. 5.10**).[34,39]

To create a bridge construct, suture limbs from the medial row are retrieved, overlaid atop the lateral tendon, and affixed into the greater tuberosity with a lateral anchor(s) (**Figs. 5.7, 5.8**).[3,28,40–42] If more than one lateral anchor is to be used, a cruciate bridging pattern can be conferred atop the tendon. As biomechanical data and clinical experience has accumulated in support of smaller implants, we now commonly use 4.75mm Swivelock anchors (rather than 5.5mm) for lateral fixation of bridged constructs. This allows for increasing the size of the implant as needed if the bone turns out to be suboptimal.[43] **Tip**: If a dog-ear is anticipated, a FiberLink or SutureTape luggage-tag of this tissue can be added for subsequent incorporation into a lateral anchor, as this will help in the initial fixation strength of the.[42] The end result should be a watertight repair construct with maximized cable suspension function, footprint apposition, load-sharing, and interconnectivity (**Figs. 5.7, 5.8**).[3,21,25,45]

Upon completion of the repair, the shoulder should be copiously irrigated to remove debris. All instruments and cannulas are removed, and the skin is then cleansed with Chloraprep prior to closure. The portals are closed with 3-0 nylon suture in a simple interrupted fashion, and a sterile dressing is placed. The arm is carefully secured in a sling and abduction pillow.

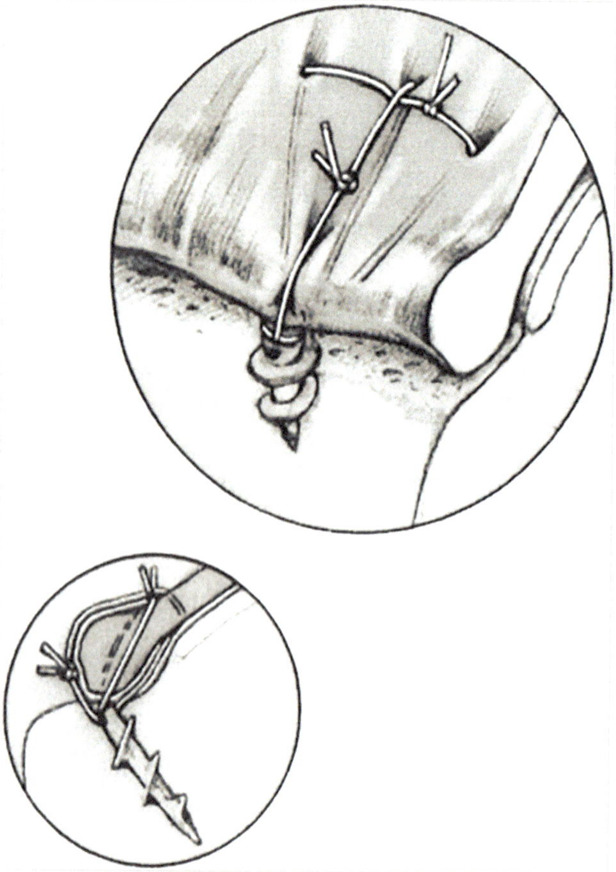

Fig. 5.10 Schematic of the modified Mason–Allen technique using a suture anchor. (Reprinted with permission: Scheibel MT, Habermeyer P. A modified Mason-Allen technique for rotator cuff repair using suture anchors. Arthroscopy. 2003; 19 (3):330–333.)

Application of a bioelectrical silver-zinc dressing, such as the "Jumpstart" dressing (Arthrex) has recently been shown to reduce skin bacterial load, which may decrease the risk for surgical site infection.[46]

5.7 Tips and Pearls/Expert Suggestions

- Perform bilateral shoulder examination under anesthesia prior to patient positioning to evaluate range of motion and stability.
- Epinephrine may be added to the local anesthetic to reduce portal site bleeding.
- Intra-articular evaluation of the subscapularis is critical, and if repair is required, it must be done first.
- After distal clavicle excision, advance a 7-mm cannula in the ASP into the acromioclavicular joint to ensure complete and symmetric resection.
- If the rotator cuff tear is not adequately visualized through the posterior portal, switch to the 70-degree scope, or make an additional posterolateral viewing portal (**Fig. 5.6**).
- It may be necessary to let down balanced suspension and rotate the arm to evaluate the integrity of the rotator cable.
- The rotator cable is the key—restoration of balanced suspension takes priority over restoration of the mediolateral footprint.
- The punch is best used to breach cortical bone, and the tap can compress and preserve bone density to follow.
- If a dog-ear forms during reduction of the rotator cuff tendon to the medial row, consider luggage tagging this tissue with a free FiberLink or SutureTape and incorporating it into the lateral row (**Fig. 5.8**).
- A free FiberLink is very helpful for passing multiple suture strands through a single tissue pass.
- Rip-stop sutures can be used to load-share and improve edge apposition.

5.8 What to Avoid

- Do not make large portals to avoid fluid turbulence.
- Avoid violation of the deltoid fascia, which can lead to extravasation of fluid.
- Do not rush the bursectomy, as remaining bursal tissue can lead to continued pain and poor visualization during anchor placement.
- Avoid injury to the coracoclavicular ligaments as well as the posterosuperior acromioclavicular capsule during distal clavicle resection.
- Do not perform rotator cuff releases 2.5 cm medial to the glenoid to avoid injury to the suprascapular nerve.
- Footprint preparation should be gentle, so as to not compromise anchor fixation.
- Avoid repair constructs that do not match the tear pattern. No one size fits all.

5.9 Complications/Bailout/Salvage

- In the setting of a large **U**-shaped tear, reduction of the tear apex to the bone may be difficult. Consider converting the

U-shaped tear to a crescent tear through side-to-side repair, and then repairing the construct to the lateral bone.
- If anchor pullout is encountered, select a new anchor site or upsize the anchor. If neither is able to be performed, consider leaving the anchor in situ and stacking a second anchor adjacent to the original.
- In the case of a greater tuberosity fracture upon implant insertion, consider incorporating a TOE tension-band suture construct that spans the fracture site and reduces the fractured fragment to its native location.
- If a complete repair is unable to be performed, emphasis should be placed on reestablishing the rotator cuff cable to its native footprint.
- If surgery is unable to be performed or completed arthroscopically, surgeons must be comfortable with transitioning to a mini-open or open approach.

5.10 Postoperative Care

Postoperative management of rotator cuff surgery is individualized to the patient and depends on several factors, including tear size, quality of tendon and bone, strength of the repair, age of the patient, and patient comorbidities. The primary goal of postoperative care is to protect the repair site and permit biologic healing while promoting early passive motion to prevent stiffness and reduce pain.

In the postoperative unit, the patient is instructed to perform gentle range-of-motion exercises of their elbow and wrist. Passive range of motion (PROM) of the operative shoulder to 90 degrees in the scapular plane is permitted. The first follow-up in clinic is scheduled for 7 to 10 days after surgery, at which point wounds are cleaned, sutures are removed, and Steri-Strips are applied. Examination during this visit verifies that the patient can achieve PROM to 90 degrees in the scapular plane. **Tip:** Ask the patient to gently provide this passive motion with assistance from their contralateral extremity. Often PROM done by a physician or therapist results in reflexive inhibition and an inaccurate assessment of motion. Patients are instructed to remain in the sling and pillow when sleeping and when out of the house, but are permitted to remove these and interpose a bedside pillow between their arm and body when comfortable at home. Home PROM exercises are continued until 4 weeks postoperatively, at which point formal physical therapy is prescribed to help assist full passive motion in the scapular plane. The patient is again evaluated in clinic at the 6-week postoperative time point, verifying continued improvements in motion. At this juncture, the patient is weaned out of the sling, and active assist as well as gentle active motion is permitted. Light resistance exercises are begun at 3 months postoperatively, and patients are sequentially evaluated every 6 weeks thereafter to monitor progression.

Establishing clear communication with patients during their postoperative visits is instrumental to the overall success of their rehabilitation. Often citing alleviation of their preoperative pain, patients may proceed with shoulder activities prematurely, consequently putting undue stress through their repair sites. Conversely, excessive pain, inadequate rehabilitation, or poor compliance with therapy can often lead to shoulder stiffness. As both of these instances are best remedied in the early phases of rehabilitation, compliance with follow-up visits should be emphasized. Return to daily overhead activity is typically permitted at 6 months postoperatively, and reserved for 6 to 9 months for those wishing to return to activity involving heavy manual labor or high-level athletics. It is important to counsel patients that ultimate maturation of the repair site and full restoration of strength may take upward of 12 months.[47]

References

1. Liem D, Buschmann VE, Schmidt C, et al. The prevalence of rotator cuff tears: is the contralateral shoulder at risk? Am J Sports Med 2014;42(4):826–830
2. Yamaguchi K, Ball CM, Galatz LM. Arthroscopic rotator cuff repair: transition from mini-open to all-arthroscopic. Clin Orthop Relat Res 2001(390):83–94
3. Cole BJ, ElAttrache NS, Anbari A. Arthroscopic rotator cuff repairs: an anatomic and biomechanical rationale for different suture-anchor repair configurations. Arthroscopy 2007;23(6):662–669
4. Gartsman GM. Arthroscopic management of rotator cuff disease. J Am Acad Orthop Surg 1998;6(4):259–266
5. Gartsman GM. All arthroscopic rotator cuff repairs. Orthop Clin North Am 2001;32(3):501–510, x
6. Norberg FB, Field LD, Savoie FH III. Repair of the rotator cuff. Mini-open and arthroscopic repairs. Clin Sports Med 2000;19(1):77–99
7. Oh LS, Wolf BR, Hall MP, Levy BA, Marx RG. Indications for rotator cuff repair: a systematic review. Clin Orthop Relat Res 2007;455(455):52–63
8. Stollsteimer GT, Savoie FH III. Arthroscopic rotator cuff repair: current indications, limitations, techniques, and results. Instr Course Lect 1998;47:59–65
9. Wolf BR, Dunn WR, Wright RW. Indications for repair of full-thickness rotator cuff tears. Am J Sports Med 2007;35(6):1007–1016
10. Murray MR, Saltzman MD, Gryzlo SM, Terry MA, Woodward CC, Nuber GW. Efficacy of preoperative home use of 2% chlorhexidine gluconate cloth before shoulder surgery. J Shoulder Elbow Surg 2011;20(6):928–933
11. Saltzman MD, Nuber GW, Gryzlo SM, Marecek GS, Koh JL. Efficacy of surgical preparation solutions in shoulder surgery. J Bone Joint Surg Am 2009;91(8):1949–1953
12. Blaine TA, Cote MA, Proto A, Mulcahey M, Lee FY, Bigliani LU. Interleukin-1. stimulates stromal-derived factor-1. expression in human subacromial bursa. J Orthop Res 2011;29(11):1695–1699
13. Gotoh M, Hamada K, Yamakawa H, Inoue A, Fukuda H. Increased substance P in subacromial bursa and shoulder pain in rotator cuff diseases. J Orthop Res 1998;16(5):618–621
14. Fukuda K, Craig EV, An KN, Cofield RH, Chao EY. Biomechanical study of the ligamentous system of the acromioclavicular joint. J Bone Joint Surg Am 1986;68(3):434–440
15. Klimkiewicz JJ, Williams GR, Sher JS, Karduna A, Des Jardins J, Iannotti JP. The acromioclavicular capsule as a restraint to posterior translation of the clavicle: a biomechanical analysis. J Shoulder Elbow Surg 1999;8(2):119–124
16. Lee KW, Debski RE, Chen CH, Woo SL, Fu FH. Functional evaluation of the ligaments at the acromioclavicular joint during anteroposterior and superoinferior translation. Am J Sports Med 1997;25(6):858–862
17. Salter EG Jr, Nasca RJ, Shelley BS. Anatomical observations on the acromioclavicular joint and supporting ligaments. Am J Sports Med 1987;15(3):199–206

18. Jerosch J, Steinbeck J, Schröder M, Castro WH. Arthroscopic resection of the acromioclavicular joint (ARAC). Knee Surg Sports Traumatol Arthrosc 1993;1(3–4):209–215
19. Strauss EJ, Barker JU, McGill K, Verma NN. The evaluation and management of failed distal clavicle excision. Sports Med Arthrosc Rev 2010;18(3):213–219
20. Ficklscherer A, Loitsch T, Serr M, et al. Does footprint preparation influence tendon-to-bone healing after rotator cuff repair in an animal model? Arthroscopy 2014;30(2):188–194
21. Taniguchi N, Suenaga N, Oizumi N, Miyoshi N, Yamaguchi H, Inoue K, Chosa E. Bone marrow stimulation at the footprint of arthroscopic surface-holding repair advances cuff repair integrity. J Shoulder Elbow Surg. 2015 Jun; 24 (6):860–6. doi: 10.1016/j.jse.2014.09.031. Epub 2014 Dec 2
22. Jo CH, Shin JS, Park IW, Kim H, Lee SY. Multiple channeling improves the structural integrity of rotator cuff repair. Am J Sports Med. 2013 Nov;41(11):2650–7 doi: 10.1177/0363546513499138. Epub 2013 Aug 13
23. Burkhart SS, Esch JC, Jolson RS. The rotator crescent and rotator cable: an anatomic description of the shoulder's "suspension bridge". Arthroscopy 1993;9(6):611–616
24. Denard PJ, Koo SS, Murena L, Burkhart SS. Pseudoparalysis: the importance of rotator cable integrity. Orthopedics 2012;35(9):e1353–e1357
25. Nguyen ML, Quigley RJ, Galle SE, et al. Margin convergence anchorage to bone for reconstruction of the anterior attachment of the rotator cable. Arthroscopy 2012;28(9): 1237–1245
26. Mesiha MM, Derwin KA, Sibole SC, Erdemir A, McCarron JA. The biomechanical relevance of anterior rotator cuff cable tears in a cadaveric shoulder model. J Bone Joint Surg Am 2013;95(20):1817–1824
27. Park MC, Tibone JE, ElAttrache NS, Ahmad CS, Jun BJ, Lee TQ. Part II: Biomechanical assessment for a footprint-restoring transosseous-equivalent rotator cuff repair technique compared with a double-row repair technique. J Shoulder Elbow Surg 2007;16(4):469–476
28. Park MC, Elattrache NS, Ahmad CS, Tibone JE. "Transosseous-equivalent" rotator cuff repair technique. Arthroscopy 2006;22(12):1360.e1–1360.e5
29. Park MC, ElAttrache NS, Tibone JE, Ahmad CS, Jun BJ, Lee TQ. Part I: Footprint contact characteristics for a transosseous-equivalent rotator cuff repair technique compared with a double-row repair technique. J Shoulder Elbow Surg 2007;16(4):461–468
30. Burkhart SS. The deadman theory of suture anchors: observations along a south Texas fence line. Arthroscopy 1995;11(1):119–123
31. Denard PJ, Burkhart SS. The evolution of suture anchors in arthroscopic rotator cuff repair. Arthroscopy 2013;29(9):1589–1595
32. De Carli A, Lanzetti RM, Monaco E, Labianca L, Mossa L, Ferretti A. The failure mode of two reabsorbable fixation systems: Swivelock with Fibertape versus Bio-Corkscrew with Fiberwire in bovine rotator cuff. J Orthop Sci 2012;17(6):789–795
33. Mall NA, Lee AS, Chahal J, et al. Transosseous-equivalent rotator cuff repair: a systematic review on the biomechanical importance of tying the medial row. Arthroscopy 2013;29(2):377–386
34. Jung SW, Kim DH, Kang SH, Lee JH. Arthroscopic modified Mason-Allen technique for large U- or L-shaped rotator cuff tears. Knee Surg Sports Traumatol Arthrosc 2016
35. MacGillivray JD, Ma CB. An arthroscopic stitch for massive rotator cuff tears: the Mac stitch. Arthroscopy 2004;20(6):669–671
36. Nelson CO, Sileo MJ, Grossman MG, Serra-Hsu F. Single-row modified mason-allen versus double-row arthroscopic rotator cuff repair: a biomechanical and surface area comparison. Arthroscopy 2008;24(8):941–948
37. Denard PJ, Burkhart SS. A load-sharing rip-stop fixation construct for arthroscopic rotator cuff repair. Arthrosc Tech 2012;1(1):e37–e42
38. Burkhart SS, Denard PJ, Konicek J, Hanypsiak BT. Biomechanical validation of load-sharing rip-stop fixation for the repair of tissue-deficient rotator cuff tears. Am J Sports Med 2014;42(2):457–462
39. Scheibel MT, Habermeyer P. A modified Mason-Allen technique for rotator cuff repair using suture anchors. Arthroscopy 2003;19(3):330–333
40. Gartsman GM, Drake G, Edwards TB, et al. Ultrasound evaluation of arthroscopic full-thickness supraspinatus rotator cuff repair: single-row versus double-row suture bridge (transosseous equivalent) fixation. Results of a prospective, randomized study. J Shoulder Elbow Surg 2013;22(11):1480–1487
41. Dines JS, Bedi A, ElAttrache NS, Dines DM. Single-row versus double-row rotator cuff repair: techniques and outcomes. J Am Acad Orthop Surg 2010;18(2):83–93
42. Frank JB, ElAttrache NS, Dines JS, Blackburn A, Crues J, Tibone JE. Repair site integrity after arthroscopic transosseous-equivalent suture-bridge rotator cuff repair. Am J Sports Med 2008;36(8):1496–1503
43. Barber FA, Herbert MA, Hapa O, et al. Biomechanical analysis of pullout strengths of rotator cuff and glenoid anchors: 2011 update. Arthroscopy 2011;27(7):895–905
44. Roghani R, Snir N, Wolfson TS, Rokito AS. The importance of tear edge fixation in modified transosseous-equivalent rotator cuff repair: a biomechanical study. Bull Hosp Jt Dis (2013) 2015;73(1):10–17
45. Nassos JT, ElAttrache NS, Angel MJ, Tibone JE, Limpisvasti O, Lee TQ. A watertight construct in arthroscopic rotator cuff repair. J Shoulder Elbow Surg 2012;21(5):589–596
46. Cooke CL, Greene RS, van Eck CF, Uquilas C, Limpisvasti O. Bioelectric Silver-Zinc Dressing Equally Effective to Chlorhexidine in Reducing Skin Bacterial Load in Healthy Volunteers. Arthroscopy. 2018 Oct;34(10): 2886–2891 doi: 10.1016/j.arthro.2018.05.046. Epub 2018 Sep 5.
47. Gulotta LV, Nho SJ, Dodson CC, Adler RS, Altchek DW, MacGillivray JD; HSS Arthroscopic Rotator Cuff Registry. Prospective evaluation of arthroscopic rotator cuff repairs at 5 years: part II—prognostic factors for clinical and radiographic outcomes. J Shoulder Elbow Surg 2011;20(6): 941–946

6 Partial Articular-Sided Supraspinatus Tear Repair

Kent Rinehart, Josh Locker, Jonathan C. Riboh, and Matthew A. Tao

Abstract

Partial-thickness tears of the rotator cuff are common and often cause a significant level of pain and dysfunction. A subset of these, partial articular-sided supraspinatus tears (PASTA), are a unique entity that have become increasingly recognized over time. As techniques and instrumentation have evolved, successful utilization of a trans-tendinous repair has emerged, which avoids disrupting the intact, bursal portion of the footprint. Our indications are fairly narrow for this form of repair; however, we do believe it offers some advantages over traditional techniques. Critical evaluation of the tear is required at the time of surgery, and if amenable, our preference is to use a PASTA-specific kit that allows for precise repair and minimal disruption of the native tendon. This restores the native anatomy with the goal of returning patients to symptom-free, functional use of the shoulder.

Keywords: *partial-thickness rotator cuff tears, partial articular-sided supraspinatus tears, PASTA, trans-tendinous repair*

6.1 Introduction

Partial-thickness rotator cuff tears (PTRCT) are a common injury that can cause diminished shoulder function and pain. These injuries can be classified based on their location as articular sided, bursal sided, or interstitial. They can also be classified by the depth of the tear.[1] Those with symptomatic partial-thickness tears who have failed appropriate conservative management may benefit from surgical treatment.

Historically, those patients requiring operative intervention typically underwent either debridement alone or surgical completion of the tear followed by repair. However, techniques, instruments, and implants are now available that allow for transtendinous repairs of partial articular-sided supraspinatus tears (PASTA) without disruption of the intact bursal component. Initial studies show equivalent outcomes at short- and mid-term follow-up with traditional repair versus transtendinous techniques.[1]

Goals of this technique are to improve pain and function by allowing healing of articular-sided tears back to the anatomic footprint without disturbing the normal bursal portion of the tendon. A theoretic advantage of the transtendinous technique is that it allows maintenance of the otherwise normal lateral insertion of the tendon so as to maintain a normal insertional footprint and normal length–tension relationship of the tendon. However, this has not necessarily demonstrated improved outcomes over tear completion and repair in the literature to date.[1,2] One prospective comparative study did demonstrate a decreased rate of postoperative bursal-sided tears in patients undergoing transtendinous repair.[3]

Although the indications for this technique are fairly narrow, we do feel that it provides a solution to an anatomic problem with some advantages over traditional techniques. Our algorithm and surgical technique are detailed below.

6.2 Surgical Technique

Our indication for the transtendinous technique is limited to isolated articular-sided tears of approximately 50% of the insertional width of the supraspinatus alone with an otherwise normal bursal surface. While this is initially diagnosed preoperatively on MRI, a thorough diagnostic evaluation should be performed intraoperatively to both visually and palpably confirm the aforementioned situation. It is useful for those tears that have failed conservative management and are of sufficient depth that they warrant surgical repair but not those that represent a near full-thickness tear.

Our algorithm for all rotator cuff surgery begins in preoperative holding with a single-shot, regional nerve block under ultrasound guidance; this can be done in either a supraclavicular or interscalene location at discretion of the anesthesiologist. Our preference is for the addition of steroid to the local anesthetic as this can significantly potentiate the duration of the block (almost twofold) and has not been shown to have negative effects on the nerve.[4] Patient positioning in the operating room, either lateral decubitus or beach chair, is dictated by the surgeon, and our preference is for beach chair in a fairly vertical position with the aid of an arm positioner. A standard diagnostic arthroscopy is performed viewing through a standard posterior portal with an anterior working portal through the rotator interval.

The depth, size, and extent of involvement of the PASTA tear can then be thoroughly evaluated with the arm in multiple positions. After inspection for additional pathology, the undersurface of the supraspinatus is gently debrided with the use of a 4.5-mm arthroscopic shaver (Dyonics Bonecutter Platinum; Smith & Nephew, Andover, MA). We prefer the use of a smooth (as opposed to serrated) blade on both sides of the shaver to avoid being overly aggressive with tissue removal. This blade also allows for precise eburnation of the underlying bone to remove any unstable bony fragments and facilitate a healing footprint. The center of the tear is marked with the use of a spinal needle and no. 0 monofilament suture (Maxon; Covidien, Minneapolis, MN).

We then move into the subacromial space and an anterolateral portal is established adjacent to the region of the tear with a double-flanged cannula (PassPort; Arthrex, Naples, FL). We remove significant bursitis that impairs visualization or would impede our repair with the use of a shaver and radiofrequency ablation wand (Super Turbovac 90; Arthrocare, Austin, TX). If a type 2 or 3 acromial spur is noted along with an impingement lesion (fraying of the coracoacromial ligament), an acromioplasty is performed with a 5.5-mm shaver (Dyonics Bonecutter Platinum; Smith & Nephew). The previously placed suture is the identified, and the bursal side of the supraspinatus is carefully inspected both visually and by palpation with a probe.

Once the decision to attempt a transtendinous repair has been made, a PASTA-specific kit (PASTA Bridge; Arthrex) is opened onto the field. The arm is placed in slight forward flexion and abduction with neutral rotation. The included 17-gauge spinal needle is used to template the anterior suture anchor angle and position at the anterior edge of the tear and immediately lateral to the articular margin. A small stab incision is made in line with the spinal needle, and the inner trocar from the needle is removed. A 1.1-mm guidewire is placed through the needle, and the wire is held carefully in place while needle is removed. The included dilator and spear are placed in sequential fashion, and the spear is impacted to the level of the laser-etched line. The wire and dilator are removed, and a 2.4-mm biocomposite suture anchor (SutureTak; Arthrex) is placed through the spear and impacted into position. The sutures are left in place coming out of the anterolateral stab incision. This process is then repeated for the posterior anchor. Both limbs of the no. 2 high-tensile strength suture from each anchor are brought out of the anterolateral cannula. One suture limb from each anchor is taken and securely tied together outside of the body using a standard surgeon's knot, and the tails are cut. We prefer to do this on top of a blunt instrument (metal arthroscopic trocar) to ensure a solid knot. The free limbs from each anchor are then tensioned simultaneously such that pretied knot is shuttled down on top of the medial, bursal side of the tendon, which compresses the tendon down to bone. It is critical to note that all bursal tissue must be cleared between the repair site and the cannula to prevent a tissue bridge from occurring. The free limbs are then loaded into a 4.75-mm biocomposite lateral row anchor (SwiveLock; Arthrex), clamped and allowed to hang out of the anterolateral cannula. A bone socket is prepared just off the lateral most edge of the greater tuberosity using the included bone punch. Proper tension on each suture limb is maintained as the anchor is inserted flush with the bone, and the suture ends are then cut.

We prefer to evaluate the repair both statically and dynamically to ensure that good compression is visible across the repair site and that it moves well in continuity. We also then reevaluate the repair from the glenohumeral joint to confirm that the anatomic footprint has been restored.

6.3 Postoperative Care

Patients are placed in a shoulder sling with an abduction pillow following the procedure. Assuming no concomitant procedures have been performed that would limit rehabilitation, such as biceps tenodesis, formal physical therapy begins at 4 weeks with gentle passive motion. Patients begin to start weaning out of the sling at this point. Motion is progressed steadily to active-assisted and eventually full active range of motion against gravity under the guidance of a therapist. Given that this is a relatively small repair with maintained healthy tendon surrounding the repair, we feel that early passive motion is appropriate and safe; however, we still avoid true resistance or strengthening for 3 months.

6.4 Conclusion

True PASTA lesions with intact and normal bursal-sided tendon present a unique scenario with multiple surgical options. Although we feel that the indications for a transtendinous repair, as described earlier, are fairly narrow, it does serve a defined role and allow for a solid, anatomic repair. This technique offers some advantages over other described methods and has been shown to have equivalent outcomes in the literature.

References

1. Ono Y, Woodmass JM, Bois AJ, Boorman RS, Thornton GM, Lo IK. Arthroscopic repair of articular surface partial-thickness rotator cuff tears: transtendon technique versus repair after completion of the tear: a meta-analysis. Adv Orthop 2016;2016:7468054
2. Kim YS, Lee HJ, Bae SH, Jin H, Song HS. Outcome comparison between in situ repair versus tear completion repair for partial thickness rotator cuff tears. Arthroscopy 2015;31(11):2191–2198
3. Johnson JMD, Caldwell PE III, Pearson SEArthroscopic transtendinous modified double-row suture bridge repair of a bony PASTA lesion. Arthrosc Techn 2014;3(4):449–453
4. Choi S, Rodseth R, McCartney CJL. Effects of dexamethasone as a local anaesthetic adjuvant for brachial plexus block: a systematic review and meta-analysis of. randomized trials. Br J Anaesth 2014;112(3):427–439

7 Arthroscopic Subscapularis Repair

Michael H. McGraw, Tim Wang, and Answorth A. Allen

Abstract
Subscapularis repair has increased in popularity as its significant role in rotator cuff function has been better understood. This repair may be achieved either with open approach or arthroscopically. There are several techniques described to achieve adequate repair, but the underlying principle is to properly identify the tear and subsequently achieve secure fixation of the tendon back to its footprint. We present our technique for arthroscopic subscapularis repair. The described technique provides reduction of the retracted tendon, sufficient pullout strength, and compression of the tendon to the footprint to facilitate healing.

Keywords: *subscapularis, rotator cuff tear, arthroscopic subscapularis repair, coracoplasty, arthroscopy*

7.1 Goals of Procedure

Historically, most of the rotator cuff literature was devoted to the repair of the supraspinatus, infraspinatus, and teres minor tendons.[1–4] However, over the last decade, it has become clear that subscapularis tendon tears are more prevalent than previously reported, and play an important role in shoulder function.[5–7]

The subscapularis is the largest and most powerful of the rotator cuff muscles and is more important for arm elevation than either the supraspinatus or infraspinatus.[8] It is the only anterior rotator cuff muscle, and as a result, repairs must be accomplished to balance the posterior forces of the rotator cuff.[9] The upper portion of the subscapularis is particularly important because this is the part of the insertion that is broadest superiorly, and this site serves as the anterior attachment of the rotator cable.[5,10] Finally, for tears extending into the supraspinatus, repair of the upper subscapularis decreases the stress on the adjacent repair of the supraspinatus.[11]

Therefore, restoration of subscapularis function is essential for long-term maintenance of acceptable clinical results for both traumatic and nontraumatic rotator cuff tears. The goals of surgery are to restore the subscapularis back to its native anatomical footprint. As a result, its biomechanical function will be restored. The described technique provides reduction of the retracted tendon, sufficient pullout strength, and compression of the tendon to the footprint to facilitate healing.

7.2 Advantages

The arthroscope is minimally invasive and may allow a quicker recovery with less postoperative pain than an open approach. It also allows the surgeon to address other intra-articular pathology that may be encountered, including labral pathology and posterior superior rotator cuff tears. Potential disadvantages include the need for advanced arthroscopic skills, especially in patients with full thickness retracted subscapularis tendon tears.

7.3 Indications

A thorough history and physical examination should be performed to diagnose subscapularis tendon tears, as well as other concomitant pathology in the shoulder. Particularly useful tests include the lift-off test and bear-hug test. After correct diagnosis, subscapularis repair, whether open or arthroscopic, should be considered in any patient with functional limitations such as internal rotation weakness and pain who have not responded to conservative management. Repair of this tendon is integral to maintaining the dynamic stabilization of the shoulder through balancing of the force couple. In addition, other studies have highlighted that the integrity of the subscapularis tendon plays a key role in reducing the recurrences of rotator cuff tears.[12]

The role of nonoperative treatment in patients with symptomatic subscapularis tears is limited. Oftentimes these injuries are unrecognized and patients with chronic tears can present with a long history of pain and dysfunction.[6] Furthermore, most patients will eventually fail nonoperative treatment modalities. In rare instances, when the patient is a poor surgical candidate, nonsurgical management is necessary. Nonoperative treatment modalities typically consist of activity modification with gentle stretching, progressive strengthening of the shoulder, and anti-inflammatory medications.

Subscapularis repair should also be considered in cases of medial subluxation of the long-head of biceps tendon, as the upper subscapularis contributes to the medial sling of the bicipital pulley.

7.4 Contraindications

Relative contraindications to surgery are lack of pain, severe atrophy, and retraction or significant fatty degeneration on MRI.

7.5 Preoperative Preparation/ Positioning

The history, physical examination, and imaging (plain films and MRI) should be reviewed before the procedure. The preoperative imaging should be used to confirm the presence of a subscapularis tendon tear and the degree of fatty atrophy and retraction, and to identify pathology to the biceps tendon.

Axial sections of the shoulder should be scrutinized to evaluate disruption of the subscapularis tendon on the lesser tuberosity.

7.5.1 Anesthesia and Positioning

Arthroscopic subscapularis repair can be achieved successfully in the lateral decubitus or beach-chair position. Position is largely based on surgeon preference. The senior author prefers the beach-chair position due to the ease of mobility of the extremity and the option to convert to an open procedure if necessary. The patient is aligned on the edge of the table so that

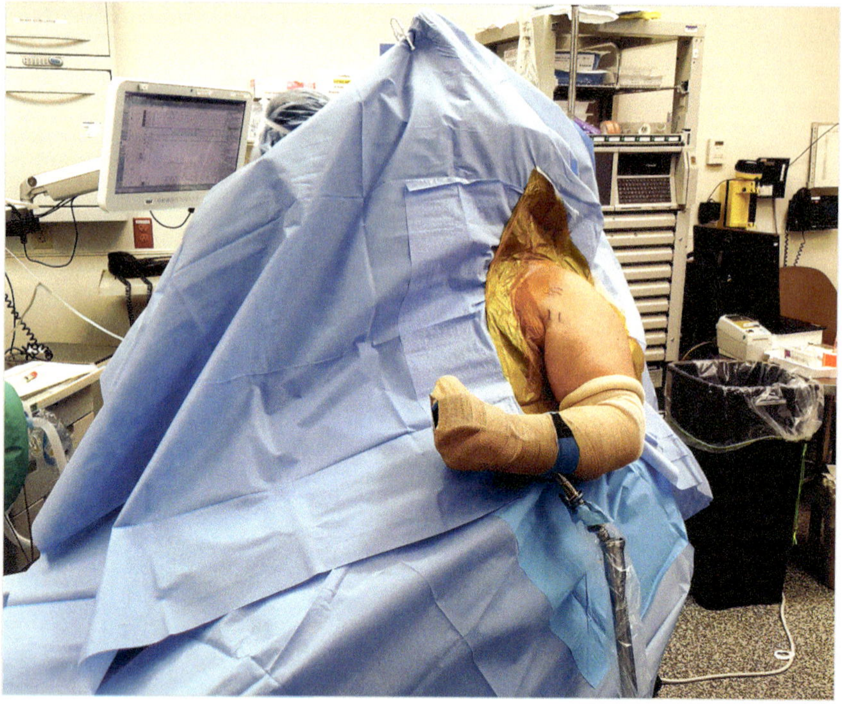

Fig. 7.1 Beach-chair position.

the affected shoulder and scapula are exposed. The back of the table is elevated so that the acromion is parallel to the floor. The head is secured to the operating table with a headrest device. Care is taken to prevent excessive neck flexion or extension.

The anesthesiologist administers regional anesthesia with intravenous sedation and applies protective eyewear to the patient. An articulating arm holder holds the extremity and allows for easy manipulation of the extremity (**Fig. 7.1**).

7.6 Operative Technique (Table 7.1)

7.6.1 Portal Placement (Fig. 7.2)

Our standard posterior portal is approximately 2 cm inferior and 1 cm medial to the posterolateral edge of the acromion. However, we adjust the portal by small amounts as needed after feeling for the "soft spot." An anterior portal is then established with an outside-in technique using a spinal needle. This portal is placed as to approach the lesser tuberosity at a 45-degree angle to facilitate anchor placement. A cannula is placed through this portal. A systematic diagnostic arthroscopy is performed looking for other intra-articular pathology, paying particular attention to the other rotator cuff and biceps tendons.

After the diagnostic arthroscopy is complete, an anterosuperolateral (ASL) portal is established via an outside-in technique. This portal should be superior and lateral in the rotator interval, and serves as the predominant working portal during the procedure but may also be used for visualization during mobilization of the tendon. The spinal needle should enter just off the anterolateral edge of the acromion and be directed into the glenohumeral joint. Appropriate placement of this portal facilitates a parallel approach to the footprint and subscapularis tendon for mobilization and suture passage. We place an additional 8.25-mm cannula through the ASL portal.

Table 7.1 Surgical steps
1. Visualization of the tear
2. Proper portal placement
3. Address the biceps tendon
4. Subcoracoid space—coracoplasty if interval < 6 mm
5. Mobilization of subscapularis
6. Bone bed preparation
7. Anchor placement
8. Suture passage
9. Knot tying

7.6.2 Visualization

The first step in repairing a subscapularis tendon tear is identifying it. To achieve this, it is helpful to minimize the differential between the patient's blood pressure and the arthroscopic pump pressure. Maintenance of a mean arterial pressure of 70 to 90 mm Hg or a systolic pressure near 100 mm Hg allows maximal visualization and minimizes bleeding. Also, judicious use of electrocautery to cauterize bleeding vessels is valuable.

The subscapularis is initially viewed with the 30-degree arthroscope from the posterior portal. The subscapularis tendon can be difficult to visualize because it is in a very confined space that may be unfamiliar to the surgeon. Placing the extremity in flexion and internal rotation lifts the tendon off its footprint and is helpful for evaluation of a partial tear. Also, the "posterior lever push," where a posterior force is placed on the proximal humerus with a simultaneous anterior force on the distal humerus, aids in visualization. Finally, the 70-degree arthroscope should be utilized interchangeably as needed and is often necessary to adequately visualize the footprint (**Fig. 7.3**).

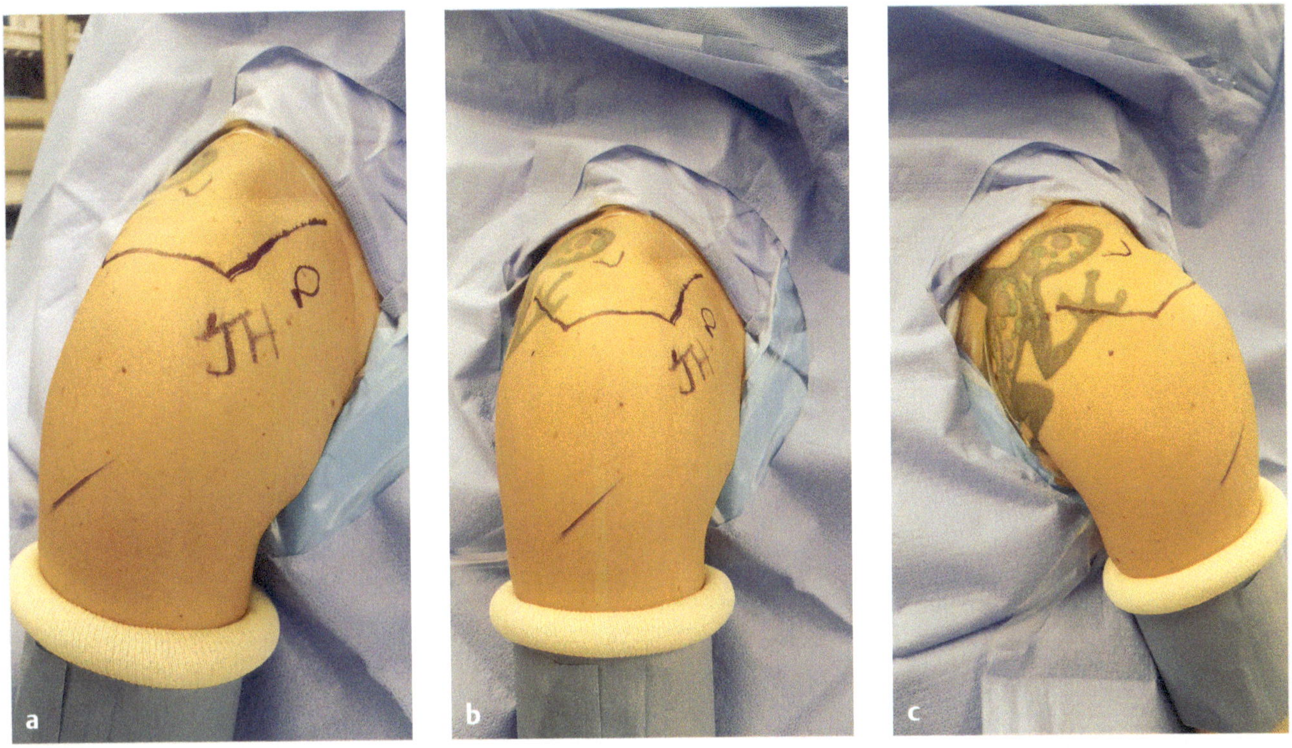

Fig. 7.2 Portal placement.

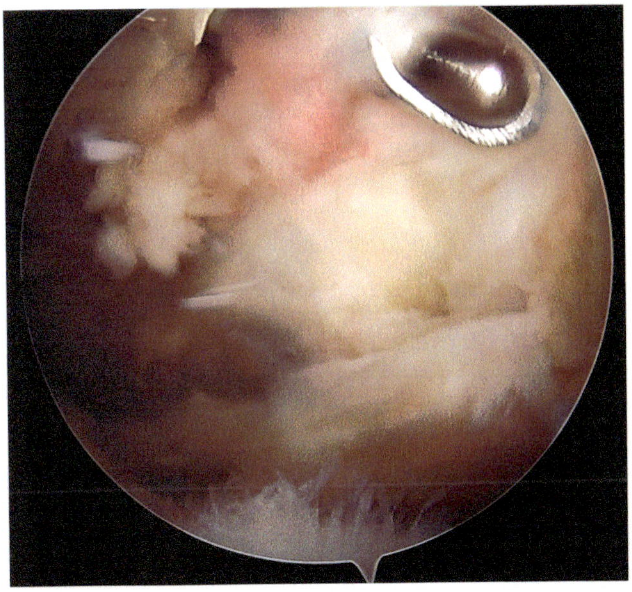

Fig. 7.3 View of the subscapularis tendon with a 70-degree arthroscope.

7.6.3 Biceps Tendon

Subscapularis tears are often associated with tearing or medial subluxation of the long head of the biceps tendon. Inferior results have been reported when the biceps is left in place in the setting of a subscapularis repair.[13] As a result, we routinely perform a subpectoral tenodesis to address the biceps tendon. Tenodesing the tendon in this position eliminates the possibility of persistent pain from recurrent biceps subluxation or pain from the bicipital groove. The role of tenotomy versus tenodesis is controversial. Our technique for biceps tenodesis is beyond the scope of this chapter; however, it is our belief that some treatment of the biceps tendon should be performed.

7.6.4 Subcoracoid Space

Assessing the subcoracoid space is an important component of subscapularis repair. Following accurate portal placement, the coracoid should be identified. The 30-degree arthroscope should be used from the posterior portal to maintain proper orientation. The 70-degree arthroscope may cause the surgeon to be disoriented and subsequently cause the surgeon to stray inferiorly to the coracoid tip, risking neurovascular injury. With partial subscapularis tears, the coracoid tip can reliably be found anterior to the upper border of the subscapularis. Through the ASL portal, the surgeon should make a window in the rotator interval just above the upper border of the subscapularis tendon using an electrocautery device or shaver. In making this window, the medial sling of the biceps should be preserved.

However, when the tear is retracted, the coracoacromial ligament can be used to direct the surgeon toward the coracoid. A blunt instrument can be used to palpate and confirm the location of the coracoid tip.

Once identified, the undersurface of the coracoid is skeletonized. If necessary, a coracoplasty is performed to create adequate working space. To determine the need for coracoplasty, the coracohumeral interval can be measured using an instrument with known dimensions (such as a probe) through the ASL portal. If the coracohumeral interval is less than 6 mm, there is evidence of subcoracoid stenosis and a coracoplasty should be performed with the goal of increasing the interval to 10 mm.

7.6.5 Mobilization

Retracted subscapularis tendon tears require a three-sided release to mobilize the tendon. To accomplish this, traction suture can be placed at the superolateral aspect of the tendon (comma tissue). The "comma tissue" is a fibrous band of tissue that is located at the superolateral border of the subscapularis tendon, and is composed of the coracohumeral ligament and superior glenohumeral ligament. The traction suture can be placed in this tissue through the ASL portal using a Scorpion suture passer (Arthrex, Naples, FL). If not performed earlier in the procedure during the coracoplasty, the posterolateral corner of the coracoid should be skeletonized using a combination of a thermal device and an arthroscopic shaver. This constitutes the "anterior" release. Using a 30-degree arthroscopic elevator or electrocautery device, the "superior" release is completed between the coracoid neck and the tendon. The release should only be done to the midpoint of the undersurface of the coracoid neck to prevent inadvertent damage to the neurovascular structures. The posterior release is performed by clearing the tissue posterior to the subscapularis tendon and the anterior to the glenoid neck (**Fig. 7.4**). Furthermore, a traction suture using a linked stitch can be placed and used for added mobilization of the subscapularis tendon.

7.6.6 Bone Bed Preparation/Anchor Placement

Next, the bone bed needs to be prepared. To remove soft tissue off the subscapularis anatomic footprint on the lesser tuberosity, the ASL portal is particularly useful. An electrocautery device and ring curette should be used to clear all soft tissue from the bone. Then an arthroscopic burr can be used gently to achieve a bleeding bone bed for tendon healing. It is always the goal to place the anchor anatomically on the lesser tuberosity; however, if this will lead to excessive tension on the repair, we medialize the anchor up to 5 mm without deleterious effects.[14] The anchors should be placed inferior to superior from the anterior portal. Rotation of the arm may allow for better exposure. Alternatively, a percutaneous portal can be established using an outside-in technique to achieve a better trajectory. We typically place one anchor for a partial tear and two anchors for a full-thickness tear. We prefer triple-loaded PEEK anchors (5.5-mm Biocomposite Corkscrew FT; Arthrex Inc., Naples, FL) to decrease the stress on the individual sutures (**Fig. 7.5**).

7.6.7 Suture Passage

We prefer to pass the sutures through the tendon with the FastPass Scorpion suture passer (Arthrex). This instrument facilitates easy and efficient antegrade passage of sutures and allows for blind capture. One strand of suture is retrieved from the anchor, pulled out the ASL cannula, and loaded in the suture passer. Tension is placed on the traction suture which is in the ASL portal but outside of the cannula. The suture is passed about 10 mm from the lateral edge of the subscapularis tendon (**Fig. 7.6**). The sutures are placed in a horizontal mattress fashion and brought out through the anterior portal. The process is repeated for all sutures of the same anchor. Knot tying then proceeds in an inferior to superior fashion using a single-row technique (**Fig. 7.7**).

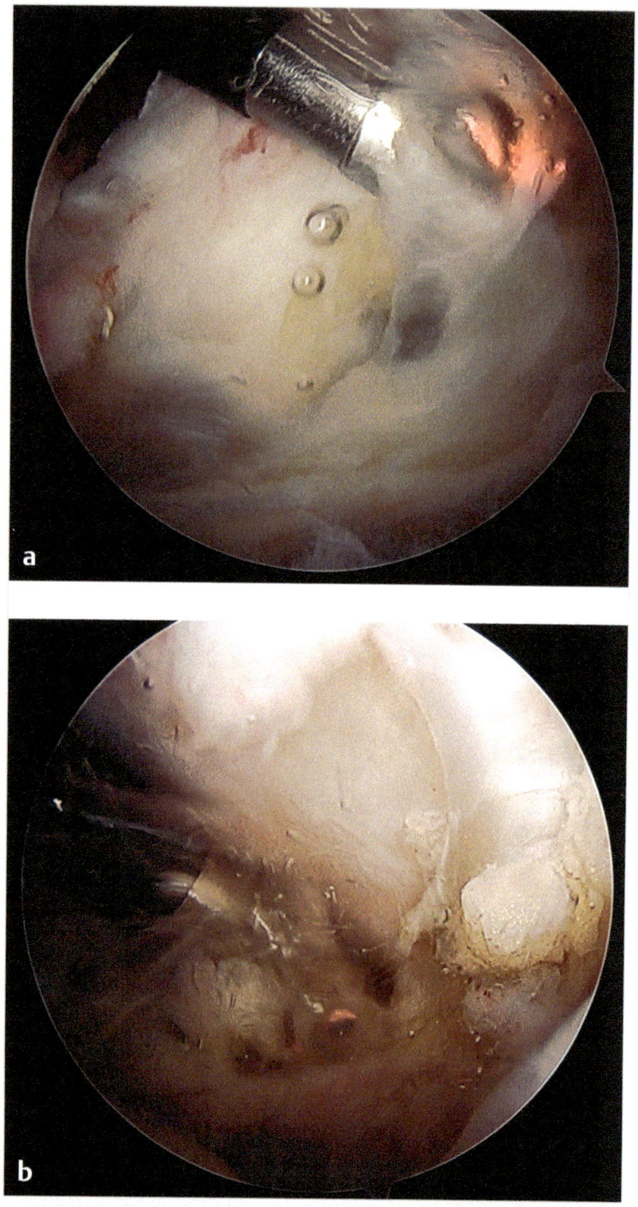

Fig. 7.4 Subscapularis mobilization: the electrocautery device is used to perform a three-sided mobilization of the tendon.

7.7 Tips and Pearls/Expert Suggestions

7.7.1 Know the Anatomy

The anatomy around the coracoid can be intimidating. The axillary nerve and artery, musculocutaneous nerve, and the lateral cord of the brachial plexus are near the coracoid. However, anatomic dissections have demonstrated these structures are on average 2.5 cm from the coracoid tip.

7.7.2 Portal Placement

Proper placement of the anterior and ASL portal can make subscapularis repair much easier. The anterior portal should be placed more medial than the standard anterior portal as

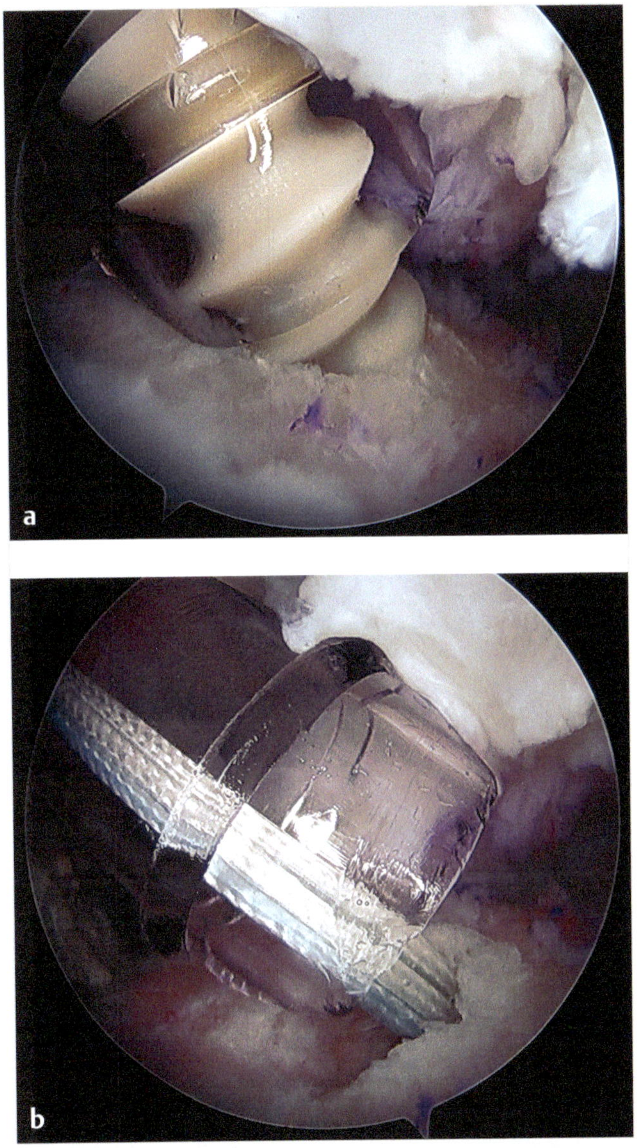

Fig. 7.5 Anchor placement: a triple-loaded 5.5-mm PEEK corkscrew anchor (Arthrex, Naples, FL) being placed in the subscapularis footprint through the anterior portal.

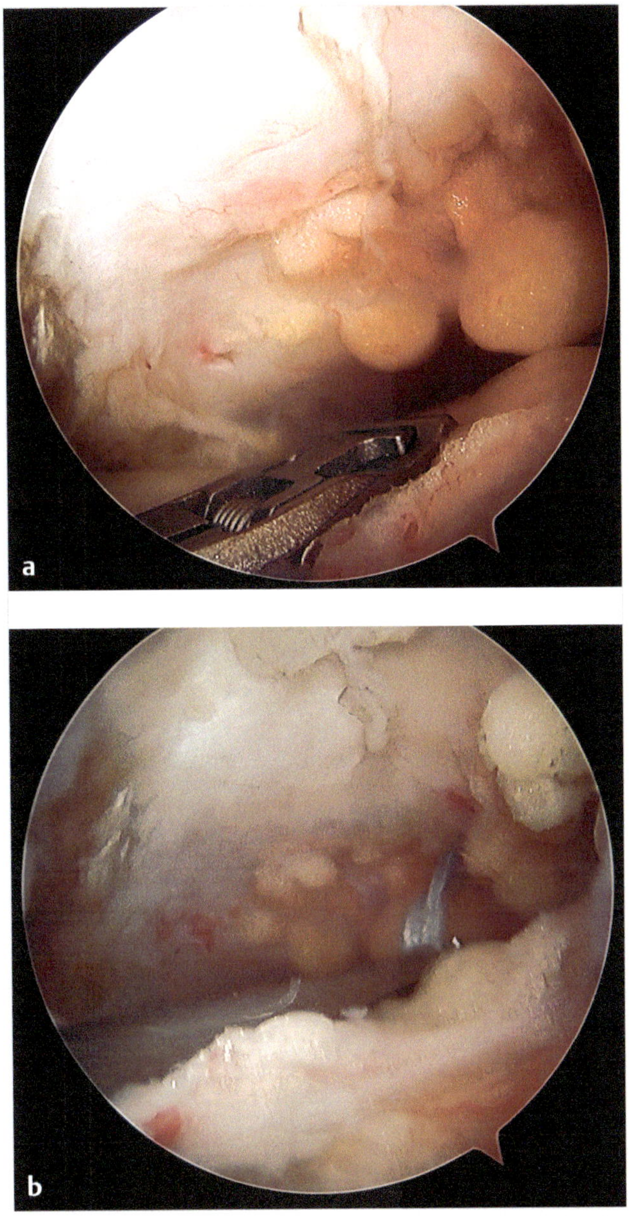

Fig. 7.6 Suture passage using FastPass Arthrex suture passer (Naples, FL).

to approach the lesser tuberosity at a 45-degree angle. The ASL portal should be inserted off the anterolateral tip of the acromion. When placed correctly, the cannula should approach the lesser tuberosity at a 5-to 10-degree angle and should be parallel to the subscapularis tendon. This is beneficial when mobilizing the tendon and performing antegrade suture passage.

7.7.3 Visualization

The subscapularis tendon should be thoroughly scrutinized for tears. The 70-degree arthroscope can be useful in visualizing the tear and the footprint. The "posterior lever push" technique is a helpful maneuver to aid in visualization when the subcoracoid space is tight.

7.7.4 Finding the Subscapularis Tendon

Lo and Burkhart described the "comma sign," which is a marker of the torn subscapularis stump and can be useful even when tackling chronic retracted subscapularis tears.[15] Locating the "comma sign" is useful in differentiating the subscapularis from the conjoined tendon and the coracoacromial ligament. The humeral insertion of the subscapularis, superior glenohumeral ligament, and the coracohumeral ligament are in close proximity and are interconnected, so the entire complex is torn together when the subscapularis tears from the lesser tuberosity. A portion of it remains attached to the superolateral corner of the subscapularis tendon. This residual tissue appears as a comma-shaped area of tissue at the superolateral border of the muscle and reliably

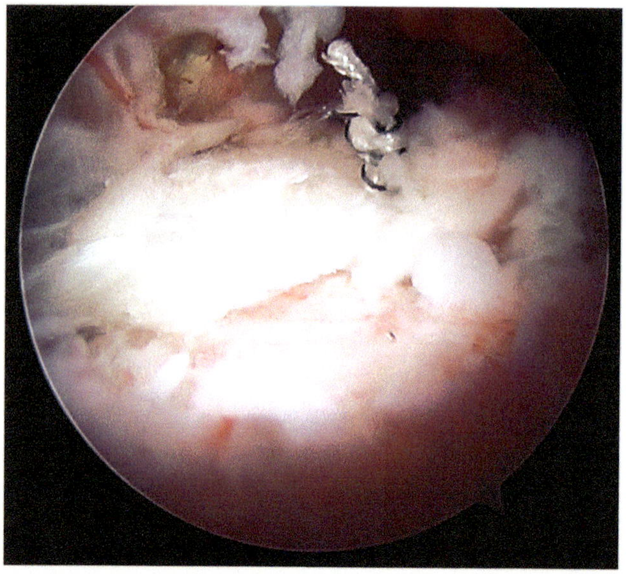

Fig. 7.7 Completed subscapularis repair.

directs the surgeon to the superolateral portion of the subscapularis.

7.8 What to Avoid

1. Avoid dissection inferior or medial to the coracoid tip to avoid damage to neurovascular structures.
2. Avoid placing the anterior and anterolateral portals in close proximity to each other.
3. Avoid tension at the repair site. If excessive tension is present, medialize the repair by up to 5 mm.

7.9 Complications/Bailout/Salvage

The complication rate after shoulder arthroscopy, in general, is very low. There is a small risk of damage to the neurovascular structures when working around the coracoid process. However, studies have documented that these structures are greater than 2.5 cm from the coracoid tip.[16] It is important to exercise caution when working in this area.

The main intraoperative difficulty when addressing the subscapularis tendon is inability to repair it arthroscopically. Open subscapularis repair can be performed if there is difficulty visualizing or mobilizing the tear arthroscopically. Furthermore, in chronic situations the tendon quality may not be sufficient for repair. Bailout options in this situation include use of an allograft tendon or performing a pectoralis major transfer.[17]

7.10 Postoperative Care

Postoperatively, the patient is protected in a sling for 6 weeks. For the first 6 weeks, external rotation is restricted to 30 degrees for partial tears. If there was a complete tear, then external rotation is restricted to neutral. No overhead motion is allowed for 6 weeks. Elbow flexion, wrist exercises, and hand exercises are encouraged. At 6 weeks, the sling is discontinued and passive external rotation and forward flexion with a rope and pulley is allowed. Strengthening is initiated at 12 weeks, progressing from resistance bands to light weights. Unrestricted activity is allowed at 6 to 12 months, depending on the size of the tear.

References

1. Codman E. The Shoulder. 2nd ed. Boston, MA: Thomas Todd Co.; 1934
2. Cofield RH. Rotator cuff disease of the shoulder. J Bone Joint Surg Am 1985;67(6):974–979
3. Iannotti JPRotator Cuff Disorders: Evaluation and Treatment. Rosemont, IL: American Academy of Orthopaedic Surgeons; 1991
4. Matsen F, Arntz C, Lippitt SRotator cuff. In: Rockwood CA, Matsen FA, eds. The Shoulder. Philadelphia, PA: W.B. Saunders; 1998:755–839
5. Richards DP, Burkhart SS, Tehrany AM, Wirth MA. The subscapularis footprint: an anatomic description of its insertion site. Arthroscopy 2007;23(3):251–254
6. Burkhart SS, Tehrany AM. Arthroscopic subscapularis tendon repair: Technique and preliminary results. Arthroscopy 2002;18(5):454–463
7. Denard PJ, Burkhart SS. Arthroscopic recognition and repair of the torn subscapularis tendon. Arthrosc Tech 2013;2(4):e373–e379
8. Kuechle DK, Newman SR, Itoi E, Morrey BF, An KN. Shoulder muscle moment arms during horizontal flexion and elevation. J Shoulder Elbow Surg 1997;6(5):429–439
9. Kelly BT, Williams RJ, Cordasco FA, et al. Differential patterns of muscle activation in patients with symptomatic and asymptomatic rotator cuff tears. J Shoulder Elbow Surg 2005;14(2):165–171
10. Burkhart SS, Esch JC, Jolson RS. The rotator crescent and rotator cable: an anatomic description of the shoulder's "suspension bridge". Arthroscopy 1993;9(6):611–616
11. Ticker JB, Burkhart SS. Why repair the subscapularis? A logical rationale. Arthroscopy 2011;27(8):1123–1128
12. Osti L, Rizzello G, Panascì M, Denaro V, Maffulli N. Full thickness tears: retaining the cuff. Sports Med Arthrosc Rev 2011;19(4):409–419
13. Edwards TB, Walch G, Sirveaux F, et al. Repair of tears of the subscapularis. J Bone Joint Surg Am 2005;87(4):-725–730
14. Denard PJ, Burkhart SS. Medialization of the subscapularis footprint does not affect functional outcome of arthroscopic repair. Arthroscopy 2012;28(11):1608–1614
15. Lo IK, Burkhart SS. The comma sign: An arthroscopic guide to the torn subscapularis tendon. Arthroscopy 2003;19(3):334–337
16. Lo IK, Burkhart SS, Parten PM. Surgery about the coracoid: neurovascular structures at risk. Arthroscopy 2004;20(6):591–595
17. Resch H, Povacz P, Ritter E, Matschi W. Transfer of the pectoralis major muscle for the treatment of irreparable rupture of the subscapularis tendon. J Bone Joint Surg Am 2000;82(3):372–382

8 Massive Rotator Cuff Repair (Mobilization Techniques, Slides)

Jonathan Berkowitz and David M. Dines

Abstract

When repairing massive rotator cuff tears, it is essential to avoid overtensioning the repaired tissue. Extensive releases of scarred and adherent tissue and interval slide techniques are essential tools to optimize the repair viability. The fixation method chosen is important, but is often secondary to proper tissue management.

Keywords: *interval slide, double row, tissue mobilization, margin convergence, L-type tear*

8.1 Goals of Procedure

- To adequately mobilize adherent and scarred rotator cuff tendons in massive tears.
- To optimize fixation of the repaired tissue.
- To improve the milieu of healing in the most difficult cases by increasing tendon-to-bone fixation and making it possible to perform double-row constructs to improve healing.

8.2 Advantages

- Allows for a tension-free repair in order to maximize repair success.
- Increases tendon-to-bone interface in the repair construct.
- Allows for double-row fixation when possible.

8.3 Indications

Massive reparable rotator cuff tears, chronic retracted tears with no evidence of muscle atrophy.

8.4 Contraindications

- Irreparable tears, fatty atrophy of the rotator cuff muscles (Goutallier 3 or above).[1]
- Severe comorbidities that can adversely affect outcomes such as diabetics and smokers.

8.5 Preoperative Preparation/ Positioning

- A detailed history and physical examination are essential for proper patient evaluation. Specifically, a history of prior trauma or previous surgeries should be elucidated.
- Standard X-rays including anteroposterior (AP), true shoulder AP, scapula Y lateral, and axillary views should be routinely obtained to evaluate for any glenohumeral arthritis, superior migration of the humeral head, and classification of the type of acromion.
- MRI is the preferred imaging modality in order to visualize any soft-tissue pathology. Standard T1 and T2 sequences as well as short tau inversion recovery (STIR) sequences can help identify fatty atrophy of muscle versus edema. Sagittal STIR sequences are especially useful in evaluating the extent of muscle atrophy of the rotator cuff musculature.
- MR arthrography is helpful for visualizing labral pathology, but is less useful for rotator cuff pathology and as such is not routinely obtained.
- CT scans are helpful in evaluating glenoid or humeral bone loss but are not routinely obtained for suspected rotator cuff pathology.

8.6 Expert Suggestions/ Comments

- Depending on the surgeon's preference, the patient should be positioned in the beach-chair or lateral decubitus position. Prior to starting the procedure, it is essential to ensure that all equipment and implants are available, including both tied and knotless technology, to ensure the best fixation options for single- or double-row lateral fixation.
- The mobilization and fixation techniques are dependent on proper visualization, evaluation, and classification of the rotator cuff tear.

8.7 Operative Technique

8.7.1 Anesthesia/Positioning

We prefer regional interscalene block with relaxation or general anesthesia. We routinely use the beach-chair position for rotator cuff pathology.

8.7.2 Portals

Standard posterolateral viewing portal is made, followed by the anterior rotator interval working portal. Once in the subacromial space, the standard direct lateral portal is made. After evaluating the rotator cuff tear type and mobility, additional portals are made as needed to serve as working portals or percutaneous anchor insertion portals. Multiple working portals are routinely used for large, retracted tears.

8.7.3 Debridement and Bursectomy

A significant bursectomy and debridement should be performed for the dual purpose of visualization and cuff mobilization as the bursal adhesions between the rotator cuff and the local tissue can be a significant inhibitor of rotator cuff mobility (specifically, adhesions to the acromion and subdeltoid fascia/

lateral shelf). In massive tears, retention of the coracoacromial ligament should be considered in order to prevent postoperative superior migration of the humeral head. However, in cases where there is significant acromial pathology, we perform an acromioplasty in routine fashion. The biceps tendon functions as both a dynamic and static humeral head depressor. However, its role in the case of massive rotator cuff tears is unclear. If there is any evidence of biceps pathology, it should be tenotomized and tenodesed.

Debridement should not be limited to the subacromial space, as an intra-articular release between the cuff tissue and superior labrum/capsule can greatly improve cuff mobility.

8.7.4 Assessment of Tear Type

After the initial debridement is performed, a thorough assessment of the rotator cuff tear and its mobility can be made. Soft-tissue graspers should be placed through the lateral portal, as well as through the anterior and posterior portals as necessary, and reduction of the rotator cuff tendon to its anatomic footprint should be trialed. The mobility of the rotator cuff should be assessed after each successive release.

The type of tear (**U**-shaped vs. **L**-shaped) should then be assessed. **L**-shaped tears should be reduced to its footprint in a different manner than **U**-shaped tears. Misidentification of the tear type can result in unnecessary releasing of an **L**-shaped tear. Margin convergence of **L**-shaped tears using a side-to-side repair technique can transform an **L**-shaped tear to a crescent-type tear (**Fig 8.1**).[2]

With the camera in the posterior portal, the interval limb of the **L**-shaped tear (anterior or posterior) should be mobilized with the shaver or cautery to release any adhesions and tissue contractures. Next, viewing through the lateral portal, arthroscopic piercers are used through the anterior and posterior portals to pass a nonabsorbable no. 2 suture through the medial and lateral leaflets of the tear. The suture is then tied down with either a locking sliding knot or half hitches. This technique significantly reduces tension at the most lateral edge of the repaired tendon and allows for a more stable repair.

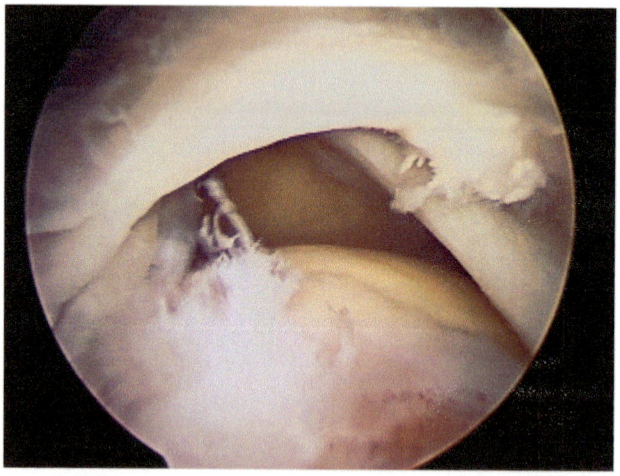

Fig. 8.1 An **L**-shaped tear: a large **L**-shaped tear as viewed from the lateral portal. Note the intact posterior attachment of the supraspinatus, with medial retraction of the anterior portion of the tendon.

8.7.5 Interval Slides

Interval slides can be the most effective mobilization technique. Anterior interval slides are used more frequently than posterior slides, and are an essential tool in the management of massive rotator cuff repairs. In large chronic tears, the supraspinatus tendon is tethered to the coracohumeral ligament and contracted tissue of the rotator interval. Releasing this tether with electrocautery or sharp dissection will release this anterior tether and improve the mobility and gliding of the supraspinatus tendon.[3] The posterior interval slide is made between the supraspinatus and infraspinatus tendons along the axis of the scapular spine. However, this is not a well-defined anatomic interval, and it can damage intact tendon if it is performed too aggressively. Additionally, if a posterior slide is combined with an anterior interval release, there is a potential risk of devascularizing the rotator cuff tissue between the two slides (**Figs. 8.2–8.4**). In the setting of a concomitant subscapularis tear, repairing the

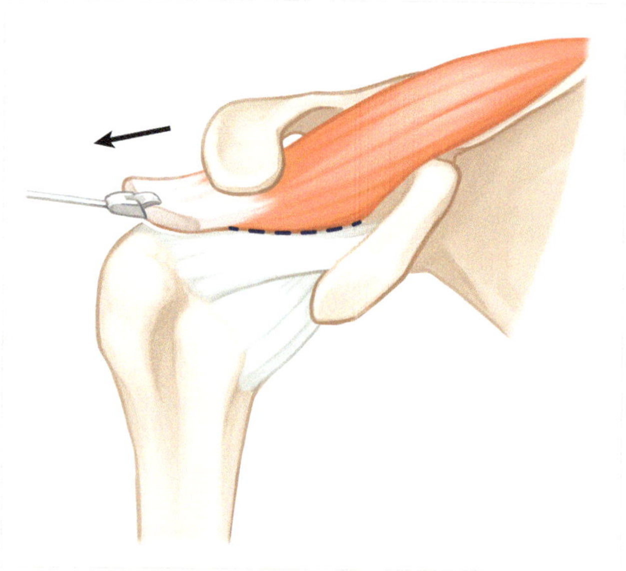

Fig. 8.2 An artist's representation of an anterior interval slide. Traction sutures are placed in the rotator cuff and lateral traction is applied, while sharp dissection or electrocautery separates the anterior supraspinatus from rotator interval tissue.

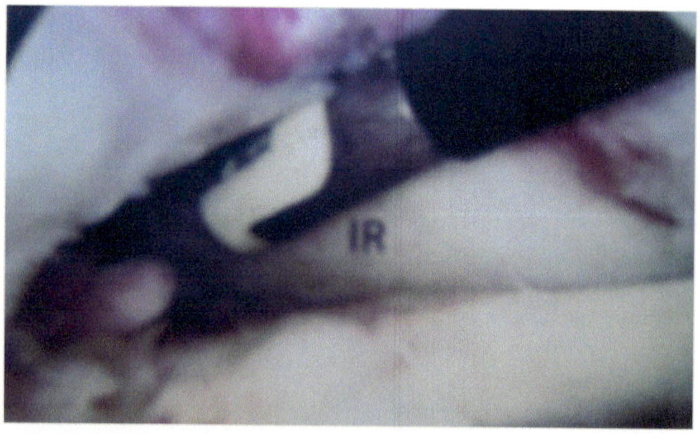

Fig. 8.3 Interval release being performed with electrocautery device.

subscapularis first can help transform a larger supraspinatus tear into a more easily manageable crescent-type tear.

After using the above techniques, if the cuff is still not mobile enough to reach its anatomic footprint, the articular cartilage at the medial border of the footprint can be resected using a burr. It is generally safe to medialize the footprint up to 1 cm; any further medialization may result in a significantly reduced moment arm of the rotator cuff.

8.7.6 Repair Technique and Anchor Configuration

There is still no consensus regarding the optimal repair technique and anchor configuration. While double-row fixation is biomechanically stronger, in the setting of a massive tear it may overtension the repaired rotator cuff tissue. To keep tension low, a single suture row at the articular margin may be preferred. Only after thoroughly assessing the mobility of the released rotator cuff can the surgeon decide between a single- and a double-row technique.

If double-row fixation is chosen, the authors prefer using a double-row technique with medial knotless anchors.[4] First, two knotless anchors preloaded with sutures are placed along the articular margin. Next, a self-retrieving suture passing device is used to pass the preloaded suture through the rotator cuff tendon. These passed sutures are then brought to a lateral row of knotless anchors in a transosseous equivalent manner (**Fig. 8.5**).

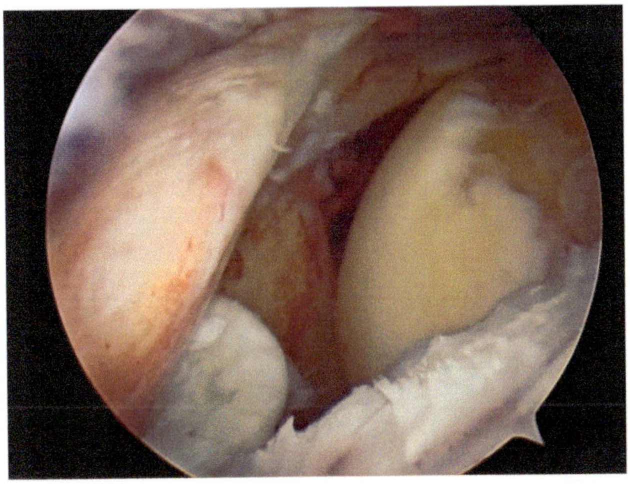

Fig. 8.4 After interval release.

8.8 Tips and Pearls/Expert Suggestions

While the arthroscopic techniques described here are amplified in other chapters, it is important to evaluate each rotator cuff tear configuration in the context of mobilization, fixation, and potential for healing. In cases where after maximal release the tendon is still unable to reach its anatomic footprint without maximal tension, the likelihood of success is minimal. Other options such as partial repair, debridement, biceps tenotomy, or even superior capsule reconstruction should be considered.

8.9 What to Avoid

When releasing the supraspinatus from its inferior capsular adhesions to the superior labrum and glenoid, excessive medial releasing must be avoided as the suprascapular nerve runs approximately 2 cm medial to the glenoid rim.

It is important to avoid the temptation of incompletely releasing the torn rotator cuff, which would result in leaving tension on the repair.

8.10 Complications/Bailout/Salvage

8.10.1 Complications

Suprascapular nerve injury from overresecting the adhesions between the supraspinatus and superior labrum/glenoid.

8.10.2 Bailout

Although most massive tears can be repaired after all appropriate releases, there are still those that will be irreparable. Simple debridement may be enough for some of these patients. For those patients who continue to have pain and loss of function, superior capsular reconstruction should be considered.

8.10.3 Salvage

In a young laborer, latissimus dorsi or lower trapezius transfer to the greater tuberosity is indicated. In older, low-demand patients, reverse total shoulder arthroplasty is the treatment of choice to restore function and reduce pain.

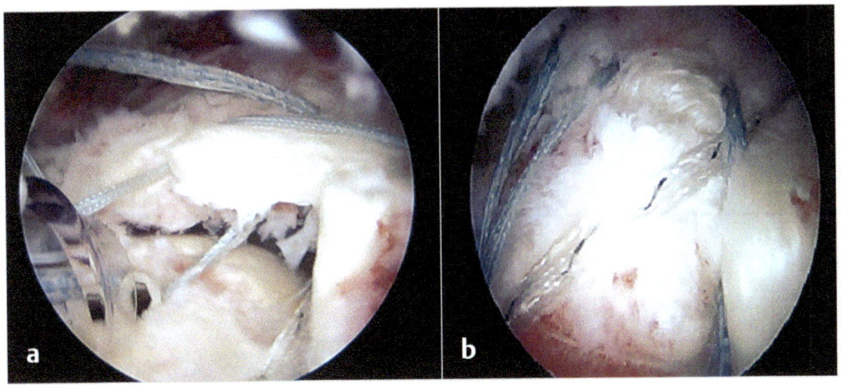

Fig. 8.5 Distal suture bridge construct with interval repair.

8.11 Postoperative Care

Prolonged immobilization in a sling for 2 to 6 weeks is preferred after repair of massive rotator cuff tears to allow time for tendon-to-bone healing.

References

1. Goutallier D, Postel JM, Bernageau J, Lavau L, Voisin MC. Fatty muscle degeneration in cuff ruptures. Pre- and postoperative evaluation by CT scan. Clin Orthop Relat Res 1994;304(304):78–83
2. Burkhart SS, Athanasiou KA, Wirth MA. Margin convergence: a method of reducing strain in massive rotator cuff tears. Arthroscopy 1996;12(3):335–338
3. Tauro JC. Arthroscopic "interval slide" in the repair of large rotator cuff tears. Arthroscopy 1999;15(5):527–530
4. Meier SW, Meier JD. The effect of double-row fixation on initial repair strength in rotator cuff repair: a biomechanical study. Arthroscopy 2006;22(11):1168–1173

9 Massive Rotator Cuff Repair: Margin Convergence

Robert U. Hartzler, Andrew J. Sheean, and Stephen S. Burkhart

Abstract
Rotator cuff tear patterns vary. Consequently, surgeons should be prepared to employ different repair techniques based on individual tear characteristics. The term *margin convergence* refers to side-to-side suturing of a posterosuperior rotator cuff tear. A margin convergence technique can be the key to an anatomic and biomechanically sound repair in appropriate tear patterns. Longitudinal rotator cuff tears (U, L, or reverse L) have significant anteroposterior mobility and often require side-to-side suturing for reduction without undue tension on the repair. In this fashion, margin convergence can convert a seemingly irreparable tear into an easily reparable one. From a biomechanical perspective, side-to-side suturing of an appropriate rotator tear (classically, the U pattern) carries the advantage of decreasing strain along the free margin of the tear by decreasing the length and increasing the cross-sectional area of the tear. In a traditional margin convergence technique, a series of individual side-to-side sutures is placed from anterior to posterior across the tear. As these are sequentially tied from medial to lateral, the margin of the tear converges toward the greater tuberosity bone bed. The repair can subsequently be completed using anchor-based fixation of the tendon to the greater tuberosity. The newer *shoestring-to-bone* construct gives the surgeon a knotless option for margin convergence to bone.

Keywords: *shoulder arthroscopy, rotator cuff repair, margin convergence, shoestring*

9.1 Introduction

Burkhart coined the phrase "margin convergence" and described the biomechanical rationale for this surgical technique[1]; however, the concept of using side-to-side sutures in rotator cuff repair dates back to Codman[2] and McLaughlin.[3] Knowledge of the principles, indications, techniques, and limitations of margin convergence techniques for arthroscopic rotator cuff repair will greatly aid shoulder surgeons in the care of their patients.

9.2 Goals of Procedure

Margin convergence techniques in arthroscopic rotator cuff repair serve the ultimate purpose of obtaining *anatomic tendon-to-bone healing* to restore pain-free and functional use of the shoulder.

9.3 Advantages

When used for appropriate rotator cuff tear patterns, margin convergence repair techniques achieve two goals: decreased strain along the free margin of the rotator cuff and increased likelihood of an anatomic repair construct. These advantages have led to excellent clinical results.[4–6] When significant anteroposterior mobility of the cuff tear exists, use of side-to-side suturing will counteract the deforming forces and make the reduction and repair construct more anatomic.

Biomechanical principles concerning the impact of strain and strain reduction on the rotator cuff have been laid out in detail by Burkhart previously[1,7] and have also been confirmed with biomechanical testing.[8–10] In short, margin convergence by side-to-side suturing creates a modified tear margin that has reduced strain for a given force from the cuff musculature. The reduced strain results from a smaller tear length at the apex and an increased cross-sectional area at the apex of the tear (**Fig. 9.1**). Decreased strain is hypothesized to decrease pain, protect a tendon-to-bone repair construct, and prevent tear propagation.[8]

9.4 Indications

In the authors' opinion, repair of large to massive rotator cuff tears should be attempted for nearly all patients who do not have significant glenohumeral arthrosis (Hamada[11] stages 4 to 5). Margin convergence techniques are then utilized as determined by the tear pattern as assessed intraoperatively. In Davidson and Burkhart's geometric classification of rotator cuff tears,[12] longitudinal (**L**-, reverse **L**-, or **U**-shaped) tears require some degree of anterior-to-posterior reduction and often require side-to-side suturing for reduction and/or repair. In particular, **U**-shaped tears, which have roughly equal anterior-to-posterior mobility of the tear leaves (**Fig. 9.2**), often evolve from seemingly irreparable to easily reparable after side-to-side suturing (**Fig. 9.3**). Finally, massive, contracted (immobile) tears repaired using interval slides or superior capsular reconstruction (SCR) often require reinforcement using side-to-side suturing after fixation of the tissue to the bone bed.[13]

9.5 Contraindications

Margin convergence techniques should not be used for rotator cuff tear patterns for which they are not suited. For example, in a massive, contracted (immobile) tear, the surgeon might be able to "force" a few side-to-side sutures and be quickly done with the case when the best repair construct might instead be a well-done partial repair or SCR after mobilizing the tear fully with interval slides. Margin convergence should not be thought of as a panacea for all large to massive rotator cuff tears.

9.6 Preoperative Preparation/ Positioning

Although intraoperative assessment should be the gold standard for assessing tear and repair patterns, preoperative MRI can be helpful for predicting these.[14] When planning for repair of large to massive cuff tears or in the revision setting, we

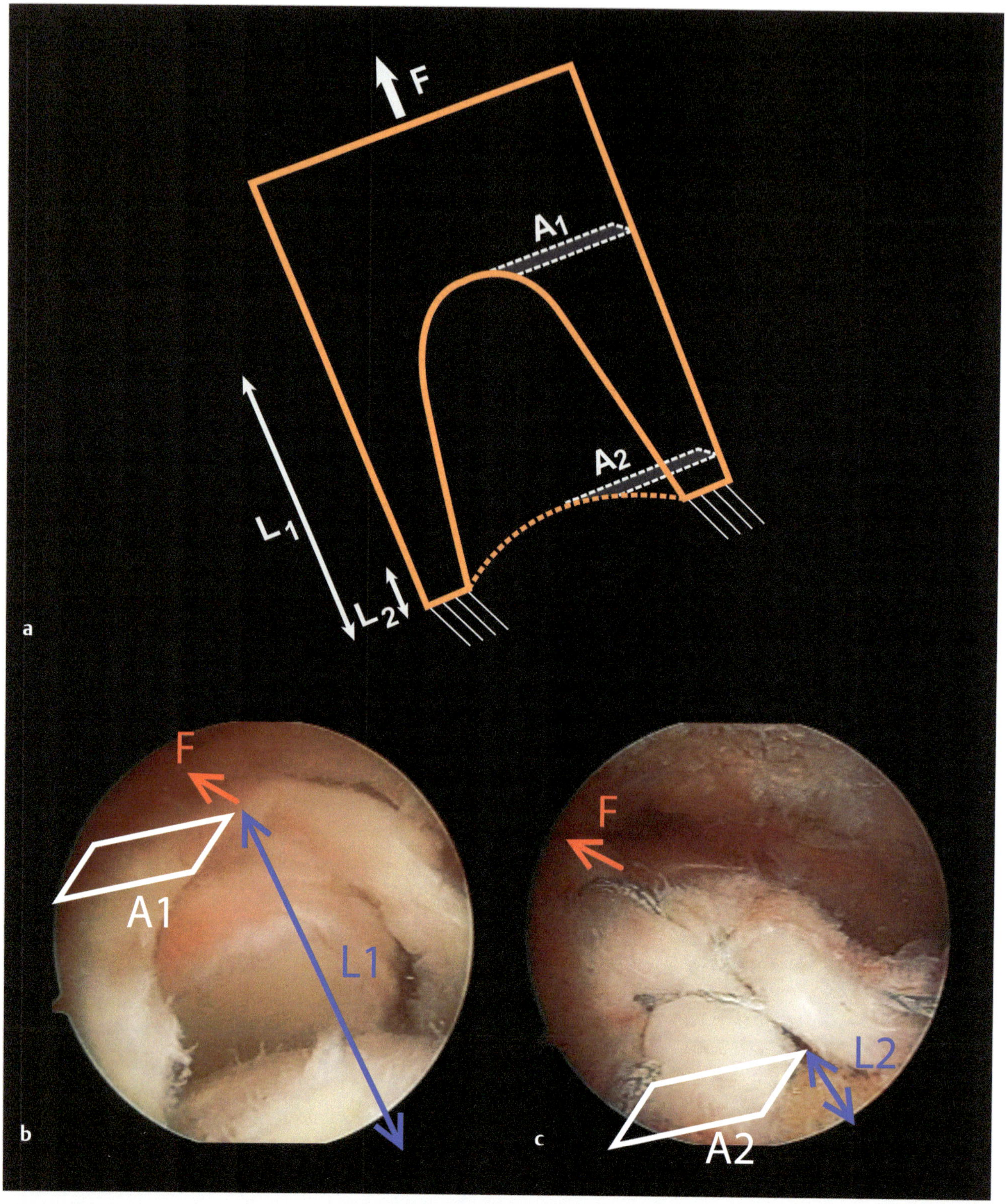

Fig. 9.1 **(a)** Diagram of a rotator cuff tear with a U-shaped tear margin (*solid line*) having length *L*1 from apex to greater tuberosity and cross-sectional area *A*1 at the apex. After side-to-side suturing, the "converged margin" (*dotted line*) has a much smaller length (*L*1) from new apex to tuberosity and larger cross-sectional cuff area (A2) at the new apex. For a given force on the cuff (*F*), the strain will be reduced by a factor of $\frac{L_1 A_2}{L_2 A_1}$.[1] If *L*2 is a third of *L*1 and *A*2 is twice *A*1, strain will be reduced at the new apex by a factor of 6. **(b)** Illustration of a **U**-shaped rotator cuff tear with apex length *L*1 and cross-sectional area *A*1 at the apex. **(c)** After margin convergence by a running tape suture (shoestring technique), the new margin has apex length *L*2 and cross-sectional area *A*2 at the apex, which results in much less strain at new tear margin.

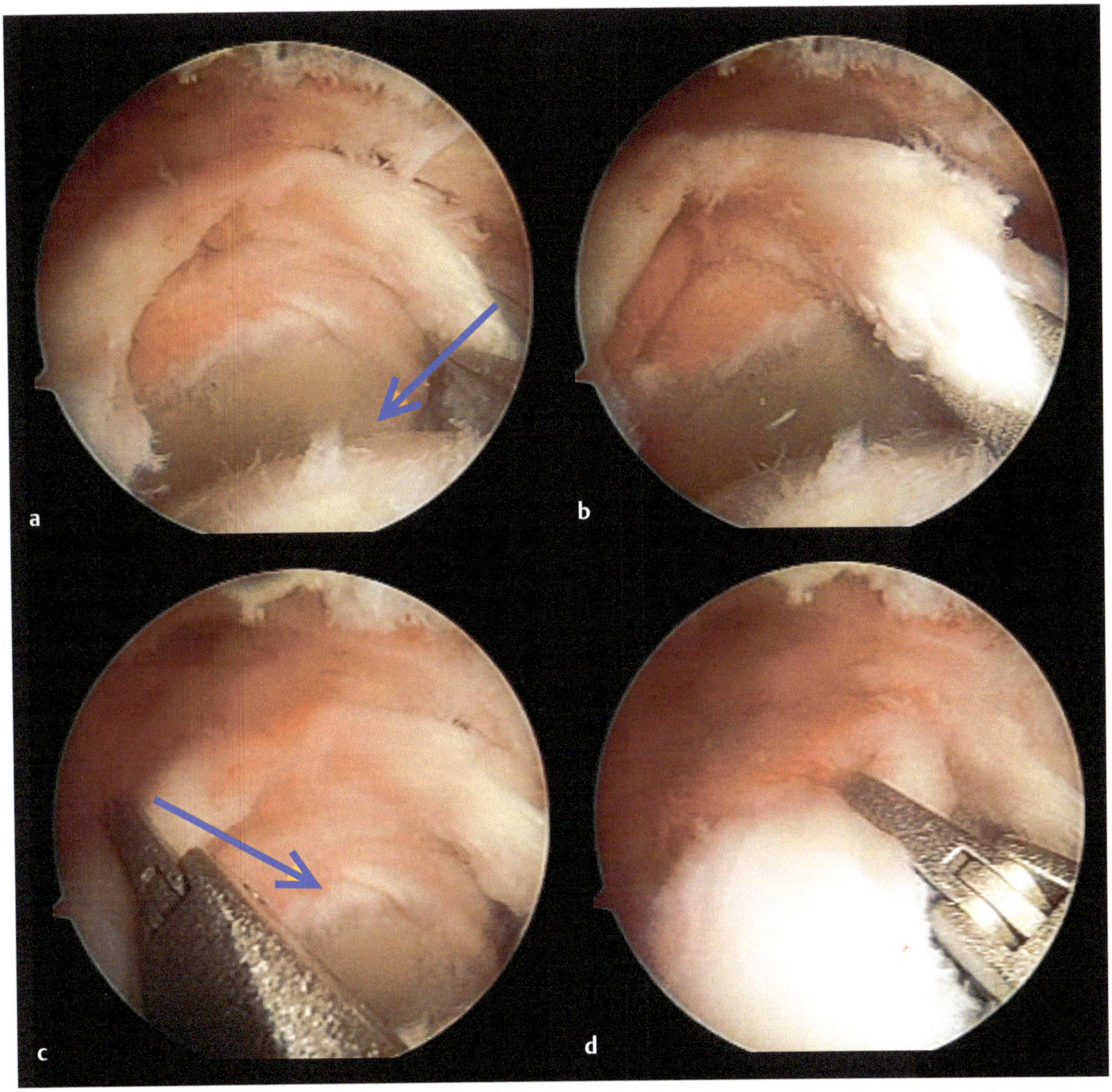

Fig. 9.2 Right shoulder 70-degree posterior viewing portal showing a massive, **U**-shaped rotator cuff tear. The mediolateral dimension is usually longer than the anteroposterior dimension in a **U**-shaped tear. The anterior leaf **(a)** has good posterior mobility **(b)** upon reduction with a tendon grasper. The posterior leaf **(c)** has approximately equal anterior mobility **(d)**.

prepare for the possibility of addressing an irreparable tear with arthroscopic dermal allograft SCR.[13]

We perform all arthroscopic rotator cuff surgery in the lateral decubitus position with a standard operating room setup that includes a second assistant standing opposite the surgeon to provide adjustments to the arm, such as the posterior lever push.[15] We have found the lateral decubitus position to provide the best arthroscopic visualization, a critical factor for performing complex arthroscopic rotator cuff surgery.

9.7 Operative Technique

Rotator cuff tear patterns amenable to repair using margin convergence techniques are typically large to massive and should be carefully assessed for associated subscapularis tears and biceps tendon pathologies, as these are common.[16] In complex arthroscopic rotator cuff surgery, the order of performing each step in the operation is important.[17] Prior to working on the posterosuperior portion of the tear, we perform other indicated procedures in the following order: (1) diagnostic 70-degree arthroscopy of the subscapularis tendon and bicipital groove,[18] (2) biceps tenotomy and whipstitch,[19] (3) subscapularis repair,[20] and (4) arthroscopic biceps tenodesis.[19]

Next, the surgeon should take care to adequately prepare the subacromial space and rotator cuff for assessment of the tear pattern, as this assessment will be the key to whether margin convergence techniques will be used. First, place the arthroscope in the subacromial space from the posterior portal and

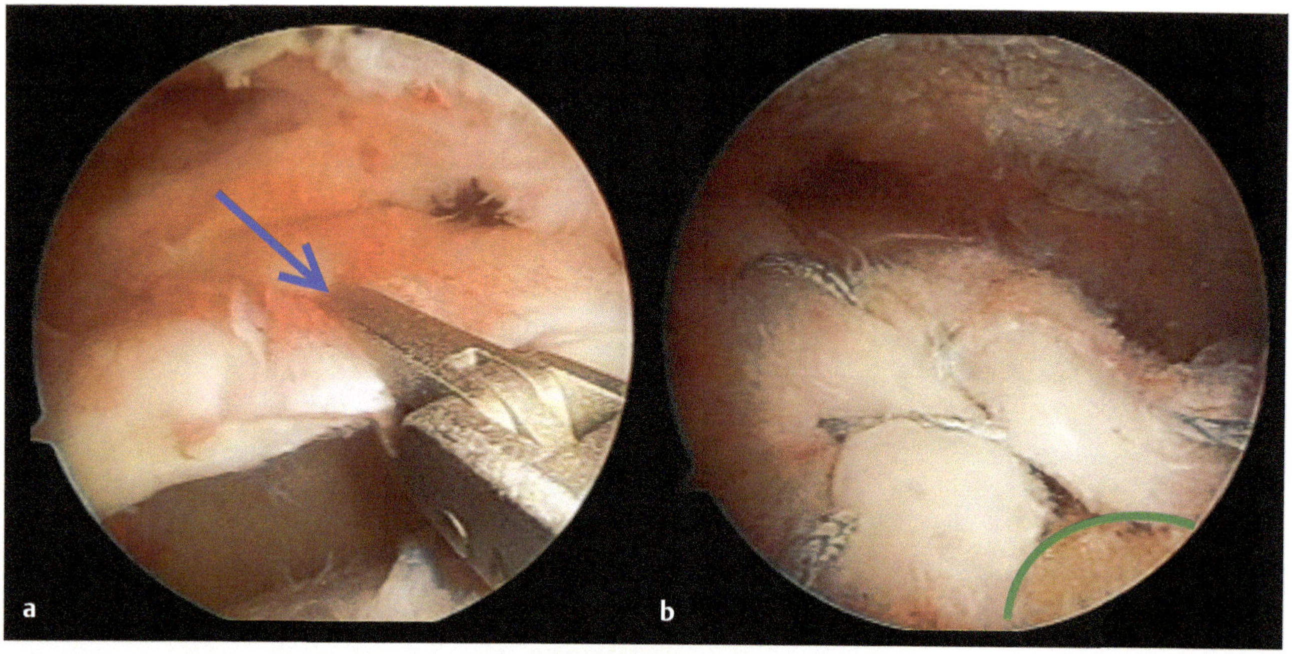

Fig. 9.3 The massive, **U**-shaped tear seen in **Fig. 9.2** will appear to be irreparable **(a)** if the surgeon only attempts to reduce the apex directly laterally (*blue arrow*). After side-to-side suturing using the shoestring technique **(b)**, the converged margin of the tear (*green line*) now sits directly over the bone bed under no tension.

view laterally. Instead of using anatomic landmarks (e.g., a specified distance from the acromion), use a spinal needle to establish a lateral portal using an "outside-in" technique. Ensure that this portal is "low enough" by placing the spinal needle at an angle and location that gives good access to the entire subacromial working space. Leave the spinal needle in place until after the shaver has been introduced into the working space.

After an initial debridement of the anterolateral subacromial bursa to improve visualization, use a cautery device to incise the internal deltoid fascia at the lateral portal superiorly up to the lateral acromial margin and inferiorly toward the bottom of the blind pouch of the lateral gutter. Incision of the internal deltoid fascia at both lateral and posterior portals allows the surgeon to identify bony landmarks, facilitates easier switching of the scope and instruments between portals, and provides better freedom of movement of instruments in the subacromial space.

The end points of preparation of the subacromial space include clear visualization of bony landmarks (the spine of the scapula, acromioclavicular joint, anterior and lateral acromion), the individual muscle-tendon units of the posterosuperior cuff, and the true margin of the rotator cuff tear. To achieve these end points, alternate between using electrocautery and shaver to remove the subacromial bursa and fibrofatty tissue in the subacromial space including in the lateral and posterior gutters. Alternate between working and viewing from lateral and posterior portals. Finally, alternate as needed between 30- and 70-degree arthroscopes for visualization.

In massive rotator cuff surgery (especially in revision cases), a particularly difficult task can be delineation of the true rotator cuff tear margin from "bursal leaders," which are bands of scar tissue that insert into the internal deltoid fascia instead of into the humerus. Often, maximally internally rotating the humerus while viewing from a lateral portal can bring the true insertion of the posterior tear margin into view. If bursal leaders are significant, switching multiple times between different viewing and working portals using both 30- and 70-degree arthroscopes often becomes necessary.

Finally, we perform any bony work on the distal clavicle (resection or coplaning) or acromion (smoothing or anterior/lateral acromioplasty) prior to proceeding with the posterosuperior rotator cuff assessment and repair. For massive tears, we most often preserve the coracoacromial (CA) ligament and perform subacromial smoothing with lateral acromioplasty (lateral). For smaller tears, we formally resect the CA ligament arthroscopically, convert the acromion to type 1 using a cutting block technique,[21] and perform lateral acromioplasty, as indicated.[22]

Assessment of the rotator cuff tear pattern is performed most often viewing from a posterior or posterolateral portal using a 70-degree arthroscope. An arthroscopic tendon grasper is used from a lateral portal to assess the mobility of the entire tear margin (**Video 9.1**). Longitudinal (**L**-, reverse **L**-, or **U**-shaped) tears have a significant component of anterior-to-posterior mobility of the tear margins. **L**- and reverse **L**-shaped tears have a "corner" that can be reduced to the anterolateral or posterolateral greater tuberosity, respectively. Conversely, **U**-shaped tears do not have a "corner" and instead have roughly equal anterior-to-posterior mobility of the tear leaves (**Fig. 9.1**).

The **U**-shaped tear is the classic pattern for a margin convergence technique.[1] In a *traditional* margin convergence technique, a series of side-to-side no. 2 FiberWire sutures (Arthrex, Inc., Naples, FL) are placed and tied sequentially between the anterior and posterior leaves of the tear (**Fig. 9.4**). These "free margin convergence" sutures can be passed anterograde or retrograde but are typically placed and tied working from medial to lateral (**Video 9.1**). After tying these sutures, the "converged margin" of the cuff usually adopts a crescent configuration (**Fig. 9.3b**), with easy lateral mobility to the bone bed amenable to suture anchor repair.

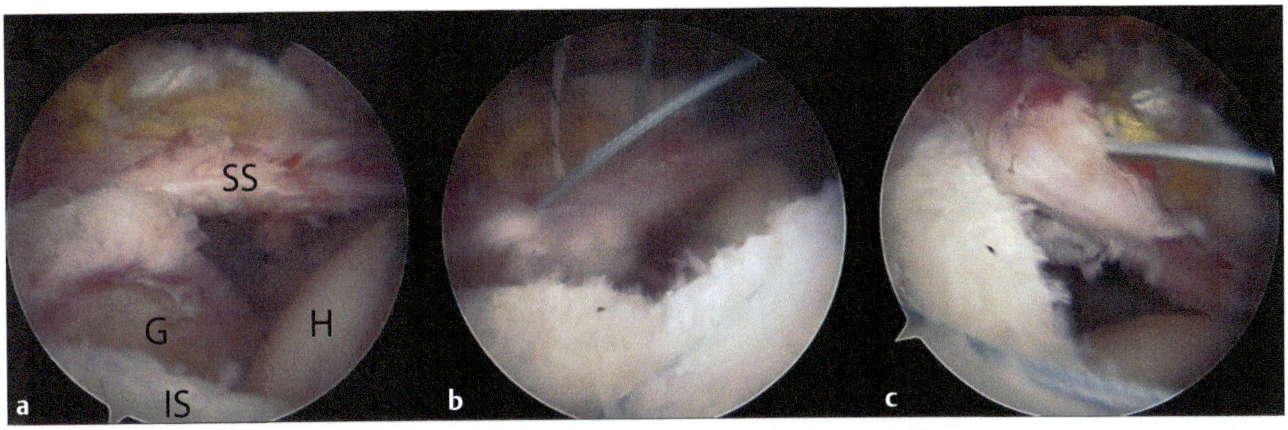

Fig. 9.4 Right shoulder 70-degree posterior viewing portal showing a large, **U**-shaped rotator cuff tear **(a)**. Three, free-margin FiberWire (Arthrex, Inc.) sutures have been placed between the anterior and posterior leaves of the tear **(b)**. The medial two sutures have been tied **(c)** and the most lateral of the free-margin sutures has been retrieved in preparation for tying. Observe how the tear margin is being converged toward the greater tuberosity under minimal tension. G, glenoid; H, humeral head; IS, infraspinatus tendon; SS, supraspinatus tendon.

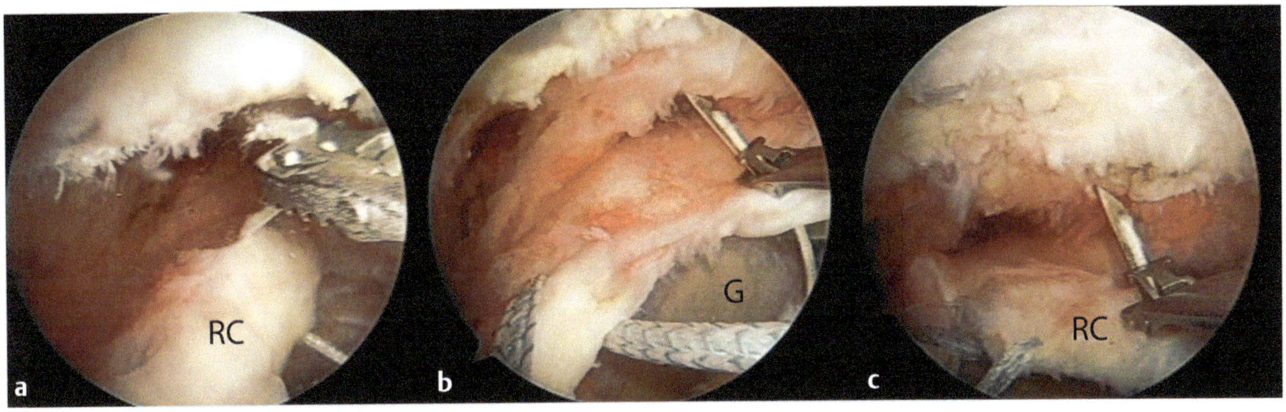

Fig. 9.5 Right shoulder 70-degree posterior viewing portal showing a massive, **U**-shaped rotator cuff tear being repaired with a shoestring margin convergence technique. A FiberTape (Arthrex, Inc.) suture converges the tear margin as it is woven using an antegrade suture passer (FastPass Scorpion, Arthrex, Inc.). **(a)** In this case, the first pass of the FiberTape is through the posterior leaf medially. **(b)** The second pass of the FiberTape is then through the anterior leaf medially. After multiple passes **(c)**, the repair begins to take the characteristic "shoestring" configuration. G, glenoid; RC, rotator cuff.

An alternative technique for **U**-shaped tears is the "*shoestring to bone*" repair, which has been made possible by the development of knotless suture anchors. To perform this repair, a FiberTape suture (Arthrex, Inc.) is woven like a shoestring between the tear leaves from medial to lateral using an antegrade suture passer (FastPass Scorpion, Arthrex, Inc.; **Fig. 9.5; Video 9.1**). The tape suture acts to converge the tear margin and allows the surgeon the freedom to plan and place additional anchors and sutures. Subsequently, fix the FiberTape to the greater tuberosity bone as single row equivalent repair, usually using a 4.75-mm biocomposite SwiveLock suture anchor (Arthrex, Inc.). Finally, tie any remaining sutures from accessory medial anchors and, if possible, secure the tails to lateral row anchors to complete a linked, double-row repair (**Video 9.1**).

Longitudinal rotator cuff tears are often suited to the technique of "margin convergence to bone."[10] In this technique, the final margin convergence sutures are anchor-based (as opposed to using a free margin suture). The knotless anchor that fixes the shoestring to the bone is an example of a margin-to-bone anchor. Margin-to-bone repairs can be useful for both **U**-shaped tears (**Fig. 9.6, Video 9.1**) and **L**-shaped tears. In the latter, the margin-to-bone anchor is placed to secure the corner of the tear, the sutures securing the tear edge to both bone and intact tendon (**Fig. 9.7**). **L**- and reverse **L**-shaped tears also often benefit from placement of one or two free-margin sutures; however, the surgeon must take care that these do not malreduce the tear. To this end, it is often best to place these as the last step in the repair.

9.8 Tips and Pearls/Expert Suggestions

Excellent visualization in the subacromial space is the key to assessing posterosuperior rotator cuff tear patterns and performing complex repairs. Our keys to improved visualization include the following:

- Lateral decubitus position so that the anesthesiologist can safely keep the systolic blood pressure low (around 100 mm Hg) and traction/manipulation of the arm can be optimized.
- Pump pressure high enough to provide good visualization (usually minimum 60 mm Hg).

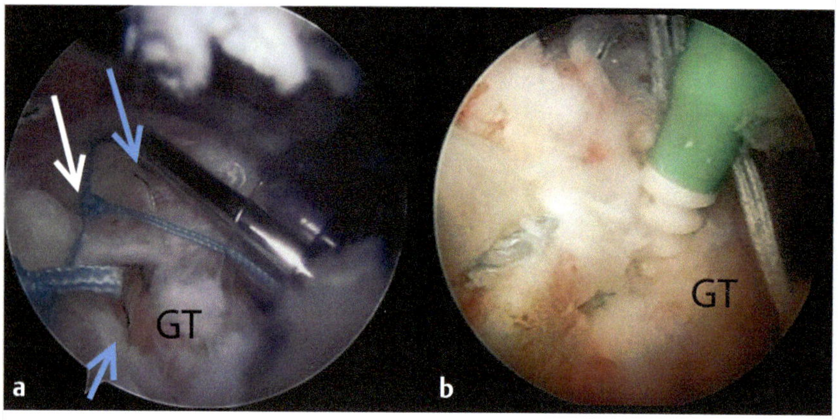

Fig. 9.6 Margin-to-bone constructs can be very useful in **U**-shaped rotator cuff tears. **(a)** In a traditional margin convergence technique, a Corkscrew FT (Arthrex, Inc.) suture anchor has been placed at the medial margin of the greater tuberosity. The white no. 2 TigerWire (*blue arrow*; Arthrex, Inc.) has been passed through the most lateral part of the tear and remains untied. The blue FiberWire suture (*white arrow*) is being tied so that the converged margin is secured to the bone via the suture anchor. **(b)** In the shoestring to bone technique, the woven FiberTape suture is fixed to the greater tuberosity (GT) using a knotless Swive-Lock (Arthrex, Inc.) suture anchor. Since the shoestring to bone is a knotless technique, it has the advantage of being faster than a traditional margin convergence technique.

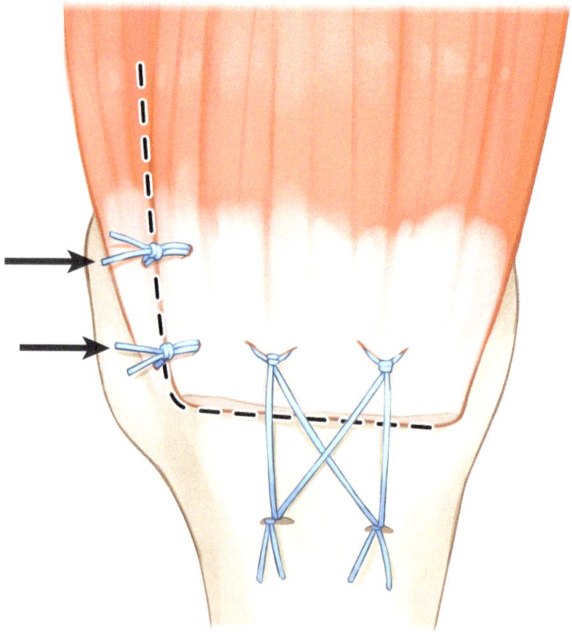

Fig. 9.7 In an **L**-shaped rotator cuff tear, a margin-to-bone construct is very useful for anatomically securing the corner of the tear to the greater tuberosity. Two FiberWire sutures (*black arrows*) from a Corkscrew FT anchor have been passed and tied with one suture limb through the intact cuff margin and the other limb through the corner of the tear.

- Eliminate rapid fluid egress by digital pressure (Dutch boy technique) on or around portals to prevent turbulence.[23]
- Incision of the internal deltoid fascia to facilitate switching instruments and the scope between portals.
- Routine use of a 70-degree arthroscope (used for the majority of the tear evaluation and repair).
- Thorough subacromial decompression including bursectomy, debridement of the posterior and lateral gutters, and resection of bursal leaders.

9.9 What to Avoid

As stated earlier, surgeons should avoid the temptation to use margin convergence techniques when they are not suited to the cuff tear pattern. When a truly irreparable primary rotator cuff tear is encountered after advanced mobilization techniques have been employed, consider a well-done partial repair or SCR instead of placing side-to-side sutures under high tension.

9.10 Complications/Bailouts/Salvage

The most common intraoperative complications we encounter during arthroscopic rotator cuff repair result from a combination of poor tissue quality and difficult tears (massive contracted, immobile) and include failure of tendon or bone to hold suture or anchor. Many techniques exist for managing poor-quality tissues,[24] and most of these can be adapted as indicated to tears that require a margin convergence construct.

9.11 Postoperative Care

After arthroscopic massive rotator cuff repair, postoperative care should prioritize tendon healing to bone. Additionally, significant postoperative stiffness after *arthroscopic* massive rotator cuff repair is very uncommon. Thus, the authors recommend sling immobilization with a small abduction bolster for the first 6 weeks after surgery. During the first 6 weeks, patients are instructed to perform active range of motion of the elbow, wrist, and hand to prevent postoperative stiffness. Patients are instructed to bend forward at the waist in order to perform axillary hygiene, dressing, and donning and doffing of the sling, and this also produces some gentle passive forward elevation at the shoulder.

At week 6, the sling is discontinued and the arm can be used for light activities of daily living below shoulder level. From weeks 6 to 12 (small, medium, or large tears) or 6 to 16 (massive tears), patients are instructed to perform passive stretching exercises to regain range of motion focusing on forward elevation and external rotation. Active and passive internal rotation is restricted to the belt line. Tendon-to-bone healing is not advanced enough at this time to allow strengthening.[25]

Starting at week 12 (small, medium, or large tears) or 16 (massive tears), patients may begin active overhead use of the arm and strengthening with rubber bands. If desired by the patient, supervised physical therapy is also allowed at this point. Throwing and golf remain restricted activities until 6 months (small, medium, or large tears) or 1 year (massive tears) postoperatively.

References

1. Burkhart SS, Athanasiou KA, Wirth MA. Margin convergence: a method of reducing strain in massive rotator cuff tears. Arthroscopy 1996;12(3):335–338
2. Codman EA. The shoulder; rupture of the supraspinatus tendon and other lesions in or about the subacromial bursa. Boston, MA: Todd Company; 1934
3. McLaughlin HL. Lesions of the musculotendinous cuff of the shoulder. The exposure and treatment of tears with retraction. Clin Orthop Relat Res 1994(304):3–9
4. Burkhart SS, Danaceau SM, Pearce CE Jr. Arthroscopic rotator cuff repair: Analysis of results by tear size and by repair technique-margin convergence versus direct tendon-to-bone repair. Arthroscopy 2001;17(9):905–912
5. Wolf EM, Pennington WT, Agrawal V. Arthroscopic side-to-side rotator cuff repair. Arthroscopy 2005;21(7):881–887
6. Kim KC, Shin HD, Cha SM, Kim JH. Repair integrity and functional outcomes for arthroscopic margin convergence of rotator cuff tears. J Bone Joint Surg Am 2013;95(6):536–541
7. Burkhart SS. The principle of margin convergence in rotator cuff repair as a means of strain reduction at the tear margin. Ann Biomed Eng 2004;32(1):166–170
8. Andarawis-Puri N, Ricchetti ET, Soslowsky LJ. Rotator cuff tendon strain correlates with tear propagation. J Biomech 2009;42(2):158–163
9. Mazzocca AD, Bollier M, Fehsenfeld D, et al. Biomechanical evaluation of margin convergence. Arthroscopy 2011;27(3):330–338
10. Nguyen ML, Quigley RJ, Galle SE, et al. Margin convergence anchorage to bone for reconstruction of the anterior attachment of the rotator cable. Arthroscopy 2012;28(9): 1237–1245
11. Hamada K, Yamanaka K, Uchiyama Y, Mikasa T, Mikasa M. A radiographic classification of massive rotator cuff tear arthritis. Clin Orthop Relat Res 2011;469(9):2452–2460
12. Davidson J, Burkhart SS. The geometric classification of rotator cuff tears: a system linking tear pattern to treatment and prognosis. Arthroscopy 2010;26(3):417–424
13. Adams CR, Denard PJ, Brady PC, Hartzler RU, Burkhart SS. The arthroscopic superior capsular reconstruction. Am J Orthop 2016;45(5):320–324
14. Davidson JF, Burkhart SS, Richards DP, Campbell SE. Use of preoperative magnetic resonance imaging to predict rotator cuff tear pattern and method of repair. Arthroscopy 2005;21(12):1428
15. Burkhart SS, Brady PC. Arthroscopic subscapularis repair: surgical tips and pearls A to Z. Arthroscopy 2006;22(9):1014–1027
16. Denard PJ, Jiwani AZ, Lädermann A, Burkhart SS. Long-term outcome of arthroscopic massive rotator cuff repair: the importance of double-row fixation. Arthroscopy 2012;28(7):909–915
17. Koo SS, Burkhart SS. Subscapularis tendon tears: identifying mid to distal footprint disruptions. Arthroscopy 2010;26(8):1130–1134
18. Sheean AJ, Hartzler RU, Denard PJ, Lädermann A, Hanypsiak BT, Burkhart SSA. A 70° arthroscope significantly improves visualization of the bicipital groove in the lateral decubitus position. Arthroscopy 2016;32(9):1745–1749
19. Lo IK, Burkhart SS. Arthroscopic biceps tenodesis using a bioabsorbable interference screw. Arthroscopy 2004;20(1):85–95
20. Denard PJ, Lädermann A, Burkhart SS. Arthroscopic management of subscapularis tears. Sports Med Arthrosc Rev 2011;19(4):333–341
21. Sampson TG, Nisbet JK, Glick JM. Precision acromioplasty in arthroscopic subacromial decompression of the shoulder. Arthroscopy 1991;7(3):301–307
22. Lädermann A, Denard PJ, Burkhart SS. Revision arthroscopic rotator cuff repair: systematic review and authors' preferred surgical technique. Arthroscopy 2012;28(8): 1160–1169
23. Burkhart SS, Danaceau SM, Athanasiou KA. Turbulence control as a factor in improving visualization during subacromial shoulder arthroscopy. Arthroscopy 2001;17(2): 209–212
24. Denard PJ, Burkhart SS. Techniques for managing poor quality tissue and bone during arthroscopic rotator cuff repair. Arthroscopy 2011;27(10):1409–1421
25. Sonnabend DH, Howlett CR, Young AA. Histological evaluation of repair of the rotator cuff in a primate model. J Bone Joint Surg Br 2010;92(4):586–594

10 Revision Rotator Cuff Repair: Patch Augmentation

Evan S. Lederman

Abstract

During revision rotator cuff repair tissue compromize is common. This chapter will discuss indications, operative technique, and challenges when utilizing a patch for rotator cuff structural and biologic augmentation.

Keywords: *rotator cuff, rotator cuff repair, graft, augmentation, patch, arthroscopic repair, revision, extracellular matrix graft*

10.1 Goals of Procedure

Improve the outcome of revision rotator cuff repair (RCR) by utilizing extracellular matrix (ECM) tissue to structurally and biologically augment rotator cuff repair procedures.

Recurrent rotator cuff tears after large RCR are still reported to be 34 to 94%. In an effort to improve the healing rates of large tears, the use of ECM grafts derived from human or animal tissues can be used to surgically augment the repaired rotator cuff by reinforcing the repair. Augmentation of RCR may increase mechanical strength at initial fixation. RCR reinforced with ECM grafts have been shown to decrease gap formation by up to 40% and increase ultimate load to failure by 35% in a human cadaveric model that was tensioned over the repair.[1] Onlay reinforcement has also been validated biomechanically to decrease gap formation and increase load to failure.[2] The best technique for reinforcement has not been defined.

10.2 Advantages

Augmentation of RCR can improve initial fixation of the rotator cuff. Graft procedures can be performed arthroscopically or by open techniques.

10.3 Indications

Augmentation of RCR is generally considered for revision cases or in large to massive tears with tissue compromise.

10.4 Contraindications

Contraindications to revision RCR include advanced fatty infiltration, glenohumeral joint degenerative change or humeral greater tuberosity deformity, advanced age, medical comorbidity, or significant tobacco use. Augmentation would be contraindicated if the patient has sensitivity or allergy to any part of the particular product chosen. Please review manufacturer information regarding possible sensitivity or allergy. The suspicion or presence of past or current infection would be considered a contraindication.

10.5 Preoperative Preparation

Preoperative evaluation should emphasize an understanding of the patient's history with regard to the original diagnosis, review of operative report and photos, circumstances of the re-tear, and pertinent medical comorbidities. Physical examination should assess motion, strength deficiencies, cervical disease, and neurologic status. The clinician should always consider infection as a cause of re-tear. Imaging is recommended to include plain X-ray and advanced imaging. MRI is the imaging of choice. In the presence of metallic hardware or when MRI is contraindicated, a CT arthrogram is indicated. The rotator cuff should be assessed for atrophy, fatty infiltration, and the location of re-tear (specifically a re-tear medial to the prior repair or type II failure) as this may influence the indication for repair. The clinician should consider that many patients can function well even when the rotator cuff is deficient and avoid surgery in functional pain-free shoulders.

10.5.1 Positioning

- Anesthesia: general, interscalene block, or combination.
- The patient is positioned in the lateral decubitus or the beach-chair position.

10.6 Operative Technique

An examination under anesthesia is important as many of the patients have contractures or adhesions and releases are frequently necessary. In cases of revision rotator cuff tears, the author prefers to insert the arthroscope directly into the subacromial space to avoid any iatrogenic injury to the residual posterior cuff. Standard posterior, lateral, and anterior portals are established. Additional portals are commonly used for anchor insertion, suture management, and graft passage including anterolateral, posterolateral, and the Neviaser portals. Use disposable working cannulas to minimize fluid extravasation. There is usually significant bursal hypertrophy, and a complete bursectomy will aid visualization and proper assessment of the tear pattern and reparability. The remainder of the shoulder pathology is addressed and additional procedures completed as needed. Loose sutures are removed and anchors are removed if needed. Anchors are only removed if loose or prominent, as the residual defects may require bone grafting and repair can be compromised.

Localizing the scapular spine and coracoid process can assist in identifying the rotator cuff tendons, and mobilization techniques to include interval slides, interval slide in continuity, and release of the articular side capsular contractions can help restore muscle tendon excursion. At this stage, reparability is assessed. For a successful ECM augmentation, the rotator must be reparable by a single- or double-row technique with or without margin convergence or side-to-side repair with minimal tension. If the rotator cuff cannot be primarily repaired, the clinician can consider debridement only, partial repair, interposition, or superior capsular reconstruction.

10.6.1 Repair

Many techniques have been described for rotator cuff augmentation. The author prefers a technique that tensions the graft independent of the RCR to assist in load sharing.[3] The greater tuberosity is debrided preserving subchondral bone. The graft will be attached medial to the repair and these sutures are placed prior to initiating the RCR. Mattress sutures (no. 2 nonabsorbable) are placed in the tendons to be repaired 5 mm lateral to the musculotendinous junction and spaced 1 cm apart. It is far simpler to place these sutures at this stage than after the cuff is repaired. The repair can be performed all arthroscopically or open. The arthroscopic technique is described below; however, the technical steps are the same for open repair.

The steps involved in repairing the rotator cuff and attaching the ECM graft depend on the type of repair the surgeon chooses. Anchors are inserted (or alternatively bone tunnels) and sutures are passed through the rotator cuff tendons for standard RCR by the surgeon's choice of method. In many cases, the bone is soft or compromised, frequently requiring larger diameter anchors. If the repair is a single-row or transosseous tunnel repair, then all sutures can be tied or secured at this time. When utilizing a double-row or transosseous equivalent (TOE) technique, all sutures should be passed but not secured laterally. Multiple accessory portals are frequently required for anchor placement and suture management.

The size of the desired graft is measured. The graft should extend beyond the defect by at least 5 mm medial, anterior, and posterior, and extend laterally 1 cm over the greater tuberosity. The ECM graft of surgeon's choice should be handled based on manufacturer's recommendation, thoroughly irrigated, and trimmed to the appropriate size. The author recommends a graft 1.5 to 2.0 mm in thickness.

The graft is brought to the patient and placed on a towel near the lateral portal. The lateral portal is exchanged for a 1-cm-diameter portal to aid in graft passage. The sutures that were previously placed for graft attachment are identified individually and one limb from each pair in placed in Mason–Allen technique and spaced equally on the medial side of the graft. If a TOE repair is utilized, the medial row sutures are also passed through the ECM graft at the appropriate spacing. Care is taken to pass all sutures individually and have an assistant maintain tension on all passed sutures to avoid tangling. The author prefers to pass no. 2 sutures with a commercial arthroscopic suture passer and punch the graft with a 2-mm skin biopsy punch for larger sutures that allow the graft to glide over the sutures for easier insertion. Once all suture passes are complete, an additional no. 2 suture is placed in the graft medially and then shuttled into the shoulder and retrieved through a Neviaser portal. This suture allows the surgeon to pull the graft into the shoulder with tensioning any of the repair sutures to avoid anchor or tissue pullout. Two additional no. 2 sutures are passed at the anterolateral and posterolateral corners. These are utilized for final tensioning during lateral fixation. The graft is then rolled anterior to posterior and a tissue grasper is used to push the graft into the shoulder. The push/pull technique minimizes the risk of tissue or anchor failure. The medial row sutures are tied completing the medial repair.

Lateral Fixation in Single-Row Technique or Transosseous Tunnels

Standard suture anchors can be utilized and the incorporated suture passed through the lateral edge of the patch by a suture passer. If tunnels are used, they need to be placed about 1 cm distal on the greater tuberosity.

Lateral Fixation in Double-Row (TOE) Technique

The lateral row is fixed by lateral row TOE type anchors. These anchors/tunnels must be placed to put the graft under gentle tension. When using a TOE method, additional sutures can be placed in the lateral edge of the graft to ensure graft tension.

The TOE sutures are retrieved in order based on the repair technique chosen. The lateral graft sutures are incorporated into the repair anchors. The TOE sutures are tensioned to properly secure the RCR and the patch sutures are individual tensioned to complete the lateral repair.

10.6.2 Arm Position During Repair

The arm is placed into 20 to 30 degrees of abduction during the repair for both techniques. Additional anterior or posterior sutures can be placed as needed to complete the repair.

10.7 Tips and Pearls/Expert Suggestions

- If visualization is compromised, consider converting to an open technique.
- Have 30- and 70-degree scopes available.
- Use multiple cannulas for suture management.
- Keep fluid pressures low to limit fluid extravasation as these procedures take longer than standard RCR.
- Preplace medial graft repair sutures before initiating RCR.
- Do not overtension RCR. Use single-row repair if needed.

10.8 What to Avoid

- Do not overtension repair.
- The graft should be under some tension at repair. Evaluate arm position during fixation.
- Manage fluid and blood pressure to limit extravasation.

10.9 Complications/Bailout/Salvage

- The arthroscopic procedure can be converted to open if visualization and suture management of fluid extravasation become an issue.
- Suture entanglement is common. Meticulous technique can minimize.
- Suture anchor stability is often compromised in revision cases due to prior surgery. Avoid removal of prior anchors unless needed. Have anchors of larger sizes available. Watch your angle of insertion and space anchors as much as possible. Bone tunnels can be used if needed. In event of anchor failure, a screw can be placed distal on the greater tuberosity and used as a suture post.
- Modern grafts in use have few reports of inflammatory reaction as reported in early experience.[4] High suspicion of infection is warranted if drainage, redness, or swelling

is present. Irrigation and debridement and graft removal should be strongly considered in suspicious cases.

10.10 Postoperative Care

A very conservative approach is recommended for rehabilitation consistent with a massive RCR protocol. An abduction sling with a pillow that provides 15- to 20-degree abduction is worn for 8 to 10 weeks. Passive range of motion (external rotation and elevation within range of motion determined at time of repair) for up to 6 weeks is advisable. At the 6-week time point, active assisted motion with pulley and wand exercises can be started. At 8 to 10 weeks, the abduction sling can be removed and isometric strength exercises started. Active range of motion is permitted at 3 months, and patients can resume normal activities at 6 months.

References

1. Shea KP, Obopilwe E, Sperling JW, Iannotti JP. A biomechanical analysis of gap formation and failure mechanics of a xenograft-reinforced rotator cuff repair in a cadaveric model. J Shoulder Elbow Surg 2012;21(8):1072–1079
2. Beitzel K, Chowaniec DM, McCarthy MB, et al. Stability of double-row rotator cuff repair is not adversely affected by scaffold interposition between tendon and bone. Am J Sports Med 2012;40(5):1148–1154
3. Lederman ES, Toth AP, Nicholson GP, et al. A prospective, multicenter study to evaluate clinical and radiographic outcomes in primary rotator cuff repair reinforced with a xenograft dermal matrix. J Shoulder Elbow Surg 2016;25(12):1961–1970
4. Iannotti JP, Codsi MJ, Kwon YW, Derwin K, Ciccone J, Brems JJ. Porcine small intestine submucosa augmentation of surgical repair of chronic two-tendon rotator cuff tears. A randomized, controlled trial. J Bone Joint Surg Am 2006;88(6):1238–1244

11 Superior Capsule Reconstruction with Fascia Lata Autograft

Teruhisa Mihata

Abstract

In 2007, we developed a new surgical treatment, "superior capsule reconstruction," to restore superior stability and muscle balance in the shoulder joint without repairing supraspinatus and infraspinatus tendon tears, consequently improving shoulder function—particularly deltoid muscle function—and relieving pain. The presence of indications for this surgery is determined by preoperative MRI. Goutallier grades 3 and 4 (fatty infiltration equal to, or more than, the muscle volume) are absolute indications. Moreover, in Goutallier grade 2, if the torn tendon is severely atrophied, degenerated, and thin, we recommend superior capsule reconstruction. During arthroscopy, the quality and mobility of the torn tendon are examined. If the tendon cannot be made to reach its original footprint (i.e., if the tear is irreducible), a preoperative decision is made for superior capsule reconstruction. If, after mobilization, the tendon can be made to reach the original footprint (i.e., if the tear is reducible), superior capsule reconstruction followed by rotator cuff repair over the reconstructed superior capsule is chosen. Factors prognostic of clinical outcome are the degree of graft healing and the level of deltoid function. Re-tear of the graft of the repaired infraspinatus tendon causes shoulder pain or decreased active elevation. In some patients, concomitant cervical spinal (C5) palsy or axillary nerve palsy worsens clinical outcomes after surgery, resulting in poor shoulder function despite graft healing.

Keywords: *autograft, fascia lata, irreparable, reconstruction, rotator cuff, shoulder, superior capsule, tear*

11.1 Goals of Procedure

In 2007, we developed a new surgical treatment, "superior capsule reconstruction" (**Figs. 11.1–11.3**), to restore superior stability and muscle balance in the shoulder joint without repairing supraspinatus and infraspinatus tendon tears,[1–4] consequently improving shoulder function—particularly deltoid muscle function—and relieving pain.[5]

11.2 Advantages

Superior capsule reconstruction restores shoulder function and results in high rates of return to work and to recreational sport, including overhead sports, with relatively low rates of postoperative complications. Furthermore, the native glenohumeral joint can be kept in the superior capsule reconstruction, resulting in better shoulder range of motion, especially external rotation and internal rotation, compared with reverse shoulder arthroplasty.

11.3 Indications

Patient suitability for superior capsule reconstruction is determined by preoperative MRI. Goutallier grades 3 and 4 (fatty infiltration equal to, or more than, muscle volume) are absolute indications. In Goutallier grade 2, if the torn tendon is

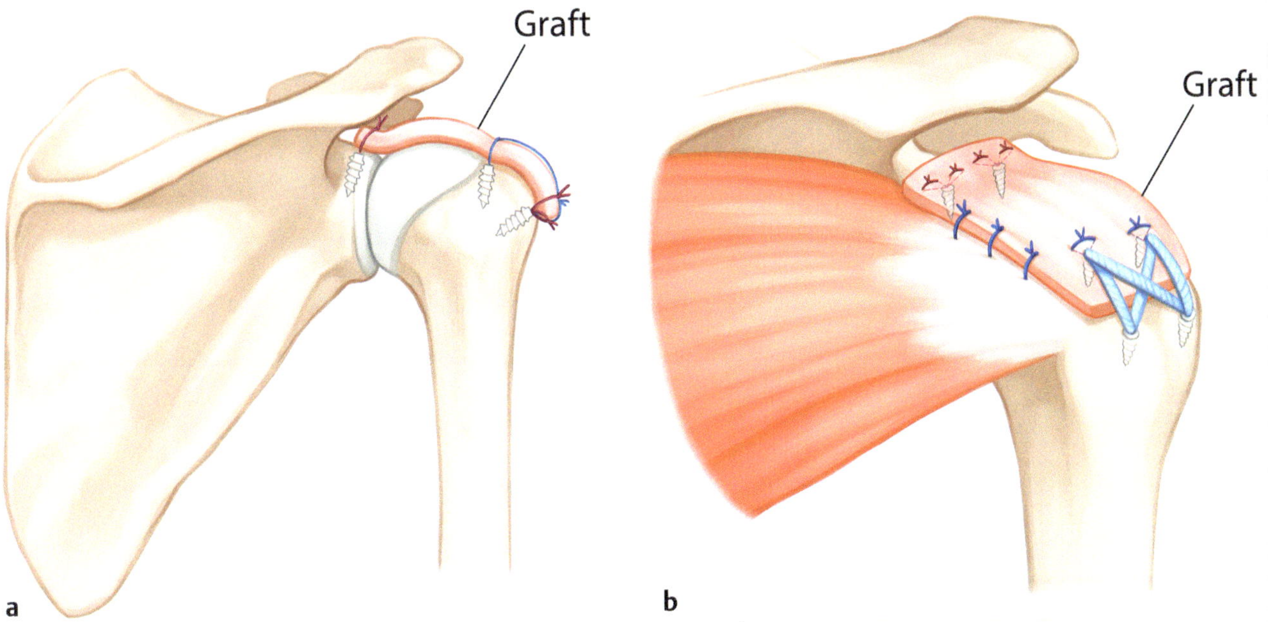

Fig. 11.1 Superior capsule reconstruction. The graft is attached medially to the superior glenoid and laterally to the greater tuberosity. This is followed by side-to-side suturing between the graft and the infraspinatus or teres minor tendon. (a) The compression double-row repair technique. (b) The SpeedBridge repair technique (Arthrex).

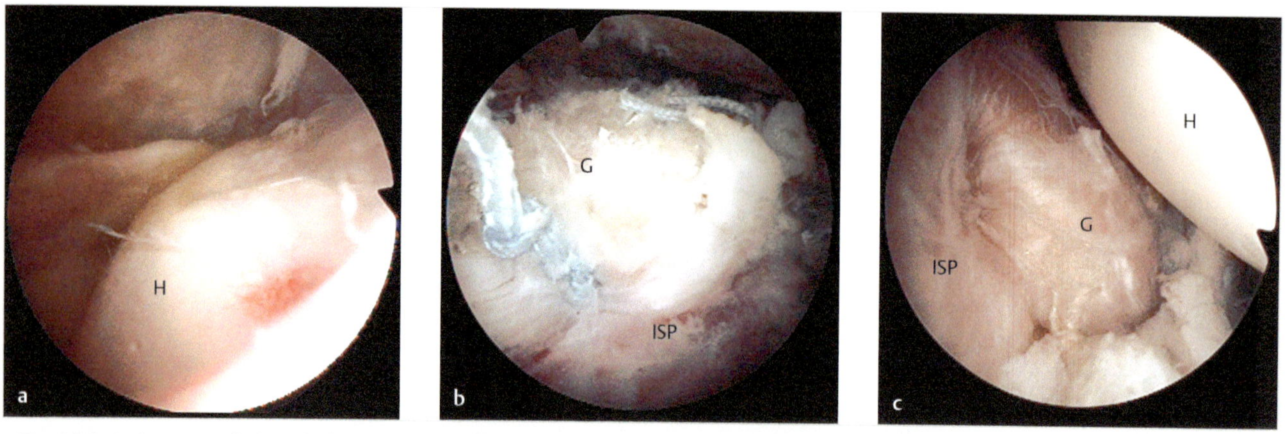

Fig. 11.2 Arthroscopic findings before and after superior capsule reconstruction. **(a)** Before surgery. **(b,c)** Just after surgery.

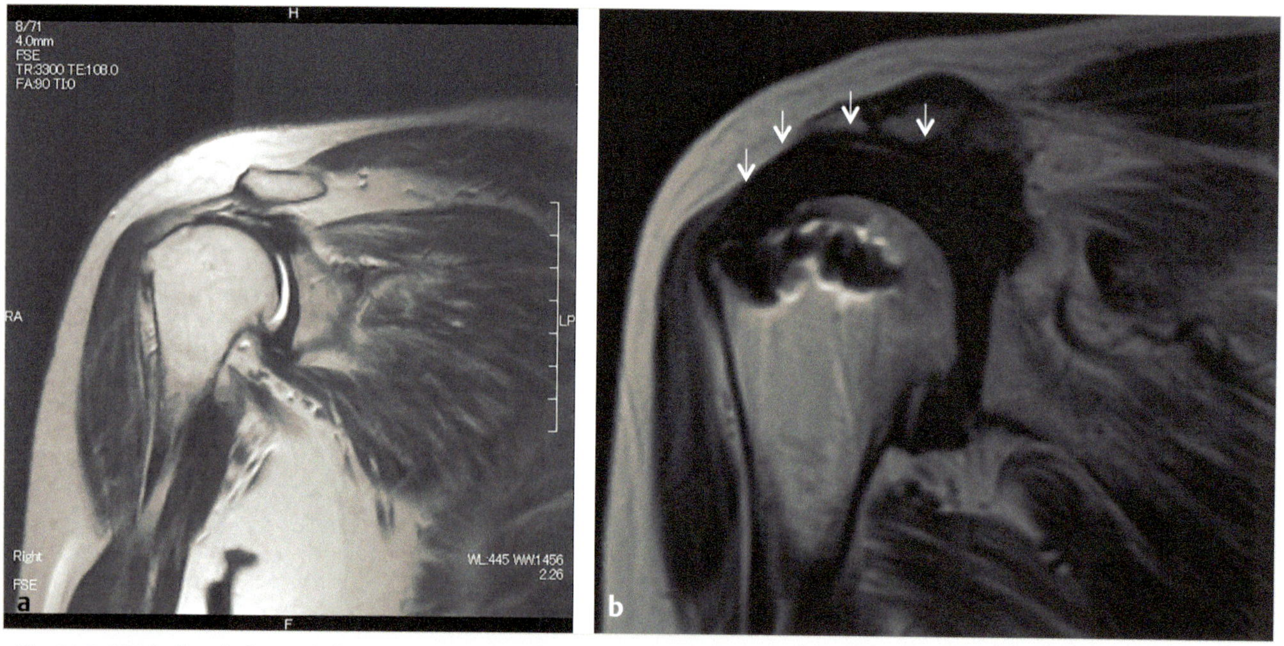

Fig. 11.3 MRI findings before and after superior capsule reconstruction. **(a)** Before surgery. The torn supraspinatus tendon is severely retracted, and the supraspinatus muscle is severely atrophied and infiltrated with fat. **(b)** One year after surgery.

severely retracted, degenerated, and thin, we also recommend superior capsule reconstruction.

Irreparable rotator cuff tears of Hamada grades 1 to 3 are an absolute indication for arthroscopic superior capsule reconstruction (ASCR). Whereas young patients with Hamada grade 4 are recommended for ASCR, elderly patients with Hamada grade 4 and all patients with Hamada grade 5 should have total shoulder arthroplasty with open surgical superior capsule reconstruction.

During arthroscopy, the quality and mobility of the torn tendon are examined. If the torn tendon cannot be made to reach the original footprint (i.e., if the tear is irreducible), a preoperative decision is made to perform superior capsule reconstruction alone. If the torn tendon can reach the original footprint after mobilization (i.e., if the tear is reducible), superior capsule reconstruction followed by rotator cuff repair over the reconstructed superior capsule is recommended.

11.4 Contraindications

When patients already have severe deltoid atrophy and weakness from concomitant cervical spinal palsy (at the C5 level) or axillary nerve palsy, we do not recommend superior capsule reconstruction because we cannot expect functional improvement after surgery, even when the graft is healed. However, we sometimes do superior capsule reconstructions in patients with slight or moderate deltoid weakness, to decrease shoulder pain.

11.5 Preoperative Preparation/ Positioning

Preoperative preparation for superior capsule reconstruction is the same as for rotator cuff repair. The surgery can be performed either arthroscopically or by an open approach, and both the lateral decubitus position and the beach-chair position are suitable.

11.6 Operative Technique

11.6.1 Measurement of Defect Size

Subacromial bursal tissue around the torn tendons is completely removed before measurement of the defect size. The defect is then measured in the mediolateral (5–6 cm in most cases: from "the superior glenoid," not the edge of the torn tendon, to the lateral edge of the greater tuberosity) and anteroposterior (from the anterior edge to the posterior edge of the torn tendon) directions (**Fig. 11.4**).

11.6.2 Deciding on Graft Size

The graft length in the anteroposterior direction is determined to be exactly the same as the length of the defect without partial repair of the torn infraspinatus tendon. In the mediolateral direction, the graft should be 15 mm longer than the distance from the superior glenoid to the lateral edge of the greater tuberosity to make a 10-mm footprint on the superior glenoid and allow for 5 mm of latitude in graft size. A biomechanical study has indicated that the appropriate graft thickness for superior capsule reconstruction using the fascia lata is 6 to 8 mm.[4] Therefore, the amount of fascia lata that we need to harvest will be at least double the estimated graft length or width.

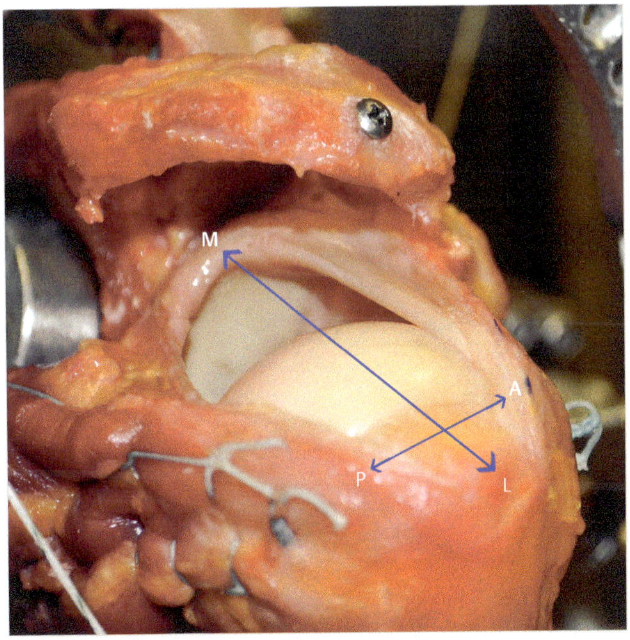

Fig. 11.4 Measurement of defect size. The size of the defect is measured in the mediolateral (from the superior glenoid [M] to the lateral edge of the greater tuberosity [L]) and anteroposterior (from the anterior edge [A] to the posterior edge [P] of the torn tendon) directions.

11.6.3 Harvesting the Fascia Lata and Making the Autograft

The fascia lata is harvested beginning 1 to 2 cm distal to the greater trochanter, with care to include the posterior, thicker tissue (**Fig. 11.5**). The average thickness of a single layer of autologous fascia lata is 2 to 4 mm. Therefore, a graft thickness of 6 to 8 mm is achieved by folding the fascia lata two or three times. Also, the fascia lata includes an intermuscular septum that consists of the tissues of two tendons and connects the fascia lata to the femur. To make a thicker graft, this intermuscular septum should be included in the graft (**Fig. 11.5**). The fascia lata is mostly thinner at its anterior aspect than posteriorly; therefore, to make a flat graft of even thickness, the intermuscular septum is usually sutured to the anterior surface of the fascia lata after being completely detached from it (**Fig. 11.6**). All fatty tissue should be removed from the graft. Finally, the layers of the fascia lata are united very closely with nonabsorbable sutures to prevent delamination after surgery.

11.6.4 Treatment of Associated Lesions

Subscapularis tears should be repaired. Biceps tenodesis or tenotomy is performed for biceps tendon subluxation or dislocation.

11.6.5 Acromioplasty

The coracoacromial ligament, and spurs on the anterior, lateral, or medial side, should be resected to prevent subacromial impingement after surgery.[2] Also, the inferior surface of the acromion is usually made flat. Although acromioplasty is performed in all cases of superior capsule reconstruction, we have had no cases of postoperative superior dislocation of the humeral head.

11.6.6 Anchor Placement on the Superior Glenoid

All soft tissue on the footprint of the superior glenoid should be removed to give a good bone bed before insertion of the suture anchors. Excessive resection of the cortical bone may lead to anchor pullout after surgery. Two 4.5-mm Corkscrew FT (Arthrex, Naples, FL) anchors are inserted, at the 10 or 11 o'clock and 11 or 12 o'clock positions on the glenoid of the right shoulder, and at the 12 or 1 o'clock and 1 or 2 o'clock positions on the left shoulder (**Fig. 11.7**).

11.6.7 Anchor Placement on the Medial Footprint

All soft tissue on the footprint of the greater tuberosity should be removed. Two 4.75-mm SwiveLock (Arthrex) anchors with FiberTape (Arthrex) are inserted on the medial footprint of the greater tuberosity to make a SpeedBridge (Arthrex). Alternatively, when we fix the graft to the greater tuberosity by using a compression double-row repair technique, two 4.5-mm Corkscrew FT (Arthrex) anchors are inserted on the medial footprint.[6,7]

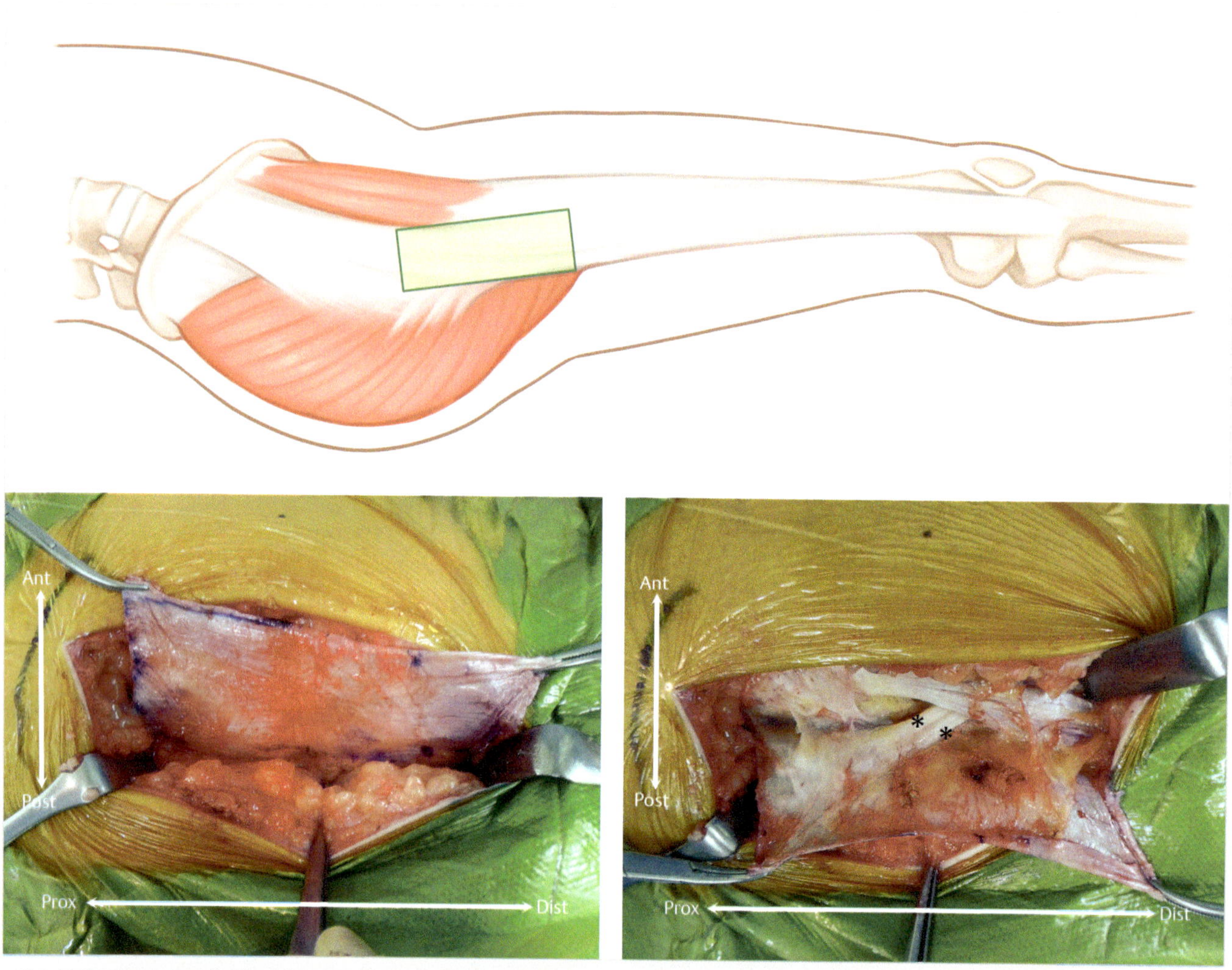

Fig. 11.5 Harvesting the fascia lata. **(a)** The fascia lata is harvested beginning 1 cm distal to the greater trochanter. **(b)** The fascia lata is cut along the proximal, anterior, and distal marks. **(c)** After the fascia lata is flipped over. The fascia lata includes an intermuscular septum (*asterisk*) that consists of the tissues of two tendons and connects the fascia lata and the femur. To make a thicker graft, this intermuscular septum should be included in the graft. Ant, anterior; Dist, distal; Post, posterior; Prox, proximal.

11.6.8 Insertion of Fascia Lata into the Subacromial Space

A 10-mL syringe is used as a cannula. FiberWires (Arthrex) from the superior glenoid suture anchors are placed through the fascia lata in a mattress fashion when the graft is still outside the body (**Fig. 11.8**). After all FiberWires have been placed through the fascia lata, one FiberWire is tied, while the graft is pushed into the subacromial space. The graft can then be inserted in its appropriate place on the glenoid. All sutures are then tied in the subacromial space.

11.6.9 Attachment to the Greater Tuberosity

To complete the SpeedBridge fixation, the additional two 4.75-mm SwiveLock (Arthrex) anchors are inserted at 5 mm distal to the lateral footprint of the greater tuberosity. The author recommends making additional medial mattress suturing using FiberWires from two SwiveLock anchors, which had been inserted on the medial footprint of the greater tuberosity.

11.6.10 Side-to-Side Suturing between the Graft and the Infraspinatus Tendon or Teres Minor

In a dynamic observational study of cadaveric biomechanics, four of seven shoulders had posterosuperior subluxation during external and internal rotations in the absence of side-to-side suturing; after the addition of posterior side-to-side suturing, the glenohumeral joint was secure and stable, and posterosuperior subluxation did not occur.[3] Therefore, two or three sutures for posterior side-to-side suturing should be placed between the graft and the infraspinatus tendon or teres minor to increase superior shoulder stability and to prevent posterosuperior subluxation.[3] Side-to-side suturing both anteriorly and posteriorly may cause postoperative shoulder stiffness, so anterior side-to-side suturing in superior capsule reconstruction using the fascia lata is not recommended.

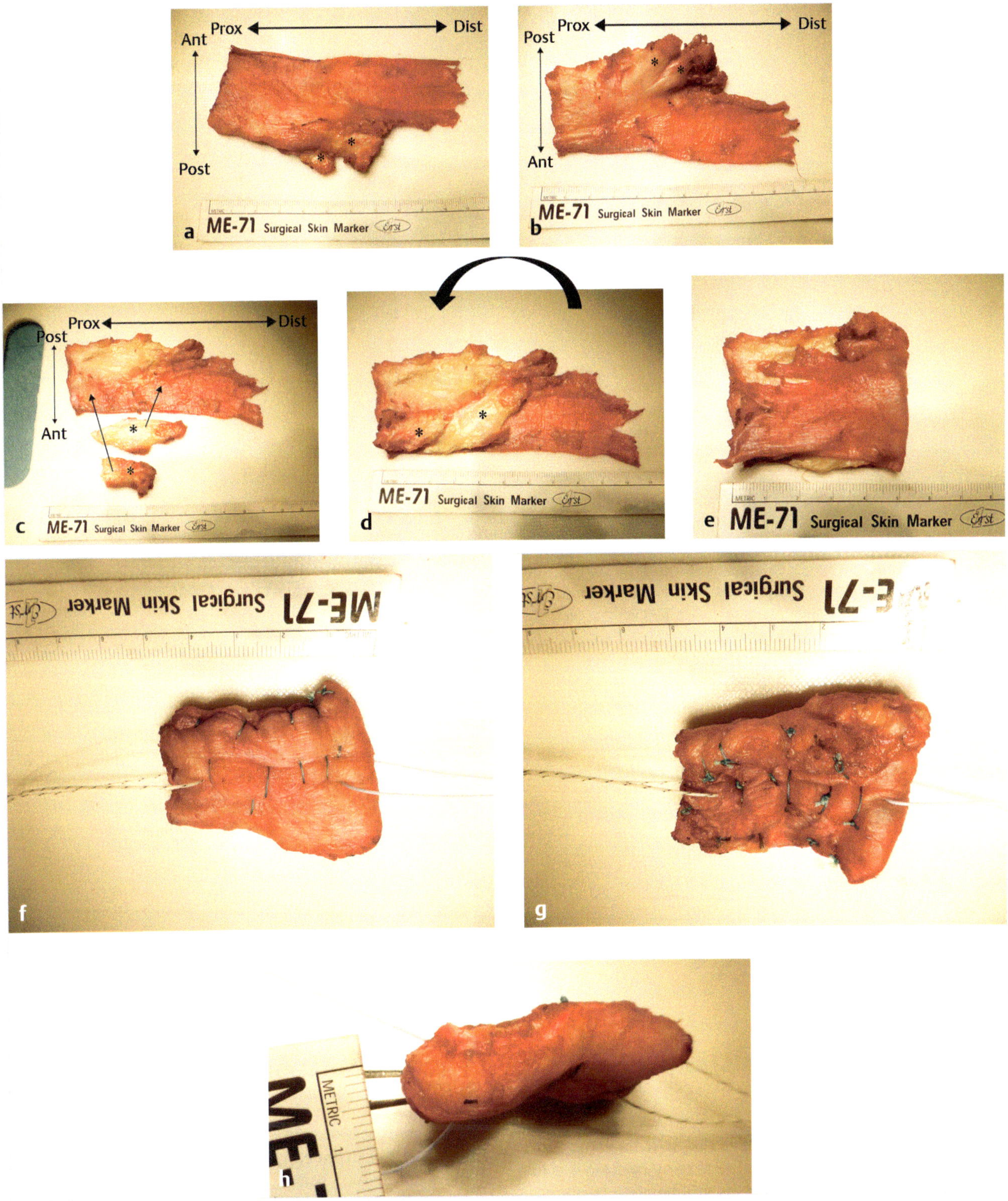

Fig. 11.6 **(a)** The obverse side of the harvested fascia lata. **(b)** The reverse side of the harvested fascia lata. **(c–e)** The fascia lata tends to be thinner anteriorly. Therefore, to make a flat graft of even thickness, the intermuscular septum is usually sutured to the anterior surface of the fascia lata after being detached from it. Then the fascia lata is folded. **(f–h)** Finally, the layers of the fascia lata are united by using nonabsorbable sutures. Ant, anterior; Dist, distal; Post, posterior; Prox, proximal.

12 Superior Capsular Reconstruction

Brandon J. Erickson and Joshua S. Dines

Abstract
Massive irreparable rotator cuff tears present a difficult problem to the treating surgeon. One relatively new option in treatment of large, irreparable rotator cuff tears is a superior capsular reconstruction (SCR). Although originally described using fascia lata autograft, this procedure is now commonly performed with dermal allograft tissue. The purpose of an SCR is to use this allograft tissue to depress the humeral head, thereby preventing superior escape of the humeral head in large, irreparable rotator cuff tears. The hope is that by depressing the humeral head and keeping it articulating properly with the glenoid, patients will maintain a functional shoulder while not progressing as quickly to rotator cuff tear arthropathy necessitating a reverse total shoulder arthroplasty. The goal of this chapter is to present the indications for an SCR as well as a step-by-step guide to performing the procedure. This safe and easy-to-learn technique will allow surgeons to perform an accurate, reproducible SCR. Tips and pearls will be provided, as will strategies to deal with difficulties during surgery. Finally, the postoperative rehabilitation will be discussed as it pertains to patients following SCR.

Keywords: *rotator cuff tear, massive, irreparable, shoulder, superior capsular reconstruction, allograft, arthroscopy, repair*

12.1 Goals of Procedure

The goal of a superior capsular reconstruction (SCR) is to anatomically reconstruct the superior capsule to allow increased function and decreased pain in a patient with a large, irreparable rotator cuff tear. The SCR functions as a humeral head depressant, thereby centering the humeral head on the glenoid and allowing the deltoid to elevate the arm.[1] Other options for these patients include a simple debridement (+ biceps tenotomy/tenodesis), partial rotator cuff repair, bridging patch graft, latissimus dorsi transfer, lower trapezius transfer, and reverse total shoulder arthroplasty. However, the SCR anatomically reconstructs the superior capsule using dermal allograft, which restores the biomechanical fulcrum of the shoulder and thereby restores function in a way that these other procedures do not.[1,2]

12.2 Advantages

- The SCR can be performed arthroscopically with a similar setup to a rotator cuff repair and accurately restores the superior stability of the shoulder.[1]
- The SCR is a reliable technique that produces excellent clinical outcomes in patients with irreparable rotator cuff tears.[3]

12.3 Indications

- Large, irreparable rotator cuff tears involving the supraspinatus and/or the infraspinatus in young patients without significant glenohumeral arthritis.

12.4 Contraindications

- Significant glenohumeral arthritis.
- Irreparable rotator cuff tears involving either the subscapularis or teres minor in addition to the supraspinatus/infraspinatus (having all these tendons involved disrupts the balanced transvers plane force couple).
- Nonfunctioning deltoid.
- Significant bone loss or bony deformity of the glenohumeral joint.
- Previous reaction to dermal allograft tissue or religious beliefs prohibiting implantation of this allograft tissue.

12.5 Preoperative Preparation/ Positioning

- This procedure can be performed in the beach-chair or lateral decubitus position:
  - The authors prefer the beach-chair position, so this technique is for the beach-chair position.
- Nonoperative arm at side and taped with a pillow around it, padding all bony prominences and the head secured.
- An arm positioner (Trimano; Arthrex, Naples, FL) is helpful to maintain various arm rotations throughout the case.
- Prep and drape in the usual sterile fashion.

12.6 Operative Technique

- Mark out shoulder:
  - Acromion, clavicle, scapular spine, acromioclavicular joint, and soft spot for Neviaser portal between clavicle and scapular spine.
- Mark portals:
  - Posterior, lateral, anterosuperolateral, Neviaser.
- A no. 11 blade to make posterior portal skin incision, introduce trocar into glenohumeral joint.
- Perform a complete diagnostic arthroscopy:
  - In the setting of a potential SCR, there should be a large rotator cuff tear allowing visualization of both the glenohumeral joint and subacromial space simultaneously.
- Move the arthroscope subacromial in the posterior portal and make the lateral portal under direct visualization, coming in at the 50-yard line of the lateral acromion:
  - Debride the subacromial bursa to improve visualization of the rotator cuff (**Fig. 12.1**):
    - Mobilize the tear using electrocautery, shaver, Bankart's elevator, arthroscopic scissors, etc., and attempt to reduce the rotator cuff to the greater tuberosity:
      - i. If the tendon reduces without significant tension, perform an arthroscopic rotator cuff repair.
        - a. If part of the rotator cuff can be repaired, this can be done after the SCR is secured.[4]
      - ii. If it does not reduce, proceed with the SCR.

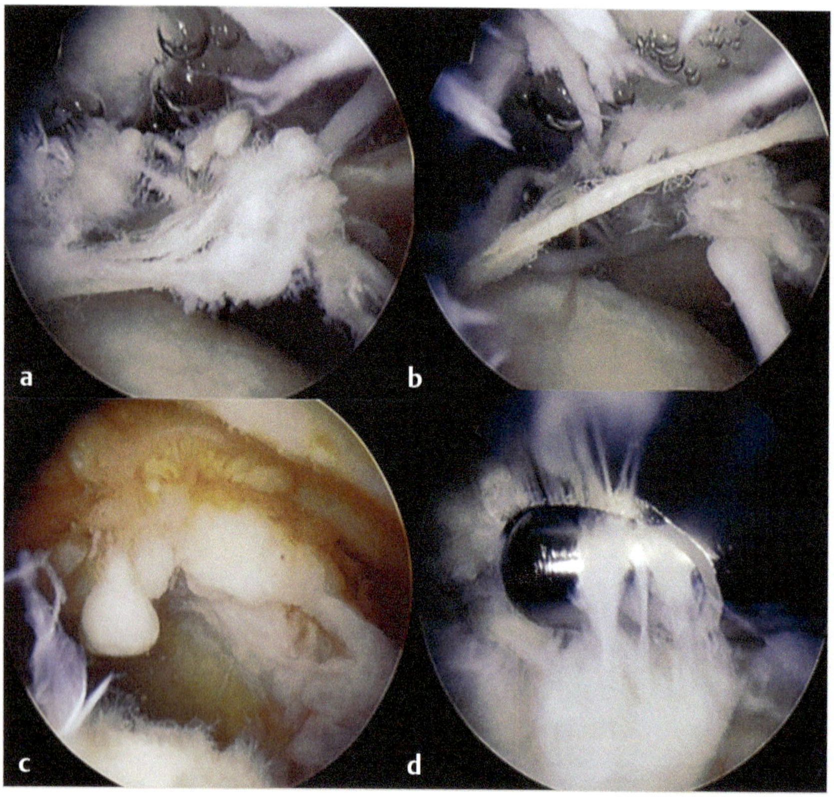

Fig. 12.1 (a–d) Arthroscopic images demonstrating subacromial decompression and debridement of the remnant rotator cuff.

- Use a combination of the electrocautery device, shaver, and burr to expose and prepare the superomedial glenoid rim and greater tuberosity:
  - Do not go too medial on the glenoid, as the suprascapular nerve can be injured.[5]
  - Do not take too much bone when preparing the glenoid and greater tuberosity as this can compromise fixation of the anchors.
- Now place in two passport cannulas (Arthrex; one is a lateral and one is an anterosuperolateral portal).
- There are now two options as to how to proceed:
  - The surgeon may place both the glenoid and humeral anchors before passing the graft into the joint, or he or she may place the glenoid anchors, pass the graft, and then place the humeral anchors.
    - This technique will be for placing the glenoid anchors, passing the graft, and then placing the humeral anchors.
- Place two single-loaded SutureTak anchors loaded with FiberWire (Arthrex) in the glenoid:
  - Make the previously marked out Neviaser portal and place a switching stick in there to help retract tissues to better expose the glenoid:
    - A small stab incision may be needed to obtain the ideal trajectory for the anchors on the glenoid rim (**Fig. 12.2**):
      i. Do not compromise anchor placement because of inability to access the glenoid rim with the current portals—make additional percutaneous stab incisions to place anchors as needed.
  - Anchors should be placed at least 1 cm away from one another.
- Now use the arthroscopic measuring tool to measure the distance between the anchors on the glenoid, and the proposed spots for the anchors on the humeral head, and then measure the distance between the anchors on the glenoid rim:
  - Then, use this tool to measure the distance from the posterior anchor on the glenoid to the proposed spot for the posterior anchor on the humeral head, and then measure the distance from the anterior anchor on the glenoid rim to the proposed spot for the anterior anchor on the humeral head:
    - Write all these measurements down:
      i. Ensure accurate recording of all measurements.
- Once all measurements are obtained, roll out the piece of dermal allograft matrix on a blue towel.
- Mark the allograft at all the measurements, and cut the allograft to be 1 cm longer in all directions from what you measured:
  - Then mark with a marking pen on the cut piece of collagen exactly where the anchors are.
  - One by one, use an arthroscopic suture passing device (author's preference is the Scorpion [Arthrex]) to pass the suture from the corresponding glenoid anchor on the piece of collagen:
    - Maintain tension on the sutures as they are passed to avoid tangling of the sutures.
  - Tie the two glenoid-side sutures (FiberWire) coming out of the superior aspect of the graft to each other.
  - Retrieve the glenoid sutures that were not passed through the graft out Neviaser portal.
- Once the sutures from the glenoid anchor are passed (you will have two pieces coming through the collagen), insert the collagen piece into the shoulder via the passport cannula.
- Gently roll this up and put it in through the cannula:
  - When placing this through the cannula, push it in rather than twisting as this can lead to the sutures becoming tangled.
  - Make sure not to drag the collagen along the patient's skin to avoid dragging skin flora into the shoulder (**Fig. 12.3**).
- Use the two strands of suture coming out Neviaser portal to help parachute the tendon graft into place on the glenoid.

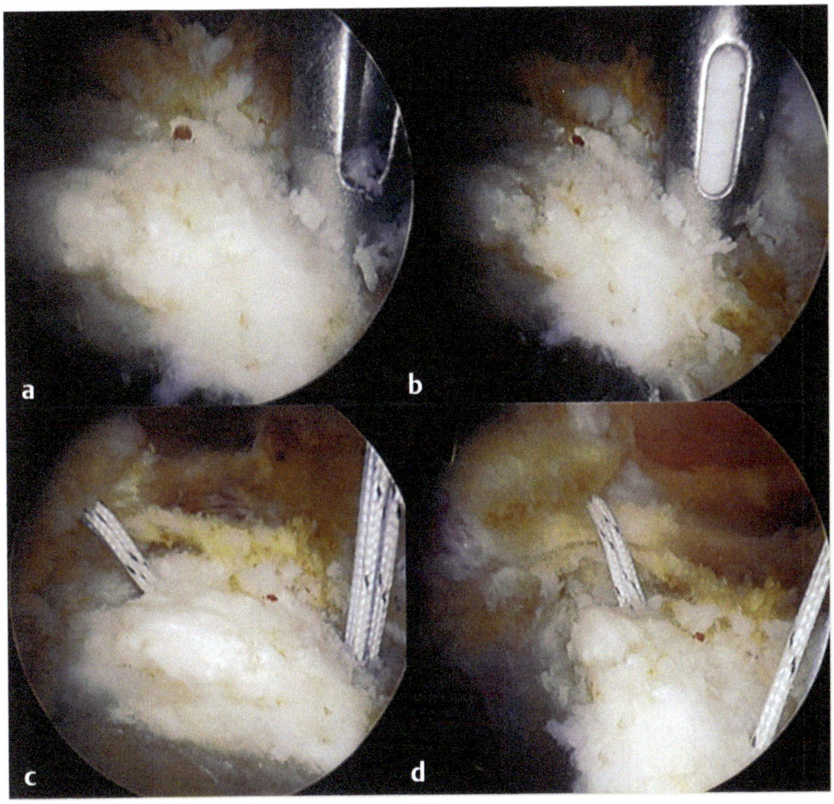

Fig. 12.2 (a–d) Arthroscopic images demonstrating percutaneous placement of the two glenoid anchors.

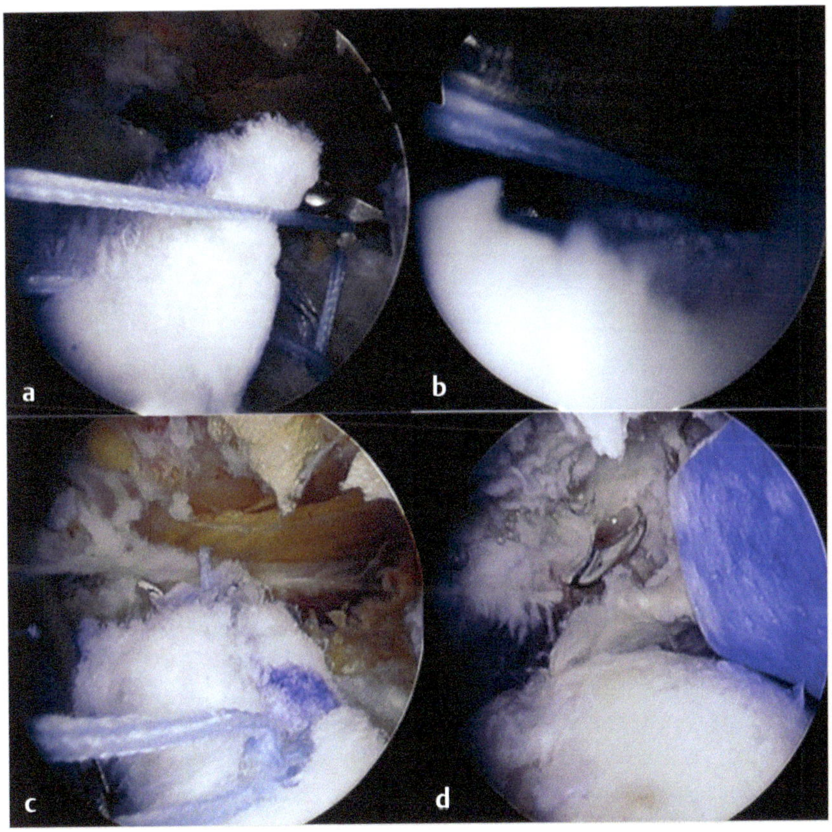

Fig. 12.3 (a–d) Arthroscopic images of the dermal allograft secured to the glenoid. Tension is maintained on the sutures to avoid tangling. The arthroscopic knot of the surgeon's choice can be used.

- Unroll the allograft with a probe once inside the shoulder and lay it flat (**Fig. 12.4**).
- Now retrieve the glenoid sutures coming out Neviaser portal through the lateral portal and tie arthroscopic knots to secure the graft to the glenoid (**Fig. 12.3c**). Do not cut these sutures after tying. Instead, to increase the load to failure of the construct and help flatten the graft over the glenoid, we incorporate these strands into a PushLock Anchor (Arthrex) posteriorly on the glenoid.
- Next, place the punches for two SwiveLock anchors loaded with either FiberTape or FiberWire in the humeral head just lateral to the articular margin (**Fig. 12.5**):

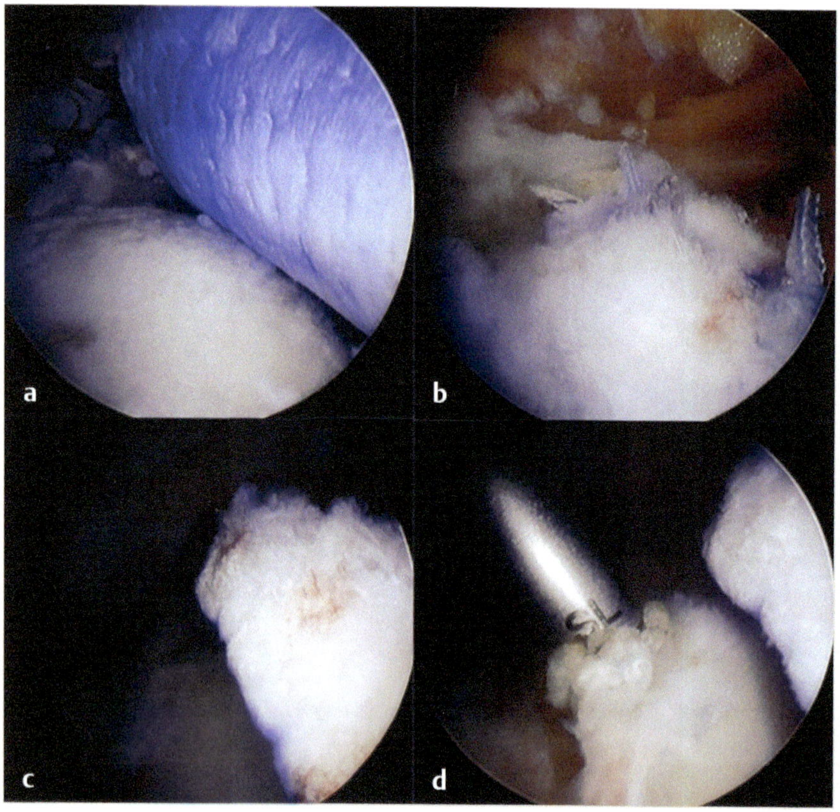

Fig. 12.4 (a–d) The allograft is rolled out to cover the humeral head, and the punch for the first humeral anchor is placed. This graft was premeasured so it should fit perfectly.

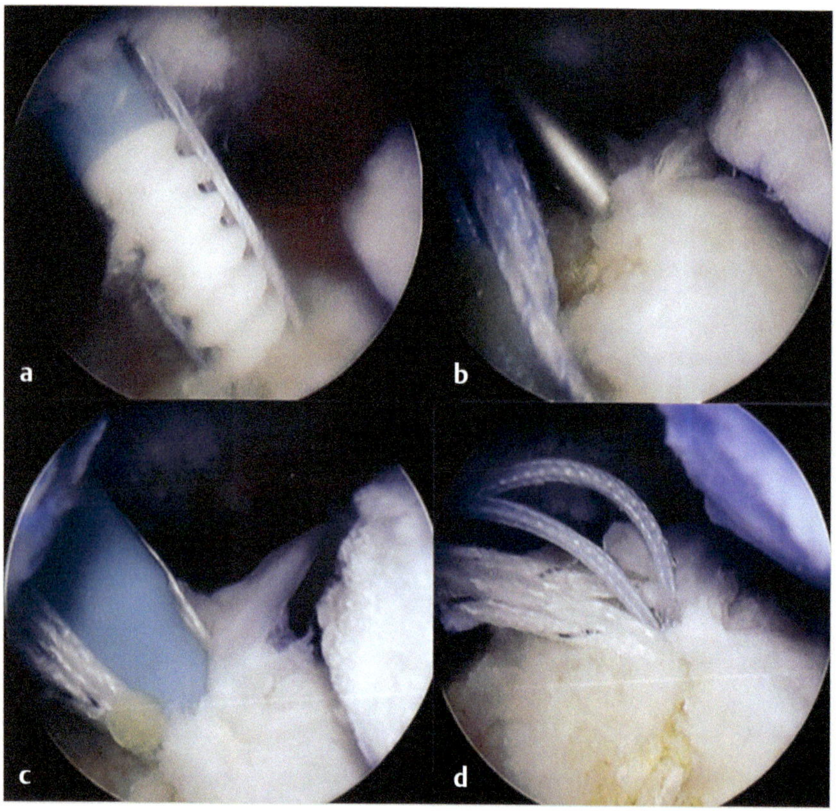

Fig. 12.5 (a–d) The rest of the humeral head anchors are placed.

- The anchors should be placed far enough apart so that when the graft is secure to them, it will cover the defect appropriately from anterior to posterior.

- The humeral fixation will be treated like a SpeedBridge double-row rotator cuff repair (**Fig. 12.6**):
  - Use an electrocautery to clean off an area on the lateral humerus.

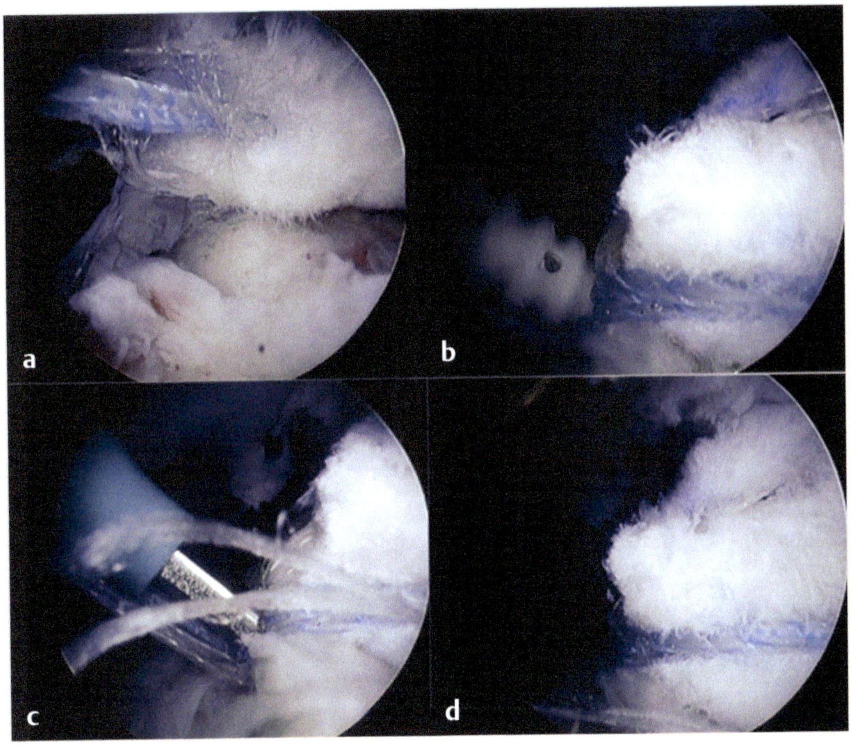

Fig. 12.6 (a–d) Sutures are passed through the allograft and these sutures are placed into a second lateral row of anchors, similar to a double-row rotator cuff repair.

- Place two unloaded SwiveLock anchors in the lateral humeral head:
  - First, with the shoulder in internal rotation, place the posterior anchor:
    i. Pass the posterior suture of each of the two humeral head anchors through this SwiveLock, and pull tension on the sutures once the anchor is seated into bone before it is malleted and screwed in to get any slack out of the system, and mallet the anchor into place.
  - Then place the anterior anchor in a similar manner.
- The allograft is now secured.
- The remaining posterior rotator cuff is now sutured to the allograft:
  - Typically there will be some posterior cuff left to sew the collagen to:
    - Anteriorly, the subscapularis should not be included in the repair, but rotator interval tissue or any anterior supraspinatus that is present should be sewn to the collagen.
  - Place two to three sutures between the collagen and cuff using a suture passing device and tie standard arthroscopic knots. This is done in a similar fashion to what is used for margin convergence sutures in massive rotator cuff repairs (**Fig. 12.7**).

12.6.1 Closure

- 3–0 Prolene for portals.
- Steri-Strips.
- 4 × 4, abdominal, Medipore tape.
- Sling.

12.7 Tips and Pearls/Expert Suggestions

- Always attempt to fix the rotator cuff before moving onto an SCR.
- Proper portal placement is key to avoid overcrowding and to allow access to all necessary parts of the shoulder (posterior, lateral, Neviaser, and anterosuperolateral):
  - Use needle localization judiciously to ensure proper trajectory for all anchors.
- Anterior glenoid anchor should be just in front of the acromioclavicular joint.
- When passing sutures through the allograft, pass from posterior to anterior, and start with the greater tuberosity.
- When parachuting the graft into the shoulder, help push the graft straight in; do not rotate your forearm as this can cause the sutures to tangle and the graft to bind up.
- Additional anchors can be placed on the glenoid to augment the fixation.
- Incorporate the posterior cuff tissue into the allograft every time using side-to-side sutures:
  - Only incorporate anterior tissue if there is rotator interval tissue (incorporating the subscapularis will overconstrain the shoulder).[6]

12.8 What to Avoid

- Make sure to add 1 cm of tissue all the way around the graft when cutting this to your measurements to avoid the possibility of the sutures cutting out of the graft.

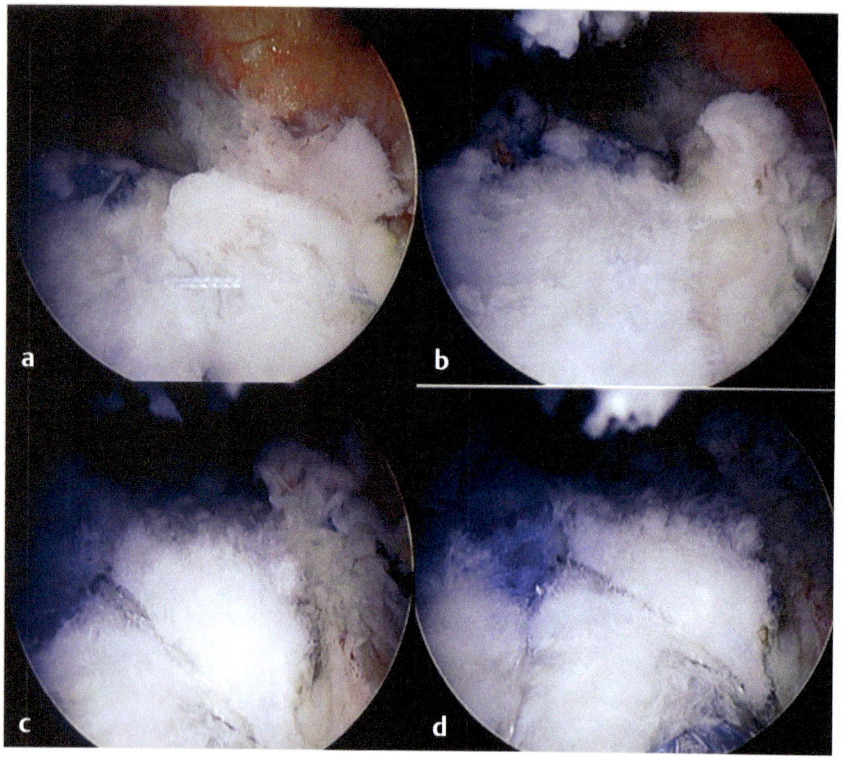

Fig. 12.7 (a–d) The final construct of the allograft in place, depressing the humeral head, securely fixed to the glenoid and humerus.

- Do not allow the sutures going through the allograft to become tangled—avoid this by having an assistant pull tension on the sutures after they are passed.
- Do not lay the graft on the patient's skin—place the graft on a blue towel when passing the sutures through it to avoid contaminating the graft with skin flora.

12.9 Complications/Bailout/ Salvage

The SCR is a salvage procedure for irreparable rotator cuff tears. If the bone quality is not good enough to hold the anchors, a debridement can provide some mild pain relief in limited patients. We find it useful to counsel the patient preoperatively about the potential need to do a reverse shoulder replacement in a small percentage of cases so that it could be done during the same operative setting, if necessary.

12.10 Postoperative Care

One must understand the biologic healing response that occurs with an SCR to properly guide patients in their postoperative protocols. A prior canine study has shown that the allograft tissue is weakest between 2 and 6 months.[7] Therefore, unrestricted activity should not be permitted until the graft has evolved to a normal tendon structure, which takes approximately 6 months.[8] The rehabilitation protocol that the authors use can be broken down into four phases:

- Phase 1: rest:
  - A sling is worn for 6 weeks to minimize shoulder motion, but patients come out of this to perform active range of motion (ROM) of the elbow, hand, wrist, and cervical spine.
  - Focus on pain management with judicious use of ice.
- Phase II: ROM:
  - Begin passive shoulder ROM in a controlled setting, often supine:
    - Progress to active-assisted motion followed by active ROM.
  - Emphasize deltoid activation.
- Phase III: strengthening:
  - At 12 weeks, patients are often allowed to begin a gentle strengthening program, provided they have regained the majority of their ROM.
- Phase IV: continued strengthening and increased activity level:
  - Patients begin to work on overhead activities and plyometric exercise.

References

1. Mihata T, McGarry MH, Kahn T, Goldberg I, Neo M, Lee TQ. Biomechanical role of capsular continuity in superior capsule reconstruction for irreparable tears of the supraspinatus tendon. Am J Sports Med 2016;44(6):1423–1430
2. Mihata T, McGarry MH, Pirolo JM, Kinoshita M, Lee TQ. Superior capsule reconstruction to restore superior stability in irreparable rotator cuff tears: a biomechanical cadaveric study. Am J Sports Med 2012;40(10):2248–2255

3. Mihata T, Lee TQ, Watanabe C, et al. Clinical results of arthroscopic superior capsule reconstruction for irreparable rotator cuff tears. Arthroscopy 2013;29(3):459–470
4. Sutter EG, Godin JA, Garrigues GE. All-arthroscopic superior shoulder capsule reconstruction with partial rotator cuff repair. Orthopedics 2017;40(4):e735–e738
5. Schon JM, Katthagen JC, Dupre CN, et al. Quantitative and computed tomography anatomic analysis of glenoid fixation for superior capsule reconstruction: a cadaveric study. Arthroscopy 2017;33(6):1131–1137
6. Mihata T, McGarry MH, Kahn T, Goldberg I, Neo M, Lee TQ. Biomechanical effect of thickness and tension of fascia lata graft on glenohumeral stability for superior capsule reconstruction in irreparable supraspinatus tears. Arthroscopy 2016;32(3):418–426
7. Adams JE, Zobitz ME, Reach JS Jr, An KN, Steinmann SP. Rotator cuff repair using an acellular dermal matrix graft: an in vivo study in a canine model. Arthroscopy 2006;22(7):700–709
8. Pogorzelski J, DelVecchio BM, Hussain ZB, Fritz EM, Godin JA, Millett PJ. Superior capsule reconstruction for massive rotator cuff tears: key considerations for rehabilitation. Int J Sports Phys Ther 2017;12(3):390–401

13 Arthroscopic Suprapectoral Biceps Tenodesis

Boris Poberaj and Benjamin Marjanovic

Abstract
Arthroscopic suprapectoral long head of the biceps (LHB) tenodesis with a new Cobra guide enables strong intraosseous fixation without implants. This technique requires standard arthroscopic portals for rotator cuff repair and additional suprapectoral portal. The suprapectoral space exploration and the LHB position in relation to the anatomical landmarks are well described. The aim of the Cobra guide is to pass shuttle sutures in the right angle fashion from anterior to lateral humeral surface and thus avoid possible axillary nerve damage. Due to precise, arthroscopic controlled technique, the final LHB fixation always maintains biceps muscle length–tension relation. This type of tenodesis can also be safely performed as the last step of a more complex shoulder procedure.

Keywords: *suprapectoral space, intraosseous biceps tenodesis, implant free*

13.1 Goals of Procedure

A new arthroscopic technique with Cobra guide (**Fig. 13.1**) was developed to enable fast, controlled, and strong intraosseous biceps tenodesis using bone tunnels and sutures without implants.

13.2 Advantages

Because it is an implant-free technique, there are no complications related to the device, either mechanical or biological failure such as implant fracture or migration, synovitis from implant degradation, and osteolysis.[1] This implant-free fixation technique has superior biomechanical properties compared to other suturing methods, including interference screw type of fixation. Proposed tenodesis of the long head of the biceps (LHB) can be performed safely even in the presence of swelling during rotator cuff repair, as it is the last step of the shoulder procedure.

13.3 Indications

This technique can be used for all kinds of symptomatic pathological conditions of the LHB that require surgical resort. Tenodesis, in general, might be preferred over tenotomy for several reasons, including improved cosmetic appearance, maintenance of elbow supination and flexion strength, and maintenance of the biceps muscle length–tension relation. Further, bony fixation techniques have shown better results than soft-tissue fixation.[2]

13.4 Contraindications

This technique is not recommended for chronic ruptures of the LHB with muscle retraction. It is also not recommended in acute ruptures with short muscle-tendon stump, because biceps muscle length–tension relation cannot be controlled.

13.5 Preoperative Preparation/ Positioning

This procedure can be done in a beach-chair or in a lateral decubitus position under general anesthesia or scalene block only.

13.6 Operative Technique

- **Step 1: Standard anteroinferior portal formation.** After insertion of the scope through standard posterior portal and inspection of glenohumeral (GH) joint, the standard outside-in anteroinferior portal is made. This portal is used for later suprapectoral suture management and the LHB tenotomy.

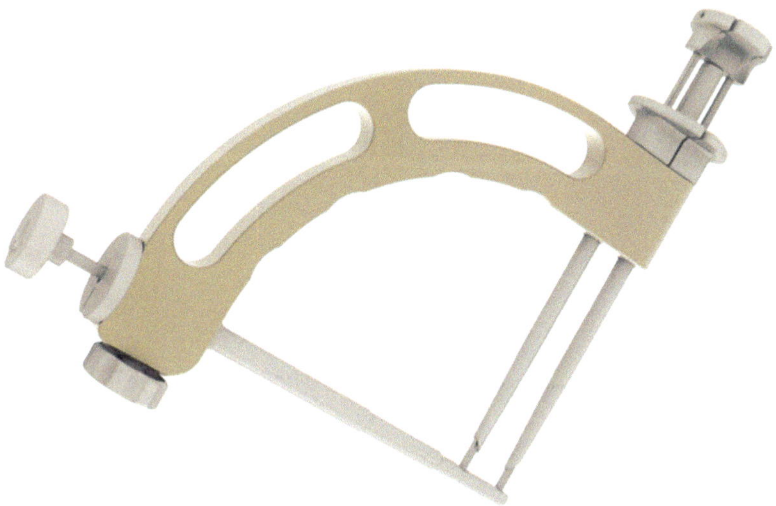

Fig. 13.1 Cobra guide.

- **Step 2: Standard lateral subacromial (SA) portal formation.** With the scope switched into the SA space, the standard lateral portal is made. This viewing portal is used for suprapectoral visualization and later knot tying.
- **Step 3: Visualization of the suprapectoral space.** With the trocar through lateral portal in the SA space, the downward shift is sited toward the superior pectoralis major insertion with the tip of trocar touching the anterolateral humeral cortical edge at the same time. Usually, there is some bursal tissue, which is removed with the electrode through the anteroinferior portal. The LHB is most frequently covered by the falciparum ligament, which is the proximal extension of the pectoralis major tendon insertion. This ligament has to be removed in order to expose the LHB.
- **Step 4: Suprapectoral portal formation.** This portal is performed with a spinal needle from outside-in, with an angle of approximately 45 degrees, against the humeral cortex toward cranial direction. Through this portal, the bony tunnel will be drilled later on.
- **Step 5: The marking stitch passage.** The marking stitch passes through the LHB at the level of the future entrance of the bony tunnel. This important step controls and prevents the final overtension of the tenodized tendon.
- **Step 6: Tenotomy of the LHB.** Classical tenotomy of the LHB at its base is done with the scope through the posterior portal inside the GH joint, and biceps scissors from the anteroinferior portal.
- **Step 7: The proximal biceps is pulled out through the suprapectoral portal.** The scope switched back to the suprapectoral space; with the grasper through the suprapectoral portal, the proximal part of the LHB is pulled out through the skin.
- **Step 8: Holding the suture passage.** The proximal part of the LHB is pulled out as much as it goes and a mosquito clamp is placed at the level of the skin to prevent slippage of the tendon back inside. A modified Kessler holding stitch is passed in order to form a distance between both strands (entry and exit) of approximately 1 cm.
- **Step 9: K-wire introduction.** The K-wire (motorized) introduced through the suprapectoral portal to the anterior humeral cortex with an angle of less than 45 degrees and pointed toward the humeral head and slightly medial. The aim is to get enough bone length to drill a 30-mm-deep bony tunnel. The entry point is at the level of the marking stitch placement.
- **Step 10: First (primary) bony tunnel drilling.** Cannulated drill over the K-wire is used to make a primary bony tunnel for the LHB (**Fig. 13.2**). The size of the drill depends on the size of the biceps tendon, but it should not be less than 6 mm. The lower part of the tunnel entrance is smoothened with the shaver blade to avoid conflict of the LHB tendon with a sharp bony edge after tenodesis.
- **Step 11: Cobra guide positioning.** The Cobra guide is introduced inside the primary bonny tunnel (**Fig. 13.3**). The depth of insertion is controlled by the scope, and it must be ensured that both holes at the end of the primary cannulated stick are inside the tunnel.
- **Step 12: Drill guides insertion.** Once the Cobra guide is placed inside the primary bony tunnel, the C-frame is rotated to the desired level to avoid axillary nerve injury. Both drill guides are then inserted through the skin incisions ("Cobra bites") to the lateral humeral cortex and tapped slightly (**Fig. 13.4**).
- **Step 13: Two parallel bony tunnels drilling.** With the drill guides in place, two parallel bony tunnels are made using 3-mm-sized drills with stoppers (**Fig. 13.5**).
- **Step 14: Insertion of the double suture loop inserter.** The double suture loop inserter is loaded with two sutures (of different colors). Then, it will be inserted through the drill guides down to the end (**Fig. 13.6**).
- **Step 15: Insertion of the locking needle and passing the suture loops (shuttles).** The locking needle is then inserted through the primary cannulated stick. The Cobra guide will be removed; finally, the two suture shuttle loops will have a common exit through the suprapectoral portal in the front and two separate exits through each of the two "Cobra bite" holes (**Fig. 13.7**).

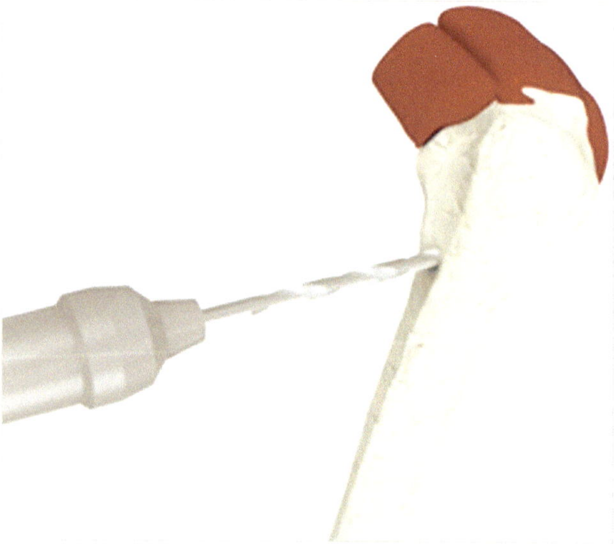

Fig. 13.2 Drilling of primary humeral tunnel. Cannulated drill over the K-wire is pointing toward humeral head and slightly medial.

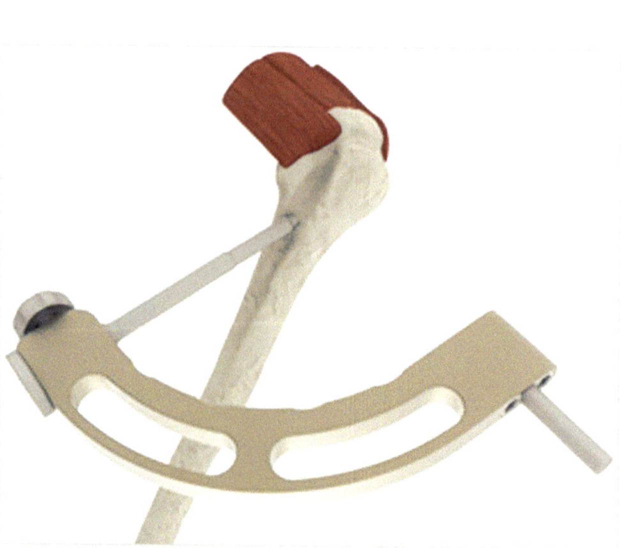

Fig. 13.3 Cobra guide positioning with the primary cannulated stick inside the primary humeral tunnel.

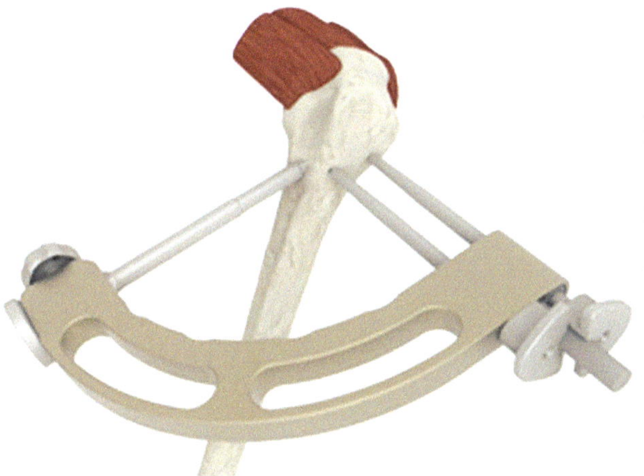

Fig. 13.4 Lateral drill guides positioning. The C-frame of Cobra guide is rotated to the desired level to avoid axillary nerve injury.

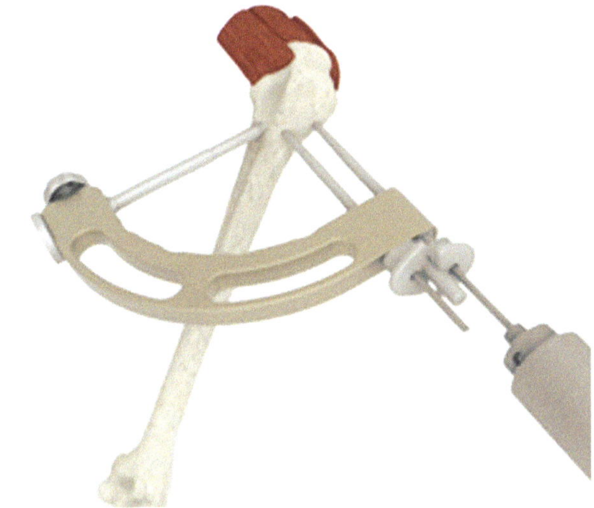

Fig. 13.5 Two lateral bony tunnels are drilled with 3-mm drills with stoppers.

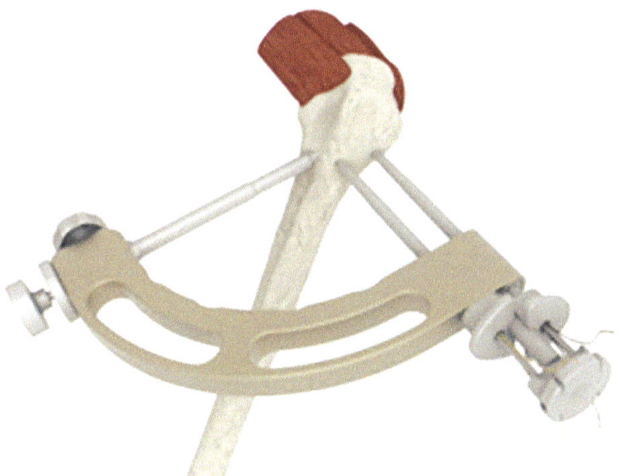

Fig. 13.6 Double suture loop inserter loaded with two sutures (#2, different colors) is inserted through lateral drill guides.

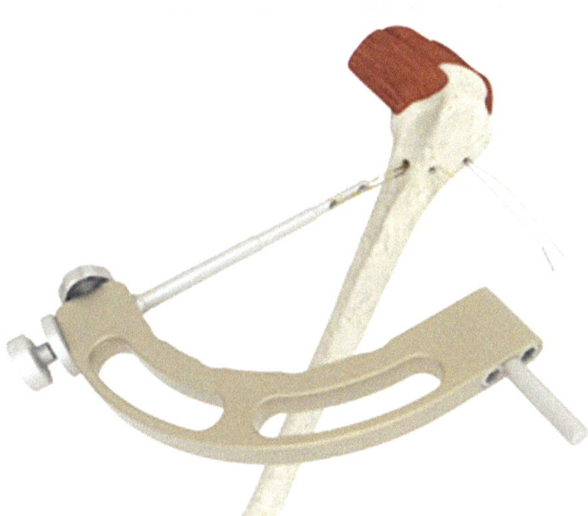

Fig. 13.7 Cobra is removed from the primary humeral tunnel and two suture loops—shuttles are passed through humerus at the right angle.

- **Step 16: Holding suture strands shuttling.** Under the scope of control through the lateral portal, each of the holding suture strands are passed through one of the shuttle loops with the suture retriever through the anteroinferior portal. Both strands are then shuttled out from the lateral "Cobra bite" incisions.
- **Step 17: Pulling the LHB inside the primary bony tunnel.** With pulling on both strands of the holding suture, the proximal part of the LHB is inserted into the primary bony tunnel up to the level of marking stitch.
- **Step 18: Final fixation with six half hitches.** Before the final knot tying, both strands should be taken out through the posterior of the two "Cobra bite" incisions. Then, six half hitches are made, the first three in the same direction and the other three in the opposite direction. Note, the scope must be in the lateral portal at all times.
- **Step 19: Removing of the marking stitch.** Finally, the scope in the lateral portal is shifted toward the suprapectoral space and pulling on the marking stitch checks biceps fixation. At the end, the marking stitch is removed and the procedure is concluded (**Fig. 13.8**).

13.7 Tips and Pearls/Expert Suggestions

Looking at the LHB outside the GH joint below the transverse ligament during the arthroscopic drive-through looks much easier than finding it under the transverse ligament. The landmarks are at the upper border of the pectoralis major tendon with its proximal extension as the falciparum ligament, which covers the LHB, and the anterolateral edge of the humeral cortex.

All steps from 1 through 8 are recommended to be done at the very beginning of the shoulder procedure, to avoid swelling of the subcutaneous tissue, which gives a hard time pulling out the proximal part of the LHB to the desired level.

In the case of marked LHB tenosynovitis inside the bicipital groove, it is recommended to open the groove and perform debridement of the inflamed tissue, to avoid persistent postoperative pain.

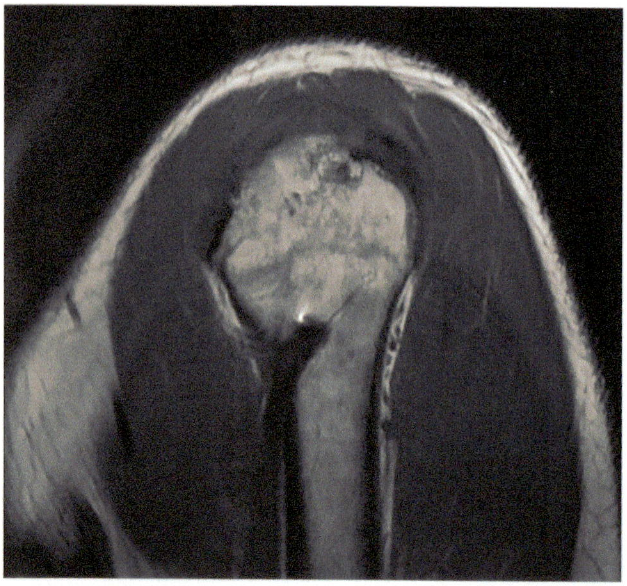

Fig. 13.8 MRI scan after an intraosseous long head of the biceps tenodesis.

13.8 What to Avoid

At the time of primary bony tunnel drilling, it is strongly recommended not to drill through the posterior humeral cortex to avoid possible axillary nerve damage.

13.9 Complications/Bailout/Salvage

In the case of a short (< 30 mm) primary humeral tunnel, only one lateral tunnel is drilled. Some of the technical steps are thus changed and the final fixation of the LHB tendon is made by using a titanium plate with two holes. Each of the holding strands are passed through each of the plate holes and six half hitches are made as described in step 18.

13.10 Postoperative Care

Special care must be taken to avoid supinating and flexing the elbow against resistance for 6 to 8 weeks. Full range of motion in the GH joint is allowed from the beginning of rehabilitation.

References

1. Park HB, Keyurapan E, Gill HS, Selhi HS, McFarland EG. Suture anchors and tacks for shoulder surgery, part II: the prevention and treatment of complications. Am J Sports Med 2006;34(1):136–144
2. Scheibel M, Schröder RJ, Chen J, Bartsch M. Arthroscopic soft tissue tenodesis versus bony fixation anchor tenodesis of the long head of the biceps tendon. Am J Sports Med 2011;39(5):1046–1052

14 Open Suprapectoral Biceps Tenodesis

Samuel A. Taylor, Jacob G. Calcei, and Matthew A. Tao

Abstract
The long head of the biceps tendon (LHBT) is a widely accepted pain generator in the shoulder, both in isolation and concomitantly with other pathologies. Recent paradigm shifts suggest a more intimate and interdependent relationship between the LHBT and the labrum, together making the biceps-labrum complex (BLC). The BLC can be broken down into three clinically relevant zones: inside (the biceps anchor and the superior labrum), junction (intra-articular segment of LHBT and the stabilizing biceps pulley at the articular margin), and bicipital tunnel. There are a number of techniques to address pathology of the BLC, both arthroscopic and open. This chapter presents a technique for open suprapectoral biceps tenodesis that effectively addresses pathologic lesions occurring inside and junction zones and within zones 1 and 2 of the bicipital tunnel. We will briefly discuss the preoperative evaluation of patients with shoulder pain and suspected BLC pathology, followed by the surgical decision-making and technique along with pearls and pitfalls of the procedure. Finally, we will outline a postoperative rehabilitation protocol to optimize outcomes and minimize postoperative complications.

Keywords: *biceps-labrum complex, long head of the biceps tendon, tenodesis, suprapectoral, bicipital tunnel*

14.1 Introduction

The long head of the biceps tendon (LHBT) is a widely accepted pain generator in the shoulder, both in isolation and concomitantly with other pathology. Historically, the LHBT and the labrum were thought of as two separate entities. However, recent paradigm shifts suggest a more intimate and interdependent relationship between the two structures, more frequently referred to as the biceps-labrum complex (BLC) today. The extra-articular segment of the LHBT is enclosed in a fibro-osseous structure known as the bicipital tunnel,[1] which can serve as a location of possible hidden lesions related to biceps tendonitis and resultant shoulder pain.[2]

The BLC can be broken down into three clinically relevant zones: inside, junction, and bicipital tunnel. "Inside" includes the biceps anchor and the superior labrum. "Junction" includes the majority of the intra-articular segment of LHBT and the stabilizing biceps pulley at the articular margin. The "bicipital tunnel" may be broken down further into three specific zones. Zone 1 represents what is traditionally considered the bicipital groove, extending from the articular margin to the distal margin of the subscapularis tendon. Zone 2, deemed "no man's land" because of its relative invisibility to standard diagnostic arthroscopy above, extends from the distal margin of the subscapularis tendon to the proximal margin of the pectoralis major tendon. Zone 3 consists of the subpectoralis region.

A large portion of the extra-articular LHBT that resides in the bicipital tunnel is not visualized during diagnostic arthroscopy. In their cadaveric study, Taylor et al found that 55% of the LHBT relative to the proximal margin of the pectoralis major insertion was not visualized by standard diagnostic glenohumeral arthroscopy.[2] Further, in the clinical portion of the same study, diagnostic arthroscopy failed to identify extra-articular bicipital tunnel lesions in 47% of chronically symptomatic patients.[2]

There are a number of techniques to address pathology of the BLC, both arthroscopic and open. Here, we present a technique for open suprapectoral biceps tenodesis that effectively addresses pathologic lesions occurring inside and junction zones and within zones 1 and 2 of the bicipital tunnel. We will briefly discuss the preoperative evaluation of patients with shoulder pain and suspected BLC pathology, followed by the surgical decision-making and technique along with pearls and pitfalls of the procedure. Finally, we will discuss a postoperative rehabilitation protocol to optimize outcomes and minimize postoperative complications.

14.2 Preoperative Evaluation

A thorough history and physical examination are imperative to arrive at an accurate diagnosis when BLC pathology is suspected, especially given the high prevalence of hidden extra-articular bicipital tunnel disease. Patients with BLC pathology will complain of shoulder pain, which is often dull and aching in nature. While predominately activity related, some may describe night pain especially in the setting of concomitant rotator cuff tear. During repetitive overhead motion such as throwing, patients with BLC pathology may complain of snapping or subluxation of the biceps tendon in and out of the groove, which they can misinterpret as shoulder instability. A careful, directed history and physical examination are important to parse this out; additionally, they will often have point tenderness along the bicipital tunnel.

Taylor et al described the "3-pack" examination: a trio of physical examination maneuvers that can be used to screen for BLC pathology.[3] The 3-pack has a high sensitivity and negative predictive value (NPV) and is therefore a good screening tool for BLC pathology. The first of the three tests is the bicipital tunnel palpation test, where the examiner manually palpates the LHBT along its extra-articular course while the arm is passively internally and externally rotated to localize pain to the LHBT tunnel. Next is the active compression test (O'Brien sign) in which the examiner places a downward-directed force onto the patient's arm that is held forward flexed at 90 degrees, adducted 10 to 15 degrees, and internally rotated such that the thumb points downward. The examination is then repeated with the palm facing upward. The test is positive when the patient has a reproduction of their clinical pain described as inside the shoulder with the thumb down and the pain is reduced with the palm up. The final test of the 3-pack is the throwing test where the examiner provides isometric resistance to the patient's arm as it is in the late-cocking position of the throwing motion: shoulder abducted to 90 degrees, elbow flexed at 90 degrees with maximal external rotation. The authors found the O'Brien sign and bicipital tunnel palpation to have sensitivities of 95.7 and 97.8% with NPVs of 92.6 and 96.4%, respectively, for bicipital tunnel disease.[3] Put another way, if these two tests were positive, one must have a high index of suspicion for bicipital tunnel

15 Open Subpectoral Biceps Tenodesis

Brian R. Waterman and Anthony A. Romeo

Abstract
Biceps-labral complex pathology is a common source of shoulder disability, particularly among overhead athletes and other active patient groups. With continued bicipital groove pain and failure of nonsurgical treatment measures such as physical therapy, oral medication, and corticosteroid injections, arthroscopic evaluation with biceps tenodesis may be considered. Contrary to other techniques, open subpectoral biceps tenodesis offers more consistent restoration of native length-tension relationship, stable fixation, and low risk of residual biceps groove pain or reoperation. After proximal biceps tendon release, a subpectoral incision may be performed in the axillary folds. After retraction of the pectoralis major tendon and conjoint tendon, the proximal biceps tendon is identified and delivered into the field. The proximal biceps tendon is repaired and stable interference screw fixation is achieved.

Keywords: *proximal, long head of the biceps tendon, tenodesis, tenosynovitis, superior labrum, SLAP*

15.1 Goals of Procedure

To effectively treat symptomatic pathology of the biceps-labral complex.

15.2 Advantages

Open subpectoral biceps tenodesis allows reproducible restoration of the native length-tension relationship of the proximal biceps tendon, while limiting perioperative complications and reoperation due to persistent biceps groove pain. Additionally, interference screw fixation affords strong biomechanical fixation in stronger cortical bone.

15.3 Indications

- Type II-IV superior labral anterior-posterior tears, proximal bicpital tendonopathy or symptomatic rupture, instability of the long of the biceps with a rotator cuff tear or biceps sling injury.
- Failed SLAP repair; persistently symptomatic intra-articular, subacromial, or suprapectoral biceps teondesis or prior tenotomy.

15.4 Contraindications

Asymptomatic, elderly, or low demand patient.

15.5 Preoperative Preparation/ Positioning

Open subpectoral biceps tenodesis can be capably performed from the beach chair or lateral decubitus position, and it is typically performed at the conclusion of other intra-articular or subacromial procedures. With beach chair positioning, the head of the bed is lowered to approximately 30 degrees with two operative lights projecting onto the field from the foot of the bed and between the operative extremity and a surgical assistant positioned at the head of the bed. The operative extremity is detached from any arm positioning device and placed on a padded Mayo stand in relative forward flexion, abduction, and external rotation of the shoulder and slight flexion of the elbow. If the patient is in a lateral decubitus position, the operative extremity is removed from the traction setup, and the beanbag is deflated. With assistance from your anesthesia provider and circulating nurse, the draw sheet is then simultaneous pulled from the opposite side of the bed while the operative team slides the patient over to center the patient on the operative bed in a supine position. As with a beach chair position, a similar setup is then arranged.

15.5.1 Operative Technique

The inferior rolled border of the pectoralis major is identified and demarcated at its attachment site on the lateral lip of the intertubercular groove. A 2- to 3-cm incision is marked in parallel with Langers lines near the axillary fold, allowing it to be relatively concealed upon wound healing (**Fig. 15.1**). After comprehensive arthroscopic evaluation and intra-articular biceps tenotomy, the planned surgical site is anesthetized using 1% lidocaine with epinephrine from proximal to distal, as standard interscalene block often spares this region. The skin is then incised starting approximately 1 cm proximal to the inferior pectoralis margin, and cutaneous bleeding vessels are cauterized with a needle point bovie. Metzenbaum scissors are utilized for sharp dissection to the overlying pectoral fascia, and the horizontal fibers of the pectoralis major are visualized. After longitudinal division of this investing fascia, gentle blunt finger dissection may be utilized to confirm the presence and location of the long head of the biceps within the intertubercular groove. To afford visualization of the biceps tendon, a

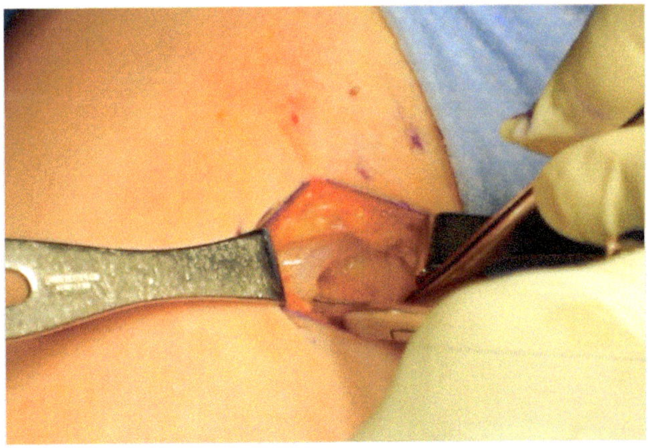

Fig. 15.1 Surgical incision with exposed overlying fascia.

small pointed Homan retractor may be placed laterally over the lateral pectoralis major footprint and a blunt Chandler retractor is placed medially and held by an assistant **(Fig. 15.2)**. The operative surgeon utilizes the deep end of an Army Navy retractor at the apex of the incision under the rolled inferior pectoralis major musculature, and the long head of the biceps is again identified. Occasionally, the bicipital sheath may need to be divided to allow mobilization of the tendon with a right-angled clamp (or gloved finger) mobilizing underneath the tendon from medial to lateral. With gentle anterior directed traction, the proximal biceps stump is delivered into the wound and clamped with an Allis clamp. A #2 high tensile non-absorbable looped suture (Fiberloop, Arthrex, Inc; Naples, FL) is utilized to prepare approximately 15-20 mm of tendon proximal to the visualized myotendinoous junction **(Fig. 15.3)**. The tendon is then sized circumferentially, amputated while leaving a small residual stump, and the interlocking sutures are clamped with a hemostat to the forearm bandage **(Fig. 15.4)**.

The retractors are then repositioned to allow optimal visualization of the intertubercular groove and periosteal tissue is cleared with a bovie electrocautery or key elevator **(Fig. 15.5)**. Greater cephalad retraction is applied to allow for proximal guidepin placement in order to restore the native length-tension relationship of the long head of the biceps, with the myotendinous junction reapproximated at the level of the inferior border of the pectoralis major **(Fig. 15.6)**. A unicortical guidepin is then drilled centrally within the intertubercular groove and directed posterior at the equator of the humerus, The cannulated reamer, typically an 8 mm size, is then reamed over the guidepin on power, with care to stay central and unicortical, and then the reamer is removed by hand to prevent unnecessary aperture widening **(Fig. 15.7)**. An appropriately-sized tap is routinely used, and the bony and periosteal debris are irrigated and debrided from the socket. A polyethylethylketone (PEEK) interference screw sized for line-to-line fit (e.g., 8 × 12 mm in length, headless PEEK screw) is then opened and assembled on the biotenodesis screwdriver. At this time, the #2 sutures are threaded into the central core of the screwdriver with use of a looped nitinol wire and clamped under tension. The unsutured stump is directed into the socket and the tenodesis driver is inserted and carefully advanced under direct visualization until flush with the surrounding cortical bone. The tenodesis driver is then removed, and direct palpation confirms that the screw is not proud and the myotendinous junction is at the level of the inferior pectoralis margin. the suture limbs are then tied with alternating half hitches and cut short, followed by removal of retractors **(Fig. 15.8)**.

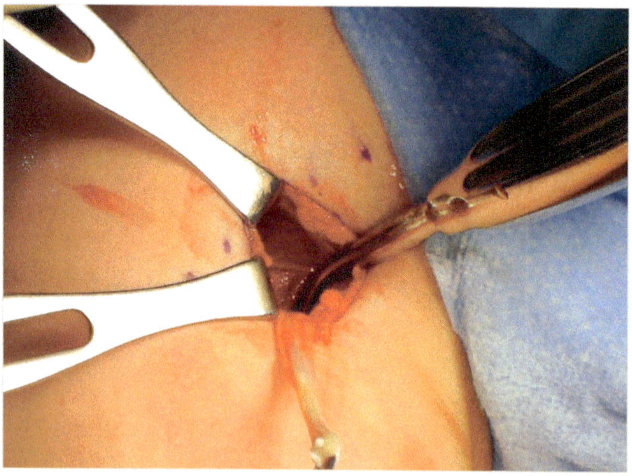

Fig. 15.2 Exposed bicipital tendon stump delivered from the intertubercular groove with retractors in place.

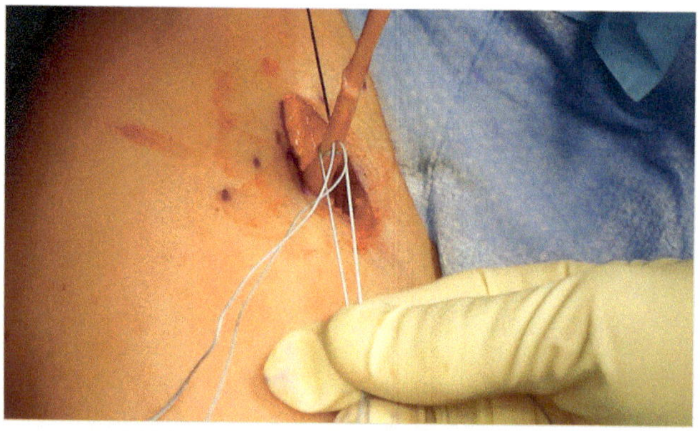

Fig. 15.3 Suture reparation of the long head of the biceps tendon.

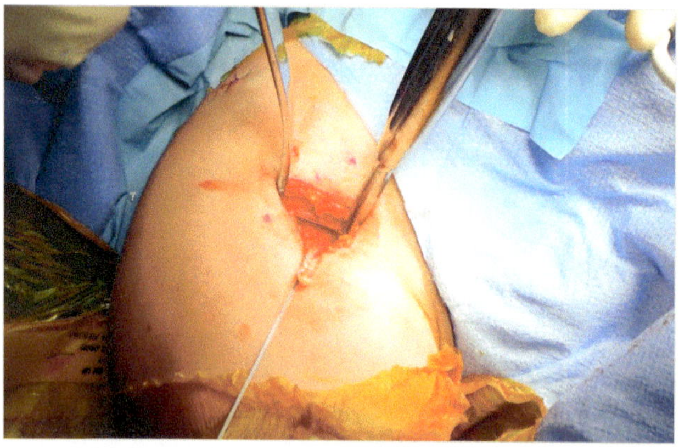

Fig. 15.4 Final preparation of the bicipital tendon with tenodesis site exposure.

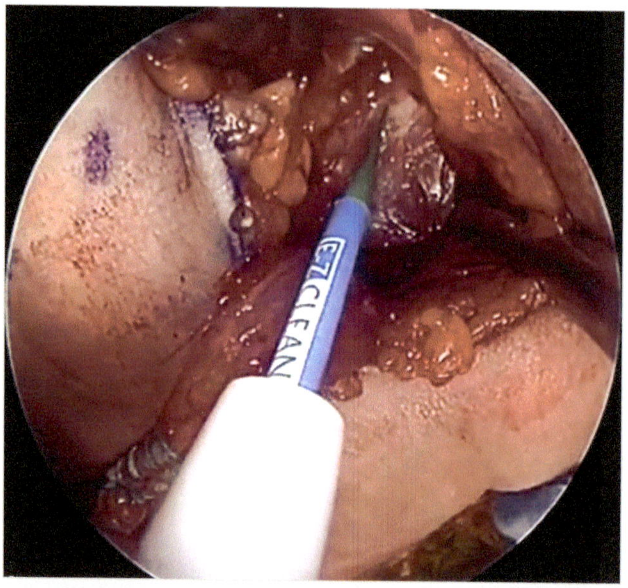

Fig. 15.5 Electrocautery preparation of the planned drilling site in the proximal intertubercular groove.

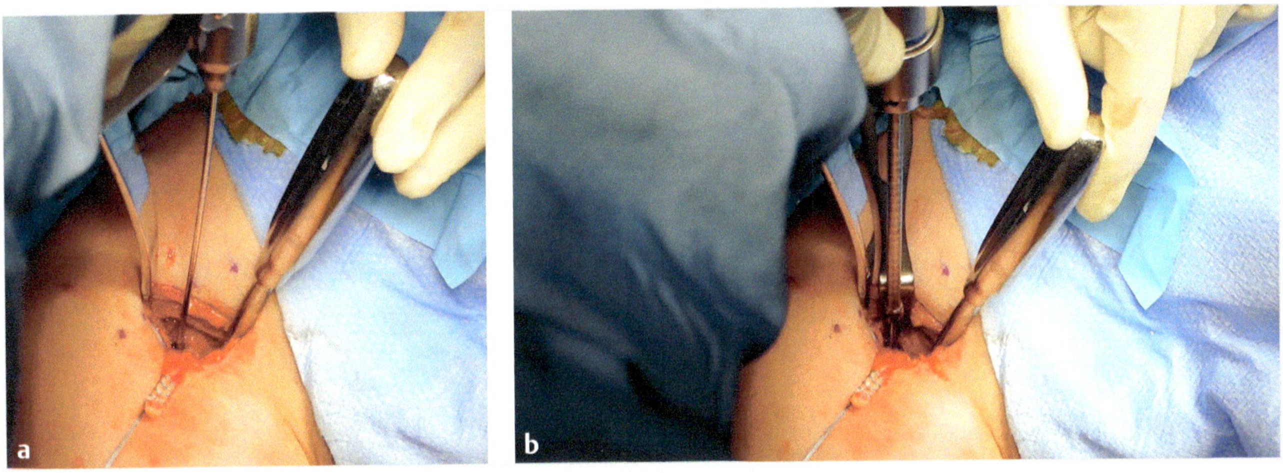

Fig. 15.6 (a) Guidepin placement and (b) cannulated reaming for subsequent screw placement.

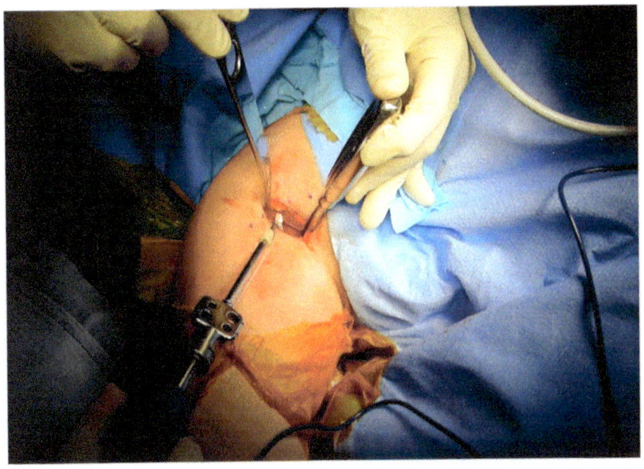

Fig. 15.7 Aperture fixation of the proximal biceps tendon using a tenodesis screw.

The wound is copiously irrigated and optional platelet rich plasma is applied at the tenodesis site. The dermal layer is reapproximated with 3-0 monocryl suture in deep interrupted fashion. Superficial subcuticular closure is performed with a 4-0 monocryl suture and reinforced with cyanoacrylate tissue adhesive. Adhesive strips may be used to hold tension on the subcuticular sutures, and a gauze dressing is applied.

15.6 Tips and Pearls/Expert Suggestions

- Reorient the patient to a supine or semi-extended position to maximize visualization and limit the effects of gravity.
- Use a strip of iodine-impregnated adhesive intraoperatively and perform water-tight closure with tissue adhesive to avoid contamination from axillary region.
- Ensure the myotendinous junction is approximated at the inferior margin of the pectoralis major to ensure restoration of the native length-tension relationship and normal bicipital contour.

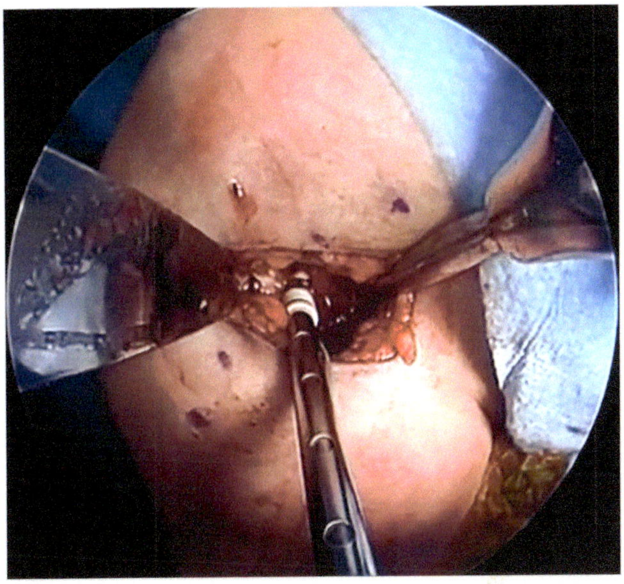

Fig. 15.8 Final fixation for the long head proximal biceps tenodesis.

- Careful 270° retractor placement can ensure direct visualization to facilitate accurate guidepin placement, reaming, and screw placement.

15.7 What to Avoid

- Avoid reapproximation of the proximal biceps tendon under excessive or insufficient tension. Insufficient tension may result in greater cosmetic deformity (i.e., Popeye deformity) and cramping, whereas excessive tension may result in increased bicipital pain.
- Limit aggressive soft tissue manipulation or sharp retractor placement to avoid iatrogenic neurovascular injury, particularly medially.
- Limit eccentric or oblique guidepin placement or reaming to prevent adjacent soft tissue injury, cortical wall blowout, or secondary humeral shaft fracture.

- Do not bridge the myotendinous junction with suture preparation of the long head of the biceps to avoid suture pullout and tenodesis failure.
- Avoid prominent tenodesis screw placement or overinsertion into the humeral canal.

15.8 Complications/Bailout/Salvage

- With eccentric reaming or compromised interference screw fixation, alternative fixation constructs may be utilized, including a cortical button, suture anchor, transosseous sutures, or bone tunnels.
- With distal tendon retraction or failed biceps tenodesis or tenotomy, the elbow may be flexed and muscle belly may be "milked" to deliver the biceps into the surgical field. Alternatively, a more extensile incision may be utilized to identify the tendon stump and dissect from any surrounding adhesions.
- With altered anatomy or excessive arthroscopic fluid extravasation, aggressive blind digital dissection or traction can lead to iatrogenic neurovascular injury. With obscured anatomy, the tendon should be directly visualized in the bicipital groove or the tendon can be traced to its myotendinous junction before traction is applied.

15.9 Postoperative Care

Without precautions related to other concomitant procedures, sling immobilization is maintained for 4 weeks postoperatively with anti-edema measures. Passive range of motion of the shoulder, elbow, and wrist may be initiated immediately and progressed to active assisted and active range of motion. Resisted elbow flexion and forearm supination and/or strengthening should be avoided for the first 6 weeks, but light isometric exercises of the rotator cuff, deltoid and periscapular musculature may begin in the second month. After full range of motion is achieved, plyometrics, closed chain, and eccentric resisted exercises are initiated at 3 months followed by more advanced conditioning and sports-specific rehabilitation, including return throwing. Collision athletics and all other activities may be resumed by 6 months.

16 Arthroscopic Biceps Transfer

Helen S. Zitkovsky, Samuel A. Taylor, and Stephen J. O'Brien

Abstract
Biceps labral complex (BLC) disease is common and can exist as isolated pathologies or concomitantly with other shoulder pathologies. Physical examination is critical to selecting the most appropriate intervention. Biceps tendon transfer to the conjoint tendon is a safe and reproducible technique that is performed arthroscopically and addresses both intra- and extra-articular BLC disease without the need for bony anchors.

Keywords: *biceps tendinitis, bicipital tunnel, biceps transfer, biceps chondromalacia, biceps tenodesis*

Arthroscopic subdeltoid biceps transfer is a soft-tissue biceps tenodesis procedure popularized by the senior author (S. J. O.) to address some of the inadequacies of both biceps tenotomy and various bony bicep tenodesis for refractory biceps tendinitis, both in isolation and in association with biceps-labral complex disorders.

Kelly et al[1] showed that although biceps tenotomy was very successful in patients older than 60 years, the cramping and cosmetic deformity noted in younger, more active patients was problematic.

Many papers have chronicled problems with biceps tenodesis, with anywhere from 10 to 20% of patients having daily pain, both with activity and rest.[2,3] In addition, we have seen some severe cases of reflex sympathetic dystrophy that have also occurred secondary to the chronic pain from proximal biceps tenodesis (Stephen J. O'Brien, personal communication).

Open subpectoral biceps tenodesis has had issues with neurovascular injuries, infection, and bony fractures.[4–7] In addition, any tenodesis to a bone construct will heal with significant scar at the bony tenodesis site.[8]

With the biceps transfer technique, the long head of the biceps tendon (LHBT) is released in the glenohumeral joint, and then transferred arthroscopically in the subdeltoid space to the conjoint tendon (NOT the coracoid process). The senior author has completed approximately 1,000 biceps transfers to date. The short- and medium-term outcomes have been published.[9,10]

There has been only one intraoperative complication, an important case to learn from, involving damage to both a branch of the axillary artery (the anterior humeral circumflex) and the median nerve, in a patient having had three prior shoulder surgeries (one complicated by a pulmonary embolus) with encasing scar surrounding anomalous anatomy of the brachial plexus and conjoint tendon not previously described (now seen twice since). This will be discussed, with the lessons learned. Although figures are provided here along with a highlight video, the entire procedure, unedited and edited, can be viewed on VuMedi.

16.1 Surgical Technique

16.1.1 Setup and Anesthesia Technique

The patient is placed in the beach-chair position (**Fig. 16.1a**), and after appropriate sedation, an interscalene block is administered to the patient with local anesthetic and steroids to help give a long-lasting block. A laryngeal mask airway is also placed by the anesthesiologist to protect the patient's airway and to allow for deepening of the anesthesia plane when going outside the block in the subdeltoid space. If this deepening does not occur, the pressure of the fluid in the subdeltoid space can stimulate the patient. This may result in increased blood pressure and subsequent bleeding, or movement of the patient as this may lighten the anesthetic plane. The blood pressure is monitored to keep the systolic blood pressure less than 110 mm Hg to control bleeding in the subdeltoid space. Although a fluid pump can be employed, the senior author prefers gravity flow (**Fig. 16.1b**).

This procedure can also be done in the lateral decubitus position for physicians who prefer this for their arthroscopic shoulder procedures.

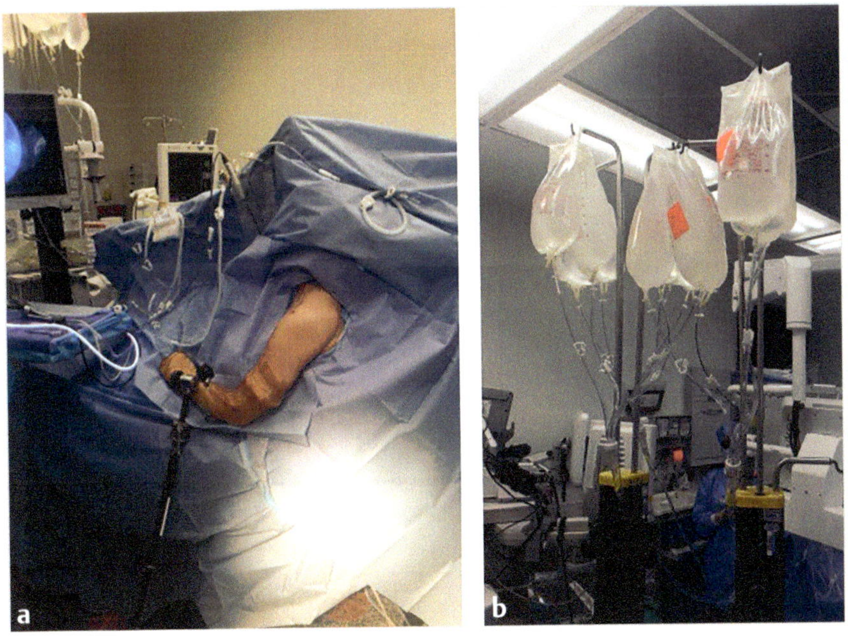

Fig. 16.1 (a) Patient in the beach-chair position with a laryngeal mask airway. (b) Gravity flow setup.

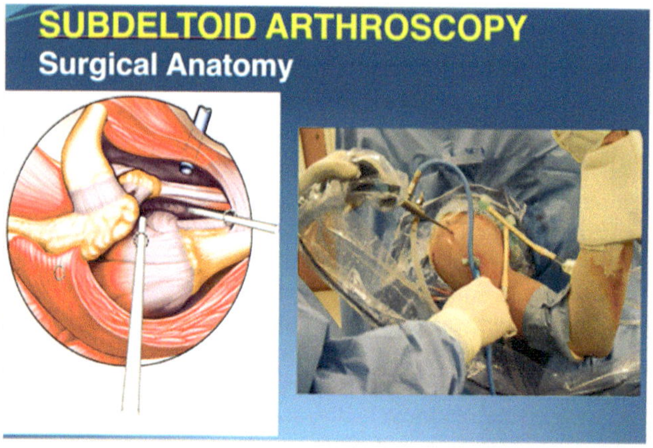

Fig. 16.8 (S) Superolateral viewing portal. (P) Pectorals working portal. (C) Conjoint portal for suture tying.

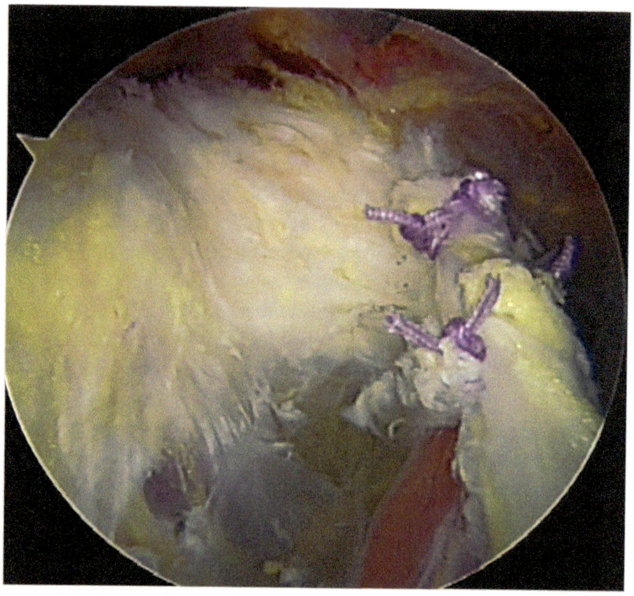

Fig. 16.9 Room with a view.

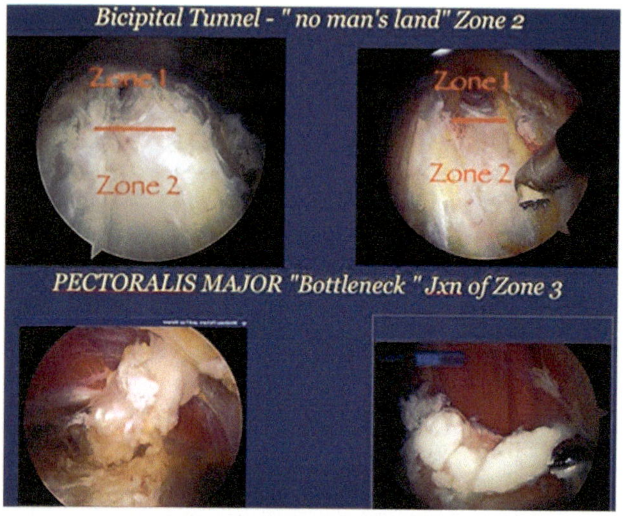

Fig. 16.10 Bicipital tunnel with zones 1, 2, and 3.

- The floor of the bicipital tunnel is the bony humerus in which you have the traditional bony bicipital groove in the proximal one-third of the bicipital tunnel, and a more flattened humerus in the second third of the bicipital tunnel to the pectoralis major tendon, which we have called "no man's land," as it becomes a graveyard for loose bodies, significant scarring, and synovitis in the bicipital tunnel above the pectoralis major tendon bottleneck (**Fig. 16.11**).
- The biceps is then delivered from zone 2 into zone 3 through an aperture created just above the pectoralis major in the bicipital hood. The LHBT is then brought out through the "PecPortal," and two Thompson stitches are used to "tag" the LHBT for passage in the subdeltoid space and tensioning the transferred LHBT.

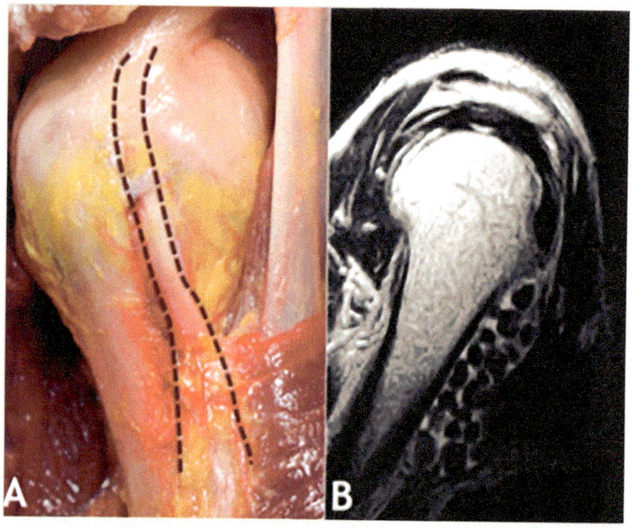

Fig. 16.11 Surgical pictures **(a)** and MRI **(b)** showing loose bodies above pectoralis major on "bottleneck."

16.1.4 Transfer of the Long Head of the Biceps Tendon

- A superior tensioning portal is then placed via spinal needle localization in line with the conjoint tendon, and the LHBT is passed through the subdeltoid space and tensioned (**Video 16.3**). We have been tensioning the LHBT by mildly "bowstringing" the LHBT and then passing sutures between the LHBT and the conjoint tendon. A "log rolling" stitch is used to place the LHBT "over" the conjoint tendon. The most inferior sutures are placed first to "lock in" the tension (or reduction), and then three to four sutures are placed distal to proximal with appropriate spacing (at 1 cm; **Video 16.4**).
- The extra tendon length above the most proximal stitch is then released and delivered out of the body via the superior portal.
- All in all, there are three extra portals are currently used for the subdeltoid part of this procedure, and these are all closed with at least two sutures per portal, and occasional deltoid fascia closure sutures to avoid "buttonholes" or inverted portals. All portals other than the first posterior glenohumeral portal are placed after spinal needle localization, and blunt passage of the cannulas to avoid damage

to any neurovascular structures. Care is also taken to only pierce the skin with the scalpel, again to avoid any damage to neurovascular structures.

16.2 Tips, Potential Pitfalls, and Anomalous Anatomy

A good way to begin becoming a subdeltoid shoulder surgeon, besides reading this chapter and viewing the videos here and on VuMedi, would be to visit us at the Hospital for Special Surgery. In addition, you may want to gradually advance your dissection arthroscopically into the subdeltoid space on subacromial procedures. Study the anatomy of the subdeltoid space. Know where the acromial branch of the thoracoacromial artery will be. Know where the ascending branch of the anterior humeral circumflex artery is, including its two veins crossing the inferior border of the subscapularis ("three sisters"; **Fig. 16.12**).

The anatomy of the musculocutaneous nerve and its variability should be known. Knowledge of the presence of the cephalic vein in the "ceiling" of this space is warranted, underlining the need for spinal needle localization for any portals, blunt trocars and cannula, and using the scalpel to only penetrate the skin. We have had two cases where the cephalic vein was injured, requiring a cut down and division of the cephalic vein with suture ligation of the divided ends.

Care should be taken to maintaining a "steady state" of inflow and outflow to avoid excessive swelling of the shoulder. We have had no complications from the saline in the chest, although from the beginning, we set an arbitrary limit of 2 hours with any subdeltoid surgery. During the learning curve with this procedure, concerns were expressed at times by anesthesia about the swelling in the chest on the involved side.

However, there has never been a problem to date in ventilating any patient. In addition, expect the patient to have discomfort in the recovery room for approximately 1 to 1.5 hours from the fluid in their breast. It is important to notify the patient, family, recovery room staff, and the anesthesiologist.

Care should be taken in creating the aperture to deliver the LHBT from the bicipital tunnel from the lateral side. The bicipital hood has tremendous variability in its thickness, but it is quite easy to get into the LHBT and damage it. By far the most important tip and warning would be to clearly identify the coracoid process. We have seen three cases of anomalous anatomy where the conjoint tendon was above the deltoid fascia, and easily confused with the deltoid muscle (**Fig. 16.13**). The first

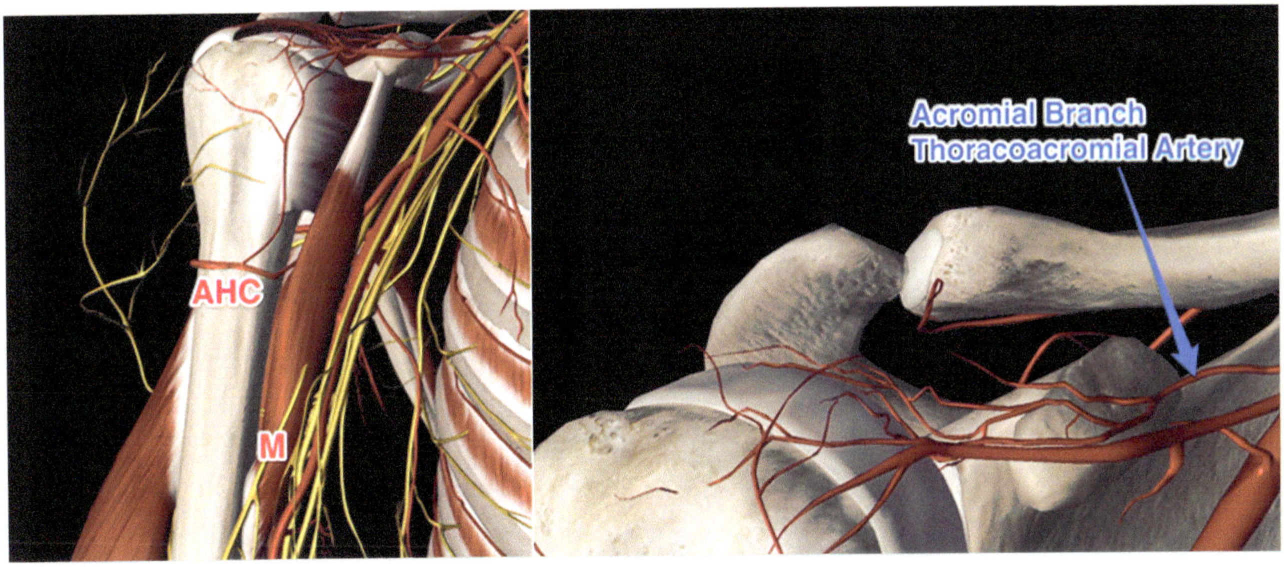

Fig. 16.12 Anterior humeral circumflex (AHC), median nerve (M), and acromial branch of the thoracoacromial artery.

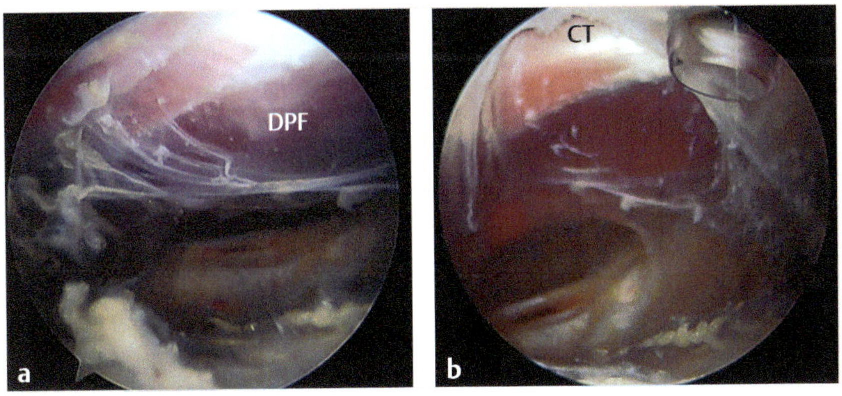

Fig. 16.13 Anatomical variant. The coracoid and conjoint tendon (CT) is above the deltopectoral fascia (DPF) leaving the "white" structures as the axillary arteries and the brachial plexus. Care must be taken to palpate the coracoid first before further exploration.

of these three cases resulted in damage to the anterior humeral circumflex artery and median nerve. The patient had had three previous shoulder surgeries with significant scar encasing the subdeltoid space. After fighting through the scar, the "white structure" we encountered in the place where the conjoint tendon had been in all previous cases, a structure identical in appearance to the conjoint tendon that turned out to be the axillary artery and brachial plexus. We had done so many of these previously; we had previously abandoned the extra step of identifying the coracoid process first. That we now know could have avoided this complication, but we had no suspicion or knowledge of this anomalous anatomy. In addition, in the two subsequent cases, we noted clearly the axillary artery, but went ahead to identify the coracoid process, and released the fascial envelopes to identify the conjoint tendon.

Please know that with the fluid pressure running in the subdeltoid space, you will only see the arterial pulsations if the fluid pressure is let down (**Video 16.5**). Do not rely on your naked eye. You are not likely to see any pulsations.

16.3 Postoperative Care

The patients are discharged home after recovery room criteria are satisfied as outpatient surgery. The sling is discontinued after all sensation and motor function is restored.

This is done on postoperative day 1. Patients are instructed in postoperative range-of-motion exercises to start day 1 in the supine position only when going overhead. Any range of motion with the arm at the side is allowed.

The patients are restricted from any pushing or pulling for 6 weeks, which we presume is the time for adequate healing. Up until recently, we have had very few injuries (less than 1%) in the first 6 weeks, but in the last 2 years, we had two college football players injure the tendon at 3 months, but both were taking "supplements" from the start postoperatively. We have since cautioned our patients against these supplements for the first 6 months postoperatively. Less than half of the patients have required early physical therapy, restoring their normal motion on their own (**Video 16.6**), and then we start formal physical therapy at 4 to 6 weeks postoperatively. Return to overhead throwing has been at 3 to 4 months.

References

1. Kelly AM, Drakos MC, Fealy S, Taylor SA, O'Brien SJ. Arthroscopic release of the long head of the biceps tendon: functional outcome and clinical results. Am J Sports Med 2005;33(2):208–213
2. Dines D, Warren RF, Inglis AE. Surgical treatment of lesions of the long head of the biceps. Clin Orthop Relat Res 1982(164):165–171
3. Becker DA, Cofield RH. Tenodesis of the long head of the biceps brachii for chronic bicipital tendinitis. Long-term results. J Bone Joint Surg Am 1989;71(3):376–381
4. Dein EJ, Huri G, Gordon JC, McFarland EG. A humerus fracture in a baseball pitcher after biceps tenodesis. Am J Sports Med 2014;42(4):877–879
5. Rhee PC, Spinner RJ, Bishop AT, Shin AY. Iatrogenic brachial plexus injuries associated with open subpectoral biceps tenodesis: a report of 4 cases. Am J Sports Med 2013;41(9):2048–2053
6. Dickens JF, Kilcoyne KG, Tintle SM, Giuliani J, Schaefer RA, Rue JP. Subpectoral biceps tenodesis: an anatomic study and evaluation of at-risk structures. Am J Sports Med 2012;40(10):2337–2341
7. Nho SJ, Reiff SN, Verma NN, Slabaugh MA, Mazzocca AD, Romeo AA. Complications associated with subpectoral biceps tenodesis: low rates of incidence following surgery. J Shoulder Elbow Surg 2010;19(5):764–768
8. Urch E, Taylor SA, Ramkumar PN, et al. Biceps tenodesis: a comparison of tendon-to-bone and tendon-to-tendon healing in a rat model. Am J Orthop 2017;46(6):E388–E395
9. Drakos MC, Verma NN, Gulotta LV, et al. Arthroscopic transfer of the long head of the biceps tendon: functional outcome and clinical results. Arthroscopy 2008;24(2):217–223
10. Taylor SA, Fabricant PD, Baret NJ, et al. Midterm clinical outcomes for arthroscopic subdeltoid transfer of the long head of the biceps tendon to the conjoint tendon. Arthroscopy 2014;30(12):1574–1581
11. Taylor SA, Khair MM, Gulotta LV, et al. Diagnostic glenohumeral arthroscopy fails to fully evaluate the biceps-labral complex. Arthroscopy 2015;31(2):215–224
12. Taylor SA, Fabricant PD, Bansal M, et al. The anatomy and histology of the bicipital tunnel of the shoulder. J Shoulder Elbow Surg 2015;24(4):511–519

17 SLAP Repair

Dean N. Papaliodis, Curtis A. Bush, and John E. Conway

Abstract

Superior labrum tears, SLAP lesions, and biceps tendon-superior labral complex injuries are among the most common injuries associated with shoulder pain and dysfunction. Numerous theories have been proposed for both overhead athletes as well as the general population. In throwing athletes, the treatment and pathogenesis remains controversial, and the structural changes encountered may be purposeful and adaptive. In the general population, pathogenesis has been related typically to degenerative processes with associated arthritis, rotator cuff disease and age. This chapter addresses the senior author (JEC)'s treatment approach and surgical indications in addressing SLAP tears as well as the preferred technique in performing surgical repair.

Keywords: *SLAP repair, superior labral complex injury, throwing athlete*

17.1 Introduction

Superior labrum tears, SLAP (superior labral tear from anterior to posterior) lesions, and biceps tendon–superior labral complex injuries are among the most common structural derangements, correctly and incorrectly associated with shoulder pain and dysfunction, especially in the thrower's shoulder. Numerous theories regarding the etiology of these superior labral lesions have been proposed, and they vary for the general population, nonoverhead athletes, and overhead athletes. For the thrower, the pathogenesis of biceps tendon–superior labral complex pathology remains both controversial and multifactorial, but in many cases, mobilization of the superior labrum may be either purposeful and adaptive, or pathologic and destabilizing. In the general population, pathogenesis is typically degenerative and has been related to rotator cuff disease, arthritis, and increased age.

The nonoperative treatment of SLAP lesions is now, or should now be, the mainstay of treatment, particularly in throwers, and has shown some success.[1] Even with initial failure of nonoperative treatment, Fedoriw et al demonstrated reasonable success with a second course of physical therapy specifically designed to address concomitant pathology such as kinetic chain disorders, glenohumeral motion deficits, scapular dyskinesia, and posterior capsular contracture.[2] The surgical treatment of SLAP lesions, whether by debridement, repair, or biceps tenotomy/tenodesis, has overall been successful in selected general population patients, but results of surgery are far less favorable in overhead athletes. Traumatic SLAP tears represent a subset in which surgery may be indicated when symptomatic. In the older degenerative population, surgical SLAP repairs have yielded worse results with increased revision rates.[3]

Initial emphasis for the majority of SLAP tears should be placed on conservative treatment, namely rest and physical therapy for this condition. Subacromial and biceps tunnel injections of anesthetic/steroid serve both therapeutic and diagnostic roles and may be of significant help in determining if the SLAP tear is indeed a pain generator. Failed nonoperative treatment may warrant surgical intervention; however, success may be largely influenced by factors independent of the quality of surgical repair, such as age, associated pathology, competitive level, and position in sport. For instance, Fedoriw et al showed that higher level pitchers return to play and at a higher level than lower level pitchers, regardless of whether they undergo nonoperative or operative treatment.[2]

Prior to the recognition of superior labral lesions as potential contributors to shoulder dysfunction in a thrower, these lesions were treated either nonoperatively or with debridement alone. After this lesion was further defined and classified, numerous repair methods were described. Unfortunately, the overall success with surgical treatment of SLAP lesion has been less than satisfactory in throwers. In the nonthrowing general population, the surgical treatment of degenerative SLAP lesions has also gained considerable attention and repair is no longer recommended in patients older than 40 years. In that setting, debridement or biceps tenotomy/tenodesis provides a more predictable and successful outcome.

17.2 Goals

The goal of treatment is to improve pain and function in all subsets of patients. In nonthrowers, in the event of a symptomatic traumatic SLAP tear, restoration of anatomy is the surgical goal. In throwers, SLAP tears may contribute to decreasing velocity and performance in conjunction with other shoulder pathology. The goal of treatment in throwers is to first restore the overhead athlete's shoulder function and return the athlete to play at his or her previous level without the need for surgery. When that fails, the surgical goal is to do as little as is needed to accomplish that aforementioned goal, understanding that undoing adaptive changes in the shoulder, whether this involves mobilizing the posterosuperior labrum or peeling away a portion of the posterosuperior rotator cuff within the rotator cable, will likely result in loss of shoulder motion, alteration in throwing mechanics, and a decrease in performance.

A better understanding of the potential purposeful and adaptive etiology of SLAP lesions as well as which SLAP lesions are potentially "good" and "bad" has left a more selective treatment algorithm in the management of SLAP lesions. The SLAP lesion should be classified as "good" or "bad" based on a number of factors, which will be discussed later in this chapter. In addition, we now understand that intra-articular long head biceps disease and biceps tunnel disease are separate entities that need to be considered independently and included in the treatment algorithm regarding superior labral tears.

Nonoperative treatment of superior labral tears in the overhead athlete is recommended as initial treatment and there are reported improved outcomes treating SLAP lesions nonoperatively when compared to treating these lesions operatively. Physical therapy should be directed toward treating concomitant pathology and kinetic chain problems. This would include quadriceps weakness, motion loss in the leg and hip, lumbo-pelvic-hip malalignment, core strength deficiencies, scapular malposition/dyskinesia, shoulder motion recovery (now based on humeral torsion measurements), shoulder stabilization including entities such as dynamic posterior instability in a thrower, and correction of known throwing mechanic factors that contribute to injury. The majority of the SLAP lesions in the thrower probably occur gradually with attrition over time and many are not symptomatic.

17.3 Indications

As part of the clinical assessment, many special shoulder tests have been described for SLAP lesions. None have been shown individually or collectively to have reliably high sensitivity and specificity. It is the opinion of the senior author that none of the tests can be expected to confirm pain caused by an intra-articular structural change until after the subacromial spaces have been injected. If there is pain on a test that is completely relieved by subacromial injection, then the pain is caused by subacromial outlet impingement. Whether that intra-articular structural change contributes to the cause of subacromial impingement is unclear. Nevertheless, it is not possible to say that a documented SLAP lesion is causing pain during a specialized test if the pain on that test is relieved by subacromial injection. Some authors advocate for intra-articular injections, but in the senior author's opinion, that is rarely indicated. More commonly, a biceps tunnel injection may be valuable in helping to sort out whether or not the pain is caused by the biceps tunnel disease. This is because many overhead athletes with shoulder pain will have some glenohumeral synovitis and the injection itself may relieve the pain caused by that synovitis and this superior labral tear may still be an asymptomatic lesion.

17.3.1 Indications for Primary Repair in a Thrower

The management of type II SLAP tears in patients without obvious intra- or extra-articular long head of the biceps tendon disease is still controversial. The biceps tendon–superior labral complex contributes to the translational and rotational stability in the shoulder. As such, preserving the biceps tendon–superior labral complex even in the presence of a superior labral tear is preferred over biceps tenodesis given its contribution to stability. Furthermore, repairing clearly degenerative and disrupted superior labral tissue or employing methods that overconstrain the biceps tendon at its base or along the posterosuperior labrum is known to cause loss of external rotation. For example, placing anchors anterior to the biceps tendon in the absence of superior glenohumeral ligament (SGHL) avulsion would not be appropriate. The overhead athlete, especially a thrower, was previously always considered for SLAP lesion repair. However, outcomes of repair in this population are concerning, as 22 to 64% of throwing athletes return to the same level of play. This rate of return for throwers was worse than for other overhead athletes.[4] It has been argued that in overhead athletes, the chronic attritional loads placed on the superior labrum in the late cocking stage of throwing may be too high even for a repaired labrum to withstand. While this may be true, some experts would argue that the method with which the superior labrum was repaired and the selection process of which lesions to repair may have contributed to the poor outcomes.

Careful assessment of SLAP tear patterns with consideration of associated intra- and extra-articular pathology allows for subclassification of an overhead athlete's lesion into "good" and "bad" SLAP tears. The "good" SLAP lesions are purposeful, beneficial adaptations in throwers that allow greater labral mobility, horizontal abduction, and external rotation with possible improvements in pitch velocity and performance. While these good SLAP lesions may become frayed and may benefit from debridement, repair would likely undo adaptive benefits conferred by the extra mobility, resulting in loss of motion and decreased performance. Laughlin et al reported an alteration in throwing mechanics in athletes undergoing SLAP repair.[5]

The "bad" SLAP lesions are pathologic changes causing translational and rotational microinstability, pain, and worsening performance. These tears have more complicated lesions of the complex with disrupted labral tear patterns and are often associated with more significant posterosuperior rotator cuff disease such as the PASTA lesion (partial-thickness articular surface rotator cuff tear occurring at the junction of the posterior supraspinatus and anterior infraspinatus). When history and the arthroscopic findings suggest that these "bad" SLAP lesions are traumatic, then repair is reasonable as these tears did not occur slowly over time as purposeful adaptations. When degenerative disruptive pathologic tears are debrided and leave behind poor-quality tissue for repair or the tear pattern extends into the biceps tendon itself, then biceps tenodesis becomes a more reasonable option. In addition, since many "bad" SLAP lesions are associated with rotator cuff disease, the surgeon needs to be confident that the anterior and posterior rotator cables are intact and that rotator cuff pathology is appropriately addressed. In most cases, a footprint repair should not be considered, and rotator cuff repair would only be added to the management of the superior labral treatment if the anterior or posterior rotator cables are detached. Additionally, the surgeon must also address the subacromial bursa. The best candidate for repair has history, physical examination, MRI, and arthroscopic findings consistent with a symptomatic "bad" SLAP lesion but no evidence of intra- or extra-articular biceps tendon pathology.[6]

The surgeon must be able to differentiate from multiple pain generators and treat pathology where it exists. By recognizing certain salient features of pain associated with SLAP tears, the surgeon is capable of treating superior labral disease and biceps tunnel disease with the appropriate operation. It is important to recognize that biceps tunnel disease does occur in throwers who have concomitant biceps tendon–superior labral complex pathology. When unrecognized, superior labral debridement and repair will fail to relieve anterior shoulder pain, resulting in continued functional limitation and loss of performance. You cannot treat biceps tunnel disease with superior labral surgery. Given our current understanding of biceps–superior labral pathology in the upper extremity athlete, debridement alone and management of other shoulder pathology, such as dynamic posterior instability with posteroinferior labral repair, subacromial outlet impingement with subacromial bursectomy, or biceps tunnel disease with suprapectoral biceps tenodesis, would be a more reasonable surgical option that superior labral repair.

17.3.2 Indications in Degenerative SLAP Lesions

Degenerative changes in the superior labrum may include mild fraying and slight hypermobility and may be treated conservatively if the patient does not have biceps-related pain. If this pathology exists in conjunction with biceps pain or instability of the biceps tendon, tenotomy or tenodesis is indicated. In symptomatic type I lesions with a nondiseased biceps tendon, arthroscopic debridement with preservation of the anchor is recommended. Additionally, age may be a consideration, with many authors advocating for biceps tenotomy/tenodesis in middle-aged and older patients, but establishing an age cut-off remains controversial.

17.4 Preoperative Preparation/ Positioning/Surgical Findings

In the operative treatment of SLAP lesions, a preoperative exam with the patient awake and one under anesthesia are important diagnostic tools and should be incorporated into the operative plan. Common findings might include increased anteroinferior laxity, increased or decreased external rotation at 90-degree abduction, increased or decreased internal rotation at 90-degree abduction, total arc of motion difference relative to contralateral side, and diminished horizontal (cross-body) adduction at 90 degrees of forward flexion (representing posterior capsular contracture). In the evaluation of range of motion, the surgeon must also take into account humeral torsion, as external/internal rotation and total arc of motion differences may be in part attributable to humeral torsion, which may be different between the thrower's dominant and nondominant upper extremity.

The arthroscopic evaluation may be performed in either the beach-chair or lateral decubitus position using traditional posterior and anterior portals. The surgeon may encounter several different tear types, which were initially described using a classification by Snyder et al.[7] The Snyder classification has since been modified by others with the addition of several tear patterns.[8,9] The biceps–labrum complex may be evaluated for the "peel back" phenomenon indicating glenoid detachment and loss of washer and bumper effect.[7,10–12] One should be familiar with the anatomic variants such as sublabral foramina, Buford complex, or meniscoidlike labral attachment without evidence of "peel back."[13] Other associated findings may include articular cartilage damage indicating increased translation of the humeral head[14]; anterior inferior capsular laxity; loss of tension in posteroinferior glenohumeral ligament; increased posterior labral thickness and fraying indicated by increased translation and consequent shear and compression on the labrum (**Fig. 17.1a, b**); posterior capsular thickness, representative of the capsular changes that contribute to motion loss; and biceps tenosynovitis (**Fig. 17.2**). SLAP tears and rotator cuff tears are linked by their pathological mechanisms in overhead-throwing athletes, and as a result, rotator cuff pathology is commonly present as well. Morgan et al found 31% incidence of partial-thickness rotator cuff tears in association with SLAP tears,[9] and Fedoriw et al found that 12/45 (27%) professional pitchers with a SLAP tear had a rotator cuff tear of at least 30% thickness.[2] In these circumstances, the challenge for the treating physician is to differentiate which is the true etiology of pain for the elite overhead-throwing athlete.

17.5 Operative Technique

The labral repair begins with appropriate portal placement. A traditional posterior portal is used in conjunction with a 1 o'clock rotator interval portal. Some surgeons utilize a second anterior portal through either the superior rotator interval or a transtendinous (through supraspinatus) portal. We prefer to use a 1 to 2 o'clock rotator interval portal for glenoid preparation and suture management, and we prefer an 11 o'clock, no cannula, 3-mm transtendinous/transmuscular portal through the supraspinatus for suture passage, anchor site drilling, and anchor/labral fixation. While we believe that a transtendinous portal is essential to proper anchor placement, we strongly discourage the use of a transtendinous cannula.

The sequence of repair is as follows. First, the surgeon should evaluate for the "peel back" phenomenon. The meniscoid rim, often frayed, is debrided. The superior and posterosuperior glenoid bony rim is then exposed and prepared with a shaver and/or curette. Knotless anchor drill sites are placed on the rim of the glenoid but not onto the face. A typical repair will incorporate three to four knotless anchors, spaced approximately 4 to 6 mm apart. Sutures are passed through the labrum only, remaining lateral to the biceps tendon fibers, in order to avoid capturing or strangulating the biceps tendon. It is important to avoid capturing or causing any trauma to the superior capsule to avoid postoperative fibrosis within the superior glenoid recess. Suture knots on the superior labrum have been shown to cause chondral and/or rotator cuff abrasion and therefore contraindicated. Knotless anchors are preferred (**Fig. 17.3**) except for cases where the SGHL/MGHL avulsion and instability are thought to contribute to symptoms. Sutures are avoided anterior to the 12 o'clock position as this has been shown to decrease external rotation in abduction. Following repair, the biceps is re-evaluated for mobility to make sure it is not overconstrained in abduction and external rotation. Special attention is paid to ensure that no

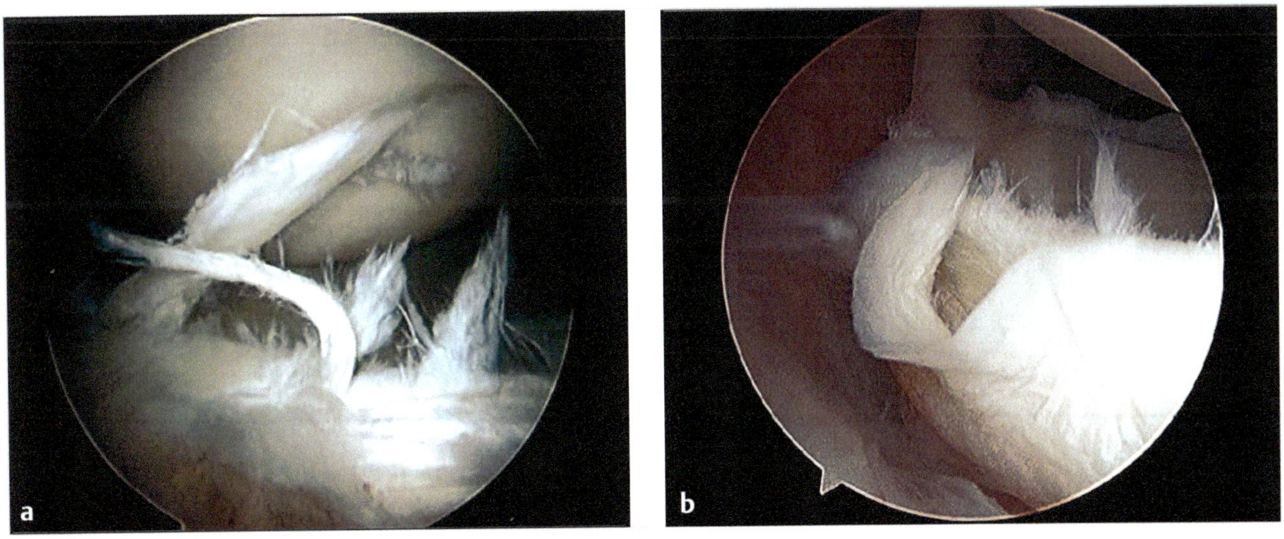

Fig. 17.1 (a, b) Posterior superior labral tear with fraying and increased thickness.

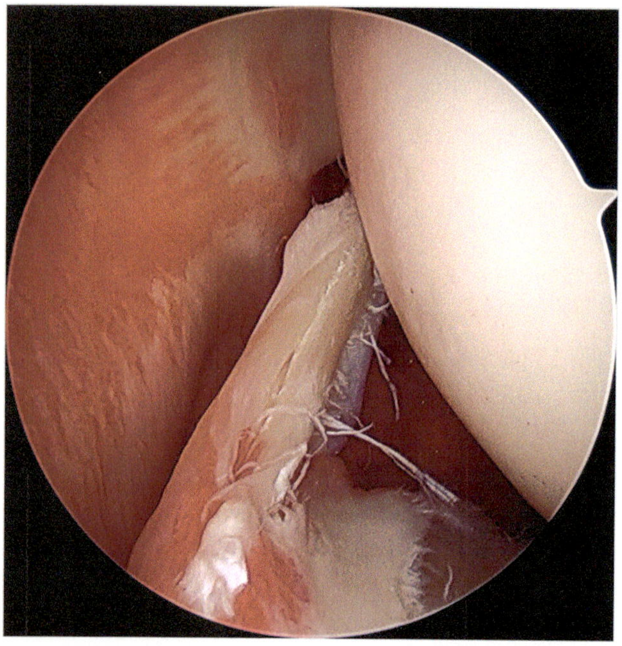

Fig. 17.2 Posterior capsular thickness with changes that contribute to motion loss.

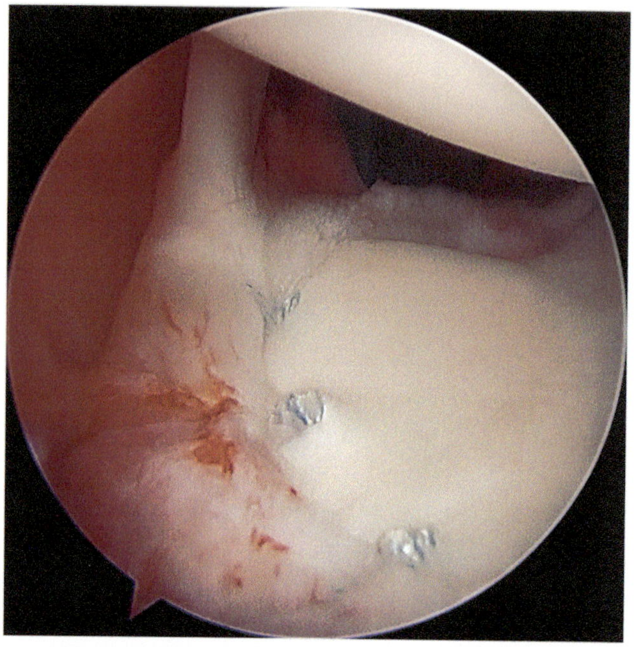

Fig. 17.3 SLAP repair using knotless anchors in the posterior superior positions.

external rotation is lost compared to preoperative assessment.[15] In the thrower's shoulder, it is commonly held that "too loose" is better than "too tight."

17.6 Tips and Pearls/Expert Suggestions

In general, the authors attempt to treat superior labral disease with superior labral surgery (debridement or repair) and to treat biceps or biceps tunnel disease with biceps tunnel surgery. Accordingly, our approach is to perform a biceps tenodesis if there is obvious pathology in the biceps tendon, such as frank tear or marked tenosynovitis (**Fig. 17.2**). In such a case, we would typically perform an arthroscopic suprapectoral tenodesis, using an arthroscopic modified Caspari–Weber method. Biceps tenodesis may also be considered for revision SLAP surgery in some cases. Among the potential risks of biceps tenodesis relevant to the throwing athlete is proximal humerus fracture due to the stress riser created in the proximal humerus, but this is primarily related to the axis of drilling and subpectoral fixation.[16] Further research on the benefits and risks of biceps tenodesis in throwers is needed.

When labral disease exists and the surgeon is to perform a SLAP repair, the authors choose to emphasize the following pearls:

1. Do not do a bad SLAP repair.
2. A bad SLAP repair includes sublabral hole repair, superior sulcus repair, asymptomatic SLAP repair, irreparable SLAP repair, poor method/poor skill SLAP repair, and missed biceps tendon or biceps tunnel disease.
3. Superior labrum debridement and biceps tenodesis are both better than a bad SLAP repair.
4. The patient must have good quality labrum and biceps tendon.
5. Avoid any contact with the superior glenoid capsule.
6. Debride/remove compromised tissue and do not repair disrupted delaminated avascular tissue.
7. Prepare the glenoid rim.
8. Use a noncannulated transtendinous/transmuscular portal; do not place transtendinous cannulas.
9. Avoid anterior sutures except for SGHL/MGHL avulsion injuries. In the absence of a clear avulsion of the MGHL/SGHL, no suture should be placed anteriorly to the biceps tendon.
10. Primarily repair posterior superior tears. Anterior repairs for instability only. Posteriorly, the decision needs to be made whether to fully capture the labrum or only stabilize that part which seems to be creating an unstable anchor for the biceps tendon.
11. Utilize a knotless method with tight loops that do not limit normal biceps tendon translation and rotation or strangulate the tendon.
12. Remove excess meniscoid labrum. There is some controversy regarding repair of a large meniscal segment. Some argue that the segment may actually be a contributor to the cause of the superior labral pathology. Others suggest it still plays a role in the joint. In those cases where repair seems to be poorly advised, debridement alone or biceps tenodesis become reasonable.

17.7 What to Avoid

Poor surgical outcomes after SLAP repair can be attributed to a number of causes. The surgeon must question why the primary intervention failed before directing further treatment. First, inadequate or incomplete assessment may explain why the intervention failed. For example, the failure to understand that the SLAP is not the problem; instead, it is a result of another or combination of other derangements along the kinetic chain. If the problems leading to the superior labrum tear are not identified and corrected, no surgical method is likely to have long-term success.

Contributing problems include kinetic chain issues, kyphothoracolumbar posture, hamstring tightness, hip rotation loss, pelvic malrotation, poor dynamic stability of the scapular spine and shoulder, scapular malposition and dyskinesia, and shoulder rotational deficits. Other nonlabral problems that may go unrecognized or incompletely treated include missed extra-articular biceps tendon pathology and subcoracoid stenosis.

17.8 Complications/Bailout/Salvage

Complications associated with SLAP repair include general complications of shoulder arthroscopy including infection, brachial plexus traction injury (lateral position traction and distraction) in addition to refractory pain, and failed repair. Stiffness of the shoulder joint with motion loss may result in a longer rehabilitation period with persistent pain and dysfunction. If there is persistent pain after SLAP repair, consider other causes and treat appropriately. Higher revision rates have been reported in patients older than 40 years treated with SLAP repairs,[17] but there are some authors who report comparable results in patients in younger and older patients with repair.[18] As a salvage procedure and based on other concomitant shoulder issues, revision SLAP repair or biceps tenotomy/tenodesis may be considered.

17.9 Postoperative Care

In the postoperative period, the arm is placed in a sling for 3 to 4 weeks. Internal rotation is allowed, as well as external rotation to neutral position, 0 degrees, in weeks 2 to 4. Additionally, true glenohumeral abduction to 90 degrees in the scapular plane is allowed. Sling wear is discontinued at 4 weeks with therapy for passive range of motion and posterior capsular stretching. At 6 weeks, passive external rotation with abduction is allowed. After 3 months, the patient may begin active strengthening with weights. Return to sporting activity is allowed between 3 and 6 months, except for throwers who return based on throwing program progression.

17.10 Conclusion

A better understanding of the potential purposeful and adaptive etiology of SLAP lesions as well as which SLAP lesions are potentially "good" and "bad" has left a more selective treatment algorithm in the management of SLAP lesions. In addition, we now understand that intra-articular long head biceps disease and biceps tunnel disease are separate entities that need to be considered independently and collectively in the treatment algorithm regarding superior labral tears. This has led to return of nonoperative treatment of superior labral tears in the overhead athlete as an initial treatment, and furthermore, studies have shown improved outcomes treating SLAP lesions nonoperatively when compared to treating these lesions operatively.

It is also important to note that the outcomes that are reported on superior labral repair reflect old surgical methods and an outdated understanding of superior labral disease. Current surgical knotless techniques that avoid use of transtendinous cannulas, superior capsule abrasion, biceps tendon strangulation, and anteriorly placed sutures are more likely to provide an effective repair that does not create more problems than it was designed to correct.

References

1. Edwards SL, Lee JA, Bell JE, et al. Nonoperative treatment of superior labrum anterior posterior tears: improvements in pain, function, and quality of life. Am J Sports Med 2010;38(7):1456–1461
2. Fedoriw WW, Ramkumar P, McCulloch PC, Lintner DM. Return to play after treatment of superior labral tears in professional baseball players. Am J Sports Med 2014;42(5):1155–1160
3. Huri G, Hyun YS, Garbis NG, McFarland EG. Treatment of superior labrum anterior posterior lesions: a literature review. Acta Orthop Traumatol Turc 2014;48(3):290–297
4. Gorantla K, Gill C, Wright RW. The outcome of type II SLAP repair: a systematic review. Arthroscopy 2010; 26(4):537–545
5. Laughlin WA, Fleisig GS, Scillia AJ, Aune KT, Cain EL Jr, Dugas JR. Deficiencies in pitching biomechanics in baseball players with a history of superior labrum anterior-posterior repair. Am J Sports Med 2014;42(12):2837–2841
6. Burns JP, Bahk M, Snyder SJ. Superior labral tears: repair versus biceps tenodesis. J Shoulder Elbow Surg 2011;20(2, Suppl):S2–S8
7. Snyder SJ, Karzel RP, Del Pizzo W, Ferkel RD, Friedman MJ. SLAP lesions of the shoulder. Arthroscopy 1990;6(4):274–279
8. Maffet MW, Gartsman GM, Moseley B. Superior labrum-biceps tendon complex lesions of the shoulder. Am J Sports Med 1995;23(1):93–98
9. Morgan CD, Burkhart SS, Palmeri M, Gillespie M. Type II SLAP lesions: three subtypes and their relationships to superior instability and rotator cuff tears. Arthroscopy 1998;14(6):553–565
10. Burkhart SS, Morgan CD, Kibler WB. The disabled throwing shoulder: spectrum of pathology. Part II: evaluation and treatment of SLAP lesions in throwers. Arthroscopy 2003;19(5):531–539
11. Bankart AS, Cantab MC. Recurrent or habitual dislocation of the shoulder-joint. 1923. Clin Orthop Relat Res 1993(291):3–6
12. Veeger HE, van der Helm FC. Shoulder function: the perfect compromise between mobility and stability. J Biomech 2007;40(10):2119–2129
13. Burkhart SSUnderstanding and recognizing pathology. In: Burkhart S, Lo IKY, Brady PC, eds. Burkhart's View of the Shoulder: A Cowboy's Guide to Shoulder Arthroscopy. Philadelphia, PA: Lippincott Williams & Wilkins; 2006
14. Savoie FH III, Field LD, Atchinson S. Anterior superior instability with rotator cuff tearing: SLAC lesion. Orthop Clin North Am 2001;32(3):457–461, ix
15. Kibler WB, Kuhn JE, Wilk K, et al. The disabled throwing shoulder: spectrum of pathology-10-year update. Arthroscopy 2013;29(1):141–161.e26
16. Dein EJ, Huri G, Gordon JC, McFarland EG. A humerus fracture in a baseball pitcher after biceps tenodesis. Am J Sports Med 2014;42(4):877–879
17. Erickson J, Lavery K, Monica J, Gatt C, Dhawan A. Surgical treatment of symptomatic superior labrum anterior-posterior tears in patients older than 40 years: a systematic review. Am J Sports Med 2015;43(5):1274–1282
18. Alpert JM, Wuerz TH, O'Donnell TF, Carroll KM, Brucker NN, Gill TJ. The effect of age on the outcomes of arthroscopic repair of type II superior labral anterior and posterior lesions. Am J Sports Med 2010;38(11):2299–2303**Fig. 17.2**

greater muscular development compared to the nondominant shoulder.[6] The scapulae should be evaluated for positioning, dyskinesias, and winging. Patients with internal impingement may also have asymmetric microinstability. Distinguishing between pathologic and adaptive laxity, however, may be difficult. However, we have found the "relocation" test to be an extraordinarily sensitive sign for pathologic anterior instability in throwers. Symptoms reflective of "dead arm," shoulder weakness after throwing, or a subjective sense of a slipping shoulder may indicate pathologic microinstability. Apprehension in 90 degrees of abduction and external rotation is not uncommon. While the posterior impingement test is frequently positive,[25] the impingement sign as described by Neer[11] is typically absent.

Rotator cuff strength should be assessed. Rotator cuff pathology may range from undersurface fraying and partial articular-sided tears to full-thickness tears. The infraspinatus is most commonly involved; therefore, assessment of external rotation strength is critical. As mentioned earlier, internal impingement often occurs in the setting of concomitant injuries, including superior labral anterior and posterior (SLAP) and biceps lesions, bursal-sided rotator cuff tears, and tendinitis, and the patient should be examined accordingly.

18.3 Radiographic Evaluation

Standard radiographs, including internal and external rotation anteroposterior, scapular Y, axillary, and West Point views, are obtained. Radiographs are most often normal, but may show a "Bennett lesion" (exostosis of the posteroinferior glenoid rim), greater tuberosity sclerosis, posterohumeral osteochondral cysts, and rounding of the posterior glenoid rim.[26,27]

MRI is critical to a thorough radiographic evaluation. MRI has a high sensitivity for rotator cuff, labral, and capsular pathology.

Table 18.1 Jobe's clinical classification of internal impingement

Stage	Presentation/symptoms
I: early	Shoulder stiffness and need for prolonged warm-up, no pain with ADLs
II: intermediate	Pain localized to the posterior shoulder in the late-cocking phase, no pain with ADLs
III: advanced	Same as stage II, but refractory to a period of adequate rest and rehabilitation

Abbreviation: ADL, activities of daily living.

We prefer a noncontrast MRI, as it has demonstrated to have equivalent or superior sensitivity to MR arthrogram when specific pulse sequences are employed.[28] Common MRI findings in patients with internal impingement are partial-thickness articular-sided rotator cuff tears, posterosuperior labral tears, and cystic changes in the posterior humeral head[24,29] (**Fig. 18.1**). Patients may also display a Bennett lesion, posterior capsular contracture and thickening at the level of the posterior band of the inferior glenohumeral ligament, and subchondral fracture and possible remodeling of the posterosuperior glenoid.[15] In particularly severe cases, this remodeling may produce narrowing of the spinoglenoid notch adjacent to the suprascapular neurovascular bundle. As MRI may reveal lesions that are asymptomatic, radiologic findings must be correlated with clinical signs and symptoms. Halbrecht et al[4] found that 4 of 10 collegiate baseball players had abnormal signal change in the rotator cuff tendons despite the absence of symptoms. Other studies have also shown that MRI findings do not always correlate with the athlete's symptoms.[30,31]

While CT may be useful in assessing humeral and glenoid version, CT is rarely used for the evaluation of internal impingement of the shoulder.

18.4 Treatment

18.4.1 Nonoperative Management

Patients may be treated according to the stages outlined by Jobe. Patients with early stages of the syndrome describe poorly localized pain with stiffness.[5] These patients are almost always treated with rest and nonsteroidal anti-inflammatory medications. Patients with more localized posterior shoulder pain typically require 4 to 6 weeks of rest and may benefit from physical therapy.[15] Physical therapy has demonstrated to be both therapeutic and protective against injury in numerous studies.[13,14,32]

Therapy is directed to primarily stretch the posterior capsule and correct scapular dyskinesia. Posterior capsular stretching is achieved largely with the "sleeper stretch," which has been proven to improve motion and prevent injury in high-level tennis and baseball players.[13,14] The anterior capsule, on the other hand, should not be stretched, as that may exacerbate anterior laxity. Because anterior laxity may be a potential cause of internal impingement, strengthening of the dynamic shoulder stabilizers should be emphasized. Additionally, core

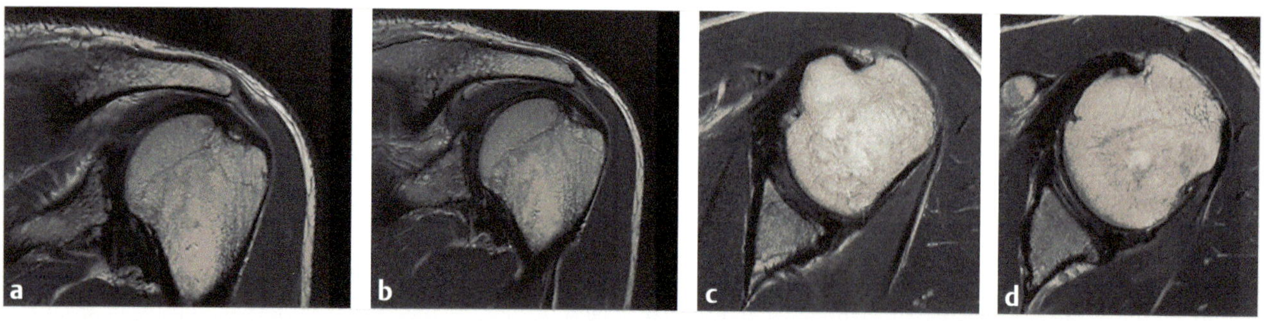

Fig. 18.1 **(a,b)** Coronal proton density sequence demonstrates rotator cuff tendinosis with an articular-sided partial-thickness tear at the interface between the supraspinatus and infraspinatus footprints. **(c)** Axial image shows thickening of the posteroinferior glenohumeral ligament and capsule, consistent with glenohumeral internal rotation deficit. **(d)** A Bennett lesion, or mineralization of the posteroinferior glenohumeral ligament, is seen. (These images are provided courtesy of Hollis G. Potter, MD.)

and lower body strengthening should be targeted to maximize efficiency in the kinetic chain. Proper throwing mechanics should also be reviewed.[32]

Injections into Bennett lesions have been described.[33] These injections, however, have served diagnostic, rather than therapeutic, purposes. There are no convincing data to endorse injections for internal impingement in young throwers and these injections should therefore be used carefully due to the potential risk of permanent tendon damage.

18.5 Operative Treatment

18.5.1 Indications and Contraindications

Arthroscopic evaluation and treatment is indicated in throwing athletes with a prolonged history of pain and mechanical symptoms that correlate with radiologic findings and are refractory to nonoperative care. Contraindications include infection or concomitant medical illness that precludes surgery.

18.5.2 Surgical Planning

Treatment of the associated pathologies described earlier must be anticipated. To this end, all instruments and materials needed for the surgery should be available and/or be on the surgical field. With adequate planning, arthroscopic treatment of internal impingement should be accomplished in under 1 hour.

18.6 Surgical Technique

The goal of surgery is to treat only the pathologic entities without changing the osseous and soft-tissue adaptations required to throw at maximal velocity. Operative management includes a comprehensive diagnostic arthroscopy, labral debridement versus repair, biceps-labral complex debridement versus repair, rotator cuff debridement versus repair, and appropriate treatment of other associated lesions, if necessary.

18.6.1 Anesthesia and Positioning

Patients are administered sedation and a regional nerve block (intrascalene, supraclavicular). Patients are placed in a modified beach-chair position with a beanbag at the medial border of the scapula, which serves to elevate the ipsilateral trunk and allow maximal clearance posterior to the shoulder (**Fig. 18.2**). The position is a slight modification of the usual beach-chair position in that the patient is more upright and the acromion is parallel to the floor. A sterile articulated arm holder is used to aid in arm positioning throughout the procedure. Prophylactic antibiotics are given and the skin is cleaned with ChloraPrep.

18.6.2 Surgical Landmarks and Portals

- Posterior: viewing portal.
- Anterior: anchor placement for anterior labral repair, if necessary, and intra-articular rotator cuff debridement.
- Anterolateral: accessory portal; viewing and suture passage for anterior labrum or capsule; and intra-articular rotator cuff debridement.
- Posterolateral (portal of Wilmington): anchor placement and suture passage in posterior labrum. Ensure that this portal is medial to the tendinous portion of the posterosuperior rotator cuff.

18.6.3 Diagnostic Arthroscopy

Prior to arthroscopy, an examination under anesthesia is performed to assess passive range of motion in all planes and joint stability in the anterior, posterior, and inferior directions. A standard posterior portal is established roughly 2 cm inferior and 2 cm medial to the posterolateral border of the acromion, and the glenohumeral joint is entered using a 30-degree arthroscope. An anterolateral portal is placed in the superolateral aspect of the rotator interval directly anterior to the leading edge of the supraspinatus tendon. A thorough diagnostic arthroscopy is then performed with special consideration given to the clinical and radiological findings. A comprehensive evaluation includes assessment of the following:

- Circumferential labrum.
- Long head of the biceps and the biceps-labral anchor.
- Humeral head and glenoid cartilage.
- Rotator cuff interval.
- Subscapularis, supraspinatus, and infraspinatus tendons.
- Anterior and posterior capsuloligamentous complex.

Provocative tests, such as the drive-through sign and the peel-back test, may be performed. In a normal shoulder, capsular

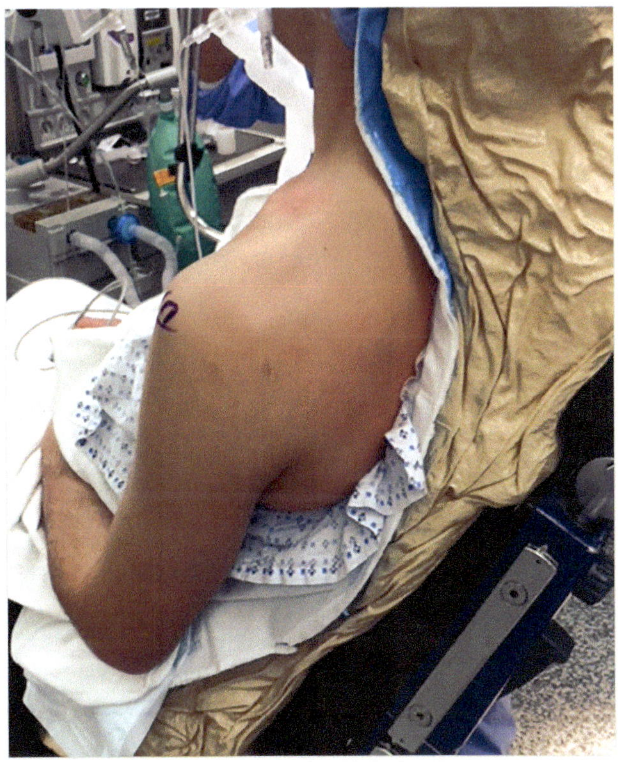

Fig. 18.2 Modified beach-chair position with a beanbag. The beanbag is positioned at the medial border of the scapula and elevates the arm in line with the scapular plane.

restraints prevent easy passage of the arthroscope from posterior to anterior at the midlevel of the humeral head, or sweeping of the arthroscope from superior to inferior along the anterior glenoid rim. The drive-through sign may signify anterior capsular laxity or pseudolaxity in the presence of a SLAP tear. The peel-back test is performed with the arm in an abducted and externally rotated position. The posterosuperior labrum is peeled medially along the glenoid neck in throwers with a posterior SLAP lesion. Isolated anterior SLAP lesions will have a negative peel-back test.

Finally, and although often unnecessary, the subacromial space may be inspected if subacromial pathology is suspected.

18.6.4 Labral Surgery

After diagnostic arthroscopy, particular attention is given to the "kissing lesion" that develops between the posterosuperior labrum and undersurface of the rotator cuff (**Fig. 18.3**). While the circumferential labrum must be viewed, the SLAP region should be of particular interest. The SLAP region contains several normal anatomic variants, such as a sublabral foramen, Buford complex, and meniscoid labrum, and these entities must be distinguished from true pathology. Hemorrhage or granulation tissue beneath the biceps-labral complex suggests injury compared to normal variance. A destabilized biceps-labral complex must be evaluated in the context of the thrower's history and physical examination. Overhead athletes with an unstable biceps anchor typically describe anterior shoulder pain.

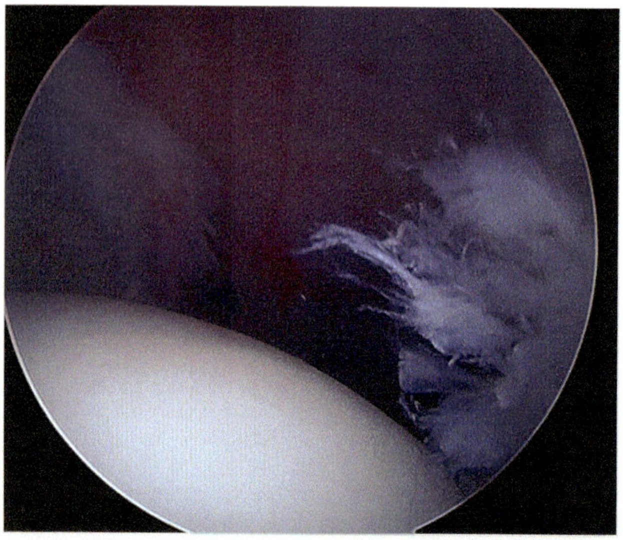

Fig. 18.3 Arthroscopic view from superior anterolateral portal showing "kissing lesion," or posterosuperior labral tear and undersurface rotator cuff tear.

The SLAP type and location (anterior, posterior, and combined) must be identified, as this will dictate accessory portal placement. A posterior type II SLAP lesion is most common in throwers. Type I lesions are degenerative and therefore rare in the thrower. SLAP types II, III, and IV are unstable and often require surgery. Type II SLAPs are most commonly treated with labral refixation. The bone bed deep to the avulsed labrum must first be prepared through the anterior or anterolateral portal to removed soft tissue and provide a bleeding cancellous bone bed for repair. A portal of Wilmington is then established under direct visualization using an 18-gauge spinal needle. The trajectory of the spinal needle should mimic that of the suture anchor to ensure accurate portal placement. Sutures are passed in line with and parallel to the biceps tendon using the appropriate suture-passing device (70-degree ACCU-PASS Suture Shuttle, Smith & Nephew, Andover, MA; or 20- or 45-degree Birdbeak, Arthrex, Naples, FL) and a suture-shuttling technique (**Fig. 18.4**). We prefer to avoid radial simple sutures, as these may articulate with and abrade the humeral head (**Fig. 18.5**). The labrum is transfixed to the glenoid using a 2.9-mm knotless suture anchor (PushLock, Arthrex). Most commonly, two anchors are required posterior to the biceps. Should the lesion extend anterior to the biceps, the labrum is repaired in an identical fashion, with exceptional care to not include the middle glenohumeral ligament (MGHL).

In type III labral tears, the bucket handle portion of the lesion is excised and the biceps anchor is evaluated for stability. Unstable lesions are repaired as described earlier. Treatment of type IV SLAP tears is dictated by biceps tendon involvement. Lesions with less than 30% biceps tendon involvement are treated with debridement and labral repair. Lesions with greater than 30% biceps tendon involvement are treated with a subpectoral biceps tenodesis and possible labral repair.

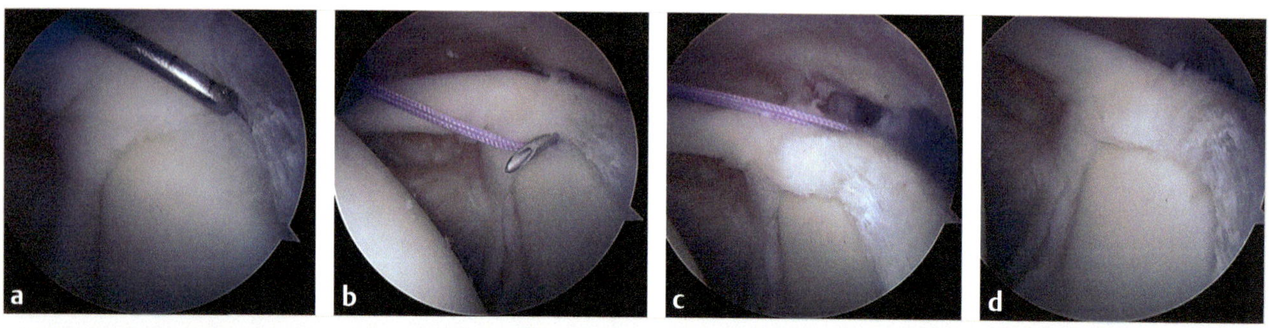

Fig. 18.4 (a) Arthroscopic view from posterior portal showing unstable superior labral anterior and posterior (SLAP) tear posterior to the biceps anchor. **(b)** High-strength suture is passed using a suture passing device and a suture shuttling technique. **(c)** Sutures are passed in a mattress configuration in line with and parallel to the biceps tendon. **(d)** Sutures are transfixed with a knotless suture anchor at the articular margin.

18.6.5 Rotator Cuff Surgery

The rotator cuff is arthroscopically evaluated with a particular focus on articular-sided partial-thickness tears, the pattern most commonly observed in overhead athletes. If a full-thickness or bursal-sided tear is suspected, the tear must be evaluated from the subacromial space. An articular-sided partial-thickness avulsion tear must be examined as a percentage of its entire footprint width, commonly noted to be roughly 14 mm in the mediolateral direction.[34] Intratendinous partial-thickness rotator cuff tears must be contextualized as a percentage of the tendon torn in relation to the entire tendon depth. Our algorithm for rotator cuff surgery in a thrower is based mostly on tear depth, but also tear type, tendon quality, the thrower's specific sport, seasonal timing, physical and imaging findings, and positional demands of the athlete.

It must be emphasized that while we present a general algorithm for the treatment of partial rotator cuff tears in throwers with internal impingement, each athlete should be treated individually and only clinically relevant pathology should be addressed. We first quantify the depth of the partial-thickness rotator cuff tear. Tears that constitute less than roughly 90% of the tendon depth are treated with debridement; tears that constitute more than roughly 90% of the tendon are treated with repair. Clearly, debridement is strongly favored compared to repair (**Fig. 18.6**).

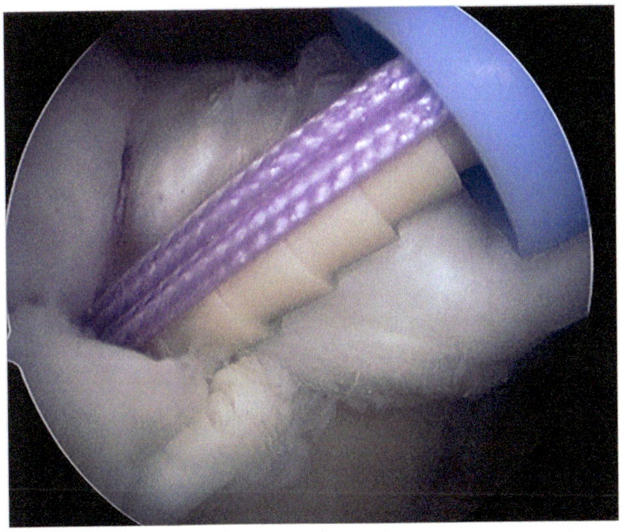

Fig. 18.5 Radial sutures passed circumferentially around the superior labrum should be avoided.

If a full-thickness tear is suspected, but not readily visualized, a spinal needle with a monofilament suture is passed through the intra-articular tear via the subacromial space. This marking suture and area of concern is then visualized from the subacromial space, and the integrity of the remaining tendon is inspected.

There is a paucity of literature on clinical outcomes in professional baseball players with full-thickness rotator cuff tears. Surgical repair of these injuries has resulted in unpredictable outcomes.[35,36] For this reason, we firmly believe that partial-thickness rotator cuff tears in overhead athletes should be treated with arthroscopic debridement, if at all possible. Nonetheless, full-thickness (or > 90%) tears that correlate with the clinical symptoms and physical examination must be repaired. The supraspinatus and infraspinatus insertions relative to the articular surface, bicipital groove, and the bare area of the humerus are well described.[37] The supraspinatus inserts immediately adjacent to the articular margin, while the infraspinatus and teres minor taper laterally away from the margin to form the bare area. An understanding of this anatomy is critical, as surgical repair should aim to restore normal biomechanics and increase the surface area available for healing.[38,39] Medial advancement of the posterosuperior rotator cuff insertion can alter the thrower's joint biomechanics and prevent them from achieving the hyper-rotation required for baseball pitching.[38]

Prior to rotator cuff repair, a thorough subacromial bursectomy is performed to improve visualization. An acromioplasty is only carried out in the presence of an impingement lesion, which is uncommon in this population. The tissue is provisionally grasped and mobilized to assess tendon excursion. Because these injuries are treated expeditiously, tendon retraction and poor tissue quality are rare. The greater tuberosity immediately adjacent to the articular margin is abraded using a mechanical shaver to enhance healing potential. Supraspinatus tears are treated with an anchor (4.75 loaded Arthrex SwiveLock) positioned immediately lateral to the articular margin in the region of the anterior attachment of the rotator cable. The posterior anchor (4.75 loaded Arthrex SwiveLock) is positioned roughly 10 to 15 mm lateral to the articular margin to reproduce the native infraspinatus footprint (**Fig. 18.7**). The medial row sutures are then fixed laterally with two knotless anchors (4.75 Arthrex SwiveLock) to provide a transosseous equivalent (double-row) repair. Anchors are passed through small, percutaneous portals, the positions of which are determined under direct visualization with a spinal needle.

Partial articular supraspinatus tendon avulsions, or PASTA lesions, are typically debrided, not repaired. Occasionally, however, PASTA lesions may be repaired back to bone with suture anchors if the tear is located anteriorly on the greater tuberosity. We

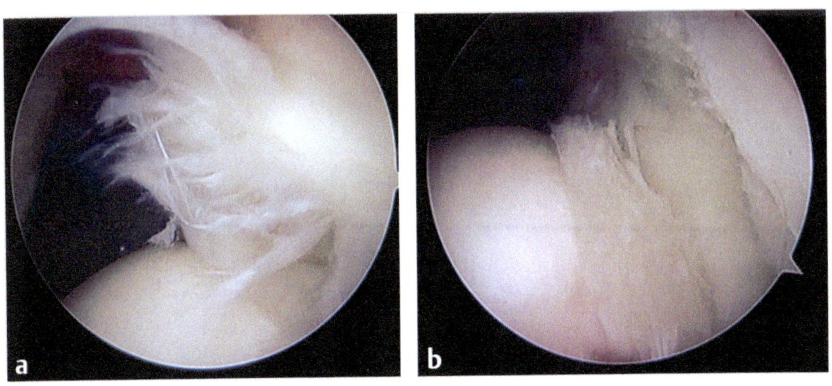

Fig. 18.6 **(a)** Arthroscopic view from posterior portal demonstrating articular-sided partial-thickness rotator cuff tear. **(b)** The tear constituted less than 90% of tendon thickness and was therefore debrided.

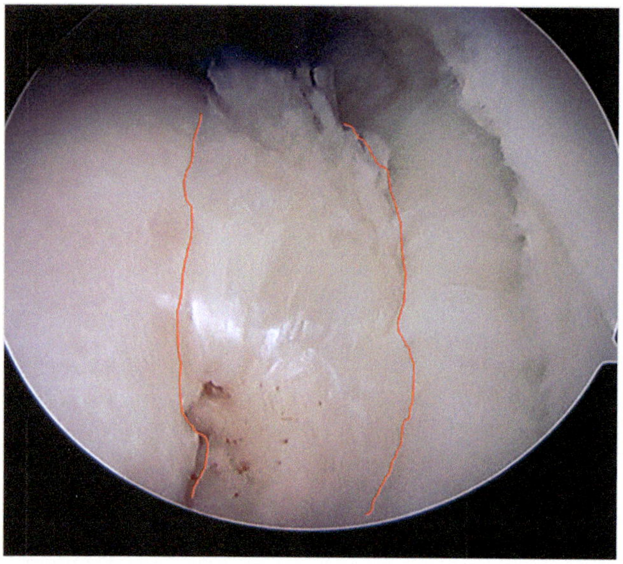

Fig. 18.7 The medial bare area between the infraspinatus footprint and articular margin should be maintained after repair.

prefer to simply debride more posteriorly located PASTA lesions, as repair may overtension the rotator cuff or obstruct normal internal impingement contact during the cocking phase of throwing. PASTA lesions that include more than 90% of the tendon depth require completion of the tear and subsequent repair, as described earlier. While it was previously recommended to repair intratendinous tears (with an intact footprint),[40] we presently advocate for simple debridement, as intratendinous repair, in our experience, has proven unpredictable.

18.6.6 Capsular Surgery

Clinical and imaging findings, along with an examination under anesthesia and intraoperative findings, are used to assess capsular laxity. It is imperative to remember that throwers must maintain a delicate balance of laxity and stability in order to generate optimal velocity. All capsular procedures, therefore, must aim to preserve sufficient stability while maintaining the obligatory mobility.

We only perform anterior capsular procedures if we perceive their instability to be the primary source of their pain. If done in the correct patient, anterior capsular procedures may resolve the symptoms related to pathologic internal impingement. These patients will almost always have a positive "relocation" test. Other signs of pathologic capsular injury or laxity include hemorrhage, midcapsular tears, or an inability to take up tension with the arm positioned in the scapular plane. Regardless of the treatment strategy employed, special care should be taken to avoid overtightening the anterior capsule, which would limit the obligatory external rotation required for competitive overhead throwers.

If anterior laxity is determined to be the chief cause of symptoms, an anterior capsular plication is performed. The location and degree of capsular plication depend largely on the desired amount of tightening. Instead of isolated capsule plication, in which the capsule is sewn to adjacent capsule, we prefer to capture the capsule and labrum and transfix them to the glenoid with suture anchors. Prior to obtaining final fixation, the arm is placed in a cocking position to confirm that the shoulder is not being overtightened.

Several standard glenohumeral joint portals are used, including a posterior viewing portal, a low anterior working portal, and a high anterolateral portal at the leading edge of the supraspinatus. The position of both portals should be placed under direct visualization using an 18-gauge spinal needle to ensure that the appropriate angles can be achieved. A blue FMS cannula (Smith & Nephew) is placed in the anterolateral portal and a PassPort cannula (Arthrex) in the low anterior portal. A large bump is positioned in the axilla and the arm is forward flexed and adducted to create space to pass instruments. A 60-degree SutureLasso (Arthrex) is used to pass PDS suture, or any monofilament suture, from the anterior portal. The capsule and labrum are captured in two bites. Standard suture-shuttling techniques are used to pass a high-strength suture (FiberWire, Arthrex) in a mattress configuration. These sutures are secured to the glenoid with knotless suture anchors (2.9 PushLock, Arthrex). In our experience, two mattress sutures and two suture anchors are sufficient.

18.7 Tips and Pearls

There are numerous tips and pearls that may aid surgeons in the treatment of internal impingement. Most importantly, however, one must only treat the pathology that directly correlates with the athlete's complaints and symptoms. Most overhead throwing athletes possess a spectrum of pathology that combines partial-thickness rotator cuff tears, posterosuperior labral injury, and anterior laxity. Appropriate recognition and treatment of each component is crucial to restoring the ability to throw without symptoms, while also recognizing that throwers maintain a delicate balance of laxity and stability. Surgical tips and pearls are listed in **Table 18.2**.

18.8 What to Avoid

There are several things, outlined in **Table 18.3**, that we believe the surgeon should avoid to ensure a predictable outcome.

Table 18.2 Tips and pearls

Procedure	Pearl
Examination under anesthesia	ROM in all planes; stability in anterior, posterior, and inferior directions
Diagnostic arthroscopy	Special attention to undersurface of posterosuperior rotator cuff, posterosuperior labrum, assess cuff in numerous arm positions, assess capsular laxity
Labral surgery	Repair with mattress suture configuration in line with biceps if unstable; debride if frayed; secure with knotless suture anchor; include anterosuperior labrum if involved
Rotator cuff surgery	Debride if tear involves < 90% tendon depth; repair if full thickness using lateralized technique, knotless transosseous equivalent repair preferred
Capsular surgery	Repair if acute capsuloligamentous injury or excessive laxity, plication incorporates capsule and labrum and secured to glenoid with knotless suture anchor, check late-cocking throwing position to avoid overtightening

Table 18.3 What to avoid

What to avoid
Avoid confusing adaptive laxity with pathologic instability
Avoid radial sutures in SLAP repair
Avoid rotator cuff repair when debridement will suffice
Avoid medialization of posterior rotator cuff footprint
Avoid overtightening of capsule and rotator cuff

Abbreviation: SLAP, superior labral anterior and posterior.

18.9 Complications: What Can Go Wrong and How to Manage It

Most complications are consistent with those associated with general shoulder arthroscopy and occur infrequently. In overhead throwers, complications include inability to return to play, persistent pain, stiffness, and recurrent instability.[1,41] Not unlike other orthopaedic operations, the keys to avoiding complications are stringent surgical indications, careful preoperative planning, visualization, and precise surgical technique. The maxim "less is more" holds true in the treatment of internal impingement in the overhead athlete. There is no predictably successful means of treating the overhead thrower. The surgeon must appreciate the "thrower's paradox," which refers to the delicate balance between mobility and stability, and allows pitchers to achieve a high level of function. The surgeon must also not surgically address normal variants or normal adaptations common to throwers.

Complications can be avoided by understanding the anatomical changes common in overhead athletes. One must also understand the rotator cuff insertional anatomy to avoid filling the bare area medial to the posterosuperior cuff. Additionally, visualization and accurate portal placement are also critical. Portal location should be confirmed using an outside-in technique with a spinal needle. This will ensure that the appropriate drilling angles can be accommodated, as poor drilling angles can result in an iatrogenic chondral shear injury.

Similar to the rotator cuff, the anterior capsule can also be overtightened. Determining the amount of capsule to plicate is challenging, but we recommend placing the arm in the throwing position prior to seating the suture anchor to confirm that the plication will not result in overtightening.

18.10 Postoperative Considerations and Rehabilitation

A well-defined rehabilitation program is a critical component of a successful recovery. The rehabilitation program is dependent on the specific procedure performed. A skilled and knowledgeable physical therapist or athletic trainer is crucial to the implementation of the program. In all rehabilitation protocols, we have found that early cryotherapy and appropriately prescribed pain and anti-inflammatory medications have allowed athletes to better participate in a physical therapy exercise program. Criteria for return to play include full and painless range of motion, return of isokinetic strength, a normal clinical examination, and successful completion of a sport-specific rehabilitation program.

In the following section, we will review common postoperative rehabilitation protocols for athletes with internal impingement.

18.10.1 SLAP and Rotator Cuff Debridement

Of course, prior to initiating a rehab protocol after SLAP and rotator cuff debridement, the size and location of the tears, along with concomitant pathology, must be considered. We emphasize early motion and prevention of muscle atrophy, all while minimizing pain and inflammation. Once the athlete demonstrates full motion, minimal pain, and good manual muscle testing in flexion, external rotation, and internal rotation, he or she may focus on regaining and improving strength, normalizing scapular and glenohumeral kinematics, along with neuromuscular control of the shoulder complex. Proprioceptive training and core, trunk, and lower extremity strength and endurance are initiated. Next, at weeks 4 to 6, the athlete prepares to throw. This includes a comprehensive throwing program, which is beyond the scope of this chapter. The final phase includes a gradual return to functional activities and beginning an interval sport-specific program.

18.10.2 SLAP, Rotator Cuff, and/or Capsular Repair

In cases in which the labrum, rotator cuff, or capsule is repaired, the rehabilitation protocol is altered to allow for healing. The approach after rotator cuff repair is more conservative, compared to that after labral or capsular repair. Nonetheless, our protocol is based very roughly on five phases: acute postoperative (phase 1), protection (phase 2), intermediate stretching and strengthening (phase 3), advanced stretching and strengthening (phase 4), and return to play (phase 5). The athlete is maintained in an abduction sling during phases 1 and 2 except while doing physical therapy. The goals of phase 1 (days 1–14) are to maintain the repair, minimize pain and inflammation, gradually increase passive range of motion, and practice dynamic stabilization to prevent muscular inhibition. In phase 2, athletes who have undergone labral or capsular surgery alone begin muscular strengthening and proprioceptive drills at weeks 3 and 4. After rotator cuff surgery, the repair is protected through week 6. These throwers focus on gravity-eliminated active motion, restoration of full passive motion, and reestablishing dynamic shoulder stability.

As dynamic strength improves, a throwing-specific protocol, such as the Thrower's Ten, is initiated. This constitutes phase 4. A comprehensive scapular program is also begun. This is continued until roughly 3 months. At this point, there is a return to more functional activities, along with improving muscular strength and power. Finally, phase 5 involves a gradual return to play through commencement of a sport-specific program. If all other parameters are met, overhead throwing may begin at roughly 5 to 6 months.

18.11 Conclusion

The complex biomechanics of the thrower's shoulder predisposes them to numerous types of shoulder dysfunction and these patients are a clinical challenge for even experienced sports medicine physicians. Internal impingement is one of the most common entities affecting overhead athletes. While the pathophysiology of this condition continues to be defined, the constellation of symptoms result largely from the abutment of the articular surface of the rotator cuff and the posterosuperior glenoid. Athletes often complain of posterosuperior shoulder pain in the late-cocking and early-acceleration phases of throwing. Accurate diagnosis requires careful correlation of history, physical examination, and imaging studies. Once the diagnosis is established, a majority of patients are successfully treated with rest and rehabilitation.

Arthroscopic evaluation and treatment, however, is indicated if exhaustive nonoperative treatment results in an inability to return to play. The thrower's shoulder undergoes numerous anatomic adaptations and the surgeon must be careful to treat only the pathology that contributes to the athlete's symptoms. The appropriate surgical treatment should be followed by a comprehensive rehabilitation program that considers the thrower's age, sport, and position.

References

1. Walch G, Boileau P, Noel E, Donell ST. Impingement of the deep surface of the supraspinatus tendon on the posterosuperior glenoid rim: An arthroscopic study. J Shoulder Elbow Surg 1992;1(5):238–245 10.1016/S1058-2746(09)80065-7
2. Jobe CM. Posterior superior glenoid impingement: expanded spectrum. Arthroscopy 1995;11(5):530–536
3. Crockett HC, Gross LB, Wilk KE, et al. Osseous adaptation and range of motion at the glenohumeral joint in professional baseball pitchers. Am J Sports Med 2002;30(1):20–26. Accessed December 6, 2016
4. Halbrecht JL, Tirman P, Atkin D. Internal impingement of the shoulder: comparison of findings between the throwing and nonthrowing shoulders of college baseball players. Arthroscopy 1999;15(3):253–258 Accessed December 6, 2016
5. Jobe CM. Superior glenoid impingement. Orthop Clin North Am 1997;28(2):137–143
6. Myers JB, Laudner KG, Pasquale MR, Bradley JP, Lephart SM. Glenohumeral range of motion deficits and posterior shoulder tightness in throwers with pathologic internal impingement. Am J Sports Med 2006;34(3):385–391 10.1177/0363546505281804
7. Osbahr DC, Cannon DL, Speer KP. Retroversion of the humerus in the throwing shoulder of college baseball pitchers. Am J Sports Med 2002;30(3):347–353. Accessed December 6, 2016
8. Wright RW, Paletta GA Jr. Prevalence of the Bennett lesion of the shoulder in major league pitchers. Am J Sports Med 2004;32(1):121–124 Accessed December 6, 2016
9. Jobe FW, Kvitne RS, Giangarra CE. Shoulder pain in the overhand or throwing athlete. The relationship of anterior instability and rotator cuff impingement. Orthop Rev 1989;18(9):963–975. Accessed December 6, 2016
10. Walch G, Liotard JP, Boileau P, Noël E. [Postero-superior glenoid impingement. Another impingement of the shoulder]. J Radiol 1993;74(1):47–50 Accessed December 6, 2016
11. Neer CS II. Impingement lesions. Clin Orthop Relat Res 1983;(173):70–77 Accessed December 19, 2016
12. Neer CS II, Craig EV, Fukuda H. Cuff-tear arthropathy. J Bone Joint Surg Am 1983;65(9):1232–1244 Accessed December 19, 2016
13. Burkhart SS, Morgan CD, Kibler WB. The disabled throwing shoulder: spectrum of pathology Part I: pathoanatomy and biomechanics. Arthroscopy 2003;19(4):404–420 10.1053/jars.2003.50128
14. Burkhart SS, Morgan CD, Kibler WB. The disabled throwing shoulder: spectrum of pathology Part III: The SICK scapula, scapular dyskinesis, the kinetic chain, and rehabilitation. Arthroscopy 2003;19(6):641–661. Accessed December 6, 2016
15. Drakos MC, Rudzki JR, Allen AA, Potter HG, Altchek DW. Internal impingement of the shoulder in the overhead athlete. J Bone Joint Surg Am 2009;91(11):2719–2728 10.2106/JBJS.I.00409
16. Paley KJ, Jobe FW, Pink MM, Kvitne RS, ElAttrache NS. Arthroscopic findings in the overhand throwing athlete: evidence for posterior internal impingement of the rotator cuff. Arthroscopy 2000;16(1):35–40. Accessed December 6, 2016
17. Grossman MG, Tibone JE, McGarry MH, Schneider DJ, Veneziani S, Lee TQ. A cadaveric model of the throwing shoulder: a possible etiology of superior labrum anterior-to-posterior lesions. J Bone Joint Surg Am 2005;87(4):824–831 10.2106/JBJS.D.01972
18. Huffman GR, Tibone JE, McGarry MH, Phipps BM, Lee YS, Lee TQ. Path of glenohumeral articulation throughout the rotational range of motion in a thrower's shoulder model. Am J Sports Med 2006;34(10):1662–1669 10.1177/0363546506287740
19. Edelson G, Teitz C. Internal impingement in the shoulder. J Shoulder Elbow Surg 2000;9(4):308–315 10.1067/mse.2000.105449
20. Burkhart SS, Morgan CD. The peel-back mechanism: its role in producing and extending posterior type II SLAP lesions and its effect on SLAP repair rehabilitation. Arthroscopy 1998;14(6):637–640
21. Andrews JR, Carson WG Jr, McLeod WD. Glenoid labrum tears related to the long head of the biceps. Am J Sports Med 1985;13(5):337–341
22. Bigliani LU, Codd TP, Connor PM, Levine WN, Littlefield MA, Hershon SJ. Shoulder motion and laxity in the professional baseball player. Am J Sports Med 1997;25(5):609–613
23. Lombardo SJ, Jobe FW, Kerlan RK, Carter VS, Shields CL Jr. Posterior shoulder lesions in throwing athletes. Am J Sports Med 1977;5(3):106–110. Accessed December 6, 2016
24. Kaplan LD, McMahon PJ, Towers J, Irrgang JJ, Rodosky MW. Internal impingement: findings on magnetic resonance imaging and arthroscopic evaluation. Arthroscopy 2004;20(7):701–704 10.1016/j.arthro.2004.06.006
25. Meister K, Buckley B, Batts J. The posterior impingement sign: diagnosis of rotator cuff and posterior labral tears secondary to internal impingement in overhand athletes. Am J Orthop 2004;33(8):412–415
26. Bennett GE. Elbow and shoulder lesions of baseball players : George E. Bennett MD (1885-1962). The 8th president of the AAOS 1939. Clin Orthop Relat Res 2008;466(1):62–73 10.1007/s11999-007-0028-z
27. Bennett GE. Shoulder and elbow lesions distinctive of baseball players. 1947. Clin Orthop Relat Res 2012;470(6):1531–1533 10.1007/s11999-012-2335-2

28. Connell DA, Potter HG, Wickiewicz TL, Altchek DW, Warren RF. Noncontrast magnetic resonance imaging of superior labral lesions. 102 cases confirmed at arthroscopic surgery. Am J Sports Med 1999;27(2):208–213
29. Giaroli EL, Major NM, Higgins LD. MRI of internal impingement of the shoulder. AJR Am J Roentgenol 2005;185(4):925–929 10.2214/AJR.04.0971
30. Connor PM, Banks DM, Tyson AB, Coumas JS, D'Alessandro DF. Magnetic resonance imaging of the asymptomatic shoulder of overhead athletes: a 5-year follow-up study. Am J Sports Med 2003;31(5):724–727. Accessed December 26, 2016
31. Matava MJ, Purcell DB, Rudzki JR. Partial-thickness rotator cuff tears. Am J Sports Med 2005;33(9):1405–1417 10.1177/0363546505280213
32. Wilk KE, Meister K, Andrews JR. Current concepts in the rehabilitation of the overhead throwing athlete. Am J Sports Med 2002;30(1):136–151
33. Yoneda M, Nakagawa S, Hayashida K, Fukushima S, Wakitani S. Arthroscopic removal of symptomatic Bennett lesions in the shoulders of baseball players: arthroscopic Bennett-plasty. Am J Sports Med 2002;30(5):728–736
34. Dugas JR, Campbell DA, Warren RF, Robie BH, Millett PJ. Anatomy and dimensions of rotator cuff insertions. J Shoulder Elbow Surg 2002;11(5):498–503 10.1067/mse.2002.126208
35. Tibone JE, Elrod B, Jobe FW, et al. Surgical treatment of tears of the rotator cuff in athletes. J Bone Joint Surg Am 1986;68(6):887–891. Accessed January 28, 2017
36. Mazoué CG, Andrews JR. Repair of full-thickness rotator cuff tears in professional baseball players. Am J Sports Med 2006;34(2):182–189 10.1177/0363546505279916
37. Curtis AS, Burbank KM, Tierney JJ, Scheller AD, Curran AR. The insertional footprint of the rotator cuff: an anatomic study. Arthroscopy 2006;22(6):609.e1 10.1016/j.arthro.2006.04.001
38. Liu J, Hughes RE, O'Driscoll SW, An KN. Biomechanical effect of medial advancement of the supraspinatus tendon. A study in cadavera. J Bone Joint Surg Am 1998;80(6):853–859
39. Lo IKY, Burkhart SS. Double-row arthroscopic rotator cuff repair: re-establishing the footprint of the rotator cuff. Arthroscopy 2003;19(9):1035–1042
40. Brockmeier SF, Dodson CC, Gamradt SC, Coleman SH, Altchek DW. Arthroscopic intratendinous repair of the delaminated partial-thickness rotator cuff tear in overhead athletes. Arthroscopy 2008;24(8):961–965. doi:10.1016/j.arthro.2007.08.016
41. Ruotolo C, Price E, Panchal A. Loss of total arc of motion in collegiate baseball players. J Shoulder Elbow Surg 2006;15(1):67–71. doi:10.1016/j.jse.2005.05.006

Part II

Instability

19 Arthroscopic Treatment of Multidirectional Instability

Diana Patterson and Leesa M. Galatz

Abstract

Multidirectional shoulder instability (MDI) continues to avoid standardized diagnosis or categorization. It can present in a wide range of situations, from macrotrauma to repetitive microtrauma accumulation to hyperlaxity with atraumatic, but pathologic, instability. Patients may complain of vague, activity-specific pain, the sensation of loose shoulders, or a variety of other symptoms, but not always with a discrete dislocation event. Examination of the shoulder should include an exam of the contralateral shoulder, as the pathologic side may not actually be more lax than the symptomatic one, an assessment of Beighton criteria, and special maneuvers to identify instability in specific directions. The main role of imaging in the diagnosis and treatment of MDI is in excluding other causes of pain or instability. Historically, treatment for MDI included a prolonged course of physical therapy and maybe an open inferior capsular shift. However, arthroscopic procedures now show comparable results to open procedures. Thermal capsulorrhaphy has been shown to be detrimental and has been abandoned. Arthroscopic capsular plication has shown equal outcomes to open inferior capsular shift. Rotator interval closure was originally thought to be critical to success, but is performed increasingly rarely, as concern for excessive loss of motion outweighs theoretical benefits. The most serious complication following arthroscopic treatment of MDI is axillary nerve injury. As surgical indications becomes refined and arthroscopic technique and technology advance, it is expected that these outcomes will continue to improve.

Keywords: *multidirectional shoulder instability, rotator interval, hyperlaxity, capsular plication*

19.1 Introduction

Multidirectional instability (MDI) of the shoulder is a diagnosis that continues to defy specific or standardized criteria. Neer and Foster first coined the term and they are widely recognized for bringing it widespread clinical attention. In 1980, they defined MDI as anterior and posterior instability associated with involuntary inferior subluxation or dislocation.[1] Others then described it as instability in two or three directions.[2] And, shortly thereafter, Matsen divided shoulder instability into two subtypes: (1) traumatic and unidirectional, containing a Bankart lesion and which is treated surgically (TUBS) and (2) atraumatic, multidirectional, and bilateral, which responds to rehabilitation but may require an inferior capsular shift for surgical treatment (AMBRI).[3] These categories are helpful for general classification, but it is important not to oversimplify and thus potentially underdiagnose multidirectional shoulder instability. For example, patients with true MDI commonly present with only unilateral symptoms, may only present following a traumatic event to the shoulder, and some do have intra-articular lesions. Such discrepancies in definition make determination of its true prevalence and comparison of clinical and research studies difficult.[4]

The etiology of MDI is multifactorial, and theories focus on anatomic, biochemical, and neuromuscular abnormalities and their interplay. The characteristic pathologic entity of MDI is increased capsular redundancy. It may be acquired, or be due to a systemic disease, such as Ehlers–Danlos, osteogenesis imperfecta, Marfan's syndrome, facioscapulohumeral dystrophy, or benign hypermobility syndrome. The capsular tissue of shoulders with MDI has qualitative and quantitative differences in the collagen when compared with controls. However, as the majority of patients with MDI do not have symptoms from birth, a component of MDI must be developed. Excessive capsular volume alone is not significant enough to cause symptoms. Acquired capsular laxity and symptomatic instability may be due to several pathologic pathways. Repeated minor injuries to the joint capsule, repetitive microtrauma during sport-specific activities, particularly overhead throwing, or work, can develop into global laxity and symptomatic instability in more than one direction, with or without labral injury. Alternatively, an isolated macrotrauma event can cause a significant circumferential injury to the capsulolabral complex, supportive structures, resulting in symptoms; this single event can be relatively minor but a "tipping point" in patients with baseline hyperlaxity.

Historically, treatment for MDI included a prolonged course of physical therapy, and, if patients failed, open inferior capsular shift. However, arthroscopic procedures are increasingly widespread and show comparable results to open procedures. Given the varied presentations of patients with MDI, from macrotrauma to repetitive microtrauma or minor injury accumulation to hyperlaxity with atraumatic but pathologic instability, it is necessary for surgeons to best identify patients who may benefit from arthroscopic interventions.

19.2 Clinical Presentation and History

Patients with MDI commonly present with complaints of vague pain without specific onset, and more rarely of instability. Patients may report degrees of painful "loose" shoulders, including the sensation of popping, clicking, grinding, pain with throwing, lifting overhead, or sleeping. In patients who present with painful or symptomatic hyperlaxity, the amount of laxity is not usually significantly different from their contralateral side; differentiating between normal laxity and instability can be intricate and requires a high level of clinical suspicion.

Cofield and Irving presented four questions to address in the workup of MDI: (1) What is the relationship to trauma? (2) Does the patient intentionally cause the instability? (3) What is the degree of instability? (4) What is the direction of instability? A single traumatic event can be responsible for tipping a patient with hyperlaxity into symptomatic instability.[5] This is particularly true if one includes repetitive use or other loss of the dynamic stabilizers in the definition of a "trauma."[6] Patients younger than 40 years with history of failed surgery for unidirectional instability should be reevaluated for MDI.[2]

Specific complaints can help provide clues as to the direction of symptomatic instability and begin to direct treatment options. Inferior instability can cause pain, numbness, and

19.9 Conclusion

Multidirectional shoulder instability can be a difficult diagnosis to make appropriately on a patient's initial presentation. It can have both vague, nonspecific complaints and a clinical history that appears at first glance to indicate straightforward unidirectional stability. Imaging is not consistently helpful. Preliminary treatment is most commonly a course of prolonged and specific physical therapy to strengthen the dynamic stabilizers of the glenohumeral joint. For those patients who do not improve with therapy or, as studies have shown, those who present with a traumatic inciting event, arthroscopic capsular
plication is an excellent option. Overall outcomes following arthroscopic plication and repair of concurrent soft-tissue pathology can provide excellent results and return to play, even in overhead athletes. As surgical indications become refined and arthroscopic technique and technology advance, it is expected that these outcomes will continue to improve.

References

1. Neer CS II, Foster CR. Inferior capsular shift for involuntary inferior and multidirectional instability of the shoulder. A preliminary report. J Bone Joint Surg Am 1980;62(6):897–908
2. Gaskill TR, Taylor DC, Millett PJ. Management of multidirectional instability of the shoulder. J Am Acad Orthop Surg 2011;19(12):758–767
3. Matsen FAGlenohumeral Instability. 2nd ed. Philadelphia, PA: WB Saunders;1998
4. McFarland EG, Kim TK, Park HB, Neira CA, Gutierrez MI. The effect of variation in definition on the diagnosis of multidirectional instability of the shoulder. J Bone Joint Surg Am 2003;85-A(11):2138–2144
5. Cofield RH, Irving JF. Valuation and classification of shoulder instability. With special reference to examination under anesthesia. Clin Orthop Relat Res. 1987 Oct;(223):32-43
6. Lee HJ, Kim NR, Moon SG, Ko SM, Park JY. Multidirectional instability of the shoulder: rotator interval dimension and capsular laxity evaluation using MR arthrography. Skeletal Radiol 2013;42(2):231–238
7. Gagey OJ, Gagey N. The hyperabduction test. J Bone Joint Surg Br. 2001 Jan;83(1):69-74.
8. Sekiya JK, Willobee JA, Miller MD, Hickman AJ, Willobee A. Arthroscopic multi-pleated capsular plication compared with open inferior capsular shift for reduction of shoulder volume in a cadaveric model. Arthroscopy 2007;23(11):1145–1151
9. Harryman DT 2nd, Sidles JA, Harris SL, Matsen FA 3rd. The role of the rotator interval capsule in passive motion and stability of the shoulder. J Bone Joint Surg Am. 1992 Jan;74(1):53-66.
10. McIntyre LF, Caspari RB, Savoie FH III. The arthroscopic treatment of multidirectional shoulder instability: two-year results of a multiple suture technique. Arthroscopy 1997;13(4):418–425
11. Gartsman GM, Roddey TS, Hammerman SM. Arthroscopic treatment of bidirectional glenohumeral instability: two- to five-year follow-up. J Shoulder Elbow Surg 2001;10(1):28–36
12. Longo UG, Rizzello G, Loppini M, et al. Multidirectional instability of the shoulder: a systematic review. Arthroscopy 2015;31(12):2431–2443

20 Arthroscopic Anterior Stabilization

Lawrence V. Gulotta and Alejandro Novoa-Boldo

Abstract

The purpose of this chapter is to review the indications, preoperative preparation, surgical technique and postoperative care in the arthroscopic Bankart repair in patients with anterior shoulder instability. When a stabilization procedure is indicated, the arthroscopic treatment is the first choice for many surgeons due to its lower morbidity and low overall complication rate. It is very important to detect and measure bone deficiency in the humerus and the glenoid to ensure better outcomes. Using knotless suture anchors allow for a technically easier and faster surgery with the advantage of not having the knot that could cause irritation to the surrounding cartilage and soft-tissue structures.

Keywords: *shoulder arthroscopy, instability, Bankart repair, operative technique, labral repair*

20.1 Goals of Procedure

- Repair the Bankart lesion and the anterior capsulolabral complex.
- Restore stability to the glenohumeral joint.
- Improve function.

20.2 Indications

- Recurrent anterior instability of the glenohumeral joint.
- Subluxation of the glenohumeral joint during sports activity that does not improve with physical therapy.
- Following a first-time dislocation in a patient in an "at-risk" population.

20.3 Contraindications

- Bony deficiencies involving more than 25% of the anteroinferior glenoid surface or large engaging Hill–Sachs lesions are better served with bone grafting procedures such as the Latarjet.
- Instability with humeral avulsion of the glenohumeral ligament (HAGL) lesion.
- Patients with brachial plexus or scapulothoracic dysfunction.
- Severe medical comorbidity burden precluding surgical intervention.
- Habitual or voluntary dislocations.

20.4 Preoperative Preparation/ Positioning

20.4.1 Clinical Evaluation

- A complete patient history is mandatory. This should include patient's age, associated conditions, such as seizures, neuromuscular disorders, or collagen deficiencies, traumatic events that resulted in instability, arm position at the moment of the accident, energy level of the lesion, how and when the reduction took place, the treatment after the reduction, and the number of dislocations.
- Physical examination should assess shoulder instability with provocative tests such as anterior apprehension, the Jobe relocation test, active compression test, load and shift test, sulcus test, and determination of generalized ligamentous laxity.

20.4.2 Imaging

- Radiographs should include anteroposterior (AP) shoulder views in internal and external rotation, a true AP Grashey view, West Point view, Stryker notch view, axillary view, and the transcapular (Y) view. The AP views in internal and external rotation demonstrate a Hill–Sachs lesion. The true AP demonstrates any erosion of the anterior glenoid rim. The West Point view is useful to study glenoid bone loss. The Stryker notch view is used to evaluate the humeral head Hill–Sachs lesions. Axillary view helps observe bony Bankart lesions and erosion of the anteroinferior portion of the glenoid rim. The transcapular (Y) view permits us to observe anterior or posterior translation of the humeral head with respect to the glenoid.
- CT is used for detecting and measuring bone deficiency in the humerus with Hill–Sachs lesions or in the glenoid with bony Bankart lesions (**Fig. 20.1**).

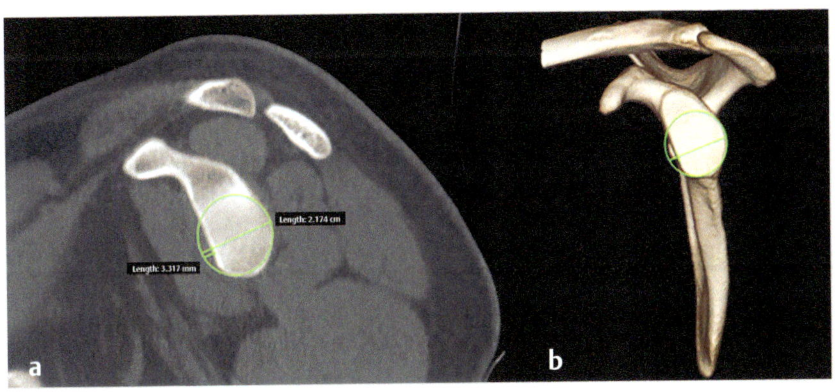

Fig. 20.1 CT sagittal **(a)** and 3D reconstruction **(b)** views used to determine glenoid bone loss.

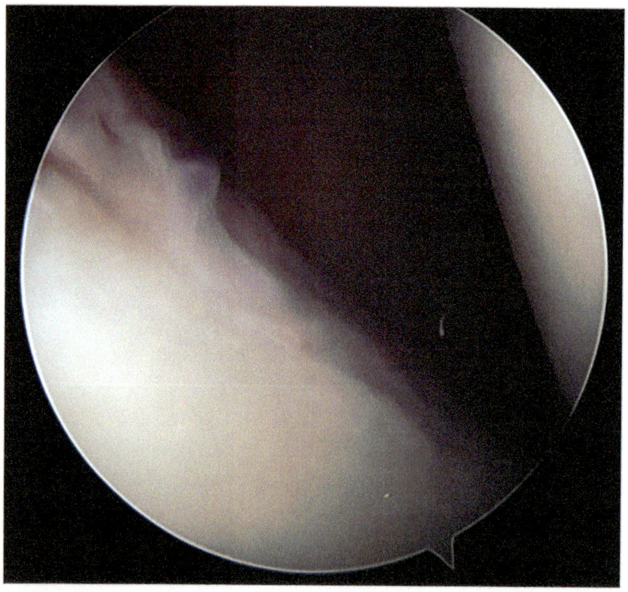

Fig. 20.9 Scarred labrum to the anteroinferior neck of the glenoid.

- An elevator or rasp from the anteroinferior portal is used to release the remaining labral and capsular tissue from the anteroinferior part of the glenoid, all the way down to the subscapularis muscle belly (**Fig. 20.12a, b**).
- The released tissue mobility is assessed with a grasper from the anteroinferior portal, to be sure it can be reduced back to the articular surface.

20.5.3 Glenoid Preparation

- The anterior rim of the glenoid is prepared with the shaver entering the joint from the anteroinferior portal leaving a decorticated bleeding bone bed that leads to a better healing of the labrum without the scar tissue and sclerotic bone left from the lesion (**Fig. 20.13**).

20.5.4 Tissue Capture and Anchor Insertion

- The first anchor is placed at the 5 o'clock position in the glenoid as follows:
  - The arthroscope will enter the joint from the anterolateral portal (**Fig. 20.14**).

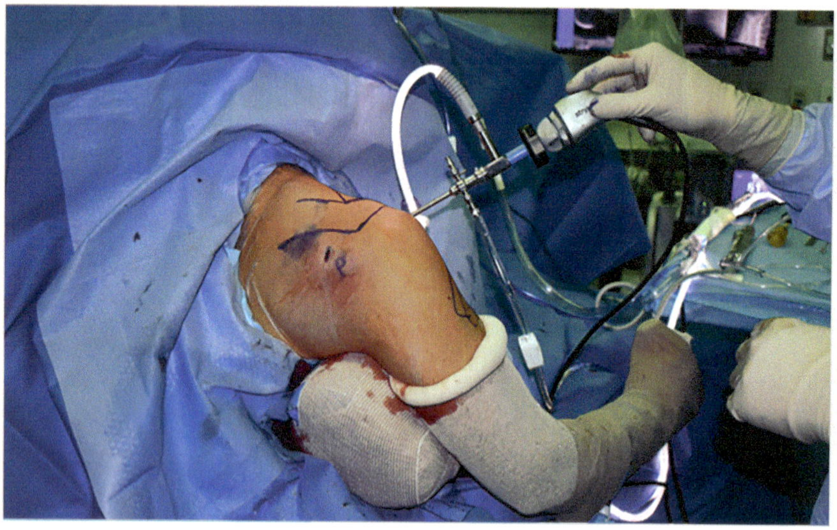

Fig. 20.10 Sterile bump situated under the armpit.

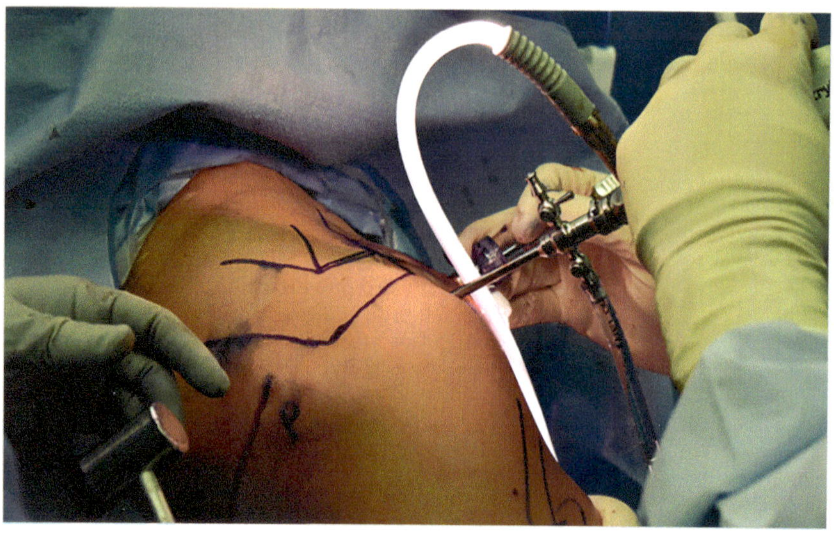

Fig. 20.11 Arthroscope situated in the (AL) portal and the elevator in the (A) portal to release the labral and capsular tissue from the glenoid.

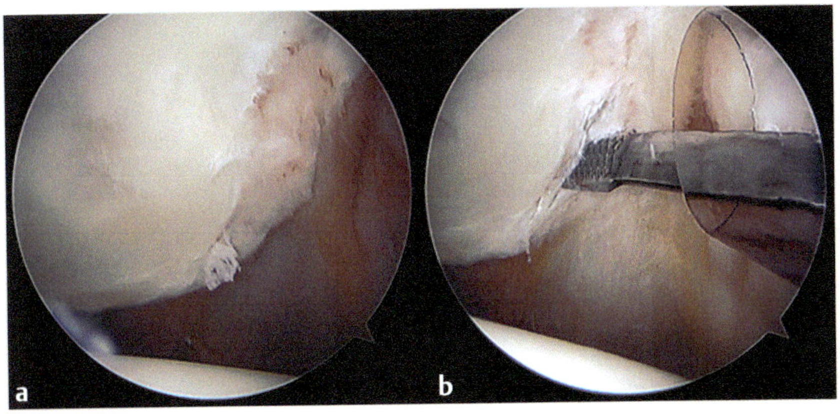

Fig. 20.12 (a) Anteroinferior labrum lesion visualized from the (AL) portal. (b) Anteroinferior labral tissue being released from the glenoid.

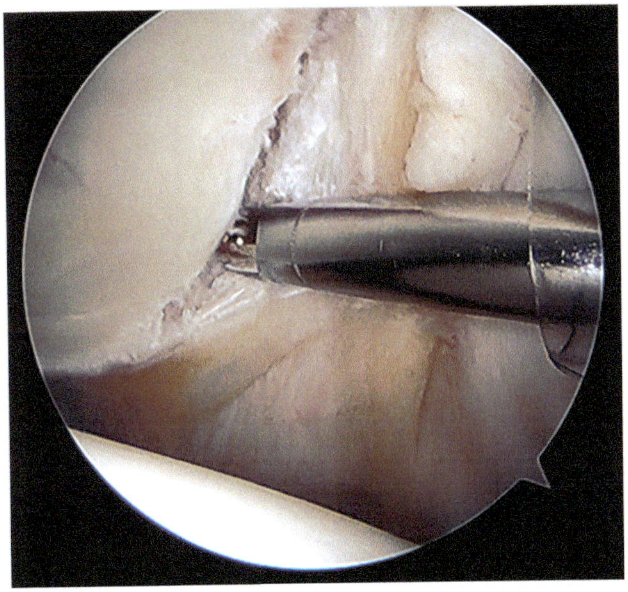

Fig. 20.13 Decortication of the glenoid rim with the shaver from the (A) portal.

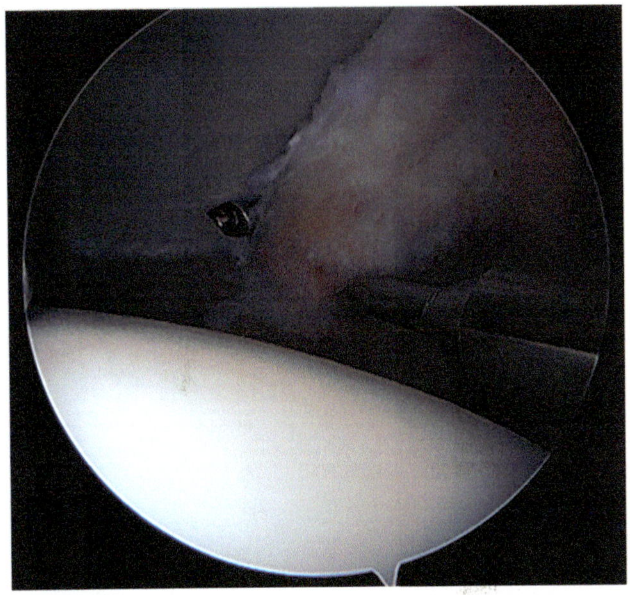

Fig. 20.15 SutureLasso passing through the capsulolabral tissue entering the joint from the (A) portal.

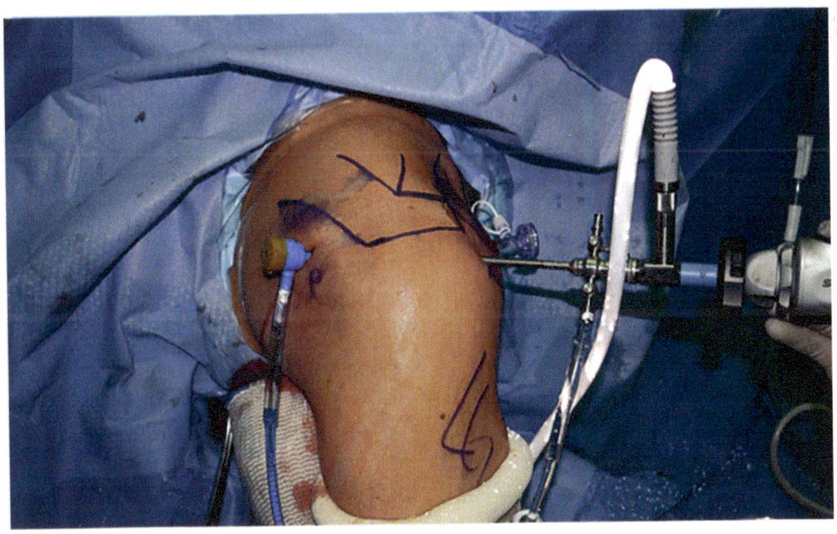

Fig. 20.14 Arthroscope entering the joint from the (AL) portal to place the most inferior anchor.

- A curved suture passing device such as a SutureLasso with a no. 2 FiberWire Suture Stick (Arthrex, Naples, FL) is placed through the anteroinferior cannula and passed through the capsulolabral tissue (**Fig. 20.15**).
- The Fiber Stick tail is retrieved through the posterior portal and secured with a Kelly clamp (**Fig. 20.16**).
- The SutureLasso is then backed out of the tissue without removing it from the joint; then it is passed through the tissue a second time to create an oblique mattress suture (**Fig. 20.17**).
- The suture is then retrieved with a suture retriever through the posterior portal (**Fig. 20.18**).

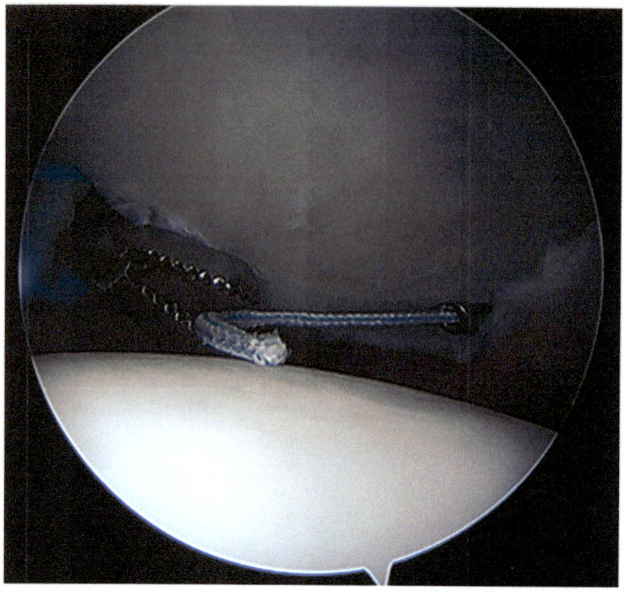

Fig. 20.16 Suture stick retrieved through the posterior portal.

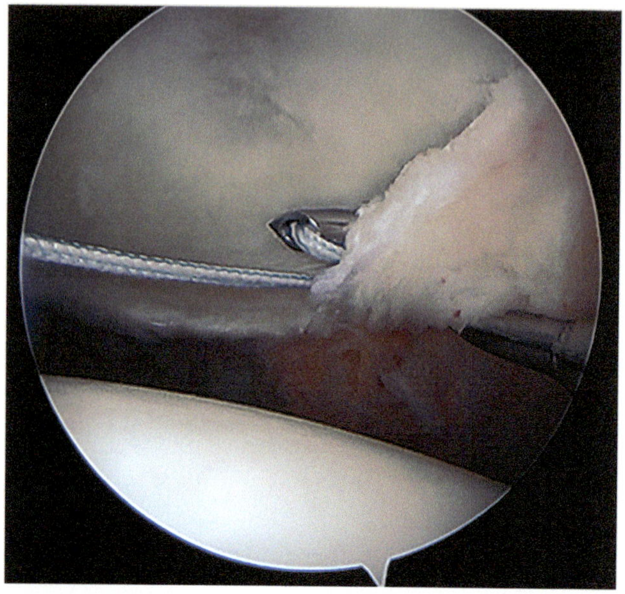

Fig. 20.17 SutureLasso passing a second time through the tissue creating an oblique mattress suture. Observe how the fiber wire is not engaged on the tip of the SutureLasso.

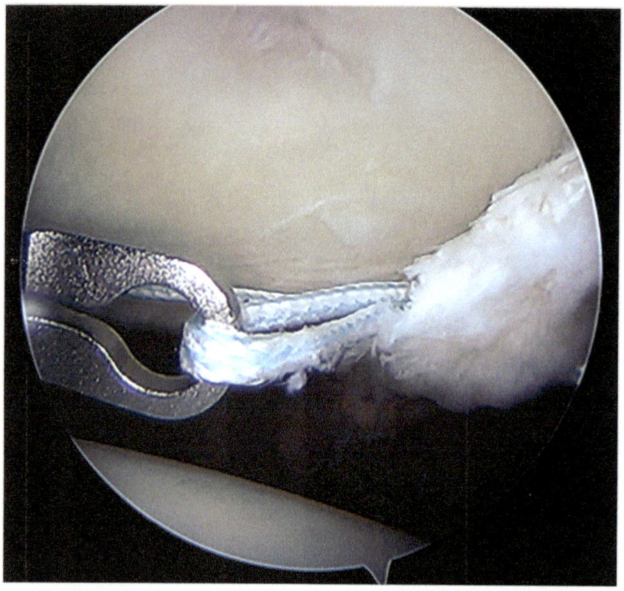

Fig. 20.18 Retrieving the suture through the (P) portal with the suture retriever.

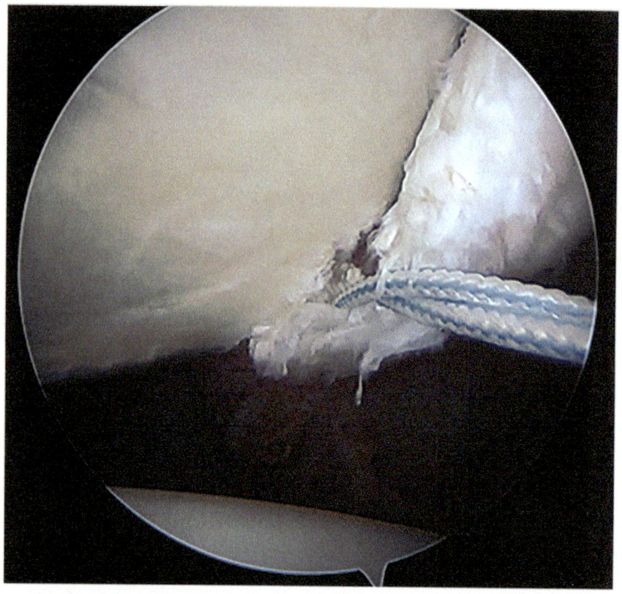

Fig. 20.19 Fiber wire shuttled through the cannula situated in the anteroinferior portal before the anchor placing.

- Both ends of the fiber wire are then shuttled through the cannula situated in the anteroinferior portal and inserted into the eyelet of the 2.9 BioComposite PushLock and secured with a Kelly clamp (**Fig. 20.19**).
- The drill guide is inserted through the cannula in the anteroinferior portal and placed in the glenoid rim to drill the bone socket. The anchor should be placed superior to where the sutures are in the tissue. This allows the tissue to be translated from inferior to superior (**Fig. 20.20**).
- The sutures are then tensioned and the anchor is slid into the joint and inside the drill hole until the anchor is in contact with the glenoid (**Fig. 20.21**). It is helpful to bring the anchor to the tissue, then as one unit move the anchor into the pilot hole and then impact and deploy the anchor.
- The sutures are then cut so as to leave as little tail as possible to avoid irritation to the surrounding cartilage and soft-tissue structures.

• Insertion of the remaining anchors: Additional anchors are placed continuously from inferior to superior advancing and retensioning the capsulolabral complex:
  - The arthroscope is moved to the posterior portal.
  - A 5.75-mm cannula is placed in the anterolateral portal (**Fig. 20.22a, b**).
  - A tissue grasper is inserted through the anterolateral portal cannula to pull the capsulolabral tissue up to advance it to the desired position.

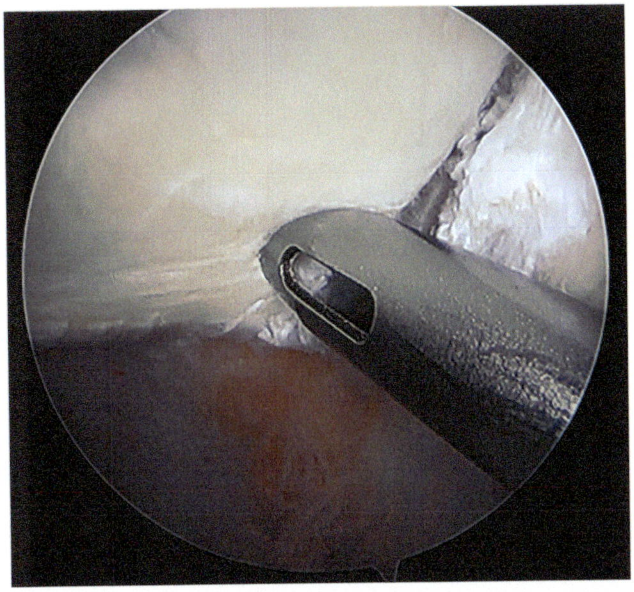

Fig. 20.20 The drill guide inserted through the (A) portal and placed on the glenoid rim.

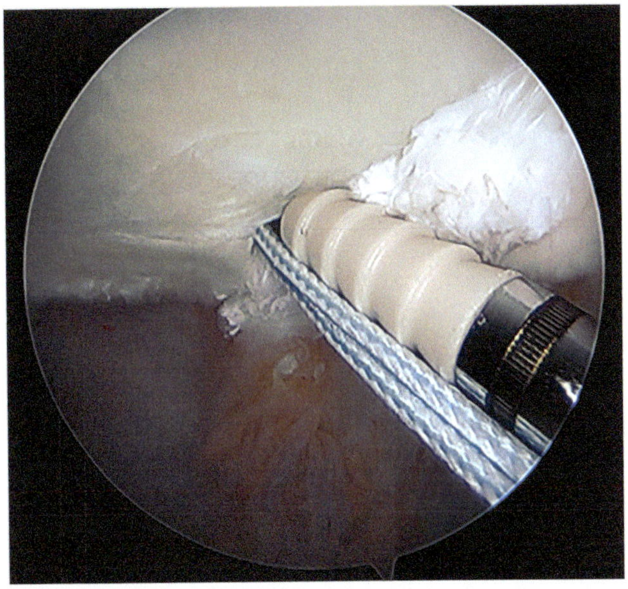

Fig. 20.21 Anchor placed from the (A) portal.

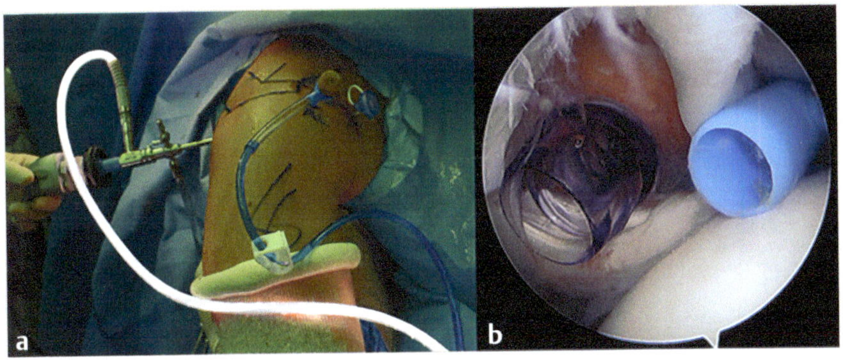

Fig. 20.22 Arthroscope entering from the (P) portal, 8.25-mm cannula in the (A) portal, 5.5-mm cannula in the (AL) portal. **(a)** Outside and **(b)** arthroscopic views.

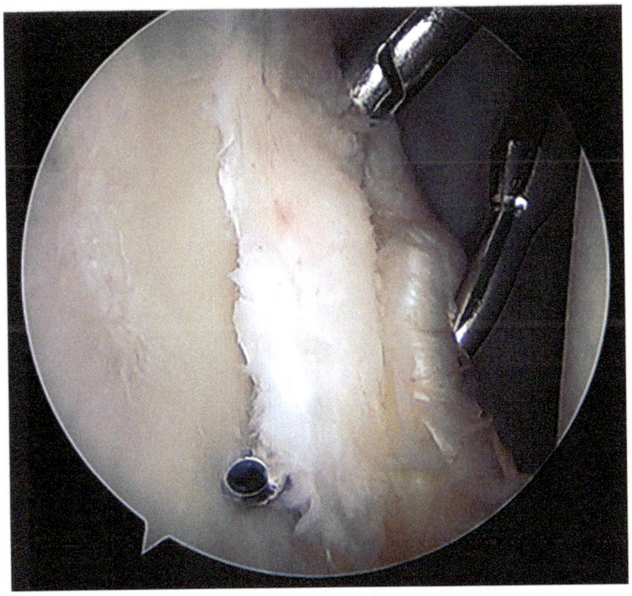

Fig. 20.23 The tissue grasper pulling up the capsulolabral tissue in order to make the first stitch with the SutureLasso.

- The SutureLasso with the no. 2 Fiber Stick is inserted through the cannula situated in the anteroinferior portal and passed through the capsulolabral tissue at approximately 5 to 7 mm from the previous anchor (**Fig. 20.23**).
- The Fiber Stick tail is retrieved through the anterolateral portal and secured with a clamp (**Fig. 20.24**).
- The SutureLasso is again moved out of the tissue without removing it from the joint, and then it is passed through a second time to create an oblique mattress suture.
- The fiber wire is retrieved with a Suture Retriever through the anterolateral superior portal.
- Both ends of the fiber wire are shuttled through the cannula situated in the anteroinferior portal and then threaded through the eyelet of a 2.9 BioComposite PushLock and secured with a clamp.
- The drill guide is again inserted through the cannula in the anteroinferior portal and placed on the glenoid rim just superior to where the sutures were placed through the labrum.
- The sutures are tensioned and the anchor is inserted and deployed.
- Sutures are cut as short as possible (**Fig. 20.25**).

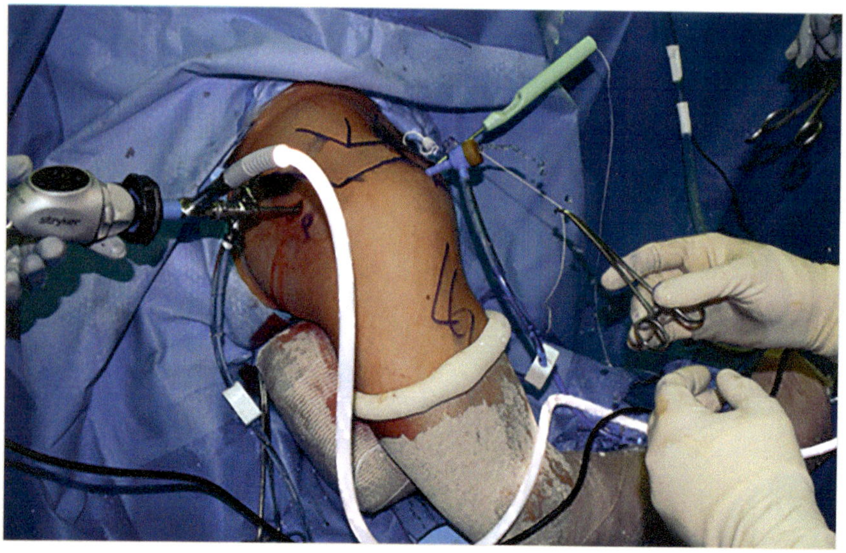

Fig. 20.24 The fiber wire is retrieved from the (AL) portal and secured with a clamp after the first stitch of the oblique mattress suture.

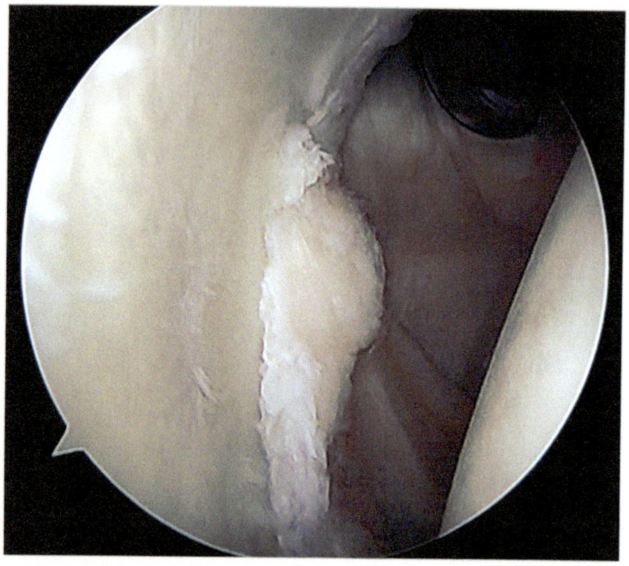

Fig. 20.25 The sutures are cut close to the bone to avoid irritation to the surrounding cartilage and soft-tissue structures.

20.5.5 Complete the Repair

- Additional anchors are placed in an identical fashion until the construct is complete.
- It is important to continue advancing the repaired labrum from inferior to superior in order to retension the capsulolabral complex.
- The final construct is then evaluated with the hooked probe.

20.5.6 Closure

- Remove all the cannulas.
- Close the portals with 3–0 Prolene.
- Cover them with sterile dressing.
- Place the arm in a sling.

20.6 Tips and Pearls/Expert Suggestions

- In order to distract the joint in the beach-chair position, a sterile bump can be placed in the axilla and the arm can be adducted. This "jacks" the joint open and creates space to work.
- Visualization through the anterolateral portal can help with mobilization of the labrum when it is scarred to the anterior glenoid neck.
- The tissue grasper should be used to manipulate the tissue when you are passing the SutureLasso through the capsulolabral tissue in order to advance the construct superiorly.
- Be sure that the fiber wire is not engaged in the tip of the SutureLasso when you are doing the second stitch of the mattress suture as it can cut the sutures.

20.7 Complications

- Recurrent instability: It can be presented in approximately 10% of the patients.
- Nerve injury: The axillary nerve can be injured when placing sutures at the 6 o'clock position.
- Stiffness: It may be present in elder patients (older than 40 years) and may be resolved with physiotherapy.
- Infection: It is very rare, but it may occur; a culture of the synovial fluid is recommended

20.8 Postoperative Care

- The arm is placed in a shoulder immobilizer for 4 weeks.
- Patients are discharged the same day of the surgery.
- The portal wounds stay covered and dry until the stitch removal (10–12 days).
- The patient is instructed on how to do distal range-of-motion exercises on their own for the first 4 weeks following surgery.

- After 4 weeks, the shoulder immobilizer is discontinued and physical therapy begins with the primary goal to achieve full active range of motion.
- Three months after the surgery, the patient may begin strength training.
- Six months after the surgery, the patient can be fully reintegrated to his daily and sports activities.

Suggested Readings

Su B, Levine WN. Arthroscopic Bankart repair. J Am Acad Orthop Surg 2005;13(7):487–490

DeFroda S, Bokshan S, Stern E, Sullivan K, Owens BD. Arthroscopic Bankart repair for the management of anterior shoulder instability: indications and outcomes. Curr Rev Musculoskelet Med 2017;10(4):442–451

Seroyer ST, Nho SJ, Provencher MT, Romeo AA. Four-quadrant approach to capsulolabral repair: an arthroscopic road map to the glenoid. Arthroscopy 2010;26(4):555–562

Matsuki K, Sugaya H. Complications after arthroscopic labral repair for shoulder instability. Curr Rev Musculoskelet Med 2015;8(1):53–58

21 Open Anterior Stabilization (Bankart/Capsular Shift)

Tim Wang

Abstract

The open Bankart procedure remains the gold standard for treating anterior shoulder instability. Though the rise of arthroscopic shoulder stabilization procedures have decreased its utilization, there remain certain clinical scenarios where traditional open techniques offer a clinical advantage over arthroscopic approaches. This chapter reviews the indications and pearls for visualization and obtaining a mechanically secure repair.

Keywords: *open bankart, shoulder stabilization, anterior shoulder surgery*

21.1 Goals of Procedure

Goals of management for shoulder instability includes achieving stable shoulder for occupational and/or sporting activities, while at the same time minimizing iatrogenic motion loss. Surgically, this includes repairing any labral tear to its native position with an associated capsular plication to reduce capsular volume.

21.2 Advantages

The open Bankart procedure remains the gold standard for treating anterior shoulder instability, with durable results at long-term follow-up. Advances in technology and techniques have led to the rise in arthroscopic management of shoulder instability.[1,2] In meta-analyses, arthroscopic methods have been shown to have similar results to open techniques for anterior instability, particularly when suture anchors are used.[3–7] Advantages of the open procedure include the ability to precisely set capsular tension for a more comprehensive shift.

However, more recent studies have found open techniques may provide longer time to recurrent instability after surgery.[8,9] These findings may be particularly relevant in the higher risk patient, such as in contact athletes, patulous capsule, or those with glenoid bone loss.[10–13] Even bone loss above 13.5% may result in unacceptably inferior clinical outcomes with isolated arthroscopic labral repair.[14] Recurrent dislocation rates for revision arthroscopic Bankart repair has been reported around 14%,[15,16] compared to 5.5 to 11.5% after open Bankart repair.[17] A recent randomized trial found lower rates of recurrent instability following open Bankart repair compared to arthroscopic Bankart repair, particularly in males younger than 25 years with a preoperative Hill–Sachs lesion.[18]

21.3 Indications

Indications for open Bankart stabilization for anterior instability include (1) revision procedure after failed arthroscopic Bankart or (2) anterior instability in a patient at high risk for recurrent instability following arthroscopic stabilization (such as moderate glenoid bone loss, 13.5–20%), presence of an engaging, "off-track" Hill–Sachs lesion, or high-risk patient (male, age less than 20 years, multiple prior dislocations, contact athlete, and excessive ligamentous laxity).

Indications for open capsular plication for multidirectional instability include revision procedure after failed arthroscopic capsular plication, or primary treatment in high-risk patients (such as excessive soft-tissue laxity in Marfan's syndrome and Ehlers–Danlos syndrome).

21.4 Contraindications

Risks of the procedure include loss of forward flexion and external rotation (ER), which are estimated at approximately 10 degrees.[17] Patients with significant glenoid bone loss (> 20 degrees) should undergo consideration for coracoid transfer procedure or glenoid reconstruction using autograft/allograft. Caution should be utilized when performing open shoulder stabilization in overhead throwing athletes, given the risk of overtensioning and possibly limiting ER.

21.5 Preoperative Preparation/Positioning

We prefer the patient to receive a general anesthetic to allow muscular paralysis for ease of exposure, particularly in young, muscular patients.

The patient is placed in the beach-chair position, with the thorax elevated approximately 45 degrees. The operating room table is rotated 90 degrees to create extra working room around the shoulder. A rolled towel is placed posteriorly along the inferior angle to stabilize the scapula. We use a pneumatic arm holder to assist in positioning of the arm. Prior to prepping and draping, maximal ER should be tested to make sure the edge of the table does not limit exposure. Examination under anesthesia is performed to assess range of motion, as well as load and shift testing.

21.6 Operative Technique

21.6.1 Superficial Dissection

Prior to making the incision, the arm should be placed in slight forward flexion and abduction to take tension off the pectoralis major and deltoid, respectively. The coracoid and axillary fold should first be identified and marked out. The skin incision is planned vertically from the center of the coracoid toward the axillary fold, approximately 6 cm (**Fig. 21.1**). Preinjection of the incision with local anesthetic with diluted epinephrine can be used to aid in both pain control and hemostasis.

The skin and dermis is incised until subcutaneous fat is identified, and the dissection is carried deep using electrocautery until the deltopectoral fascia is identified. The next step is to identify the cephalic vein, which is usually found proximally and medially in the wound. A sharp rake retractor can be used to elevate the medial skin flap, and dissection along the muscular fascia using Metzenbaum scissors will help find the vein. The plane on the medial side of the vein will be developed to allow the vein to be retracted laterally with the deltoid muscle belly. Proximally, there is often a branch from the cephalic vein diving deep in the deltopectoral interval that will require ligation to allow the vein to be fully retracted laterally. Once the vein is freed, the remainder of the deltopectoral interval can be released either bluntly or with the aid of electrocautery.

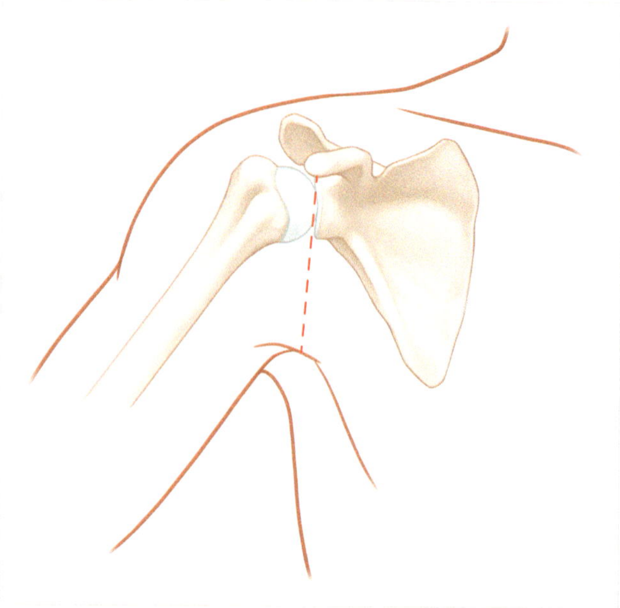

Fig. 21.1 The skin incision for open capsular shift is planned vertically from the coracoid inferiorly towards the axillary fold, approximately 6cm.

21.6.2 Deep Dissection

A Kolbel self-retaining retractor can be used to retract the deltoid laterally and pectoralis medially. The arm is then adducted and externally rotated to bring the lesser tuberosity into view. The clavipectoral fascia is incised lateral to the muscular portion of the conjoint tendon. The deep aspect of the conjoint tendon is bluntly freed with a finger, and the medial blade of the Kolbel retractor is placed deep to the conjoint tendon. Excessive retraction on the conjoint tendon should be avoided to prevent injury to the musculocutaneous nerve, which passes through the conjoint tendon 5 to 8 cm distal to the coracoid. The lesser tuberosity and subscapularis tendon should now be brought into view through arm rotation (**Fig. 21.2**). Ligation of the "three sisters" (anterior humeral circumflex artery and two accompanying veins) using electrocautery is performed at this time.

21.6.3 Subscapularis Dissection

A clean dry sponge can be used to clear off any tissue overlying the subscapularis muscle and tendon. The upper border of the subscapularis is identified by palpation. The axillary nerve should be identified medially and inferiorly along the subscapularis and protected throughout the dissection. Using a blunt elevator (Freer or small periosteal elevator), the junction between the upper two-thirds (tendinous) and lower one-third (muscular) subscapularis muscle is developed in line with the muscle fibers. The elevator is then placed in the plane between the anterior capsule (deep) and subscapularis muscle (superficial) to place tension on the upper two-thirds of the subscapularis. The upper two-thirds of the subscapularis tendon is now released 1 cm medial from its insertion on the lesser tuberosity using a needle-point electrocautery device, which aids in obtaining a more precise dissection. This is often more easily performed when starting at the level of the horizontal split and continuing

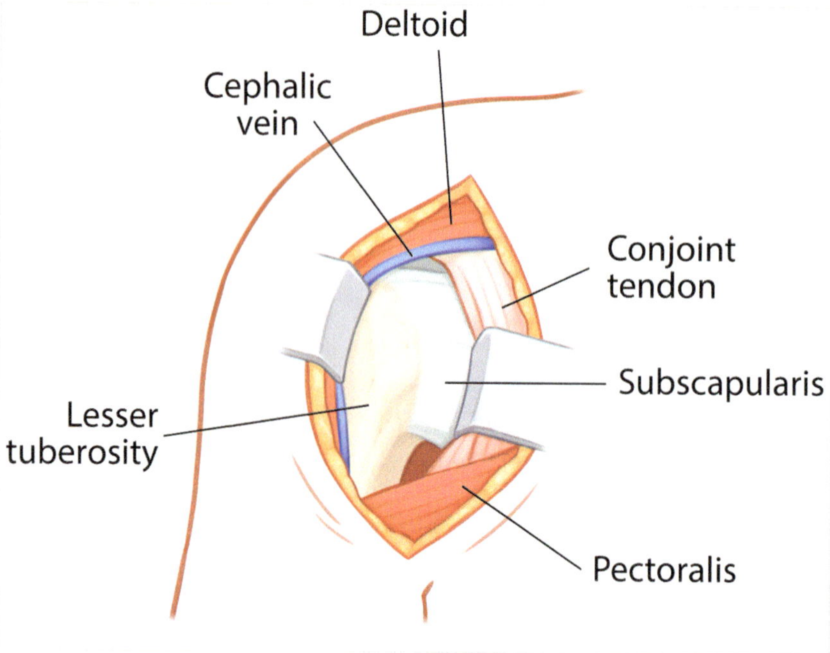

Fig. 21.2 Deep retractors are shown here, retracting the deltoid laterally and conjoint tendon medially. The clavipectoral fascia has been incised in order to visualize the subscapularis insertion onto the lesser tuberosity.

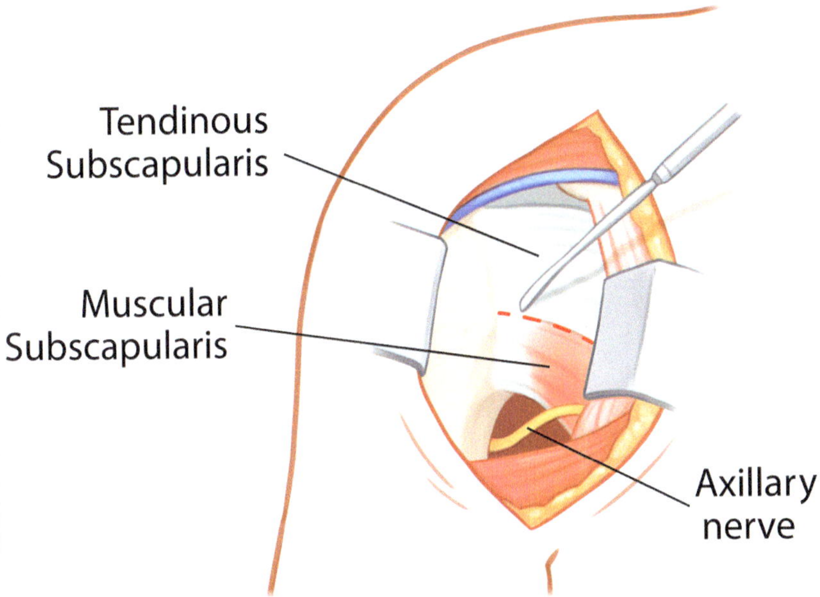

Fig. 21.3 Identification of the upper two-thirds and lower one-third of the subscapularis tendon is made using a blunt elevator.

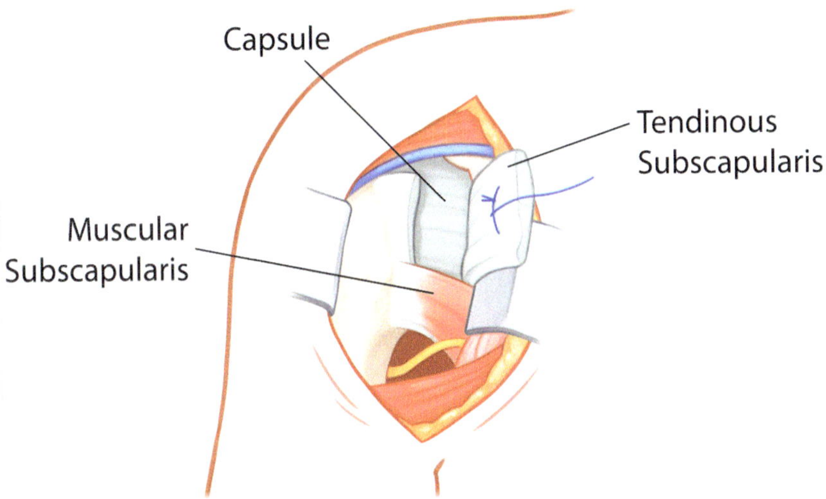

Fig. 21.4 The upper portion of the subscapularis is tagged and retracted medially, exposing the anterior capsule deep.

the release superiorly, as opposed to starting at the superolateral edge of the subscapularis tendon and working inferiorly (**Fig. 21.3**). Take care not to damage the underlying capsule with cautery. The upper portion of the tendon is then tagged with a Mason–Allen type stitch using heaving suture and retracted medially, leaving the more muscular inferior one-third intact (**Fig. 21.4**).

21.6.4 Capsular Release and Glenohumeral Exposure

Once the subscapularis has been appropriately released, the anterior capsule should be visualized. ER of the arm can aid in placing tension on the anterior capsule. A reverse L-shaped capsular release is then made. The transverse limb is through the rotator interval, along the upper border of the subscapularis, and the vertical limb is along the anatomic neck of the humerus to release the anterior capsule from its lateral attachment. The capsular release is continued inferiorly to the 6 o'clock position on the humeral head, externally rotating the arm as dissection proceeds (**Fig. 21.5**). The lateral edge of the anterior capsule is then tagged with heavy suture and retracted medially as well, to expose the anterior capsulolabral complex and glenoid.

21.6.5 Glenoid Preparation

A Fukuda retractor is placed in the glenohumeral joint and a glenoid neck retractor is placed directly on the anterior glenoid, medial to the labrum (**Fig. 21.6**). A Bankart elevator is used to free up the anterior labrum with light taps of a mallet, until it can be mobilized to its normal position along the glenoid rim. The anterior glenoid retractor is adjusted so that it is lateral to the labrum and exposes the anterior glenoid bone. The anterior glenoid rim is prepared using either a motorized shaver or rasp to optimize biologic healing. Caution should be taken to ensure the axillary nerve is not injured, where it travels from anterior to posterior along the inferior edge of the subscapularis. We place three suture anchors into the anterior glenoid (2.4-mm PEEK SutureTak with #2 FiberWire, Arthrex) spaced evenly from the 6 o'clock to the 2 o'clock position (for a right shoulder) (**Fig. 21.7**).

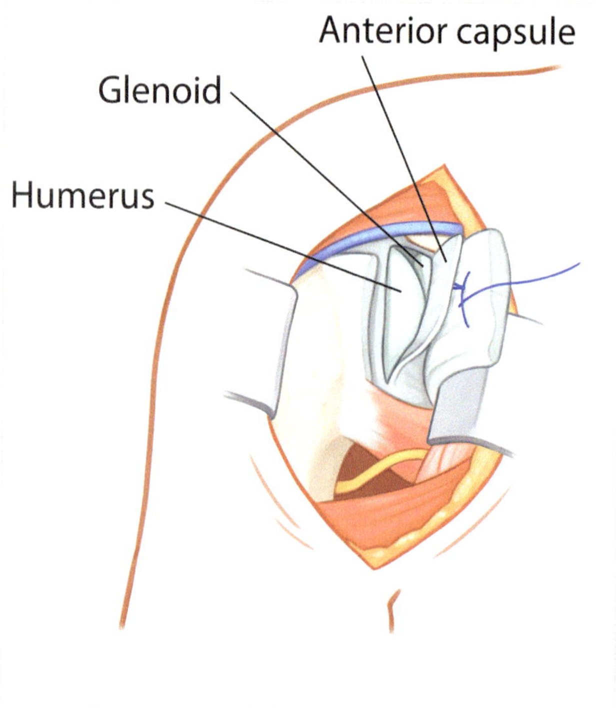

Fig. 21.5 With external rotation, tension is placed on the anterior capsule and it is released laterally along the anatomic neck of the humerus. The transverse limb is through the rotator interval. The capsulotomy continues inferiorly along articular surface of the humeral head.

21.6.6 Labral Repair and Capsular Plication

Labral tears and capsular laxity are addressed separately: the anteroinferior labrum is first repaired to its native position along the anterior glenoid (medially); then the capsular plication is completed along the anatomic humeral neck (laterally).

The anterior glenoid neck retractor is then placed medial to the anterior capsulolabral complex. Sutures from the anterior glenoid anchors are first passed through the anteroinferior labrum in a horizontal mattress fashion, either with a free needle or with the assistance of a suture shuttling device. Suture passing is performed from inferior to superior, with the goal of labral repair only without associated capsular advancement. Once all sutures are passed, they are tied sequentially. The Fukuda retractor is then removed.

Copious irrigation is performed and then the capsular shift is performed. The arm is adjusted to 30 degrees of flexion, 30 degrees of ER, and 30 degrees of abduction (the "30-30-30" position), which will serve as the position for advancement of the capsule and can be adjusted for greater (more internal rotation [IR]) or lesser (more ER) tensioning. The anterior anatomic neck of the humerus is exposed and three double-loaded suture anchors (3.0-mm PEEK SutureTak with no. 2 Fiberwire, Arthrex) are placed spaced evenly from the 6 o'clock to the10 o'clock position (for a right shoulder) (**Fig. 21.8**). The previously placed tagging suture in the anterior capsule is used to pull the anterior capsule maximally superiorly and laterally. Sutures from the anchors are then passed into the anterior capsule in a horizontal mattress fashion and then tied, once all sutures are passed, to complete the capsular shift.

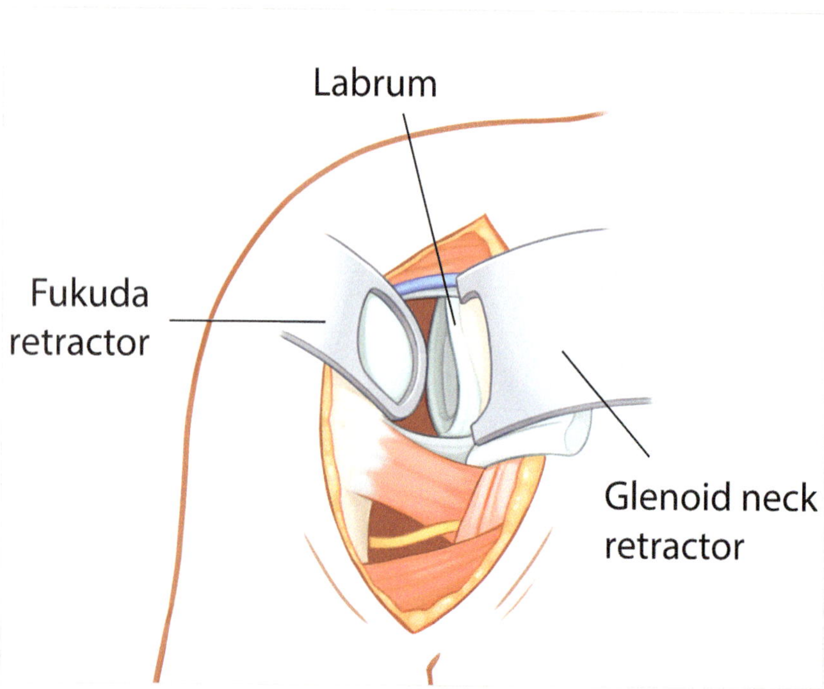

Fig. 21.6 A Fukuda retractor is placed in the glenohumeral joint to retract the humeral head laterally, and a glenoid neck retractor is placed directly on the bony anterior glenoid, medial to the labrum to expose the labrum.

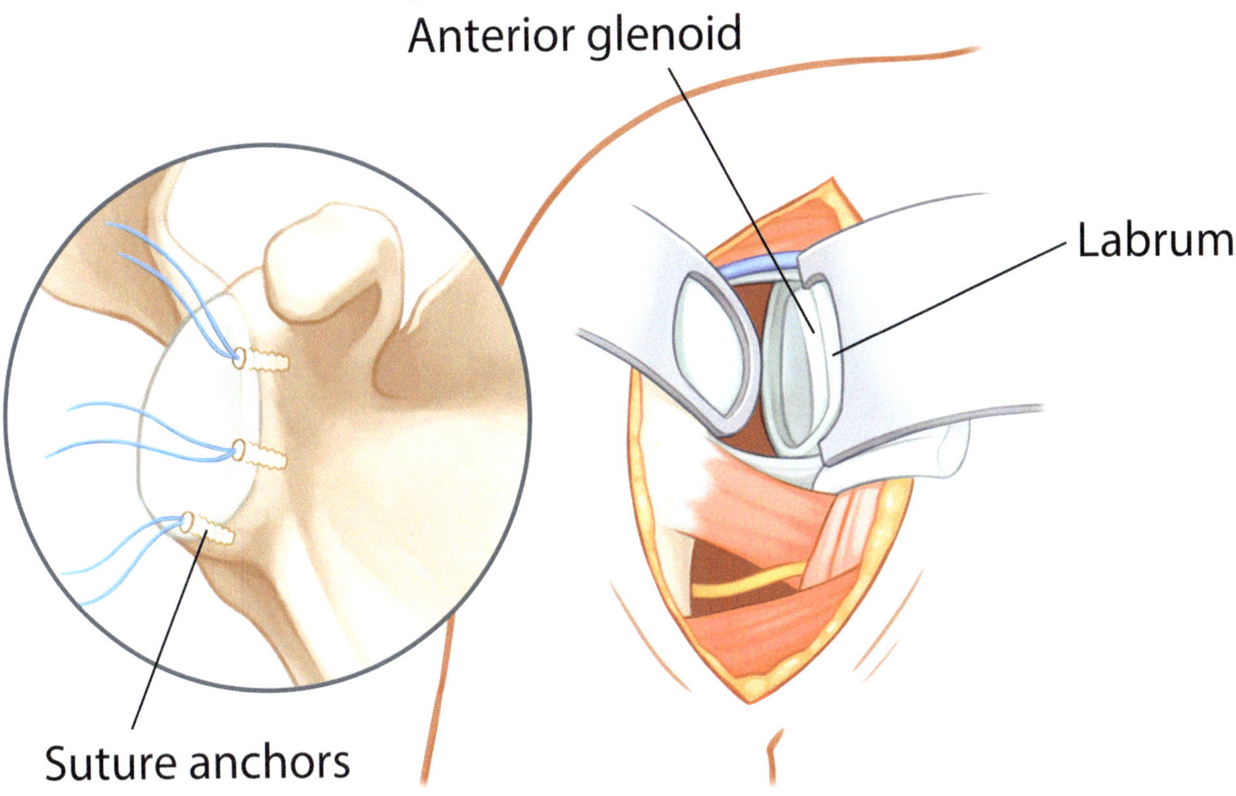

Fig. 21.7 Once the anterior glenoid is exposed, three suture anchors are placed in the antero-inferior glenoid spaced evenly from 6 o'clock to the 2 o'clock position (for a right shoulder). These sutures are then passed through and tied around the labrum for an anatomic repair.

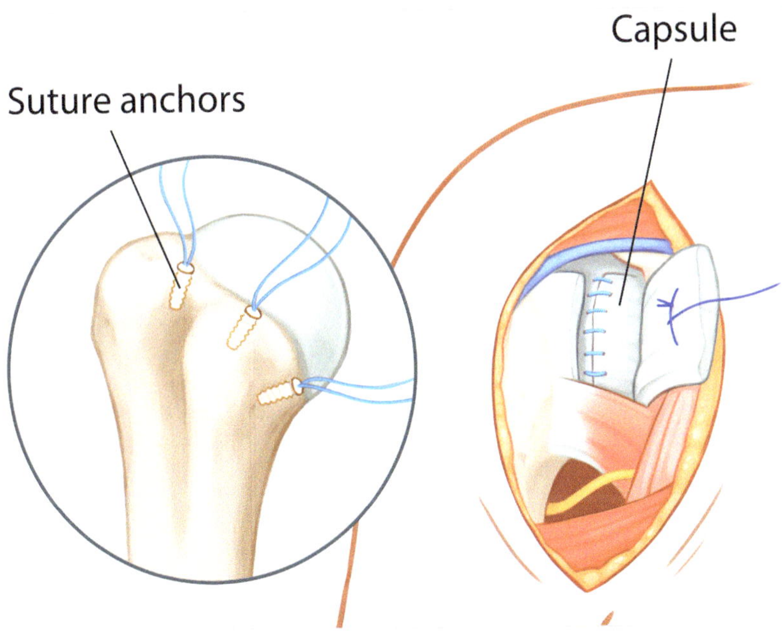

Fig. 21.8 Following labral repair, the capsular shift is performed using suture anchors in the humeral head along the articular margin. And superolateral capsular shift is performed and suture placed in horizontal mattress fashion.

21.6.7 Subscapularis Repair

The subscapularis tendon is repaired using a free needle to pass the previously placed Mason–Allen sutures through the tendon stump on the lesser tuberosity. These sutures should be passed as deep as possible along the lesser tuberosity in a horizontal mattress fashion to minimize risk of pullout. Sutures from the anchors placed in the anatomic neck can also be placed into the subscapularis tendon to reinforce the repair.

21.6.8 Final Closure

The deltopectoral interval is gently reapproximated with a running absorbable suture. Subcutaneous tissue and skin are then closed according to surgeon's preference. The dressings are placed and patients are placed into a sling without an abduction wedge.

21.7 Tips and Pearls/Expert Suggestions

- We have found that it is very helpful to place a rolled towel bump under medial scapula, to prevent protraction of the scapula and improve glenoid visualization.
- When defining the plane between the upper and lower subscapularis, this is typically easier to define medially, where the subscapularis is more muscular, as the subscapular tendon and anterior capsule tend to coalesce more laterally near the insertion.
- During the approach, the numerous tagging sutures in the subscapularis and anterior capsule may become tangled. It is often helpful to keep the color of sutures different between the subscapularis and anterior capsule, as well as use a straight clamp secured to the drape to help organize sutures.
- The subscapularis must be adequately mobilized during the dissection to ensure that it will be repairable to the tendon stump on the lesser tuberosity. This can be checked with pulling lateral tension on the traction sutures to make sure it is sufficiently released.
- Passing and tying sutures for the labral repair may be difficult due to limited exposure to the anterior glenoid through the wound. In this situation, instead of using a free needle, an arthroscopic-style curved suture lasso can be used to shuttle sutures through the labrum through the open wound. An arthroscopic-style knot pusher can also be used to tie sutures if exposure is limited as well.

21.8 What to Avoid

Ensure that the arm position when performing lateral capsular shift does not overtighten the lateral capsule and constrain ER. Gentle range-of-motion check after capsular tensioning to ensure adequate mobility can help prevent overtensioning.

21.9 Complications/Bailout/Salvage

If small-sized suture anchors have poor fixation in the lesser tuberosity, these can be salvaged with a traditional, larger metal suture anchor (G4 Titanium, Mitek Sports Medicine). The use of tape-style sutures can aid in the subscapularis repair.

21.10 Postoperative Care

21.10.1 Postoperative Rehabilitation

Goals for early postoperative rehabilitation include avoiding stretching of the anterior capsule and protecting the subscapularis healing.

- Weeks 0 to 2:
  - Immobilization in sling for 2 weeks.
  - Elbow, wrist, hand range of motion, and strengthening.
  - No active IR until 6 weeks.
- Weeks 2 to 4:
  - Start pendulums.
  - Start passive forward flexion in the plane of scapula to 90 degrees.
  - Limit ER to neutral.
- Weeks 4 to 6:
  - Passive forward flexion in the plane of scapula to 120 degrees.
  - Allow gentle ER to 30 degrees.
  - Avoid rotator cuff inflammation.
- Weeks 6 to 12:
  - AAROM (active-assisted range of motion) forward flexion, ER, and IR. Avoid forced passive ER stretching. The goal is to attain full range of motion by 12 weeks.
  - At 6 to 8 weeks: ER to 45 degrees with arm at side.
  - At 8 to 10 weeks: ER to 60 degrees with arm at side.
  - At 10 to 12 weeks: ER to 45 degrees with arm at 45-degree abduction.
  - Begin to restore deltoid, rotator cuff strength and normal scapulohumeral rhythm.
- Weeks 12+:
  - Scapular control and upper extremity strengthening.
  - Active range of motion to restore full range.
  - IR/ER in 90 degrees of abduction for overhead athletes.
  - Begin plyometric training, sports-specific activity.
  - Limited return to sport at 16 weeks

References

1. Bonazza NA, Liu G, Leslie DL, Dhawan A. Trends in surgical management of shoulder instability. Orthop J Sports Med 2017;5(6):2325967117712476
2. Zhang AL, Montgomery SR, Ngo SS, Hame SL, Wang JC, Gamradt SC. Arthroscopic versus open shoulder stabilization: current practice patterns in the United States. Arthroscopy 2014;30(4):436–443
3. Cole BJ, L'Insalata J, Irrgang J, Warner JJ. Comparison of arthroscopic and open anterior shoulder stabilization. A two to six-year follow-up study. J Bone Joint Surg Am 2000;82-A(8):1108–1114
4. Fabbriciani C, Milano G, Demontis A, Fadda S, Ziranu F, Mulas PD. Arthroscopic versus open treatment of Bankart lesion of the shoulder: a prospective randomized study. Arthroscopy 2004;20(5):456–462
5. Harris JD, Gupta AK, Mall NA, et al. Long-term outcomes after Bankart shoulder stabilization. Arthroscopy 2013;29(5):920–933
6. Karlsson J, Magnusson L, Ejerhed L, Hultenheim I, Lundin O, Kartus J. Comparison of open and arthroscopic stabilization for recurrent shoulder dislocation in patients with a Bankart lesion. Am J Sports Med 2001;29(5):538–542
7. Petrera M, Patella V, Patella S, Theodoropoulos J. A meta-analysis of open versus arthroscopic Bankart repair using suture anchors. Knee Surg Sports Traumatol Arthrosc 2010;18(12):1742–1747
8. Hohmann E, Tetsworth K, Glatt V. Open versus arthroscopic surgical treatment for anterior shoulder dislocation: a comparative systematic review and meta-analysis over the past 20 years. J Shoulder Elbow Surg 2017;26(10):1873–1880
9. Virk MS, Manzo RL, Cote M, et al. Comparison of time to recurrence of instability after open and arthroscopic

Bankart repair techniques. Orthop J Sports Med 2016;4(6):2325967116654114
10. Cho NS, Hwang JC, Rhee YG. Arthroscopic stabilization in anterior shoulder instability: collision athletes versus non-collision athletes. Arthroscopy 2006;22(9):947–953
11. Cole BJ, Warner JJ. Arthroscopic versus open Bankart repair for traumatic anterior shoulder instability. Clin Sports Med 2000;19(1):19–48
12. Rhee YG, Ha JH, Cho NS. Anterior shoulder stabilization in collision athletes: arthroscopic versus open Bankart repair. Am J Sports Med 2006;34(6):979–985
13. Yamamoto N, Kijima H, Nagamoto H, et al. Outcome of Bankart repair in contact versus non-contact athletes. Orthop Traumatol Surg Res 2015;101(4):415–419
14. Shaha JS, Cook JB, Song DJ, et al. Redefining "critical" bone loss in shoulder instability: functional outcomes worsen with "subcritical" bone loss. Am J Sports Med 2015;43(7):1719–1725
15. Abouali JA, Hatzantoni K, Holtby R, Veillette C, Theodoropoulos J. Revision arthroscopic Bankart repair. Arthroscopy 2013;29(9):1572–1578
16. Friedman LG, Griesser MJ, Miniaci AA, Jones MH. Recurrent instability after revision anterior shoulder stabilization surgery. Arthroscopy 2014;30(3):372–381
17. Cho NS, Yi JW, Lee BG, Rhee YG. Revision open Bankart surgery after arthroscopic repair for traumatic anterior shoulder instability. Am J Sports Med 2009;37(11):2158–2164
18. Mohtadi NG, Chan DS, Hollinshead RM, et al. A randomized clinical trial comparing open and arthroscopic stabilization for recurrent traumatic anterior shoulder instability: two-year follow-up with disease-specific quality-of-life outcomes. J Bone Joint Surg Am 2014;96(5):353–360

22 Role of Remplissage in Anterior Shoulder Instability

Ryan M. Degen, George S. Athwal, and Robert B. Litchfield

Abstract

Engaging Hill–Sachs defects frequently contribute to recurrent anterior glenohumeral instability. When a substantial defect is present, an isolated labral repair is often insufficient at stabilizing the shoulder. Remplissage is an augmentative arthroscopic procedure that can be performed concurrently with an anterior labral repair. This arthroscopic procedure involves filling the humeral head defect with the infraspinatus tendon and the posterior joint capsule, preventing further engagement with the glenoid rim and subsequent instability. With predictable healing, recurrence rates have been low with many patients returning to preinjury activity levels. Remplissage is best reserved for patients with engaging Hill–Sachs defects with minimal glenoid bone loss.

Keywords: *shoulder, arthroscopy, glenohumeral instability, Hill–Sachs defect, remplissage*

22.1 Introduction

The contribution of osseous lesions to recurrent anterior glenohumeral instability has been well described by Burkhart and De Beer.[1] Focusing on the humeral head, the "glenoid track" concept, proposed by Yamamoto et al, improved our understanding of potentially significant Hill–Sachs defects that may contribute to further episodes of instability.[2] Continual study of critical defect sizes with retrospective clinical studies and biomechanical cadaveric studies has altered treatment guidelines in recent years.[3] With an increasingly large, "off-track" Hill–Sachs defect and limited glenoid bone loss, isolated arthroscopic Bankart repair is often insufficient in stabilizing the shoulder. Consequently, augmentative procedures, such as Remplissage, are required to stabilize the joint and reduce failure rates of isolated soft-tissue stabilizations. This chapter will review the technical pearls associated with performing a Remplissage procedure for an engaging Hill–Sachs defect, in conjunction with a Bankart repair.

22.2 Goals of Procedure

As initially described by Purchase et al, the technical goal of the procedure is to prevent further engagement between the Hill–Sachs defect and the anterior glenoid rim, preventing recurrent instability episodes.[4] This is accomplished by performing a posterior capsulodesis and infraspinatus tenodesis into the Hill–Sachs defect to "fill" the defect (**Fig. 22.1a, b**). As a result, the defect is converted from an intra-articular defect to an extra-articular one, which then limits engagement.

22.3 Advantages

An advantage of this procedure is that it can be performed arthroscopically. The technical ease and limited associated surgical morbidity allows the procedure to be easily performed in conjunction with an arthroscopic Bankart repair. Additionally, while it represents a "nonanatomic" stabilization technique,

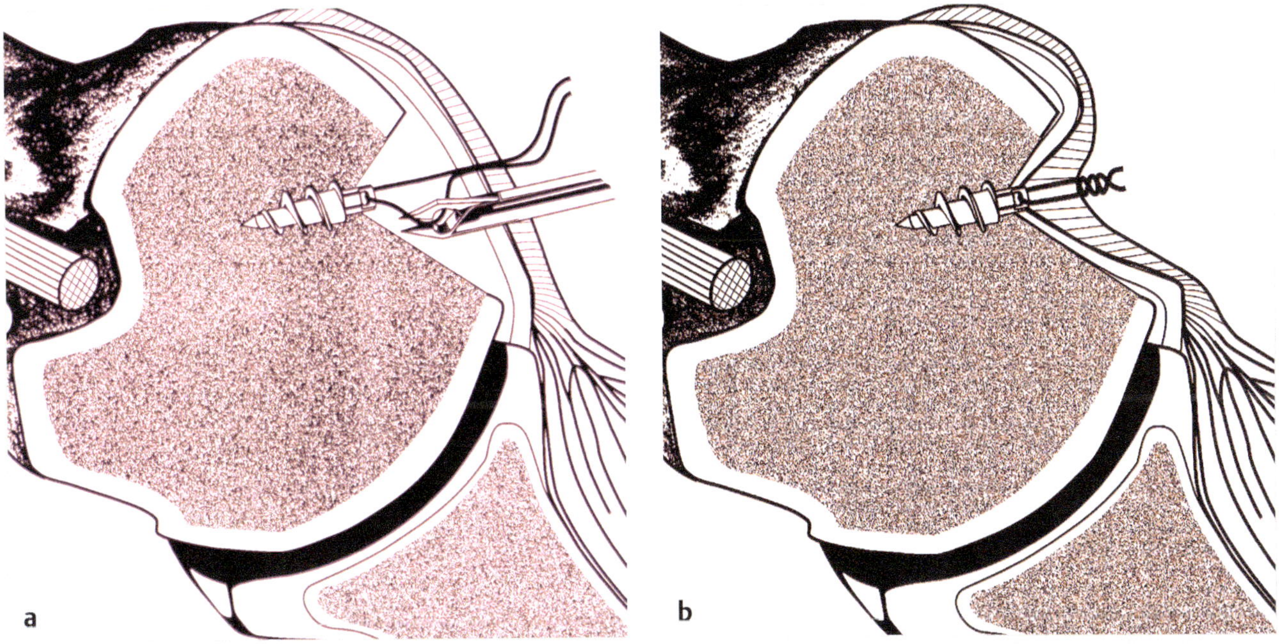

Fig 22.1 (a) Schematic axial drawing of a glenohumeral joint with a Hill–Sachs (HS) defect. A suture anchor has been placed into the base of the HS defect, and a penetrating suture grasper is being utilized to pierce through the posterior rotator cuff and capsule to pass the sutures in a horizontal mattress configuration. **(b)** Schematic axial drawing of a glenohumeral joint following completion of a remplissage, with imbrication of the overlying rotator cuff and capsule.

it is significantly less invasive and expensive when compared to osteochondral allograft reconstruction, Latarjet coracoid transfer, or partial humeral head resurfacing.

22.4 Indications

Currently, indications for performing a remplissage procedure continue to evolve. However, absolute indications include anterior glenohumeral instability with an engaging Hill–Sachs defect. Historically, a defect size of 15 to 30% of the humeral head width was also considered an indication. However, recent work by Di Giacomo et al[5] has resulted in a new terminology that may more appropriately quantify defect width, or the so-called Hill–Sachs interval width, in relation to the glenoid width.

22.5 Contraindications

Remplissage has few absolute contraindications, although it should not be performed in those with isolated glenoid bone loss or habitual dislocators.

A relative contraindication is the presence of significant bipolar bony lesions, specifically where the glenoid defect is greater than 20 to 25% of the glenoid width. In this scenario, a combined Bankart repair and remplissage is often insufficient in preventing subsequent dislocations. Rather, the glenoid defect must be addressed with either a coracoid process transfer or structural bone grafting.

Similarly, a Hill–Sachs defect size of greater than 30% of the humeral head width is also considered a relative contraindication. In this scenario, the defect is best managed with allograft reconstruction, rotational osteotomies, partial resurfacing arthroplasty, or hemiarthroplasty.

22.6 Preoperative Preparation/ Positioning

As part of the preoperative workup, a CT or MRI should be obtained to quantify the size of the Hill–Sachs defect, and to identify concomitant pathology that can be treated at the time of surgery (labral tear) or that would preclude success of an arthroscopic stabilization (glenoid bone loss > 25% or humeral avulsion of the glenohumeral ligament [HAGL] lesion).

Once it has been confirmed that the patient's injury satisfies all indications/contraindications, preparation for an arthroscopic stabilization procedure is begun. Typically, this involves an arthroscopic labral repair (Bankart repair) in conjunction with remplissage. We favor the beach-chair positioning for this procedure.

Necessary equipment includes the following:

- Standard arthroscopic setup with shoulder instruments.
- Two large-diameter cannulas.
- Knife rasp/elevator.
- Suture anchors of choice for labral repair.
- Curved suture passer.
- Two double-loaded suture anchors for remplissage (rotator cuff anchors).
- Penetrating suture retriever.

22.7 Operative Technique

We prefer to perform all shoulder arthroscopy procedures under general anesthesia with an interscalene block for postoperative pain control. After induction and patient positioning in the beach-chair position, we perform an examination under anesthesia to assess glenohumeral translation and Hill–Sachs defect engagement in various positions of abduction and external rotation. After confirming the presence of grade 3 translation and an engaging Hill–Sachs defect, we also examine and document passive motion, including external rotation, for postoperative comparison.

At this stage, a standard diagnostic arthroscopy is performed through a posterior viewing portal. A dynamic evaluation is performed to assess for Hill–Sachs defect engagement with the arm in various positions of abduction and external rotation, with engagement evaluated with glenohumeral rotation rather than forced anterior humeral head translation. After confirming engagement and ruling out any concomitant pathology not identified on imaging that may change the treatment approach (i.e., HAGL lesion), attention is turned to the anterior labrum. The glenoid rim is prepared after mobilizing the labrum and suture anchors placed inferiorly to superiorly. Sutures are passed around the labrum; however, they are not tied until completion of the remplissage procedure.

To perform the remplissage, the arthroscope is positioned in the anterior, rotator-interval portal. The Hill–Sachs defect can be visualized by translating the humeral anteriorly and externally rotating the humeral head, while advancing the camera up over the superolateral humeral head with the light source pointed downward (**Fig. 22.2**). A shaver can be introduced through the standard posterior portal and used to debride the Hill–Sachs defect. A spinal needle is then used for localization to identify suture anchor trajectory into the valley of the Hill–Sachs defect. Once identified, an accessory posterolateral portal is created and a cannula is placed into the subacromial space, staying superficial to the posterior rotator cuff.

At this stage, the arthroscope is redirected into the subacromial space and a thorough subacromial bursectomy is completed around this cannula to allow visualization during suture tying later in the case.

After switching back to the intra-articular view from the anterior portal, two suture anchors are then passed, via the posterolateral cannula, percutaneously through the posterior rotator cuff and capsule into the valley of the Hill–Sachs defect (**Fig. 22.3**). The anchors should penetrate the rotator cuff and capsule immediately adjacent to the Hill–Sachs defect to avoid overmedialization of sutures, risking restricted postoperative external rotation or posterior shoulder pain secondary to myodesis.[6] The superior anchor is placed first. A penetrating grasper is then used to percutaneously penetrate the infraspinatus tendon to retrieve one limb from each pair of sutures approximately 0.5 to 1 cm above and below the anchor location, effectively creating a horizontal mattress configuration for both pairs of sutures (**Fig. 22.4**). These sutures can then be docked through a percutaneous posterior incision for suture management. The entire process is subsequently repeated for the inferior anchor, which should be placed a minimum of 1 cm inferior to the superior anchor in the base of the Hill–Sachs defect. Sutures are passed again in a horizontal mattress configuration. At this stage, with all sutures positioned, the arthroscope is re-

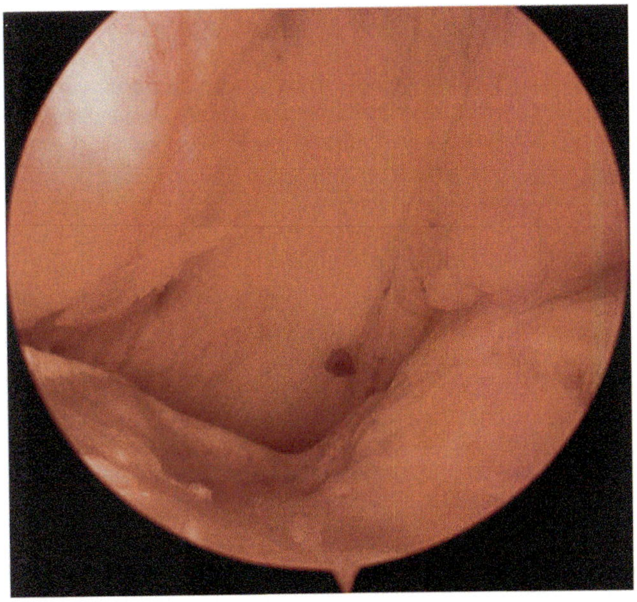

Fig. 22.2 Arthroscopic view of the Hill–Sachs defect, viewing from the anterior, rotator interval portal with the humeral head externally rotated.

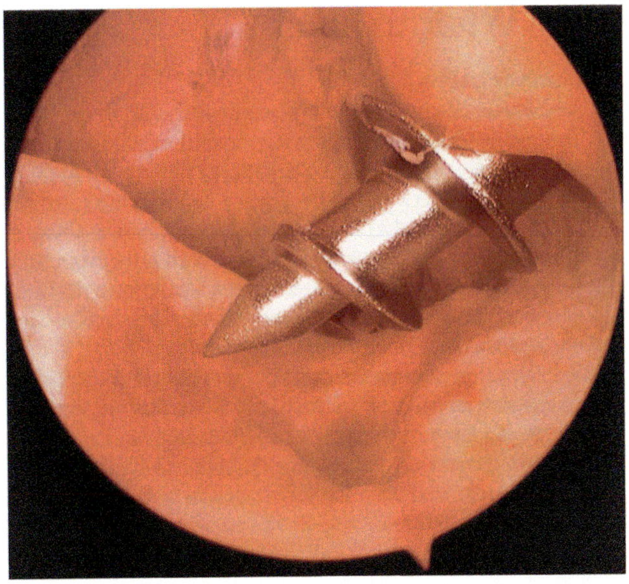

Fig. 22.3 Arthroscopic view of the Hill–Sachs defect with percutaneous insertion of a suture anchor into the base of the defect.

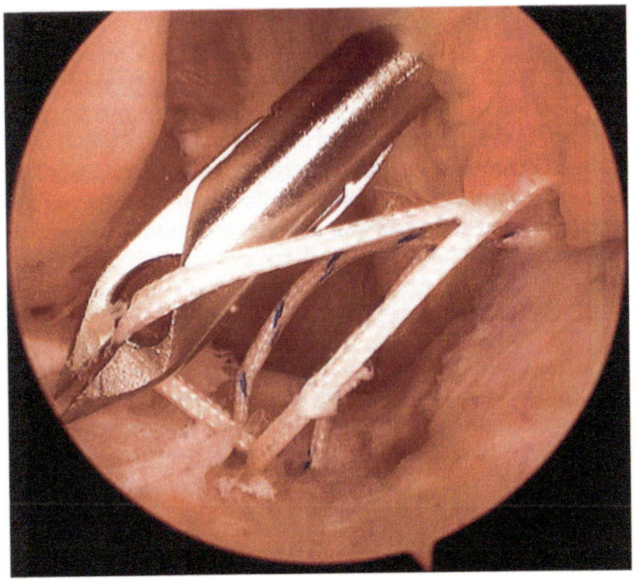

Fig. 22.4 Arthroscopic view of the Hill–Sachs defect with a penetrating suture retriever utilized to pass sutures in a horizontal mattress configuration.

turned to the subacromial space to visualize the posterior cannula and sutures. The arm is positioned in neutral rotation and the sutures are sequentially tied from inferior to superior. The scope can then be placed into the anterior portal again to visualize and confirm infraspinatus tenodesis (**Fig. 22.5**).

After completing the remplissage, the scope is then placed into the posterior portal and the previous anterior sutures for the labral repair are tied from inferior to superior.

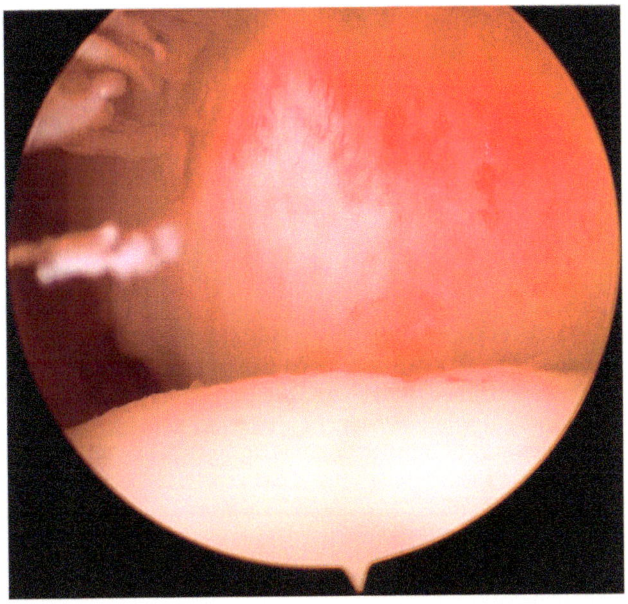

Fig. 22.5 Arthroscopic view of the Hill–Sachs defect following completion of the remplissage procedure with imbrication of the infraspinatus/posterior capsule.

22.8 Tips and Pearls/Expert Suggestions

- Arm positioning with anterior humeral translation and external rotation can significantly improve arthroscopic visualization of the Hill–Sachs defect.
- Use of cannula posteriorly assists in suture management/retrieval.
- A 70-degree scope may be helpful in viewing the Hill–Sachs defect from anterior (rarely used).

Diagnostic Arthroscopy

From the posterior portal, a 30-degree scope is used to assess the glenohumeral joint. An assistant may adduct the humerus to improve visualization. The articular surface of the rotator cuff, long head of the biceps, and entirety of the labrum are assessed. The capsule is assessed for an HAGL lesion, and the anteroinferior glenoid is assessed for bone loss, presence of a bony Bankart lesion, and quality of capsulolabral tissue. The most inferior aspect of the labral tear is visualized, to the point where normal labral tissue is seen, to indicate a reference point for placement of the most inferior anchor.

Anchor Placement, Suture Management, and Capsular Plication

An elevator is used to free the anteroinferior capsulolabral tissue from the glenoid. The labral tissue and bone are debrided using an arthroscopic shaver to create a surface for optimal healing. Care is taken to debride the anterior glenoid 10 mm medial to the rim, since the point of the double-row repair is to facilitate healing of the capsulolabral tissue to its entire footprint.

There are multiple anchor configurations that achieve the goal of repairing the capsulolabral tissue to its footprint. There are trade-offs regarding implant costs, operative time, technical difficulty, and quality of repair that must be considered when evaluating each technique. Lafosse et al described a five-anchor repair in a W configuration, with two medial row and three lateral row anchors.[7] Simple knots were tied for each anchor and knotless anchors were not used. One of the more technically difficult aspects of this procedure is that a trans-subscapularis portal was placed medially and inferiorly to place the medial row anchors, and the knots were tied medially, anterior to the capsule.

Ahmad et al described a technique using two to three 2.4-mm anchors placed 10 mm medial to the glenoid rim.[8] The two suture limbs from each anchor were anchored into a corresponding 2.9-mm knotless anchor on the glenoid rim, similar to a transosseous-equivalent double-row rotator cuff repair.

Iwaso et al described a technique that usually uses 6 anchors, placing a medial row double loaded anchor 10 mm medial to the glenoid, and anchoring each set of sutures into two lateral row knotless anchors on the glenoid rim, creating a V-configuration.[9] Usually two of these configurations are used.

The technique described in this chapter is a hybrid four-anchor technique, designed to limit technical difficulty, cost, and operative time while still obtaining compression of the capsulolabral complex to its footprint. After freeing up the capsulolabral tissue and debriding the anterior glenoid bone, a 1.6-mm double-loaded soft anchor is placed through a curved cannula at the 4 o'clock position, 10 mm medial to the glenoid rim. Using a curved drill guide prevents skiving on the anterior glenoid, and allows the anchor to be placed through a standard anterior portal. Next, a 1.6-mm soft anchor is placed on the glenoid rim at the 5:30 o'clock position. Both suture limbs from this most inferior anchor are passed through the anteroinferior labrum, tying them in a mattress fashion, keeping the knot out of the joint. This allows for anatomic reduction of the labrum to the glenoid in the most inferior position before shuttling the sutures for the double-row portion of the repair. A suture lasso is then used to shuttle two of the suture limbs from the medial row anchor around the capsulolabral complex, and they are then anchored into a 2.9-mm knotless anchor on the glenoid rim at the 4:30 o'clock position. This is then repeated, anchoring the other two suture limbs into a 2.9-mm knotless anchor on the rim at the 3:30 o'clock position. Benefits of this technique are that it only requires four anchors and four passes with the suture lasso, so the increase in cost, operative time, and technical difficulty is modest compared to a single-row repair with three anchors.

23.6.2 Open Repair Technique

Patient Positioning

After placement under general anesthesia, the patient is placed in a 30-degree modified beach-chair position. The upper body is shifted laterally so that the arm is free, with the scapula stabilized on the table with a small bump underneath it. The head is secured resting in a gel donut on a headrest.

Approach and Subscapularis Management

An anterior axillary incision followed by a deltopectoral approach is used, using a self-retaining Kolbel retractor in the deltopectoral interval. Care is taken to preserve the cephalic vein, retracting it laterally with the deltoid. The subscapularis can be approached in one of two manners. It can be split in line with its fibers starting at the musculotendinous juncture and working medially. A glenoid neck retractor is placed and a blunt-tip Gelpi is used to retract the muscle fibers. The underlying capsule is incised horizontally from the labrum to the capsule/tendon insertion laterally. A Darrach or glenoid neck retractor is then moved inside the labrum and capsule along the glenoid neck exposing the bony anterior glenoid neck. Alternately, the subscapularis is incised vertically and tagged, leaving a cuff of tissue for later repair. It is carefully dissected from the anterior capsule. The capsule is incised from the humerus and "T'd" toward the labrum, opening the joint. The anteroinferior capsulolabral tissue is visualized and dissected from the glenoid neck. A Fukuda retractor can be used to retract the humeral head. A pitchfork retractor is placed deep to the capsule exposing the glenoid neck and rim (**Fig. 23.1**).

Anchor Placement, Suture Management, and Capsular Plication

Two double-loaded 3-mm suture anchors are placed 10 to 15 mm medial to the glenoid rim at the 4:30 and 5:30 o'clock positions on the glenoid neck (in a left shoulder, the 7:30 and 6:30 o'clock positions are used). Soft anchors of 1.6 mm can also be used here. The pitchfork retractor is then placed between the subscapularis and the capsule. With a free needle, the suture limbs are shuttled through the capsule in a horizontal mattress fashion and tied but not cut. Suture anchors of 3 mm are placed along the glenoid rim in a like manner and the suture limbs pass in a vertical mattress fashion (around the labrum) and tied but not cut. One of each corner suture is crisscrossed and tied one to the diagonal limb and one to the corresponding medial or lateral anchor (**Fig. 23.2**). The lateral capsule is then repaired to the humerus, performing a capsular shift if indicated.

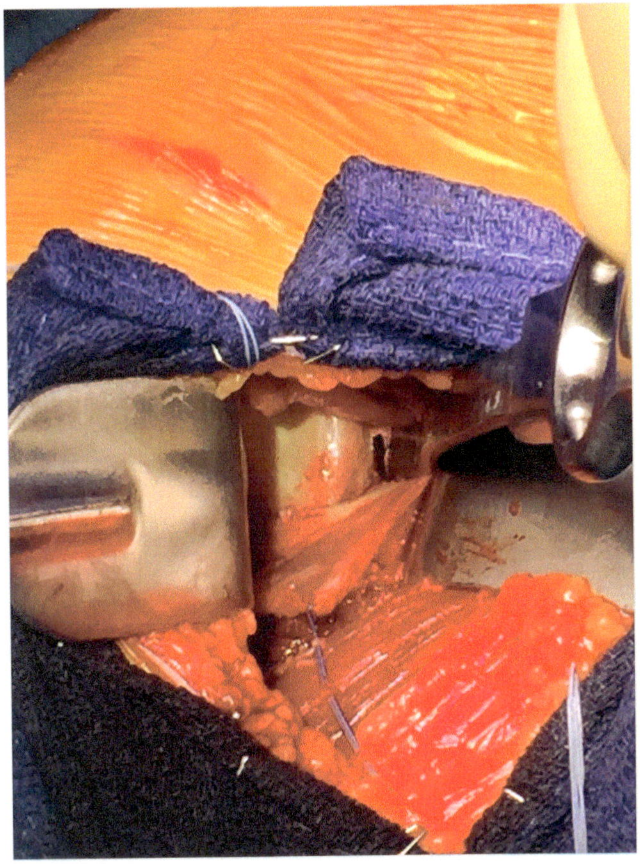

Fig. 23.1 Glenoid exposure.

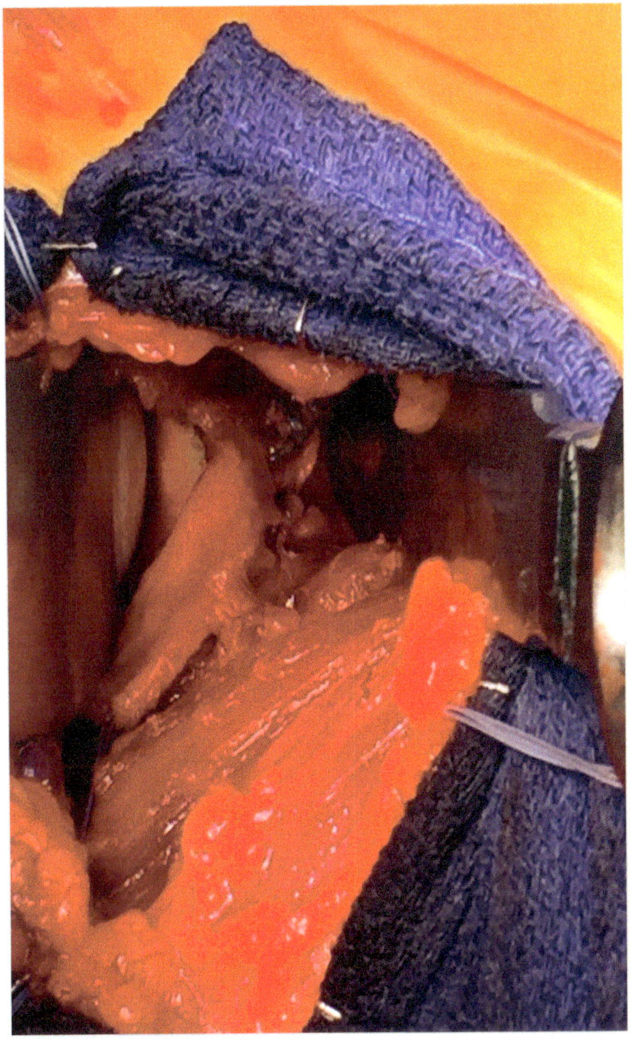

Fig. 23.2 Open double-row labral repair.

23.7 Tips and Pearls

- When inserting the medial row anchors, a curved drill guide is helpful to prevent skiving off the anterior glenoid.
- For the arthroscopic technique, inserting the medial row anchor as the first step is recommended because the capsulolabral tissue is more mobile and can be retracted anteriorly while placing the anchor.
- Using smaller soft anchors (1.6 mm) for the medial row results in less overall bone loss due to drilling. In the arthroscopic technique, a 1.6-mm soft anchor is used for the inferior glenoid rim anchor as well.

23.8 What to Avoid

As with any anterior stabilization procedure, evaluation for glenoid bone loss, HAGL lesion, and large Hill–Sachs deformity should be done to select an appropriate operative plan. Double-row repair is not recommended in lieu of a bony reconstruction procedure in cases with greater than 20 to 25% glenoid bone loss.

23.9 Complications/Bailout/Salvage

Medial row anchors can be placed using a straight drill guide, though if difficulty is encountered due to skiving off the anterior glenoid bone, there are a couple of solutions. First, the drill guide can be gently tapped with a mallet to secure its position. Second, a curved drill guide can be used instead. This requires that proper instrumentation be available, including the corresponding flexible drill bit and anchor insertion device. If there is still difficulty placing medial row anchors, the procedure can be converted to a standard single-row repair.

23.9.1 Postoperative Management

The postoperative protocol for a double-row repair is the same as for a single-row repair. The arm is placed in a sling, allowing pendulums, wrist, and elbow motion immediately postoperatively. For the first 6 weeks postoperatively, passive, active-assist, and active range of motions are progressed under the guidance of a physical therapist, taking care to protect external rotation. After 6 weeks, the sling is discontinued, and range of motion and strengthening are progressed, avoiding forceful movements into abduction and external rotation. At 3 to 4 months postoperatively, gradual return to sports-specific and strenuous activities is initiated.

References

1. McDonald LS, Thompson M, Altchek DW, et al. Double-row capsulolabral repair increases load to failure and decreases excessive motion. Arthroscopy 2016;32(11):2218–2225
2. Ahmad CS, Galano GJ, Vorys GC, Covey AS, Gardner TR, Levine WN. Evaluation of glenoid capsulolabral complex insertional anatomy and restoration with single- and double-row capsulolabral repairs. J Shoulder Elbow Surg 2009;18(6):948–954
3. Kim DS, Yoon YS, Chung HJ. Single-row versus double-row capsulolabral repair: a comparative evaluation of contact pressure and surface area in the capsulolabral complex-glenoid bone interface. Am J Sports Med 2011; 39(7):1500–1506
4. Spiegl UJ, Smith SD, Todd JN, Coatney GA, Wijdicks CA, Millett PJ. Biomechanical comparison of arthroscopic single- and double-row repair techniques for acute bony Bankart lesions. Am J Sports Med 2014;42(8):1939–1946
5. Moran CJ, Fabricant PD, Kang R, Cordasco FA. Arthroscopic double-row anterior stabilization and Bankart repair for the “high-risk” athlete. Arthrosc Tech 2014;3(1):e65–e71
6. Castagna A, Garofalo R, Conti M, Flanagin B. Arthroscopic Bankart repair: have we finally reached a gold standard? Knee Surg Sports Traumatol Arthrosc 2016;24(2):398–405
7. Lafosse L, Baier GP, Jost B. Footprint fixation for arthroscopic reconstruction in anterior shoulder instability: the Cassiopeia double-row technique. Arthroscopy 2006;22(2):231.e1–231.e6
8. Jiang KN, Byram IR, Hsu SH, Ahmad CS. Double-row labral repair: knotless suture-bridge technique. Tech Shoulder Elbow Surg 2012;13(3):107–110
9. Iwaso H, Uchiyama E, Sakakibara S, Fukui N. Modified double-row technique for arthroscopic Bankart repair: surgical technique and preliminary results. Acta Orthop Belg 2011;77(2):252–257

24 Anterior Humeral Avulsion of the Glenohumeral Ligament Repair

Nirav K. Patel, Kathryn Crum, and Christopher C. Dodson

Abstract

Humeral avulsion of the glenohumeral ligament (HAGL) occurs in 1 to 9% of patients,[1] usually from anterior subluxations or dislocations causing avulsion of the capsule and inferior glenohumeral ligament (IGHL) from the humerus. They are an important and often difficult-to-diagnose cause of anterior shoulder instability, occurring in slightly older patients (>30–35 years) and with a higher risk of recurrent instability than those with Bankart lesions. Surgical repair of HAGL lesions can be performed via open or arthroscopic techniques in some cases, but open repair provides better access and thus remains the focus of the chapter.

Keywords: *shoulder instability, anterior, HAGL lesion, open repair*

24.1 Goals of Procedure

The goal of treatment of anterior glenohumeral joint instability is to return to stability, full range of motion, and strength. Specifically, the integrity of the anterior capsulolabral complex must be restored, with reattachment of the HAGL lesion.

24.2 Advantages

Repair of an HAGL lesion restores anterior glenohumeral stability and prevents recurrent episodes. This, in turn, reduces the long-term risks of glenohumeral arthritis or failure after operative Bankart repair.

24.3 Indications

Detached HAGL lesion and the following:

- Recurrent anterior glenohumeral instability.
- Recurrent pain despite activity modification and physical therapy.
- Young athletes or manual laborers, who are at risk of recurrent instability.

24.4 Contraindications

- Neuropathic shoulder.
- Multidirectional instability.
- Noncompliant patient.
- Glenohumeral osteoarthritis.
- Lack of symptoms.

24.5 Preoperative Preparation/ Positioning

Routine preoperative imaging of the shoulder should include true anteroposterior (neutral and internal rotation), "scapular Y," and axillary radiographs. These images allow evaluation for concentric glenohumeral alignment, glenoid hypoplasia, glenoid version, humeral head impaction fractures, and glenoid rim fractures. MRI shows the HAGL lesion best on sagittal oblique or coronal oblique T2, fat-suppressed images. An MRI arthrogram or joint effusion distends the joint and allows for better visualization of IGHL defects (**Fig. 24.1**). Specifically, there is conversion of the fluid distended "**U**-shaped" axillary pouch into a "**J**-shaped" structure and extravasation of the contrast material or joint effusion across the torn humeral attachment. Based on the MRI findings, HAGL lesions can be classified using the West Point Classification system,[2] which includes six types: anterior HAGL, anterior bony HAGL, floating anterior IGHL, posterior HAGL, posterior bony HAGL, and floating posterior IGHL.

The patient is positioned supine in the beach-chair position with the head of the bed flexed 40 to 60 degrees for an open HAGL repair.

24.6 Operative Technique

A standard deltopectoral approach is utilized with an incision from the coracoid process to toward the axillary fold. The cephalic vein is identified and protected as the deltopectoral interval is entered, and the subscapularis tendon exposed. Arciero and Mazzocca[3] described an **L**-shaped incision in the lower half of subscapularis: the vertical limb is started 0.5 cm medial to the biceps groove on the lesser tuberosity at the midpoint of the subscapularis and extended to just proximal to the circumflex vessels. The horizontal limb is made from the midpoint to 2 cm medially to complete the L. Metzenbaum scissors can be used to gently separate subscapularis from the capsule without complete detachment, and reveal the anterior HAGL lesion (**Fig. 24.2**). The axillary nerve should be protected during the creation of this plane. Bhatia et al[4] described a "subscapularis-sparing" technique that is limited to treating lesions of the anterior band and midregion of the IGHL. Here, the lower border of the subscapularis tendon is identified, and the muscular–capsular plane is dissected out using a curved hemostat

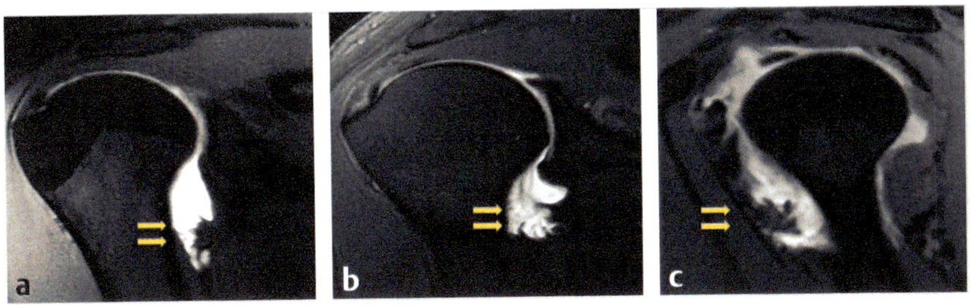

Fig. 24.1 Magnetic resonance arthrograms of anterior humeral avulsion of the glenohumeral ligament lesions. **(a)** Coronal view. **(b)** Coronal view, at another level. **(c)** Sagittal oblique view (*arrows* indicate tear location).

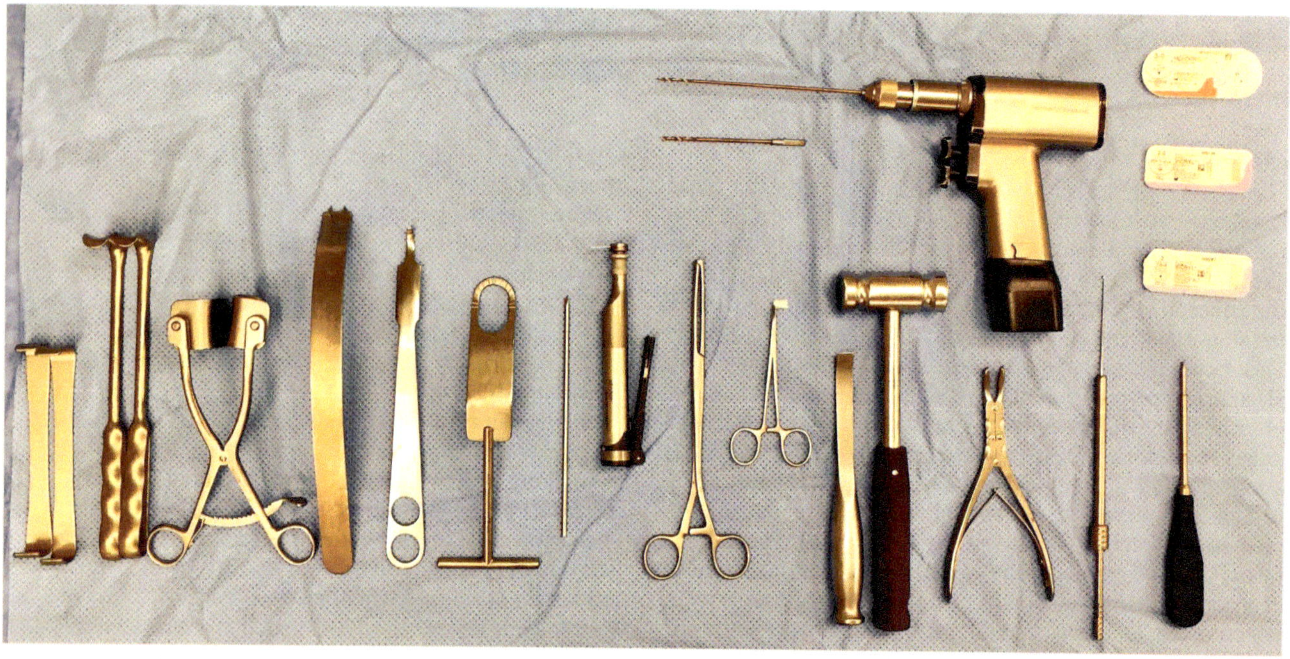

Fig. 25.2 Simple instrumentation used for the modified "one-screw" Latarjet technique.

operating theater (**Fig. 25.2**). If the Bateman retractor is not available, a Hohmann retractor can be used. If no Fukuda retractor is available, use a spoon or a Hohmann retractor at the inferior part of the joint.

25.3 Indications

The indications of Latarjet are still controversial. This procedure can be used for any case of anterior traumatic shoulder instability, as the outcomes are excellent and superior to the arthroscopic Bankart procedure.[5] However, this is not an anatomic procedure and the risk of complications is higher than that for the Bankart procedure.[6] Therefore, we recommend performing a Latarjet when there is a significant bone loss (glenoid bone loss or Hill–Sachs lesion not amenable to remplissage procedure) and in cases of contact/collision sport participation by the patient.

25.4 Contraindications

The Latarjet procedure is not indicated in case of multidirectional instability. In the rare situation of coracoid nonunion after previous coracoid fracture, we recommend assessing the quality and the size of the distal coracoid using a CT scan. We have performed some cases with success when the coracoid was usable. Otherwise, it is preferable to move to the Eden–Hybinette procedure knowing that the procedure will miss the sling effect of the coracobrachial.

25.5 Patient Preparation/ Positioning

25.5.1 Preoperative Imaging

The usual preoperative imaging assessment comprises X-rays with AP views in three rotations, Bernageau incidence, and MRI. The MRI will detect any associated lesion (cuff tear, superior labral anterior and posterior [SLAP]) that will be treated arthroscopically before the open procedure, if needed. We do not perform a CT scan routinely, except if the bone loss needs a more accurate assessment.

25.5.2 Patient Positioning

After the usual preoperative preparation to prevent surgical site infection, a general anesthesia is administered. We do not routinely perform any interscalene block as this surgery is usually well tolerated and results in less postoperative pain. The patient is situated in a beach-chair supine position (**Fig. 25.3**). Elevating the head of the table 30 to 45 degrees is usually enough to minimize bleeding and to allow the surgeon to work comfortably. Position the patient slightly toward the operative side until the lateral part of the shoulder is off of the operating room table. The arm should be stabilized with an arm holder. It should leave enough space for the surgeon to be close to the table, facing the shoulder. The assistant should be on the lateral side. A folded sheet or a sandbag is placed under the medial border of the scapula to push the affected side forward and tilt the scapula, allowing the arm to fall backward, opening the deltopectoral space and placing the coracoid process more laterally.

25.6 Operative Technique

25.6.1 Deltopectoral Approach

A short deltopectoral approach is used for exposure. The deltopectoral groove is palpated from the distal side of the coracoid. The skin incision starts from the distal tip of the coracoid process. Usually, it is easily perceptible through the skin to follow the deltopectoral groove. The length of the incision is not more than 5 or 6 cm, depending on the size and the musculature of the

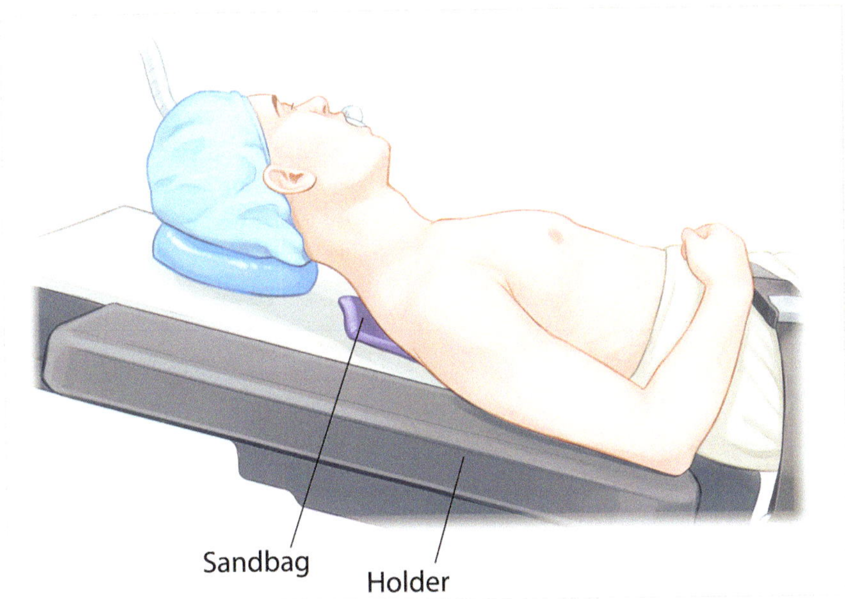

Fig. 25.3 Patient positioning. The arm will be stabilized by a holder that should be only under the shoulder and half of the arm. A folded sheet or a sandbag is placed under the spinal border of the scapula to push the affected side forward and tilt the scapula.

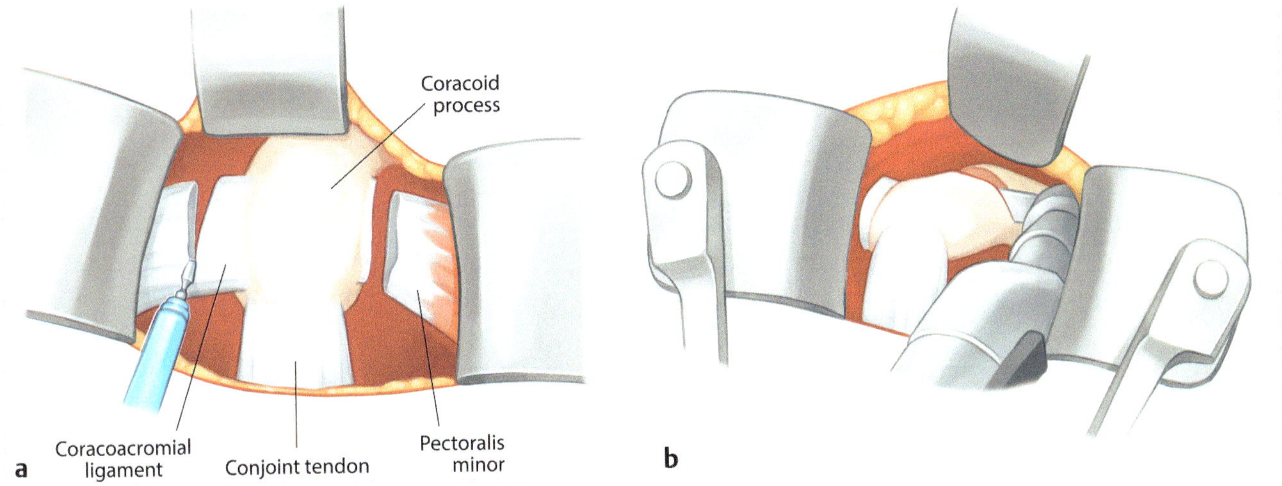

Fig. 25.4 Coracoid process exposure and harvest.

patient. After identification of the deltopectoral groove, incise the fascia over the pectoralis major, then retract the pectoralis major medially and the deltoid laterally. The cephalic vein is usually retracted laterally with the deltoid. Some branches may have to be coagulated, especially proximal to facilitate the coracoid approach. The use of the retractors is critical with this technique and the assistant has a crucial role. After using two Farabeuf retractors, a Bankart autostatic retractor can be inserted to facilitate the surgical procedure.

25.6.2 Coracoid Process Harvesting

Identify the coracoid process and the coracobrachial; then, expose the coracoid process (**Fig. 25.4**). First, use a long Farabeuf retractor; then a bone lever retractor, which is placed over the top of the coracoid process. If needed, abduction and external rotation of the arm allow the skin window to move proximally and the coracoid process approach. After identification, the coracoacromial ligament is transected 5 mm lateral to its coracoid insertion. Beware to not damage the underlying cuff. The pectoralis minor is detached from its coracoid insertion, close to the bone.

After returning the arm in adduction and internal rotation, using a 90-degree-angle blade saw, the coracoid process is cut from medial to lateral. The level of the transection is at the "knee," immediately distal to the coracoclavicular ligaments. If needed, the distal insertions of these ligaments can be palpated with the finger. A grasping forceps is used to hold the bone graft and progressively release the bone graft from the soft tissue. The coracoid process is reverted and the coracobrachial is deliberately released. Carefully attend to the musculocutaneous nerve, which is penetrating the muscle, 3 to 4 cm distal to the tip of the coracoid. Frequently, coagulation of a small artery has to be performed close and proximal to the nerve.

25.6.3 Preparation of the Coracoid Process

A Farabeuf retractor is placed at the distal end of the incision over a gauze sponge (**Fig. 25.5**). The bone block is flipped on the retractor in order to expose the deep surface, which is cleaned

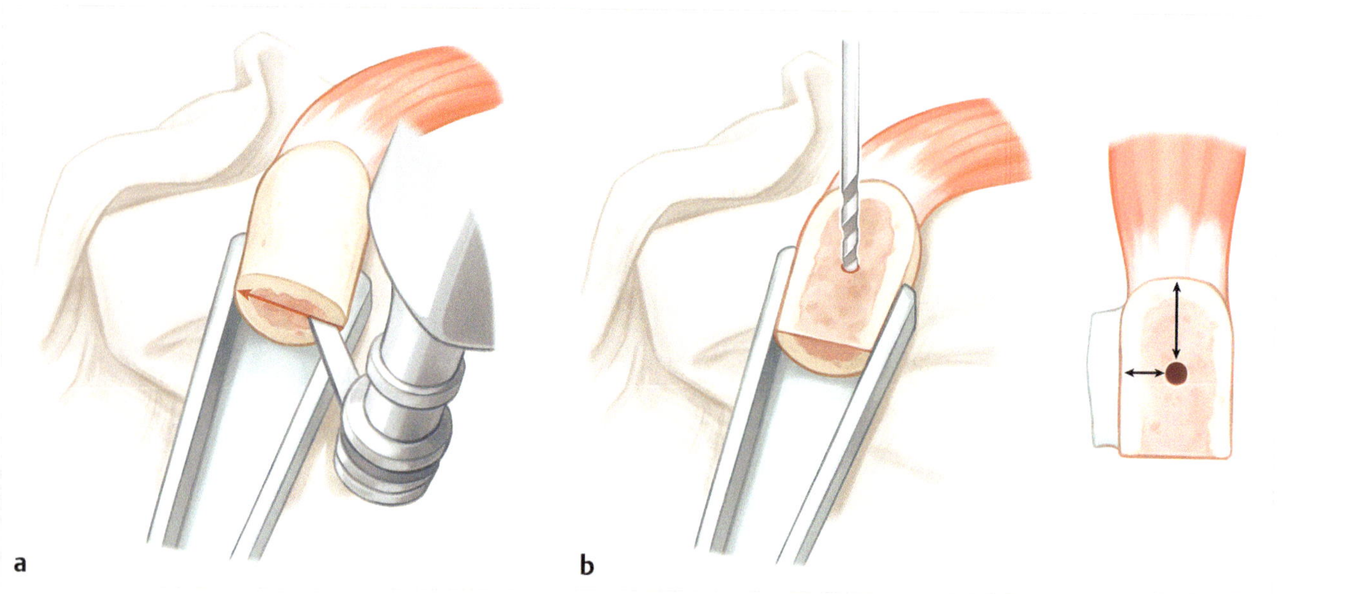

Fig. 25.5 Preparation of the coracoid process.

from the remaining soft tissue. A sagittal saw is used to decorticate the deep surface of the coracoid bone block. This step is crucial, as it must expose the cancellous bone in order to improve further consolidation. A 2.5-mm hole is performed in the center of the graft and the superficial part of the hole is cleared with an electrocautery. Using only one hole and one screw is different from the usual and traditional technique described in the literature. The purpose is to minimize the risk of intraoperative fracture of the bone block (the size of the coracoid process is variable from one patient to another one) and to maximize the cancellous bone surface and improve the consolidation of the graft. Furthermore, some coracoid has an "hourglass" shape after preparation. In that case, the unique screw will be located in the narrow portion of the bone, leaving the larger parts of cancellous bone free. Some have argued that two screws are preferable to control the rotation of the graft. In our experience, once the screw is fixed with the washer, there is no more rotational motion observed, either preoperatively or even on the CT scan systematically performed 3 months after the procedure. Once the drilling is accomplished, the distances between the hole and the lateral border and between the hole and the distal part are both measured. It will be reported on the anterior glenoid neck in a later step. The use of a plastic ruler can facilitate this measurement as shown in **Fig. 25.7.** The thickness of the hole is finally measured with a depth gauge. The Farabeuf retractor and gauze are removed, the coracoid bone block is positioned underneath a Hoesel-type retractor, and a gauze is placed at the distal part of the incision.

25.6.4 Glenoid Exposure

The superior and inferior borders of the subscapularis tendon are identified visually and through palpation (**Fig. 25.6**). At the junction of the middle and distal thirds of the tendon, the subscapularis is divided horizontally with the use of the electrocautery and scissors. The modification of the humerus rotation facilitates this step. When hyperlaxity is present, it is recommended to leave 50% proximally and 50% distally, splitting the subscapularis in the middle and increasing the sling effect.[4] Once the capsule is visualized, a gauze is pushed medially between the muscle and the capsule. An anterior glenoid neck retractor is then inserted on the anterior surface of the scapula and medial to the medial attachment of the capsule allowing to retract the medial part of the subscapularis and to expose the anterior part of the glenoid. The capsule is opened horizontally at the same level of the subscapularis split. We prefer this technique of opening instead of the "vertical technique" as it makes the capsular shift at the end of the procedure simpler (if the capsulotomy is vertical and too lateral, there is a risk of overtightening during the capsular suture). This horizontal capsulotomy allows a customized capsule retention. A Fukuda retractor is placed in the glenohumeral joint. If needed, an additional Hohmann retractor is cautiously placed at the inferior border of the glenoid allowing to expose the inferior part of the glenoid. One of the main issues in this minimally invasive technique is the retraction of the superior part of the subscapularis tendon, especially if the patient has a voluminous musculature. A Steinmann pin, impacted in the superior part of the scapular neck, usually solves this problem. The capsule, labrum, and the visible joint are inspected. The inferior portion of the labrum is resected, including the periosteum over the anterior surface of the distal half of the scapular neck. A curve osteotome is used to decorticate the bone, which will receive the coracoid graft. This is a critical step in the surgery to avoid the risk of nonunion.

25.6.5 Coracoid Fixation

The measurements previously performed on the coracoid are made on the scapular neck, with the aim of flushing the coracoid graft with the lateral border and the inferior border of the glenoid (**Fig. 25.7**). This point is marked with the electrocautery. The same 2.5-mm drill is used to create an anterior to posterior hole. The first cortex is drilled, then the second cortex is filled with the drill ("knock the door") and eventually drilled. The depth is measured with a depth gauge and added to the depth of the coracoid. The usual total length is between 30 and

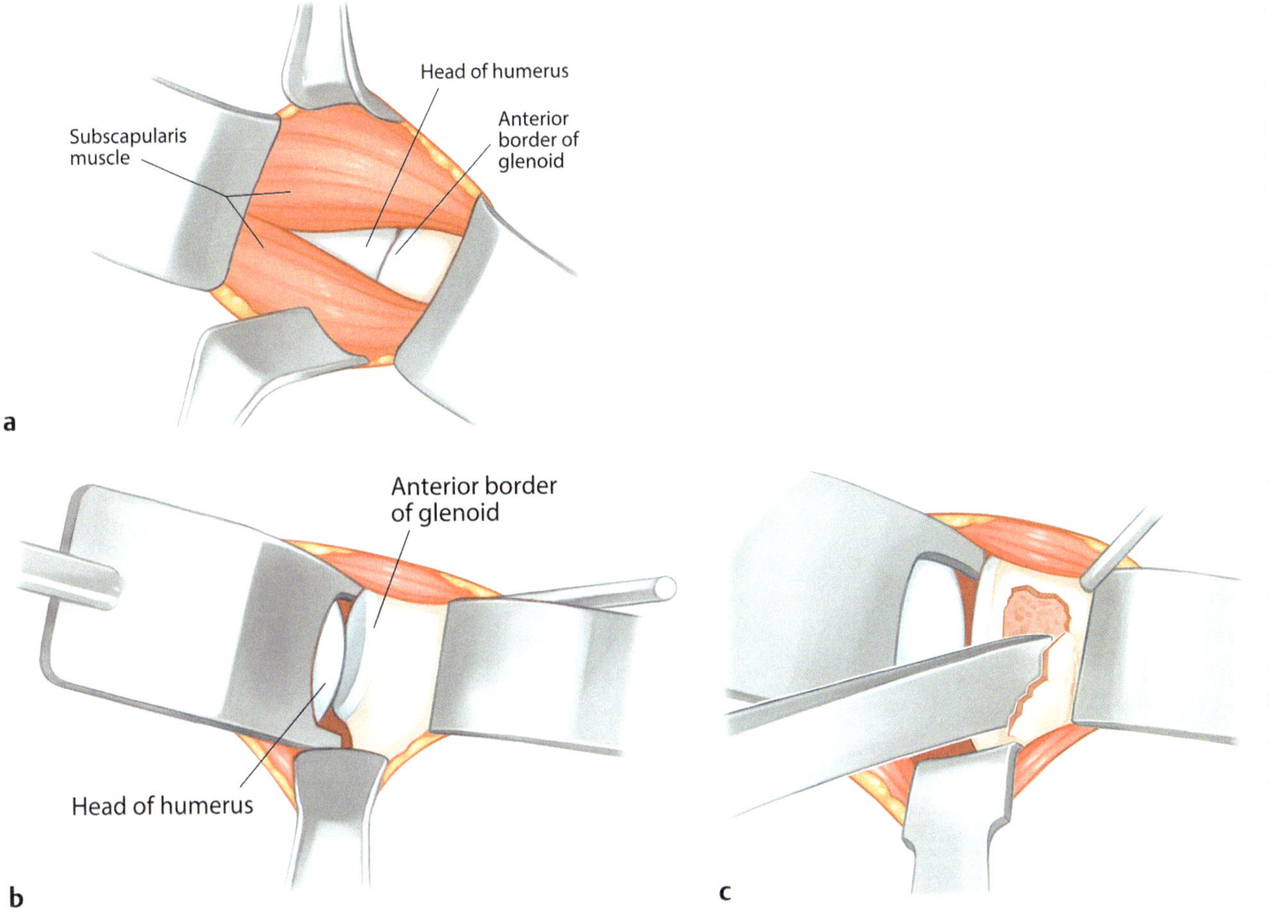

Fig. 25.6 Glenoid exposure.

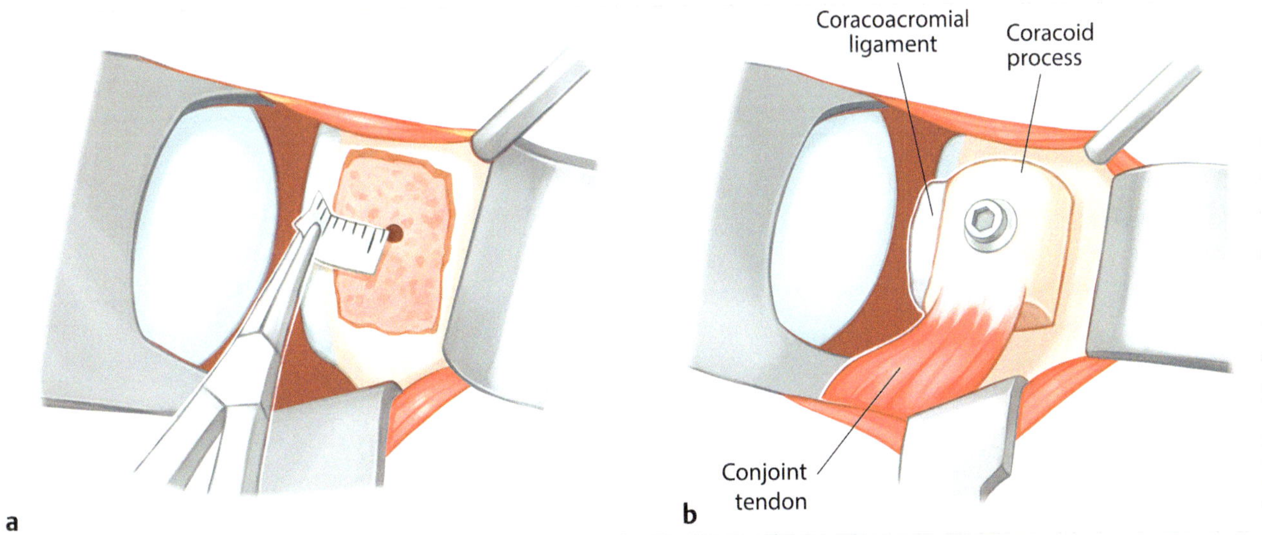

Fig. 25.7 Coracoid fixation.

40 mm. The coracoid process is retrieved from the inferior part of the incision, and the gauze is removed. The medial Bateman retractor is temporarily removed in order to remove the medial gauze, and the retractor is placed again medially at the same place. The same grasper as the one initially used holds the coracoid graft. The appropriately sized partially threaded cancellous 4-mm screw with a washer is introduced through the bone graft until the complete threaded part is passed through the graft. The tip of the screw is progressively introduced in the scapular neck hole and the grasper holding the bone graft in a correct

position is controlling the rotation. The screw must engage the posterior cortex of the scapula, with the washer, in order to get an excellent compression. The bone block must flush the anterior border of the glenoid and nerve overhang laterally to avoid the risk of osteoarthritis.[7] The finger palpation of the anterior edge of the joint and the external rotation of the humeral head allow us to assess the absence of conflict.

25.6.6 Capsular Suture and Closure

The Bankart effect is performed with a no. 2 braided absorbable suture (**Fig. 25.8**). After removal of the distal Hohmann and the Fukuda retractors, the suture is first passed in the inferior part of the coracoacromial ligament stump. The arm is in adduction and full external rotation. The arm is positioned in adduction and full external rotation, then the suture is passed to restore the capsule and inferior glenohumeral ligament tension. The medial Bateman retractor and the Steinmann pin are removed and the two parts of the subscapularis tendon are approximated with a no. 2 braided absorbable suture. No closure is performed between the deltoid and the pectoralis major. The subcutaneous and cutaneous layers are closed. If the bleeding has been significant during the procedure, a drain can be placed before closure. The patient is taken back to the recovery room with a simple shoulder sling.

25.7 Tips and Pearls/Expert Suggestions

The success of your Latarjet, in large part, depends on retractor placement and your assistant.

- Skin incision is made directly inferior to the coracoid process.
- Bone lever retractor is placed over the "coracoid knee."
- Leave the coracoacromial ligament stump.
- A coracoid osteotomy is made with a 90-degree saw at the level of the knee.
- Always be cognizant of the location of the musculocutaneous nerve.
- Decorticate the deep surface of the coracoid bone graft.
- One screw is enough, but two screws can be ok.
- Measure the position of the coracoid hole and then report to the glenoid.
- Split the subscapularis.
- Horizontal capsulotomy is preferable to vertical capsulotomy.
- Decorticate the glenoid neck.
- Place the coracoid in the "lying" position.
- Do not overhang!
- Suture the capsule in external rotation.

25.8 What to Avoid

Two main mistakes must be avoided:

- Overhanging of the coracoid graft.[7]
- Capsular suture in internal rotation.

25.9 Complications/Bailout/Salvage

25.9.1 Fracture of the Coracoid

With this technique, we never experimented an intraoperative coracoid graft fracture. In our opinion, the size of the screw (4-mm diameter) and the small washer prevent this complication.

25.9.2 Overhanging

Even with precaution, it can happen that after the fixation, the coracoid process is overhanging from the anterior border of the glenoid. It rarely concerns the total length of the graft if the

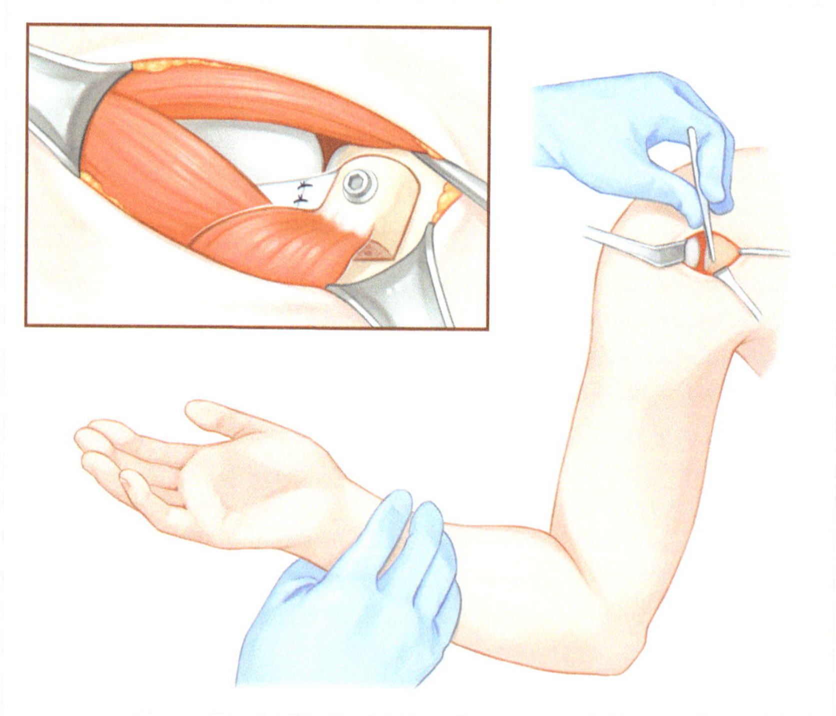

Fig. 25.8 Capsule suture.

technique has been correctly done with the report measurement. It can be the result of the anatomy of the coracoid process (hourglass shape) with only one part overhanging. In this case, it is usually not necessary to change the position of the graft and to perform a new screw hole (with the risk of low stability); just remove the overhanging part with a saw or a rongeur.

25.9.3 Missing Coracoacromial Stump

It can happen that the coracohumeral stump is too small for a correct suture passage during the capsular shift, either because the stump has been made too short or because the surgeon had to remove the distal lateral part of the graft to correct an overhanging of the coracoid graft. There are two options to solve the problem: either suture the capsule to the proximal part of the conjoint tendon, close to the inferior corner of the coracoid process, or use an anchor like in a standard arthroscopic Bankart procedure.

25.10 Postoperative Care

The patient is immobilized in a simple sling for 2 to 3 weeks for comfort. Before their discharge from the hospital, the patient is given home exercises to focus on distal range of motion (ROM) and active assisted ROM to 90 degrees. They are allowed to move immediately with no restriction in external rotation. In fact, it is our practice to encourage the patient to move their arm in external rotation, as the capsule was sutured in that position. The formal physiotherapy starts after the first 3 weeks to progressively increase the motion, especially external rotation and adduction.

The return to sport is usually possible after 3 months for noncontact sports and 4 months for contact and collision sports. We routinely perform a CT scan 3 months after surgery in order to assess the coracoid fusion and guide the return to sport.

References

1. Latarjet M. A propos du traitement des luxations récidivantes de l'épaule. Lyon Chir 1954;49(8):994–997
2. Patte D, Bernageau J, Bancel P The anteroinferior vulnerable point of the glenoid rim. In: Bateman JE, Welsch RP, eds.Surgery of the Shoulder.New York, NY: Marcel Dekker; 1985:94–99
3. Giles JW, Boons HW, Elkinson I, et al. Does the dynamic sling effect of the Latarjet procedure improve shoulder stability? A biomechanical evaluation. J Shoulder Elbow Surg 2013;22(6):821–827
4. Walch G, Boileau P. Latarjet-Bristow procedure for recurrent anterior instability. Tech Shoulder Elbow Surg 2000;1(4):256–261
5. An VV, Sivakumar BS, Phan K, Trantalis J. A systematic review and meta-analysis of clinical and patient-reported outcomes following two procedures for recurrent traumatic anterior instability of the shoulder: Latarjet procedure vs. Bankart repair. J Shoulder Elbow Surg 2016;25(5):853–863
6. Griesser MJ, Harris JD, McCoy BW, et al. Complications and re-operations after Bristow-Latarjet shoulder stabilization: a systematic review. J Shoulder Elbow Surg 2013;22(2):286–292
7. Allain J, Goutallier D, Glorion C. Long-term results of the Latarjet procedure for the treatment of anterior instability of the shoulder. J Bone Joint Surg Am 1998;80(6):841–852

26 The Arthroscopic Latarjet Procedure

Malte Holschen, Laurent Lafosse, and Jens D. Agneskirchner

Abstract
Recurrent anterior shoulder instability may be a result of an inadequate primary Bankart repair but it may also be a result of bony defects of the anterior glenoid, large and engaging Hill–Sachs defects, and insufficient tissue quality of the anterior capsule and the labrum. If bony defects or insufficient soft-tissues are responsible for recurrent anterior shoulder instability, the arthroscopic latarjet procedure may restore shoulder stability by bony augmentation of the anterior glenoid and by a soft-tissue sling provided by the attached conjoint tendons. The principle of the arthroscopic Latarjet procedure is the minimally invasive identification of the coracoid process and a consecutive osteotomy at its base. Using a positioning guide, it is then maneuvered into the joint through a horizontal split of the subscapularis tendon and fixed to the anterior glenoid with two cannulated screws. The procedure is technically demanding and associated with a considerable risk for injury to neurovascular structures. Therefore optimal visualization needs to be achieved throughout the whole procedure. The arthroscopic Latarjet procedure leads to high patient satisfaction and low recurrence rates when performed adequately. Furthermore, it is beneficial for ideal graft positioning and visualization of the neurovascular structures when performed correctly.

Keywords: *anterior shoulder instability, arthroscopic Latarjet procedure, glenoid bone-loss, engaging Hill-Sachs lesion, failed Bankart repair, bony augmentation*

26.1 Introduction

Recurrent anterior shoulder instability can be associated with bony defects of the anterior glenoid, large and engaging Hill–Sachs defects, and insufficient tissue quality of the anterior capsule and the labrum. In those cases, a sole fixation of the capsulolabral complex is related to a high risk for recurrent anterior instability.

Bony augmentation of the anterior glenoid rim using the coracoid process stabilizes the shoulder by enlarging the horizontal glenoid diameter and by the additional sling effect of the attached conjoint tendons (**Fig. 26.1**).

The principle of the arthroscopic Latarjet procedure is the minimally invasive identification of the coracoid process and a consecutive osteotomy at its base. Using a positioning guide, it is then maneuvered into the joint through a horizontal split of the subscapularis tendon and fixed to the anterior glenoid with two cannulated screws.

26.2 Indications

An arthroscopic Latarjet procedure is indicated for primary and recurrent anterior shoulder instability with the following:

- Glenoid bone loss greater than 20% of the horizontal diameter.
- Large and engaging Hill–Sachs defect.
- Combined bony defects of humerus and glenoid.
- Irreparable soft-tissue defects of the capsulolabral complex including humeral avulsion of the glenohumeral ligament (HAGL) lesions.

26.3 Contraindications

The arthroscopic Latarjet procedure is contraindicated, in case of the following:

- Adequate bone stock and soft-tissue quality allowing an arthroscopic Bankart repair.
- Adolescent patients or children.
- Relevant defects of the subscapularis tendon.
- Advanced instability osteoarthritis.

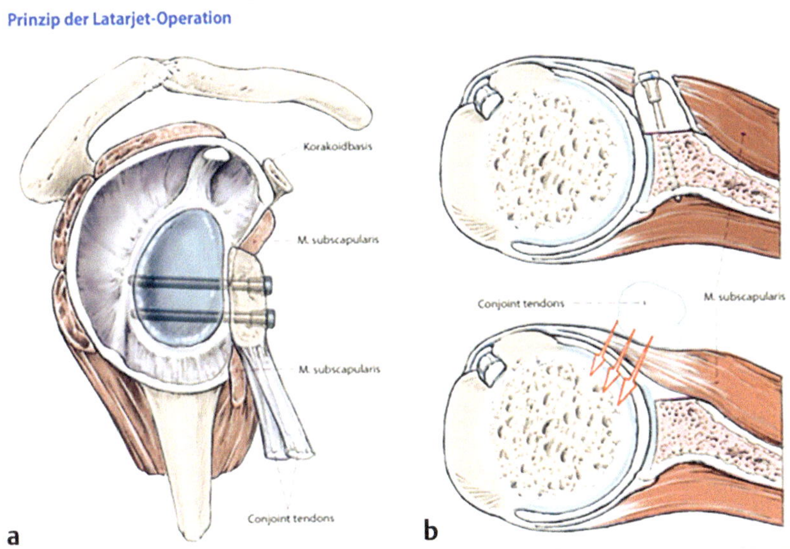

Fig. 26.1 Principle of the arthroscopic Latarjet procedure. The anterior glenoid defect is augmented with the coracoid process, which is fixed with two cannulated screws **(a)**. The inferiorly attached conjoint tendons generate dynamic compression on the subscapularis tendon and the anterior humerus (sling effect) in the abduction and external rotation position **(b)**.

26.4 Preoperative Examination

Patient history may reveal valuable clues about the severity and the risk for recurrence of anterior shoulder instability. If minor trauma causes dislocation of the affected shoulder, bone defects or severe soft-tissue damage should be considered. Recurrent dislocations after previous Bankart repair might not be addressed properly by another refixation of the capsulolabral complex. Contact sports are related to a higher recurrence rate.

Various clinical tests assess anterior shoulder instability. Most commonly, the affected shoulder is brought into an abduction and external rotation position, which causes pain or countermovement in order to avoid dislocation.

For the apprehension test the patient's shoulder is abducted into different positions and externally rotated, while the examiner applies pressure to the humerus from posterior and observes increasing pain or countermovement.

For the relocation test, the patient's shoulder is moved into abduction and external rotation in a supine position. If this causes pain, manual pressure is applied to the anterior humerus. Pain relief caused by this maneuver indicates anterior shoulder instability.

Standard anteroposterior and axial radiographs show larger glenoid substance loss and Hill–Sachs defects. Further X-ray techniques assess smaller bone lesions. The West Point view indicates glenoid defects and bone fragments, while the Stryker view projects Hill–Sachs defects.

Soft-tissue structures, cartilage lesions, concomitant lesions of the rotator cuff and the biceps tendon, as well as bone defects are revealed on MRI scans.

Bone loss and bone defects are ideally identified on CT scans. 3D reconstructions of the glenoid with a subtracted humeral head facilitate quantification and localization of glenoid defects especially when the affected glenoid is compared to the healthy contralateral side (**Fig. 26.2**).

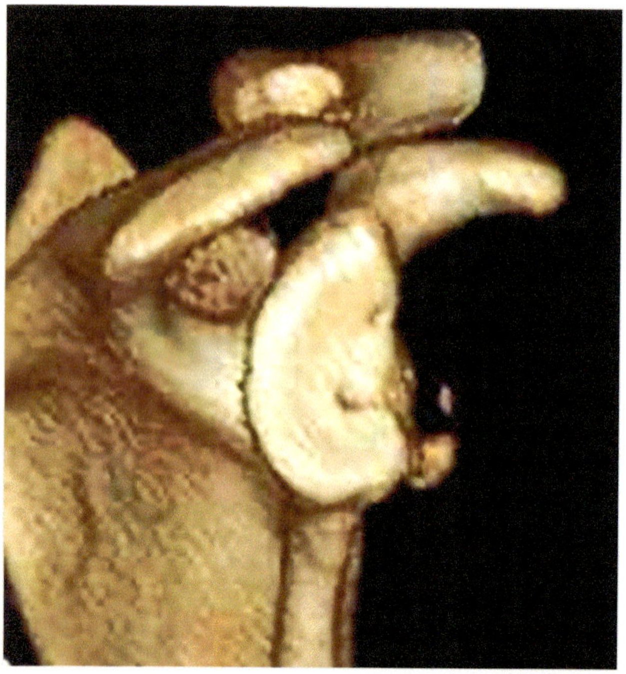

Fig. 26.2 3D CT of the glenoid. The "en face" view with a subtracted humeral head shows the extent and localization of the anterior glenoid defect.

26.5 Surgical Technique

The procedure is processed in the beach-chair position using an arm holder (e.g., Spider, Smith & Nephew). The arthroscopic Latarjet requires ideal anesthesia in combination with a nerve block of the brachial plexus. A mean arterial blood pressure between 60 and 65 mm Hg should be maintained during the coracoid transfer to avoid bleeding and poor visualization. To prevent intraoperative hypoxia, a continuous regional oximetry of the forehead should be applied (e.g., INVOS, Medtronic).

Besides a standard burr and a shaver, a radiofrequency device is mandatory (e.g., VAPR, DePuy Mitek). Laurent Lafosse has developed specific instruments for the arthroscopic Latarjet. To date, they are exclusively available from one manufacturer (DePuy Mitek; **Fig. 26.3**). Fixation of the coracoid process to the anterior glenoid is achieved through cannulated screws and sleeves (top hats).

After identification and marking of anatomical structures (**Fig. 26.4**), diagnostic shoulder arthroscopy and assessment of an engaging Hill–Sachs defect in abduction and external rotation are carried out using the posterior portal (A). Anterior labrum, capsule, and ligaments are checked for their tissue quality.

If a transfer of the coracoid process is indicated, the insufficient labrum, the medial glenohumeral ligament, and the anterior capsule are resected through an anteromedial portal (E) to visualize the anterior glenoid rim and the subscapularis muscle fibers. Bone fragments and remnants of previous Bankart repairs (sutures and anchors) have to be removed with a shaver, an elevator, or a rongeur.

The next steps are opening of the rotator interval, visualization the coracoid process by separating the coracoacromial ligament, and identification the conjoint tendons (**Fig. 26.5**).

After placing the arthroscope into the anterolateral portal, the extent of the anterior glenoid defect becomes more evident. The glenoid neck is debrided and a bone bed is prepared with a burr or a rasp through an anteromedial portal (E).

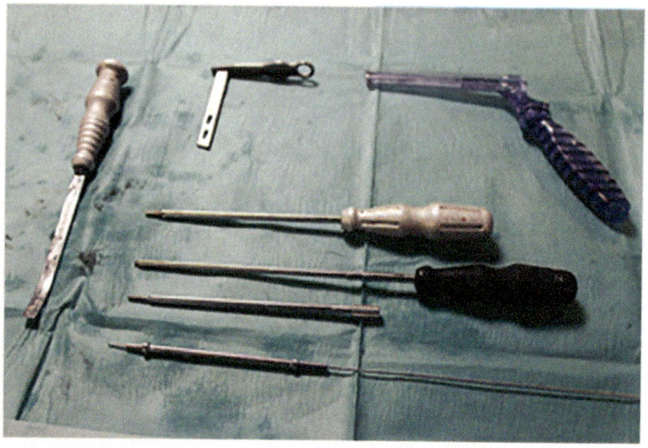

Fig. 26.3 Instruments for the arthroscopic Latarjet procedure (DePuy Mitek). Curved chisel, screwdrivers, taps, jig for K-wires penetrating the coracoid, and a positioning device with an ergonomic handle.

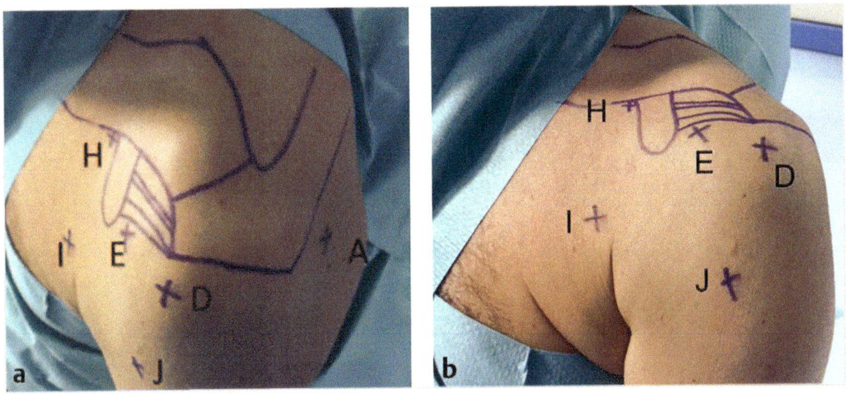

Fig. 26.4 Anatomical landmarks and portals are marked preoperatively. View from superior **(a)** and anterior **(b)**. Besides the coracoid process, the scapular spine, the acromion, the clavicle, and the required portals are marked. A, posterior portal; D, anterolateral portal; E, anteromedial portal; H, supracoracoid portal; J, deep anterolateral portal; I, deep anteromedial portal.

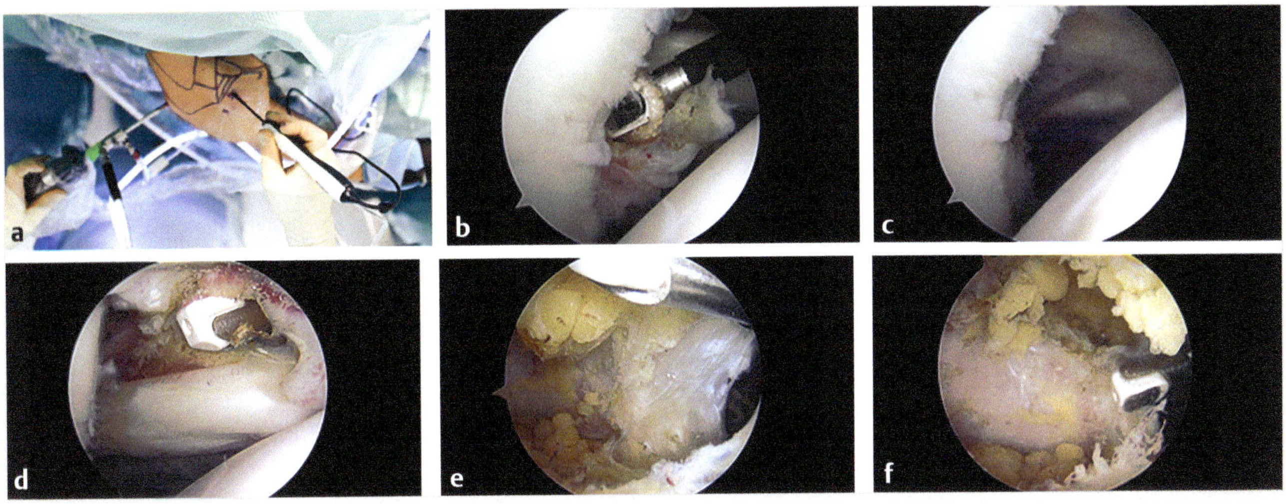

Fig. 26.5 Intra-articular preparation. The arthroscope is inserted through the posterior portal, while the radiofrequency device is passed through the anteromedial portal **(a)**. After resection of the anterior labrum and the medial glenohumeral ligament **(b)**, the glenoid defect becomes visible **(c)**. The rotator interval is opened **(d)** before the coracoacromial ligament is identified **(e)** and resected **(f)**.

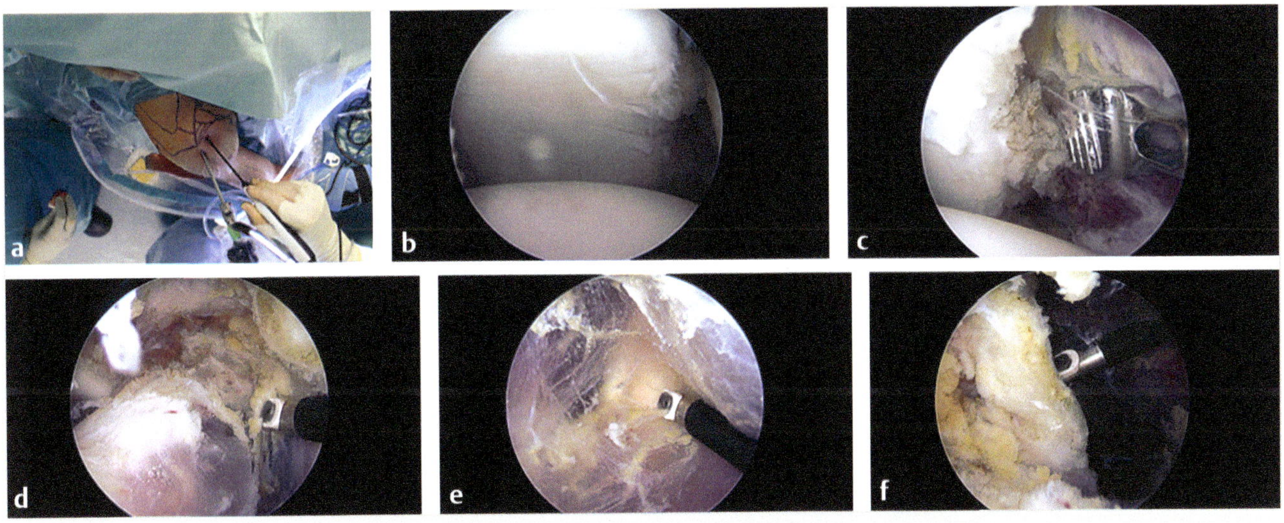

Fig. 26.6 Preparation of the glenoid and extra-articular dissection. The arthroscope is positioned anterolaterally, while the instruments are introduced anteromedially **(a)**. The glenoid defect **(b)** is prepared for the coracoid transfer with a rasp **(c)**. After careful dissection of the interval between subscapularis tendon and conjoint tendons **(d)**, the axillary nerve is identified **(e)**. The anterior side of the conjoint tendons is dissected carefully **(f)**.

After releasing the superior and lateral coracoid process, the axillary nerve can be identified with the help of careful medial preparation between the conjoint tendons and the subscapularis muscle. The conjoint tendons are also released anteriorly (**Fig. 26.6**).

The arthroscope is consecutively switched to the anteromedial portal (E). The assistant retracts the deltoid muscle cranially with a switching stick introduced through the anterolateral portal (D). After generating a medial portal superior to the coracoid process (H), the pectoralis minor tendon is detached from its insertion on the medial border of the coracoid and the conjoint tendons. Injury to the brachial plexus and to the musculocutaneous nerve has to be avoided carefully during the dissection.

Afterward, two parallel K-wires are drilled centrally through the coracoid using a jig. To evaluate the correct position of the two K-wires, the arthroscope is introduced through the supracoracoid portal. If the K-wires are both central and in the correct longitudinal coracoid axis, two holes are created using a 3.2-mm cannulated drill. After drilling, a tap is used to create threads before two sleeves (top hats) are inserted to support the threads (**Fig. 26.7**).

As a next step, the subscapularis muscle and tendon are identified utilizing a deep anterolateral portal (J). The last portal is a deep anteromedial portal, whose localization is crucial for subsequent fixation of the coracoid process. Thus, the portal needs to be in line with the glenoid surface.

In order to identify the correct level of the horizontal subscapularis split, a switching stick is inserted via the posterior portal (A) and penetrated through the subscapularis tendon under arthroscopic control right at the position of the glenoid defect (the 3 to 5 o'clock position). A radiofrequency device is inserted through the deep anteromedial portal to split the subscapularis tendon beginning at the position of the penetrated switching stick. At least one-third of the subscapularis tendon should remain superior to the split. The split should rather be extended medially into the muscle fibers than laterally, where the tendinous part should be preserved. Medially, the axillary nerve needs to be identified repeatedly in order to protect it. The size of the split needs to be large enough to provide a good view on the anterior glenoid through the deep anterolateral portal (J) and sufficient approach path for the coracoid process (**Fig. 26.8**).

The inferior breaking point of the coracoid osteotomy is determined by milling the inferior cortex of the coracoid. For

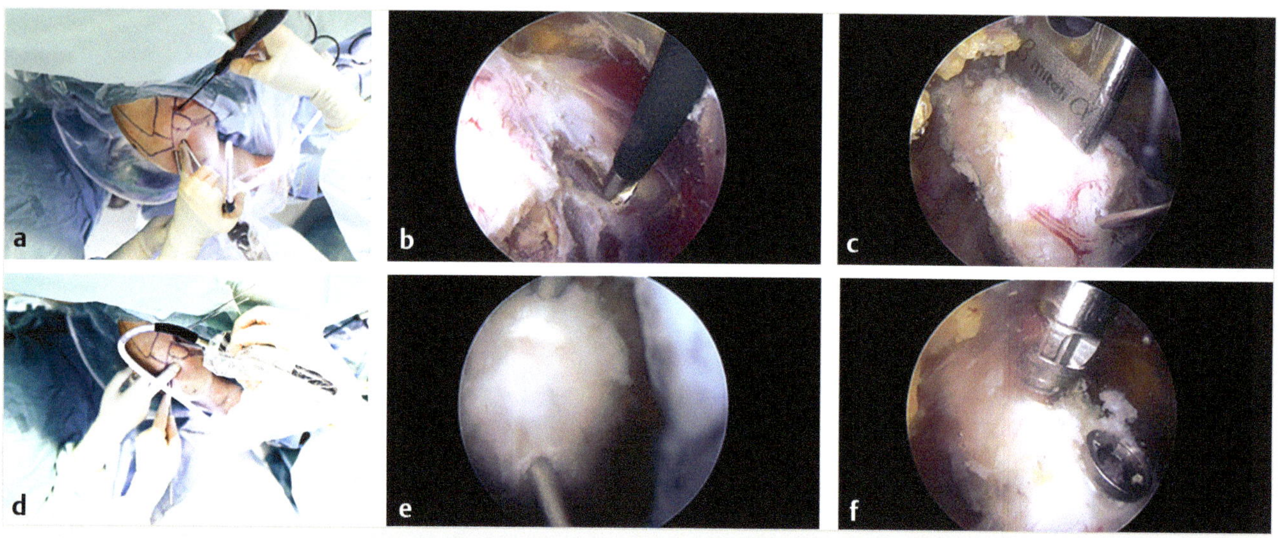

Fig. 26.7 Preparation of the coracoid process and establishment of drill holes. The assistant retracts the deltoid muscle superiorly using the anterolateral portal, while the surgeon positions the arthroscope anteromedially and the instruments into the supracoracoid portal **(a)**. After tenotomy of the pectoralis minor tendon **(b)**, two K-wires are drilled into the coracoid using a jig **(c)**. The position of the K-wires is controlled through the supracoracoid portal **(d, e)**. After drilling and tapping, two screw sleeves are inserted **(f)**.

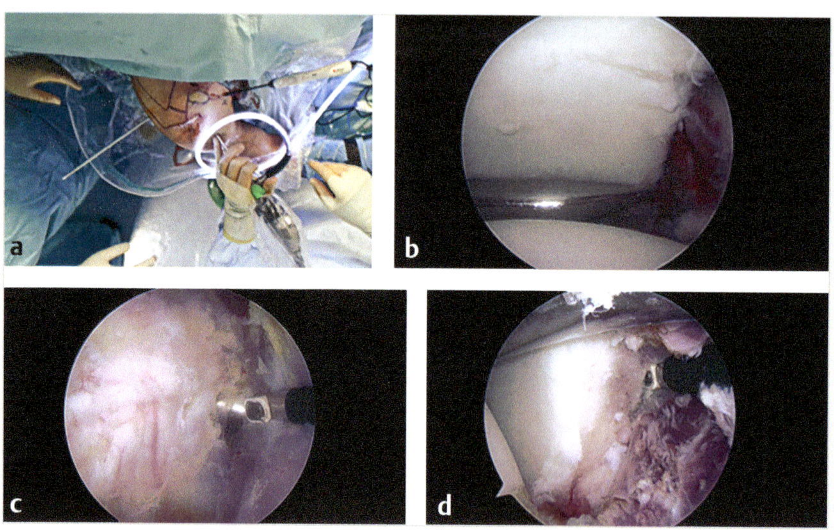

Fig. 26.8 Subscapularis split. The switching stick is introduced posteriorly. The arthroscope is positioned in the deep anterolateral portal and the radiofrequency device is passed through the deep anteromedial portal **(a)**. After the subscapularis tendon has been perforated below the upper third **(b)**, the split is extended along the course of the subscapularis fibers **(c)**. After the split has been completed, the switching stick serves as a retractor in order to open the split for the coracoid transfer **(d)**.

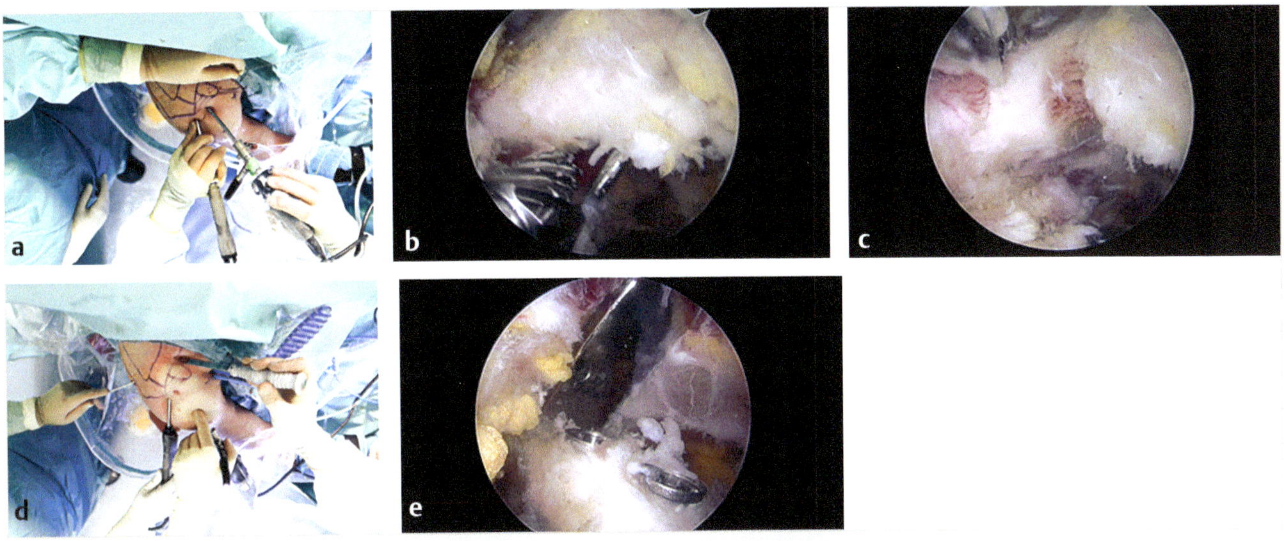

Fig. 26.9 Osteotomy of the coracoid process. The arthroscope is inserted through the anterosuperior portal, while the burr is positioned in the anterolateral portal **(a)**. After milling a breaking point into the inferior surface of the coracoid **(b, c)**, the osteotomy is carried out with a curved chisel through the supracoracoid portal **(d, e)**.

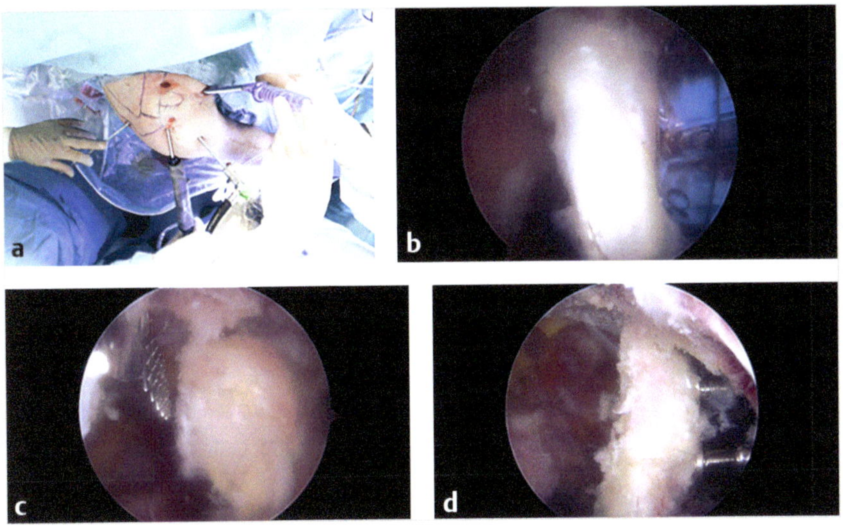

Fig. 26.10 Preparation of the coracoid transfer. The camera lies in the deep anterolateral portal. The rasp is introduced anterolaterally **(a)**. The coracoid process is fixed to the positioning device with two screws through the deep anteromedial portal **(b)**. The inferior surface of the coracoid is milled with a rasp in order to fit onto the glenoid **(c, d)**.

this procedure, a burr is inserted through the anterolateral portal (D) and visualized via the anteromedial portal (E). After the inferior cortex is weakened, the osteotomy is carried out with a curved chisel inserted through the supracoracoid portal (H; **Fig. 26.9**).

After completion of the osteotomy, the positioning device is introduced through the deep anteromedial portal (E) and the coracoid is fixed to the device with two screws. The inferior cortex of the coracoid is decorticated and shaped to fit onto the glenoid defect using a burr or a rasp via the anterolateral portal (D; **Fig. 26.10**).

The positioning device in the inferior anteromedial portal (I) is consecutively used to maneuver the coracoid through the subscapularis split and to put it onto the glenoid defect. The switching in the posterior portal (A) is used as a retractor for this step. The ideal position of the coracoid on the anterior glenoid is between the 3 and 5 o'clock positions. The graft needs to be flush with the glenoid defect and the joint level. The coracoid is then temporarily fixed with two long K-wires that pass the positioning device, the coracoid, and the glenoid in the correct level of anteversion (~30 degrees) before they penetrate the posterior skin.

The cannulated drill is used to create two drill holes. The length of the drill tunnels can be read from the drill. Afterward, two cannulated screws are tightened alternately, while the compression of the coracoid to the glenoid is checked arthroscopically via the deep anterolateral portal (**Fig. 26.11**).

The position of the graft is finally visualized from different perspectives in order to avoid parallax errors (**Fig. 26.12**). A lateral overhang of the graft can be reduced with a burr.

26.6 Postoperative Management

In order to demonstrate a correct positioning of the screws and the graft, plain radiographs (anteroposterior and Y views) and an optional CT scan with 3D reconstruction (**Fig. 26.13**) should be conducted.

The operated shoulder is immobilized in an abduction sling for 3 weeks. On the first postoperative day, assisted mobilization

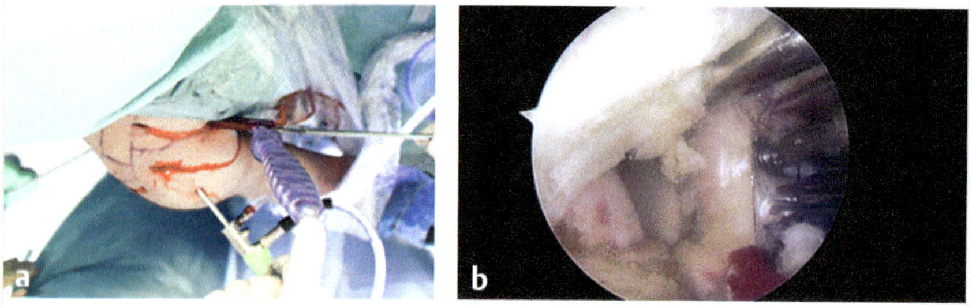

Fig. 26.11 Positioning of the coracoid. The switching stick is used to retract the superior part of the subscapularis split. The camera is inserted through the deep anterolateral portal. The positioning instrument remains in the deep anteromedial portal **(a)**. After the coracoid has been maneuvered through the subscapularis split, it is positioned onto the glenoid defect and fixed with two K-wires that are consecutively replaced by two cannulated screws **(b)**. The screws are tightened alternately.

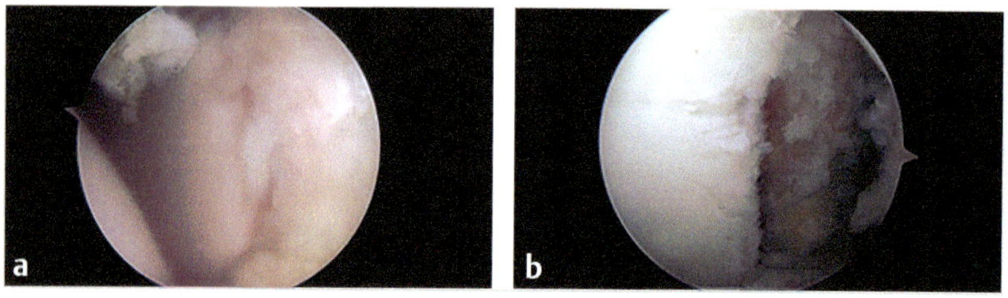

Fig. 26.12 Arthroscopic control of the transferred coracoid. The graft's position is checked from several perspectives to avoid potential parallax errors **(a, b)**.

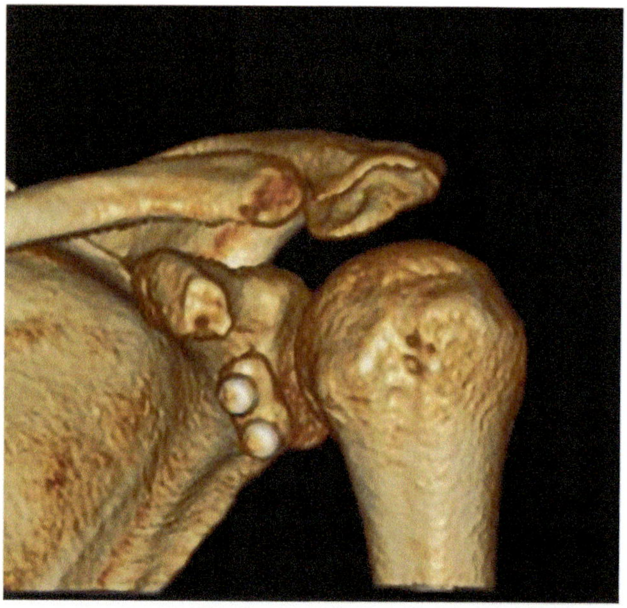

Fig. 26.13 Postoperative 3D CT. The graft is positioned ideally onto the glenoid defect and it is parallel to the glenoid surface.

is allowed until 0-degree external rotation and 60-degree abduction. From the second postoperative day until the end of the third postoperative week, assisted active mobilization until 30-degree external and 90-degree abduction is allowed.

With the beginning of the fourth postoperative week, shoulder range of mobilization is unlimited. The earliest return to sports including contact sports is recommended after 12 postoperative weeks.

26.7 Results

We investigated the clinical outcome of 50 patients after a mean of 4.5 years. The patients were satisfied subjectively (visual analog scale [VAS] for pain 1.2/10; VAS for stability 7.6/10, and VAS for overall satisfaction 8.8/10).

Clinical scores improved during the period between preoperative examination and final follow-up (Oxford Instability score from 18.7 to 40; American Shoulder and Elbow Surgeons [ASES] score from 39.4 to 86.9; Rowe score from 37 to 79; Walch–Duplay score from 35.8 to 84).

The overall rate of recurrent instability and other complications was 5%. The radiographs showed a frequent remodeling of the superior graft, which did not interfere with the clinical result.

26.8 Complications

Besides general complications and recurrent instability, specific complications of the arthroscopic Latarjet procedure involve neurovascular injury and problems around the coracoid graft and the fixation screws:

- Nerve injury (musculocutaneous nerve, axillary nerve, and brachial plexus).
- Vessel injury (axillary artery and vein).
- Medial or lateral malpositioning of the coracoid graft.
- Anterior screw impingement.
- Irritation of posterior soft tissue by screw tips.
- Screw breakage.
- Resorption or nonunion of the coracoid graft.

Suggested Readings

Allain J, Goutallier D, Glorion C. Long-term results of the Latarjet procedure for the treatment of anterior instability of the shoulder. J Bone Joint Surg Am 1998;80(6):841–852

Boileau P, Villalba M, Héry JY, Balg F, Ahrens P, Neyton L. Risk factors for recurrence of shoulder instability after arthroscopic Bankart repair. J Bone Joint Surg Am 2006;88(8):1755–1763

Hovelius L, Sandström B, Saebö M. One hundred eighteen Bristow-Latarjet repairs for recurrent anterior dislocation of the shoulder prospectively followed for fifteen years: study II-the evolution of dislocation arthropathy. J Shoulder Elbow Surg 2006;15(3):279–289

Hovelius L, Sandström B, Sundgren K, Saebö M. One hundred eighteen Bristow-Latarjet repairs for recurrent anterior dislocation of the shoulder prospectively followed for fifteen years: study I—clinical results. J Shoulder Elbow Surg 2004;13(5):509–516

Itoi E, Lee SB, Berglund LJ, Berge LL, An KN. The effect of a glenoid defect on anteroinferior stability of the shoulder after Bankart repair: a cadaveric study. J Bone Joint Surg Am 2000;82(1):35–46

Lafosse L, Lejeune E, Bouchard A, Kakuda C, Gobezie R, Kochhar T. The arthroscopic Latarjet procedure for the treatment of anterior shoulder instability. Arthroscopy 2007;23(11):1242.e1–1242.e5

Neyton L, Young A, Dawidziak B, et al. Surgical treatment of anterior instability in rugby union players: clinical and radiographic results of the Latarjet-Patte procedure with minimum 5-year follow-up. J Shoulder Elbow Surg 2012;21(12):1721–1727

Porcellini G, Campi F, Pegreffi F, Castagna A, Paladini P. Predisposing factors for recurrent shoulder dislocation after arthroscopic treatment. J Bone Joint Surg Am 2009;91(11):2537–2542

Schroder DT, Provencher MT, Mologne TS, Muldoon MP, Cox JS. The modified Bristow procedure for anterior shoulder instability: 26-year outcomes in Naval Academy midshipmen. Am J Sports Med 2006;34(5):778–786

Sugaya H, Moriishi J, Dohi M, Kon Y, Tsuchiya A. Glenoid rim morphology in recurrent anterior glenohumeral instability. J Bone Joint Surg Am 2003;85-A(5):878–884

27 The Guided All-Arthroscopic Latarjet Procedure Using Cortical Button Fixation

Pascal Boileau, Eiko Hashimoto, and David Saliken

Abstract

A coracoid bone-block transfer was first proposed by the French surgeon Michel Latarjet in 1954 as a method to treat anterior instability in the setting of glenoid bone loss or revision cases. The technique provides a triple-blocking effect by reconstructing the bone loss, reinforcing the weak inferior glenohumeral ligament by transferring the conjoint tendon closer to the joint, and lowering the inferior part of the subscapularis to create a "sling-effect." In this chapter, we describe our arthroscopic, guided surgical approach using cortical button fixation to increase the accuracy of bone-block placement, enhance the reproducibility of the procedure, and reduce the risks of complications.

Keywords: *shoulder instability, glenohumeral bone loss, arthroscopy, Latarjet, cortical button*

27.1 Goals of Procedure

In the setting of recurrent glenohumeral instability, the Latarjet procedure stabilizes the shoulder by providing a triple-blocking effect: reconstructing glenoid bone loss, reinforcing the weak inferior glenohumeral ligament by transferring the conjoint tendon closer to the joint, and lowering the inferior part of the subscapularis to create a "sling effect."[1–3] It has classically been done through an open exposure using two bicortical screws,[4] but an arthroscopic approach has been developed.[2,5,6] Our guided surgical approach using cortical button fixation increases the accuracy of bone-block placement, enhances the reproducibility of the procedure, and reduces the risks of complications.[7]

27.2 Advantages

There are many benefits to completing the Latarjet procedure arthroscopically in addition to decreased bleeding, less postoperative pain, better cosmesis, and earlier return to sport. Improved intra- and extra-articular visualization and use of a drilling guide allow accurate positioning of the coracoid bone graft. Using a guided drilling system also allows parallel placement of the cortical button fixation with the glenoid to obtain excellent bone graft compression[7] and reduces risk to the suprascapular nerve.[5,8–11] Cortical button fixation is an alternative to screws allowing equivalent bone graft union while minimizing complications reported with screw fixation.[12] The arthroscope allows effective identification of the anterior neurovascular structures reducing risk of injury. Finally, there is the ability to treat associated pathologic lesions (biceps lesions, labral tears, capsular distension, and rotator cuff disease).

27.3 Indications

Recurrent anterior shoulder instability with instability severity index score (ISIS) greater than 3; glenoid bone loss greater than 20 to 25%; and failed previous surgical stabilization (Bankart repair and/or remplissage).

27.4 Contraindications

Voluntary dislocator, painful shoulder without Bankart lesion, active infection, and surgeon inexperience.

27.5 Preoperative Preparation/Positioning

A standard history and physical examination is performed. Preoperative imaging includes X-ray (true anteroposterior in internal rotation, neutral, and external rotation, axillary, scapular Y, and Bernageau profile views) and 3D CT with particular attention to glenohumeral bone loss or associated lesions (**Fig. 27.1**). Patients receive an ISIS to guide surgical management.

Our patients receive a preoperative interscalene block and general anesthesia. The patient is positioned in the lazy beach-chair position (30–40 degrees), which allows lower systemic blood pressure to reduce intraoperative bleeding while maintaining cerebral perfusion (**Fig. 27.2**). The arm is placed on a movable support (Spider Limb Positioner, Smith & Nephew, Andover, MA) without traction. The shoulder is placed in 60 degrees of flexion (to relax the anterior deltoid) and 30 degrees of internal rotation (to increase the subcoracoid space and to relax the axillary nerve). The elbow is placed at 90 degrees of flexion (to relax the conjoint tendon). Shoulder abduction is absolutely contraindicated as it brings the neurovascular structures laterally, in front of the scapular neck, putting them at risk; this is one of the reasons why we prefer the beach-chair position instead of the lateral decubitus position. Shoulder extension is also contraindicated as it reduces the anterior subdeltoid space and puts the axillary nerve under tension.

27.6 Operative Technique

The arthroscopic Latarjet includes five major steps: (1) coracoid preparation, drilling, and osteotomy; (2) glenoid labrum preparation and anchor placement; (3) subscapularis splitting and axillary nerve protection; (4) coracoid transfer and fixation; and finally (5) Bankart repair.

We use a standard posterior portal and five anterior portals (**Fig. 27.3**). The north-west portal is used for intra-articular work; it is located at the anterolateral corner of the acromion. Four additional anterior portals will be created on each side of the coracoid during the procedure, primarily for extra-articular work.[5,7] Relative to the coracoid, the north portal is one fingerbreadth proximal, the south portal is two fingerbreadths distal (in the axillary fold), the west portal is two fingerbreadths lateral, and the east portal (passing obliquely through the

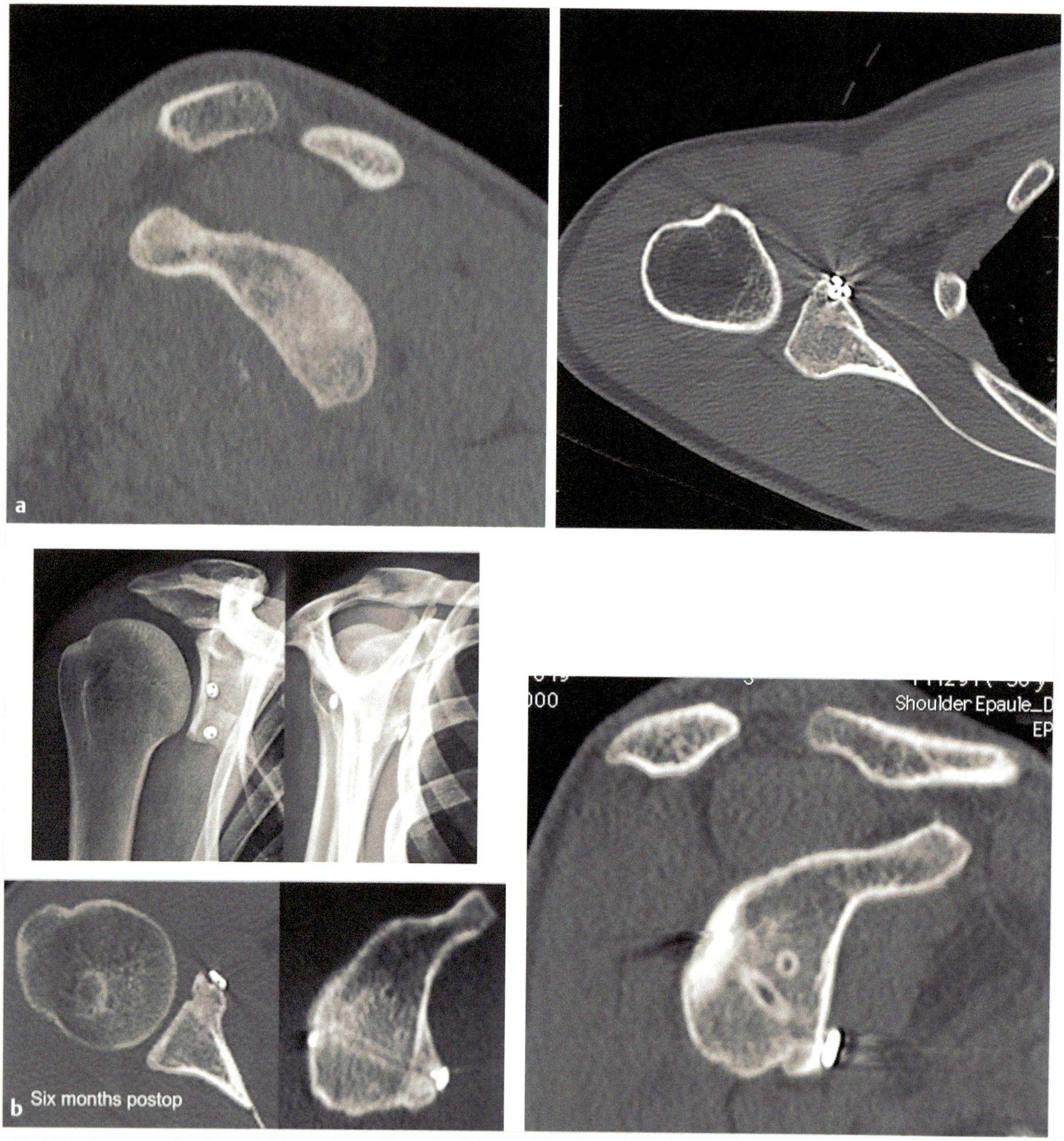

Fig. 27.1 Case example of a patient with recurrent anterior shoulder instability and significant glenoid bone loss. **(a)** Pre-op (glenoid en face view) and **(b)** 6-month post-op X-ray and CT (axillary and sagittal views) showing complete union of the coracoid bone graft.

pectoralis major muscle) is three fingerbreadths medial. A 70-degree scope is used to enhance visualization of the anterior neck of the scapula and eliminates instrument crowding as it has the capacity to view around acute angles.[13]

27.6.1 Coracoid Bone-Block Preparation, Drilling, and Osteotomy

The location of the posterior portal is crucial and is located 1 cm inferior and medial to the posterior angle of the acromion. A spinal needle is used to make sure that the scope and instruments will be flush with the glenoid surface and at the level of the equator. After a diagnostic arthroscopy, the north-west portal is created. A needle is used to ensure that instrumentation will be tangential to the anterior neck of the glenoid and perpendicular to the undersurface of the coracoid.

The scope is advanced through the rotator interval and using electrocautery and following the subscapularis tendon medially, the coracoid process is identified. The coracoacromial ligament is released from the lateral border of the acromion and the conjoint tendon is identified. The north portal is created just

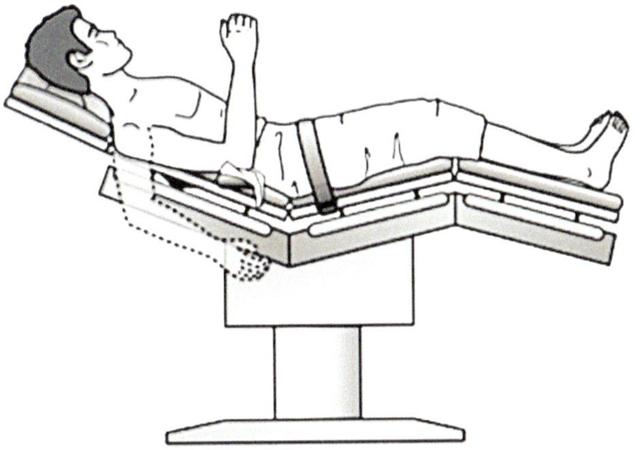

Fig. 27.2 Patient set up in a lazy beach-chair position (30–40 degrees) with mobile arm support.

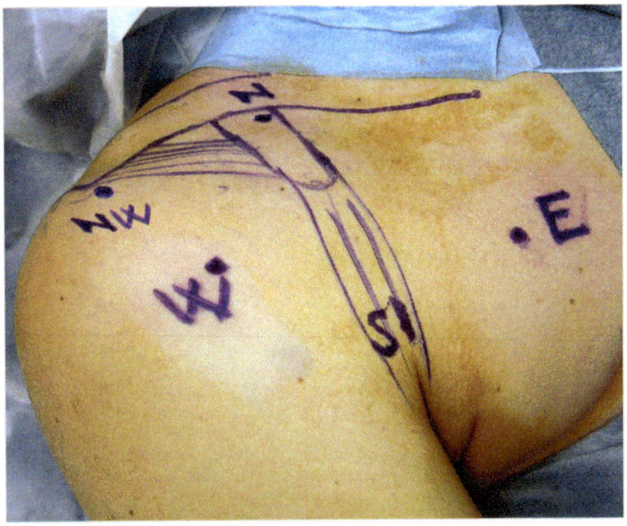

Fig. 27.3 Anterior portals: the north-west portal is located at the anterolateral corner of the acromion. Relative to the coracoid, the north portal is one fingerbreadth proximal and just medial; the south portal is distal in the axillary fold; the west portal is lateral to the conjoint tendon and midway between the north-west and south portals; and the east portal (passing obliquely at 45 degrees through the pectoralis major muscle) is three fingerbreadths medial to the conjoint tendon in line with the west portal.

medial to the coracoid process with the help of a spinal needle. Using a cautery through the north portal, the pectoralis minor is released from the medial border of the coracoid. In order to limit devascularization of the coracoid bone graft, do not dissect distal to the tip of the coracoid by more than 1 cm. A motorized rasp is introduced through the north-west portal and the undersurface of the coracoid process is abraded to create a flat surface to oppose the glenoid neck (**Fig. 27.4a**).[5]

The coracoid drill guide (Smith & Nephew) is introduced through the north portal to grasp the coracoid perpendicular to its surface (**Fig. 27.4b**). This guide ensures that the tunnel for the cortical button is equidistant to the margins and coracoid tip by 5 mm. The drill guide must be tilted 45 degrees medially to remain perpendicular to the coracoid surface; this is confirmed by visualizing the medially tine inferior to the coracoid. A drill-tipped K-wire housed inside an outer sleeve is advanced through the guide until it exits the inferior surface of the coracoid. The K-wire is replaced with a polydioxanone (PDS) suture, which is passed through the coracoid tunnel and retrieved through the west portal. The coracoid guide and sleeve are removed. The coracoid peg button (with the four-strand white suture) is pulled into place using the PDS suture as a shuttle (**Fig. 27.4c**). The blue/white Cobraid suture is retrieved through the south portal and the white sutures are retrieved through the north portal. The PDS suture is left attached to the white sutures and an alligator grasper is positioned 1 cm from its tip to be used later when passing the cortical button suture across the glenoid. It is important to protect these suture strands while performing the coracoid osteotomy. An oscillating motorized saw is introduced through the north-west portal and the coracoid is osteotomized, harvesting 15 to 20 mm of bone (**Fig. 27.4d**). The north portal is closed with a clip to avoid losing water outside the shoulder.

27.6.2 Glenoid Preparation and Drilling

A concomitant Bankart repair is important as it protects the humeral head from contact with the graft, adds shoulder stability by the "bumper effect," and preserves proprioception. Through the north-west portal, the anterior labrum is completely detached (but preserved) to visualize the glenoid bone defect. A PDS suture is passed through the labrum at the 5 o'clock position and retrieved through the west portal, allowing the labrum to be pulled away from the glenoid neck and will be used in step 5 to shuttle the Bankart suture anchor. The glenoid neck is abraded to a flat bed by use of the motorized rasp (**Fig. 27.5a**). Through the west portal, a glenoid suture anchor is inserted at the 3 o'clock position (**Fig. 27.5b**). The anchor will be used in step 5 for labrum repair and also as a landmark for coracoid bone-block positioning as the graft should be positioned below this anchor.

Using switching sticks, the scope is transferred to the north-west portal, the anterior glenoid neck preparation is confirmed, and a short half-pipe cannula is placed through the posterior portal. A glenoid drill guide, which ensures that the cortical button suture tunnel is nearly parallel and 5 mm medial to the anterior glenoid rim, is introduced inside the joint along the cannula. It is placed flush to the glenoid surface just below the suture anchor at the 5 o'clock position. Medial to the posterior portal, an incision is made to house the drill guide bullet, which is locked flush to the posterior glenoid neck (**Fig. 27.5c**). A switching stick is introduced through the west portal to retract the labrum and subscapularis allowing visualization of the anterior glenoid neck. The second drill-tipped K-wire housed inside an outer sleeve is drilled from posterior to anterior through the guide; this posterior-to-anterior drilling reduces risk of brachial plexus injury compared with anterior drilling. The hole in the glenoid should be located at the 5 o'clock position (in a right shoulder) and 5 mm medial to the glenoid rim.

The glenoid guide is removed, leaving the k-wire and sleeve in place (placing a slight bend into the k-wire will reduce the risk of it falling out posteriorly while other steps are performed). The posterior subscapularis spreader is inserted inside the joint and pushed through the subscapularis muscle

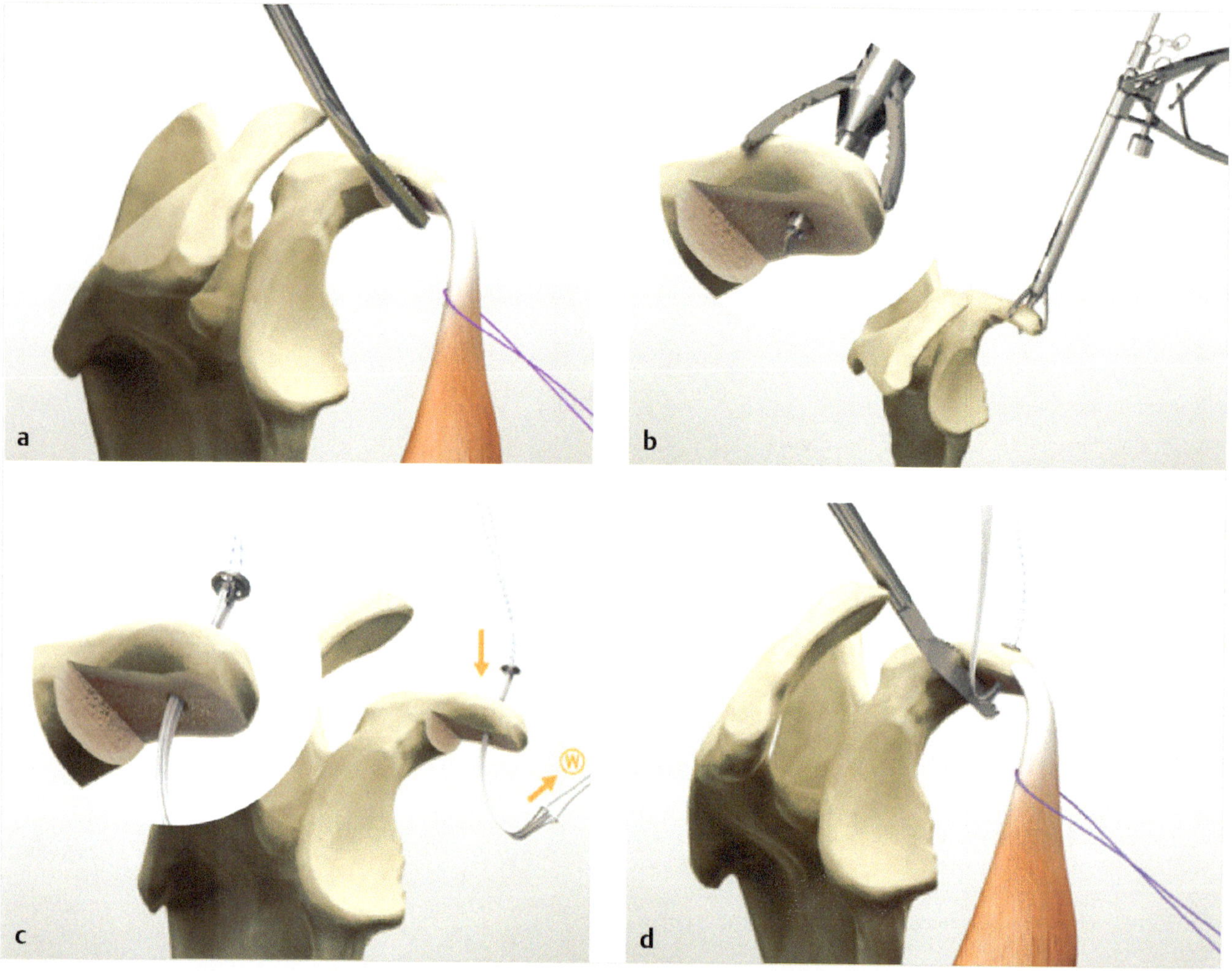

Fig. 27.4 **(a)** The coracoid rasp through the north-west portal to flatten inferior coracoid surface. **(b)** The coracoid drill guide placed through the north portal positions a drill hole 5 mm from the tip and medial and lateral edges. **(c)** The glenoid peg button is shuttled into position through the north portal in the coracoid. **(d)** The coracoid osteotomy through the north-west portal is performed 15 to 20 mm from the tip.

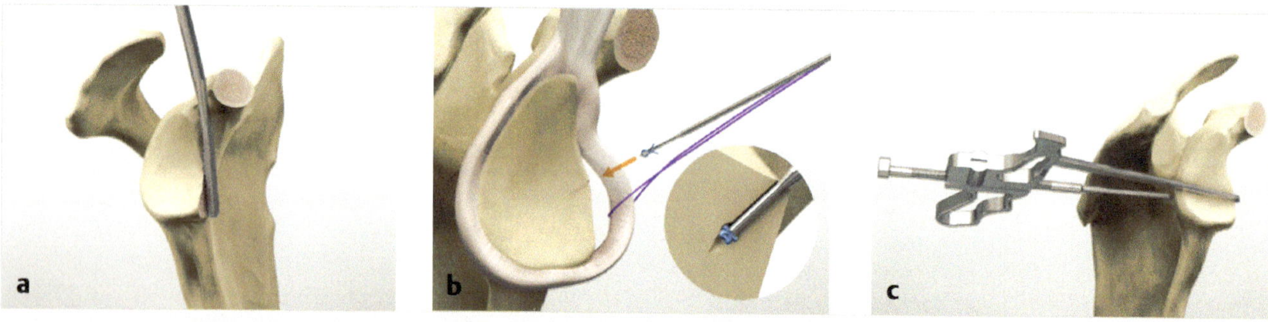

Fig. 27.5 **(a)** Glenoid preparation with rasp through the north-west portal to obtain a flat surface. **(b)** Bankart anchor placement at the 3 o'clock position for later Bankart repair. **(c)** Glenoid drill guide placed through the posterior portal along the 5 o'clock position on the glenoid (just below the 3 o'clock position suture anchor) and pierces the subscapularis at the inferior one-third subscapularis junction.

along the 5 o'clock position on the glenoid. Do not insert the spreader too deep yet as this should be done under direct vision with the scope in the west portal. This is because the tip of the spreader is typically found adjacent to the axillary nerve and the nerve must be protected. Lock the position of the spreader against the skin using the sliding tissue holder to ensure it is not inadvertently advanced.

27.6.3 Subscapularis Splitting and Axillary Nerve Protection

With the arthroscope in the west portal and the shoulder in slight internal rotation, an anterior bursectomy is performed. Following the anterior axillary vessels (the "three sisters") medially allows identification of the axillary and musculocutaneous nerves (the "two brothers"), hence our saying "The three sisters guide the surgeon to the two brothers."

Through the south portal, a straight blunt nerve retractor is used to separate the conjoint tendon from the subscapularis muscle and to mobilize and protect the nerves. With the arm by the side and slightly externally rotated, the subscapularis muscle is fully exposed and the tip of the posterior spreader is visualized. The posterior spreader position is optimized and then gently pushed anteriorly through the muscle in a lateral direction while protecting the nerves. The muscle belly should be divided parallel with its fibers, at the superior two-thirds and inferior one-third junction.[14] The spreader is opened and a cauterizing instrument replaces the nerve retractor through the south portal and is used to horizontally incise 1 cm laterally into the superficial tendon of the subscapularis (**Fig. 27.6a**). Great care is taken to incise only the tendon and not the underlying capsule (used later for Bankart repair).

The long half-pipe is inserted through the east portal just deep to the pectoralis major and advanced in a 45-degree angle toward the coracoid. The anterior spreader is introduced along the half-pipe, placed medial to the posterior spreader, and opened to visualize the abraded anterior neck of the scapula (**Fig. 27.6b**). Both spreaders create a "safe window" through the subscapularis muscle, giving access to the anterior neck of the glenoid. The anterior glenoid should now be completely exposed, and the correct position of the K-wire is confirmed.

27.6.4 Coracoid Transfer and Fixation

Using the alligator grasper, the tip of the PDS suture that is attached to the white sutures of the coracoid bone graft is advanced through the north portal to the anterior glenoid neck (**Fig. 27.7a**). Using the short half-pipe to reintroduce the grasper/PDS reduces the risk of deltoid muscle being caught. A suture retriever replaces the k-wire in the outer sleeve of the glenoid drill guide, grasps the PDS suture, and pulls the coracoid PDS suture through the glenoid tunnel (**Fig. 27.7a**). While shuttling the coracoid bone block, the posterior spreader should be rotated 45 degrees moving the inferior tine laterally to avoid catching the conjoined tendon during the transfer. The position and rotation of the coracoid graft can be controlled with the help of a coracoid grasper through the south portal. The glenoid cortical button is slid over the four white suture strands, a sliding-locking Nice knot (**Fig. 27.7b**) is tied, and the button is

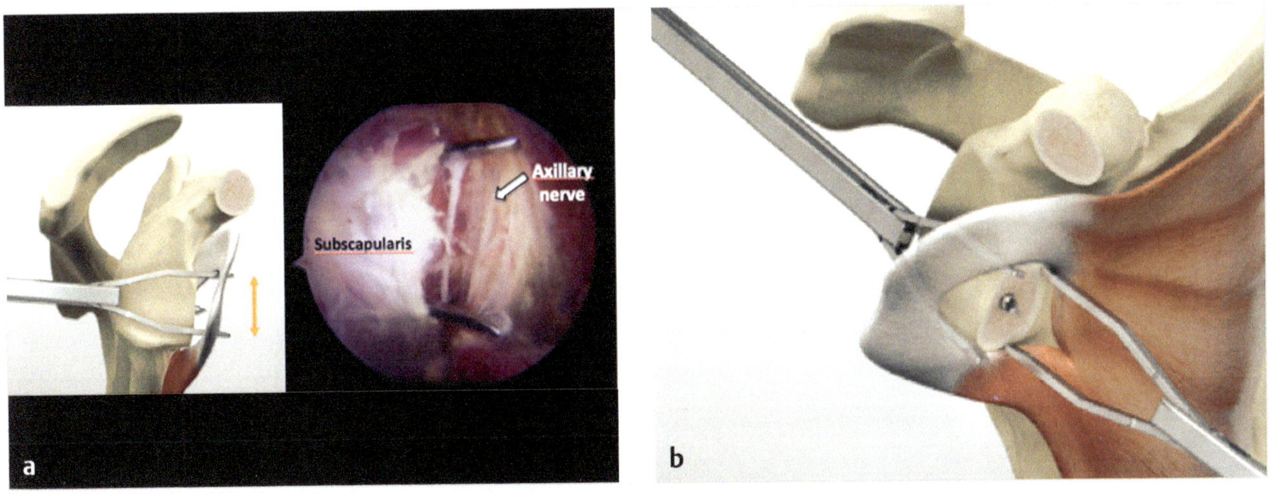

Fig. 27.6 **(a)** The subscapularis spreader is identified with the arthroscope in the west portal in the right shoulder. The axillary and musculocutaneous nerves are seen and protected with a nerve protector from the south portal. **(b)** Subscapularis split viewed anteriorly.

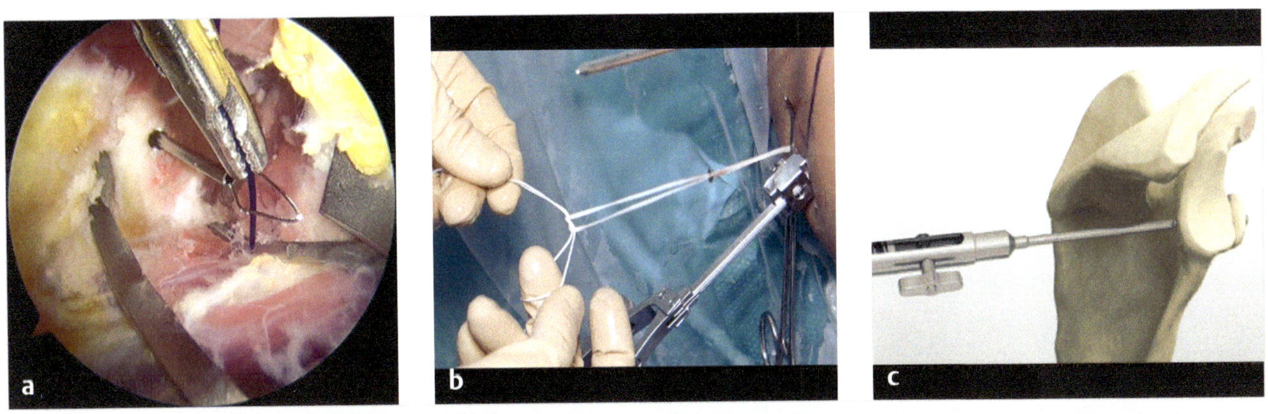

Fig. 27.7 Coracoid transfer. **(a)** A suture retriever device passed through the glenoid drill hole from posterior to anterior is used to grasp the PDS suture, which is attached to the coracoid suture. **(b)** A Nice knot is tied to secure the fixation posteriorly. **(c)** The suture tensioner is passed over the Nice knot and allows controlled tightening of the coracoid graft.

advanced onto the posterior glenoid neck. The suture tensioner (Smith & Nephew) is put in place in the back of the shoulder, and a temporary compression of 50 N is applied (**Fig. 27.7c**).

Using a switching stick and short half-pipe cannula, the scope is reintroduced into the posterior portal. Absence of glenoid overhang and subequatorial position of the graft is confirmed and rotation of the bone graft is optimized with a probe. Further compression of 100 N is obtained with the suture tensioner and solid graft fixation is confirmed.

27.6.5 Bankart Repair

The remaining capsule and labrum are now reattached to the glenoid rim, placing the graft in an extra-articular position. Use an alligator grasper through the west portal to pull the labrum from south to north performing a capsular shift. The previously placed suture anchor is used to repair the labrum through the north-west portal. Additional suture anchors should be used as necessary depending on patient anatomy.[15] The suture tensioner is removed and three square knots are tied to definitively lock the construct. The dynamic sling effect of the block can now be visualized by placing the scope in the anterior subdeltoid space through the west portal.

27.7 Tips and Pearls/Expert Suggestions

- The arthroscopic Latarjet procedure is technically demanding. We recommend a stepwise learning approach that includes training in a cadaveric lab.
- A 70-degree scope is integral in getting appropriate viewing angles and may require practice to become proficient with it.
- Appropriate arm positioning at different points in the operation is important for opening up viewing spaces (i.e., 60-degree arm flexion to relax anterior deltoid, 30-degree internal rotation to increase space under the coracoid process, and elbow flexion to relax the conjoint tendon).
- Limit bone removal during coracoid and particularly glenoid neck preparation to just enough to ensure flat, opposable surfaces.
- Take time to accurately position the Bankart anchor at the 3 o'clock position, as it will serve as a landmark for the posterior spreader and bone graft positioning.
- Follow the "three sisters" to identify the "two brothers"; identifying and protecting the axillary and musculocutaneous nerves is crucial.
- Smoking cessation is important in reducing the risk of nonunion.

27.8 What to Avoid

Shoulder abduction is contraindicated as it brings the neurovascular structures laterally in front of the glenoid neck. Shoulder extension should be avoided as it reduces the anterior subdeltoid working space and puts the axillary nerve under tension. Malposition or malrotation of coracoid block should be avoided. Use a drilling guide and prior to tensioning the button greater than 50 N, confirm rotation and position of bone block and modify accordingly. Avoid neurologic injury by identifying and protecting the axillary and musculocutaneous nerves prior to advancing and opening the subscapularis spreaders.

27.9 Complications/Bailout/ Salvage

- Coracoid bone-block fracture: take care not to rasp away too much bone and ensure proper placement of coracoid drill guide.
- In the setting of failure of arthroscopic Latarjet, revision options include a combined Bankart repair and Hill–Sachs remplissage or Eden–Hybinette procedure.

27.10 Postoperative Care

Postoperative radiographs are taken to confirm the correct graft position. The patient is discharged from the hospital the same day or the day after surgery. The arm is strictly immobilized for 2 weeks in a neutral rotation sling; this allows healing of the conjoint tendon in the muscular part of the subscapularis to reduce loss of external rotation. Pendulum exercises start after 2 weeks (5 times/d, 5 min/session). After 4 weeks, the sling is removed and formal rehabilitation with a physical therapist is started. Swimming pool therapy is encouraged. No heavy lifting is allowed for the first 12 weeks. Return to all types of sports activities, including collision and contact-overhead sports, is allowed between 3 and 6 months postoperatively.

References

1. Latarjet M. A propos du traitement des luxations récidivantes de l'épaule. [Treatment of recurrent dislocations of the shoulder]. Lyon Chir 1954;49(8):994–997
2. Boileau P, Thélu CE, Mercier N, et al. Arthroscopic Bristow-Latarjet combined with Bankart repair restores shoulder stability in patients with glenoid bone loss. Clin Orthop Relat Res 2014;472(8):2413–2424
3. Patte D, Bernageau J, Bancel P. The anteroinferior vulnerable point of the glenoid rim. In: Bateman JE, Welsh RP, eds. Surgery of the shoulder. New York, NY: Marcel Dekker; 1985:94–99
4. Walch G. Recurrent anterior shoulder instability. Rev Chir Orthop Repar Appar Mot 1991;77:177–191
5. Boileau P, Mercier N, Old J. Arthroscopic Bankart-Bristow-Latarjet (2B3) procedure: how to do it and tricks to make it easier and safe. Orthop Clin North Am 2010;41(3): 381–392
6. Lafosse L, Boyle S. Arthroscopic Latarjet procedure. J Shoulder Elbow Surg 2010;19(2, Suppl):2–12
7. Boileau P, Gendre P, Baba M, et al. A guided surgical approach and novel fixation method for arthroscopic Latarjet. J Shoulder Elbow Surg 2016;25(1):78–89
8. Young DC, Rockwood CA Jr. Complications of a failed Bristow procedure and their management. J Bone Joint Surg Am 1991;73(7):969–981

9. Zuckerman JD, Matsen FA III. Complications about the glenohumeral joint related to the use of screws and staples. J Bone Joint Surg Am 1984;66(2):175–180
10. Delaney RA, Freehill MT, Janfaza DR, Vlassakov KV, Higgins LD, Warner JJ. 2014 Neer Award paper: neuromonitoring the Latarjet procedure. J Shoulder Elbow Surg 2014;23(10): 1473–1480
11. Lädermann A, Denard PJ, Burkhart SS. Injury of the suprascapular nerve during latarjet procedure: an anatomic study. Arthroscopy 2012;28(3):316–321
12. Kodde IF, van den Bekerom MP, Eygendaal D. Reconstruction of distal biceps tendon ruptures with a cortical button. Knee Surg Sports Traumatol Arthrosc 2015;23(3):919–925
13. Bedi A, Dines J, Dines DM, et al. Use of the 70° arthroscope for improved visualization with common arthroscopic procedures. Arthroscopy 2010;26(12):1684–1696
14. Maynou C, Cassagnaud X, Mestdagh H. Function of subscapularis after surgical treatment for recurrent instability of the shoulder using a bone-block procedure. J Bone Joint Surg Br 2005;87(8):1096–1101
15. Caspari RB, Beach WR. Arthroscopic anterior shoulder capsulorrhaphy. Sports Med Arthrosc Rev 1993;1(4): 237–241

28 Eden–Hybinette for Failed Latarjet Procedure

Kyong S. Min, Neal C. Chen, Michelle J. Chang, and Jon J.P. Warner

Abstract
The Eden-Hybinette procedure is an option for treatment in patients with glenohumeral bone loss greater than 40% of the glenoid. Iliac crest bone graft is fashioned and secured to the glenoid defect. This has been a successful option in cases of failed Latarjet with 79% good or excellent results.

Keywords: *Eden-Hybinette, bone graft, Latarjet, glenoid, instability*

28.1 Introduction

Primary glenohumeral dislocations without bone loss are most commonly treated with arthroscopic anterior labral repair. However, with recurrent dislocations and/or dislocations with significant bone loss, recurrent instability after arthroscopic repair is problematic. The Latarjet procedure is the most commonly utilized procedure for recurrent dislocation or instability with critical bone loss. The Latarjet has three mechanisms of stabilization: (1) the bony support of the coracoid increasing the glenoid surface area, (2) the conjoint tendon acting as a dynamic sling on the inferior subscapularis, and (3) the repair of the capsulolabral junction.[1]

When there are larger degrees of bone loss, the Latarjet procedure may not provide sufficient stability. The Eden–Hybinette uses an iliac crest bone graft (ICBG) to reconstitute glenoid bone loss and is an alternative to the Latarjet procedure, especially in revision cases or cases of larger bone loss.

28.2 Goals of Procedure

The goal of the Eden–Hybinette is to reconstitute glenoid bone loss using autogenous ICBG.

There is continued debate on what constitutes critical glenoid bone loss. Gerber et al defined significant glenoid bone loss when the length of the defect is greater than half of the maximum anteroposterior diameter of the glenoid fossa.[2] Itoi et al concluded in a cadaveric study that a defect of greater than 21% of the superoinferior glenoid length cannot be addressed by a labral repair without bone grafting.[3] Burkhart et al reported that a defect greater than 25% of the glenoid width failed without bone grafting; in such cases, the Bankart repair alone did not yield satisfactory results.[4] Given the importance of evaluating glenoid defects in anterior shoulder instability, Jankauskas et al concluded that the loss of sclerotic glenoid line (LSGL) serves as a diagnostic indicator of anterior glenoid rim defects that cannot be treated by Bankart repairs.[5]

Yamamoto et al showed that critical bone loss in bipolar lesions is often associated with glenohumeral instability.[6] They defined the "glenoid track" in a cadaveric study as the contact zone between the glenoid and the humeral head. He concluded that if the medial margin of a Hill–Sachs lesion is more medial than the glenoid track in bipolar lesions, standard stabilization procedures such as Bankart repairs would be unlikely to restore stability of the shoulder.

Although there is debate on what defines critical bone loss, most shoulder experts agree that a soft-tissue Bankart repair is insufficient. In most situations with critical bone loss, the Latarjet is a good surgical option; however, there are situations where the Latarjet may not be adequate. The literature reports a 5 to 6% redislocation rate after the Latarjet.[7,8] Adopting the concept of the "glenoid track," Mook et al argued if there is a persistent "off-track" relationship, then there is a significantly higher probability of recurrent instability after the Latarjet.[9] This off-track relationship occurs if the Hill–Sachs lesion is medial to the track and/or if the patient has a relatively undersized coracoid process with a large glenoid defect.

When there are larger degrees of bone loss, the Latarjet procedure may not provide sufficient stability. In such situations, the Eden–Hybinette using the ICBG is an option that provides a larger amount of bone graft for stabilization.

28.3 Advantages

The Eden–Hybinette is advantageous compared to the Latarjet because it allows treatment of larger defects; however, this comes at the expense of the graft harvest site. There are advantages of healing and avoiding the risk of disease transmission when compared to distal tibia allograft.

Lunn et al reported their series on the treatment of recurrent anterior dislocation after a failed Latarjet procedure using the modified Eden–Hybinette operation.[10] In their series, 79% reported good or excellent results. Warner et al reported a case series of anatomic glenoid reconstruction using the modified Eden–Hybinette.[11] In this series, all patients returned back to preinjury level of activity. This has been reported to have good to excellent results. In using autogenous graft, there is no concern for disease transmission or graft rejection. Furthermore, the use of the autogenous graft is a cost-efficient alternative to allograft (tricortical iliac crest or distal tibia).

28.4 Indications

We perform the Eden–Hybinette in the following situations: (1) glenohumeral instability with bone loss greater than 40%, (2) revision surgery after failure of Latarjet, and (3) acute, unreconstructable glenoid fracture with subluxation or frank instability.

28.5 Contraindications

Patients with active infections, uncontrolled seizures, or the inability to follow postoperative directions are contraindications to the Eden–Hybinette procedure.

28.6 Preoperative Preparation/ Positioning

For preoperative planning of the Eden–Hybinette procedure, CT of the scapula with 3D reconstruction is obtained to calculate the amount and shape of glenoid bone loss. If available, computerized/ virtual surgical tools for patient-specific instrumentation and planning should be used to best understand the patient's anatomy and defect. If possible, obtaining a sterilized 3D printed model of the scapula will allow the surgeon to shape and position the iliac crest on to the model prior to placing it on the native scapula.

The patient is placed on the operation room table in the beach-chair position with the head elevated between 30 and 80 degrees, and the ipsilateral iliac crest is exposed. In patients with static subluxation, lower degrees of elevation may help with keeping the humeral head in a more reduced position. To obtain the ICBG, the bolsters along the iliac crest are positioned so as to support the patient, but not to impede access to the iliac crest. An electric/hydropneumatic limb positioner is utilized to manipulate and position the shoulder throughout the procedure. The shoulder, arm, and ipsilateral iliac crest are prepared and draped in the standard sterile fashion.

28.7 Operative Technique

The standard deltopectoral incision is made to visualize the deltopectoral interval. The cephalic vein is dissected and retracted laterally; dissection is taken to the level of the clavipectoral fascia. The lateral border of the conjoint tendon is identified and separated from the subscapularis. The axillary nerve is located between the conjoint tendon and the subscapularis; it runs over the inferior half of the subscapularis, under the inferior glenoid and through the quadrilateral space. It can be palpated and visualized, and it should be protected by placing a blunt retractor superior to the nerve. The circumflex vessels are isolated and ligated.

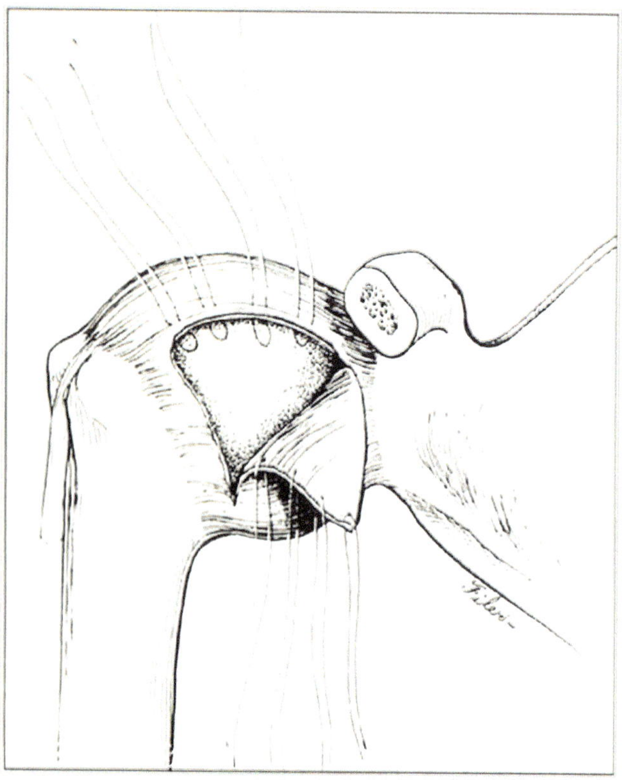

Fig. 28.1 An inverted **L**-shaped capsulotomy is created through the rotator interval to expose the glenoid. Used with permission from Warner JJP, Gill TJ, O'Hollerhan JD, Pathare N, Millett PJ. Anatomical Glenoid Reconstruction for Recurrent Anterior Glenohumeral Instability with Glenoid Deficiency Using an Autogenous Tricortical Iliac Crest Bone Graft. Am J Sports Med. 2006;34:205–212.

The subscapularis is then tenotomized off the lesser tuberosity at the lateral most margin of the tuberosity; the undersurface of the tendon is carefully dissected off the underlying capsule. At this time, the subscapularis tendon should be tagged for later repair. In most situations, three tagging sutures (no. 2 Ethibond) can be used to retract the subscapularis. Care must be taken to tag and protect the inferior subscapularis. The inferior subscapularis is more muscular and does not have much tendon. Once the subscapularis is protected, the undersurface of the tendon should be carefully separated from the glenohumeral capsule; this should be separated well medial to the anterior glenoid rim. The undersurface of the subscapularis muscle should be dissected from the subscapularis fossa. A sponge can be used to dissect and maintain hemostasis. To maximize visualization of the glenoid, a retractor can be placed deep to the subscapularis in the subscapularis fossa. This will expose the glenohumeral joint capsule.

There is commonly injury to the labrum. This labral separation can be developed. If needed for further exposure, the capsule is then released from the humeral neck (**Fig. 28.1**). An anterior glenoid neck retractor can be placed to retract the subscapularis, while a humeral head retractor (e.g., Fukuda or Fedorka retractor) can be placed to retract the humeral head posteriorly. The glenoid defect is visualized, and the bony bed is prepared to visualize bleeding bone.

Attention is turned to the bone graft. The iliac crest is exposed with an incision 2 cm posterior to the anterosuperior iliac spine and along the superior border of the iliac crest. The superior iliac crest with the inner and outer tables are exposed, and blunt retractors are used to maintain this exposure. An oscillating saw and osteotomes are used to remove a tricortical wedge-shaped graft that is approximately 3 cm in length by 2 cm in width (**Fig. 28.2**). A 90-degree oscillating saw is useful to

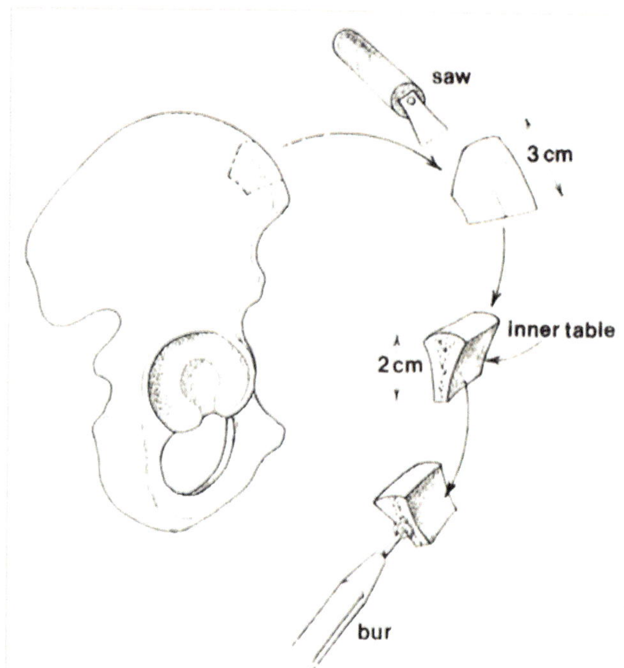

Fig. 28.2 Preparation of the iliac crest bone graft. Used with permission from Warner JJP, Gill TJ, O'Hollerhan JD, Pathare N, Millett PJ. Anatomical Glenoid Reconstruction for Recurrent Anterior Glenohumeral Instability with Glenoid Deficiency Using an Autogenous Tricortical Iliac Crest Bone Graft. Am J Sports Med. 2006;34:205–212.

complete the horizontal aspect of the osteotomy. The graft is then contoured to fit onto the anterior glenoid. It is useful to have a 3D model of the patient's glenoid and scapula to perfectly shape and fit the iliac crest. The inner table of the iliac crest is concave and will be similar in concavity to the glenoid articular surface.

Once the graft has been contoured to match the desired dimensions, it can be secured to the anterior glenoid using three 3.5-mm cortical screws. The screws are oriented parallel to the joint surface so that the screw heads are as far away from the humeral articular surface as possible. Before seating each screw, a single no. 2 ultrastrength suture is placed around the head of the screw (**Fig. 28.3**). These sutures will function as suture anchors to repair the capsular-periosteal sleeve back on to the glenoid neck.

When positioning the graft, lateralization of the graft must be avoided. The graft must be even or slightly medial to the glenoid articular surface. If necessary, a burr can be used to create a smooth congruity between the articular surface and the inner table of the iliac crest graft.

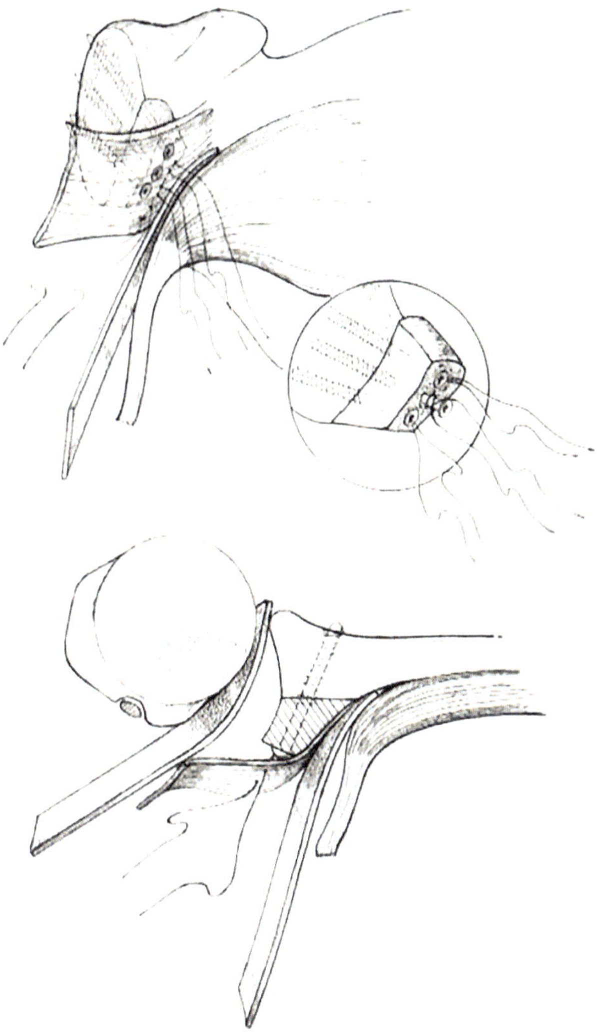

Fig. 28.3 No. 2 ultrastrength sutures are tied around the shaft of the screws to function as suture anchors. Used with permission from Warner JJP, Gill TJ, O'Hollerhan JD, Pathare N, Millett PJ. Anatomical Glenoid Reconstruction for Recurrent Anterior Glenohumeral Instability with Glenoid Deficiency Using an Autogenous Tricortical Iliac Crest Bone Graft. Am J Sports Med. 2006;34:205–212.

The humeral head retractor is then removed and the capsular-periosteal sleeve is repaired to the graft with the prepositioned no. 2 ultrastrength sutures underneath each screw head. Due to the width of the graft, lateral repair of the capsule is often limited. In such situations, the capsule can be sewn onto the undersurface of the subscapularis tendon. Then the lateral portion of the subscapularis tendon is used as an extension of the capsule (**Fig. 28.4**). The tenotomized subscapularis tendon is then anatomically repaired to its anatomic footprint using transosseous sutures or suture anchors.

28.8 Tips and Pearls/Expert Suggestions

Preoperative planning and preparation are essential to a successful procedure. A CT scan with 3D reconstruction of the affected shoulder is recommended. If possible, obtain a sterile model of the scapular for planning. During the operation, identification and protection of the axillary nerve are essential to prevent axillary nerve injuries.

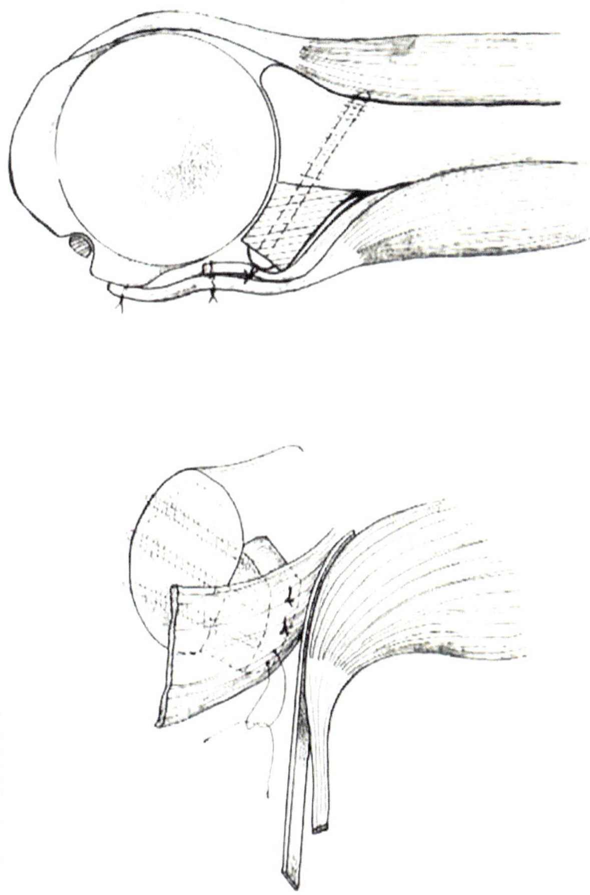

Fig. 28.4 The capsule is sewn onto the undersurface of the subscapularis, in which the lateral portion of the subscapularis tendon is used as an extension of the capsule. Used with permission from Warner JJP, Gill TJ, O'Hollerhan JD, Pathare N, Millett PJ. Anatomical Glenoid Reconstruction for Recurrent Anterior Glenohumeral Instability with Glenoid Deficiency Using an Autogenous Tricortical Iliac Crest Bone Graft. Am J Sports Med. 2006;34: 205–212.

28.9 What to Avoid

Patients who have previously sustained multiple dislocations or surgical procedures have significant scarring. Quite often, the capsule will be scarred to the undersurface of the subscapularis. With careful dissection, it is possible to separate the layers between the capsule and the subscapularis.

During the operation, it is beneficial to make an appropriately sized incision to maximize visualization and exposure. In these cases, a smaller incision may limit visualization and increase risk.

In order to maximize bone healing, smooth the glenoid to a flat surface and bleeding bone. Ensure that the iliac crest graft is sitting flush to the glenoid. Incongruent placement of the graft can lead to nonunion, graft resorption, and failure. Avoid placing the graft too laterally. Lateralization of the graft will lead to osteoarthritis. Make the graft even to the glenoid or slightly medial to the plane of the glenoid surface.

Use solid stainless steel screws to secure the graft. Titanium and cannulated screws have higher risks of hardware failure and inadequate compression.

28.10 Complications

Careful attention must be taken to protect the axillary nerve. Aggressive inferior dissection around the inferior glenoid can damage the nerve. Furthermore, meticulous dissection is necessary to identify and ligate the circumflex vessels. Failure to control these vessels can lead to uncontrolled bleeding and/or large hematoma formation, which will increase the possibility of infection.

28.11 Postoperative Care

Postoperatively, the patient is placed in a shoulder immobilizer for 4 weeks. Pendulum exercises are permitted after the first week. At the fourth week, the patient begins supervised physical therapy for passive and active regain motion. At this point, they are allowed to use the operative arm for activities of daily living. After 3 months, strengthening ensues. At 4 months, a CT scan should be attained to assess bony union. If there is evidence of union, the patient is allowed to use the arm for overhead recreational sports. Contact sports are not permitted until at least 8 months after surgery.

References

1. Patte D, Debeyre J. Luxations recidivantes de l'epaule. Encycl Med Chir Paris-Technique Chirurgicale Orthopedie 1980;44265:4.4–02
2. Gerber C, Nyffeler RW. Classification of glenohumeral joint instability. Clin Orthop Relat Res 2002(400):65–76
3. Itoi E, Lee SB, Berglund LJ, Berge LL, An KN. The effect of a glenoid defect on anteroinferior stability of the shoulder after Bankart repair: a cadaveric study. J Bone Joint Surg Am 2000;82(1):35–46
4. Burkhart SS, Debeer JF, Tehrany AM, Parten PM. Quantifying glenoid bone loss arthroscopically in shoulder instability. Arthroscopy 2002;18(5):488–491
5. Jankauskas L, Rüdiger HA, Pfirrmann CW, Jost B, Gerber C. Loss of the sclerotic line of the glenoid on anteroposterior radiographs of the shoulder: a diagnostic sign for an osseous defect of the anterior glenoid rim. J Shoulder Elbow Surg 2010;19(1):151–156
6. Yamamoto N, Itoi E, Abe H, et al. Contact between the glenoid and the humeral head in abduction, external rotation, and horizontal extension: a new concept of glenoid track. J Shoulder Elbow Surg 2007;16(5):649–656
7. Hovelius L, Sandström B, Olofsson A, Svensson O, Rahme H. The effect of capsular repair, bone block healing, and position on the results of the Bristow-Latarjet procedure (study III): long-term follow-up in 319 shoulders. J Shoulder Elbow Surg 2012;21(5):647–660
8. Mizuno N, Denard PJ, Raiss P, Melis B, Walch G. Long-term results of the Latarjet procedure for anterior instability of the shoulder. J Shoulder Elbow Surg 2014;23(11): 1691–1699
9. Mook WR, Petri M, Greenspoon JA, Horan MP, Dornan GJ, Millett PJ. Clinical and anatomic predictors of outcomes after the latarjet procedure for the treatment of anterior glenohumeral instability with combined glenoid and humeral bone defects. Am J Sports Med 2016;44(6):1407–1416
10. Lunn JV, Castellano-Rosa J, Walch G. Recurrent anterior dislocation after the Latarjet procedure: outcome after revision using a modified Eden-Hybinette operation. J Shoulder Elbow Surg 2008;17(5):744–750
11. Warner JJ, Gill TJ, O'hollerhan JD, Pathare N, Millett PJ. Anatomical glenoid reconstruction for recurrent anterior glenohumeral instability with glenoid deficiency using an autogenous tricortical iliac crest bone graft. Am J Sports Med 2006;34(2):205–212

29 Distal Tibia Allograft for Failed Latarjet

Matthew T. Provencher, Anthony Sanchez, Colin P. Murphy, Liam A. Peebles, and George Sanchez

Abstract

Recurrent shoulder instability can be a frustrating condition for both patients and surgeons alike. Following a failed Latarjet procedure in the setting of significant glenoid bone loss, bony augmentation with an osteochondral allograft is indicated, and our preferred choice of allograft for these patients is the lateral one-third of a fresh distal tibia allograft (DTA). There are several advantages of the DTA, including its accessibility, dense bone quality, and congruity with the native glenoid. In this chapter, we describe the indications and contraindications of this procedure, its associated risks and benefits, and the authors' preferred surgical technique and postoperative management.

Keywords: *shoulder, recurrent instability, dislocation, subluxation, bony defect, distal tibia allograft, Latarjet, bone augmentation*

29.1 Goals of Procedure

This procedure allows for the anatomical and biomechanical restoration of the shoulder in the setting of substantial anterior glenoid bone loss, avoiding the use of autograft.[1–3] The goals are to prevent further instability and degenerative changes while restoring normal functionality to the glenohumeral joint. This technique is performed using the lateral one-third of a fresh DTA.[3]

29.2 Advantages

Since this is an allograft technique, no autograft is required, and donor site morbidity is therefore avoided. This procedure allows for the treatment of significant glenoid bony defects, especially in the setting of a failed Latarjet revision (**Fig. 29.1a**). The distal tibial surface has a similar curvature to that of the native glenoid and an excellent congruency with the humeral head can be achieved using unmatched grafts. The distal tibia allograft (DTA) is also more readily available than glenoid allografts due to the risk of infection while harvesting the more centrally located glenoid. The dense bony quality of the DTA provides a stronger fixation for the screws in the construct. This technique is performed using the modified deltopectoral approach. Furthermore, this technique can be performed to address anterior defects on the glenoid, and has been shown to restore the anatomy and biomechanics of the glenoid with a cartilaginous surface.[3]

29.3 Indications

DTA is indicated for patients with large anterior or posterior glenoid bony defects. This technique can be used as a primary intervention or as a revision treatment option in cases with a failed Latarjet procedure (**Fig. 29.1b**).[4]

29.4 Contraindications

Global glenoid pathology is a contraindication to this procedure, as the DTA cannot augment the entire glenoid. Small glenoid defects are a relative contraindication for this procedure; in these cases, a Bankart repair is more suitable.

29.5 Preoperative Preparation/ Positioning

We recommend the use of preoperative ultrasound-guided interscalene block for regional anesthesia. The patient is then transported to the operating room, placed in a supine position, and general anesthesia is induced. Following induction, the patient is placed in the beach-chair position with all bony prominences appropriately well padded and with a bump

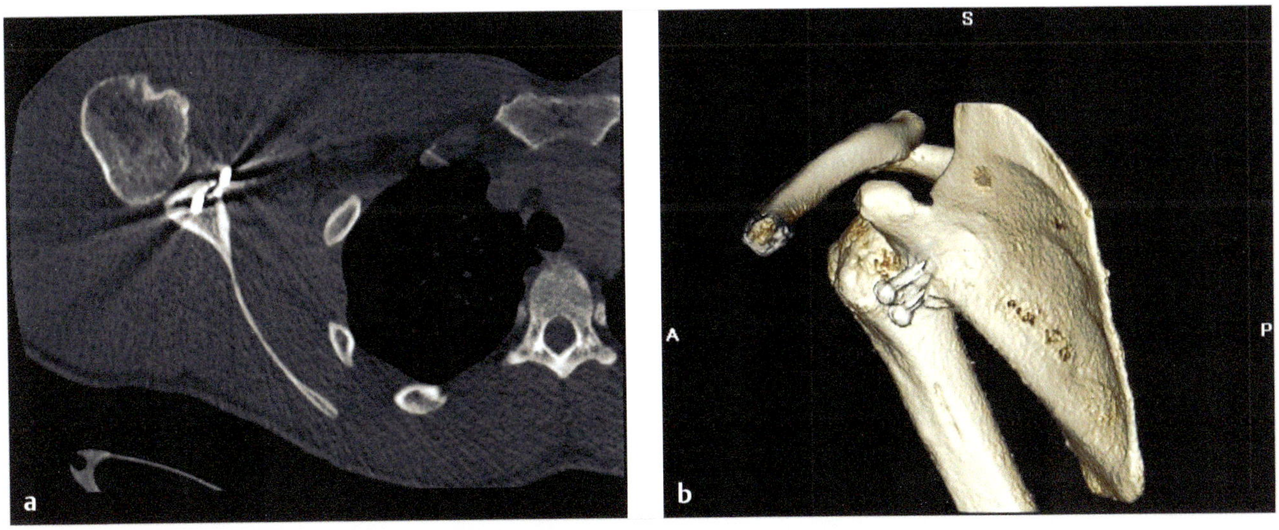

Fig. 29.1 **(a)** Postoperative 2D CT of failed Latarjet. **(b)** Postoperative 3D CT of failed Latarjet.

placed behind the medial border of the scapula. The knees are slightly flexed using a foam pad. The head must be well secured. A thorough preoperative physical examination under anesthesia is performed on the shoulder to confirm the position and degree of glenohumeral instability. The shoulder is then prepared and draped in the usual sterile fashion. Using a surgical pen, all relevant bony prominences of the shoulder are marked.

29.6 Operative Technique

29.6.1 Approach

Using a scalpel, an incision is performed starting at the tip of the coracoid process and extending inferiorly along the axillary fold for approximately 7 cm, creating a modified deltopectoral incision that is slightly more medial than the standard approach (**Fig. 29.2**). The clavipectoral fascia is identified and incised following the skin incision. The cephalic vein is identified, retracted, and protected. Gelpi or Weitlaner retractors are used to expose the fascia overlying the conjoined tendon, which is incised, and the lateral aspect of the conjoined tendon is retracted medially. The deltoid is retracted laterally using a Fukuda retractor. The subscapularis insertion on the lesser tuberosity is then identified. In primary cases, a subscapularis split can be sharply performed in line with its fibers with ease, at the junction of the superior and middle thirds. However, for revision cases, we recognize that the subscapularis tissue may not allow a split and a subscapularis takedown may be the best option for joint access (**Fig. 29.3**). The subscapularis is tagged with a no. 2 Fiberwire suture (Arthrex, Naples, FL) for easier identification and repair later on in the technique. The underlying capsule is then released from the posterior aspect of the subscapularis tendon using Metzenbaum scissors, and a T capsulotomy is performed. The remaining capsule is sharply elevated off the glenoid neck medially in a subperiosteal fashion. Attention is then turned to the evaluation of the glenoid defect. In a revision of a prior failed Latarjet, the graft and screws must be removed, as well as any soft tissue from the anterior glenoid aspect. We use a combination of coagulator, rongeur, and high-speed burr to create a bleeding anterior bone surface for the DTA. The humeral head is also evaluated for defects and, if present, the dimension and location of the defect are identified in order to evaluate the necessity for correction.

29.6.2 Allograft Preparation

A DTA, provided by a donor cadaveric source (JRF Ortho, Centennial, CO), is placed on the back table. We use a special workstation (Arthrex) designed specifically for this procedure, which we believe allows for safer, more precise cuts (**Fig. 29.4**).[5] Alternatively, an assistant can hold the graft in place with two towel clamps. The graft is cut to the specifications determined via preoperative and intraoperative imaging and measurement.[6] Constant saline irrigation is used to cool the graft while it is being cut to avoid damage. Next, two 4.0-mm drill holes are drilled in the graft, using the graft holder as a guide. Pulsatile lavage is applied to the graft for approximately 5 minutes to remove all marrow elements before graft placement (**Fig. 29.5a**). After the pulse lavage, the allograft is soaked in a combination of autol-

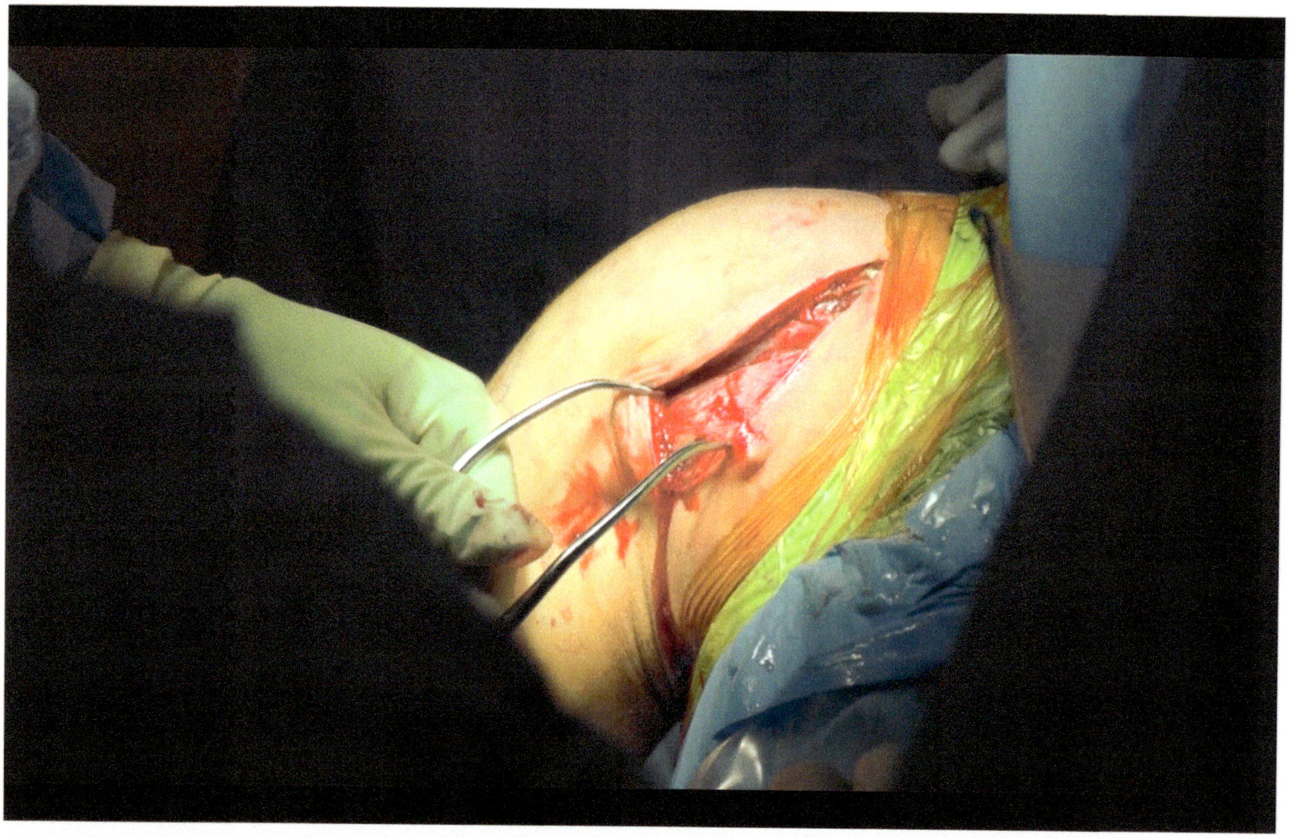

Fig. 29.2 Deltopectoral incision performed in the right shoulder with the patient positioned in the beach-chair position.

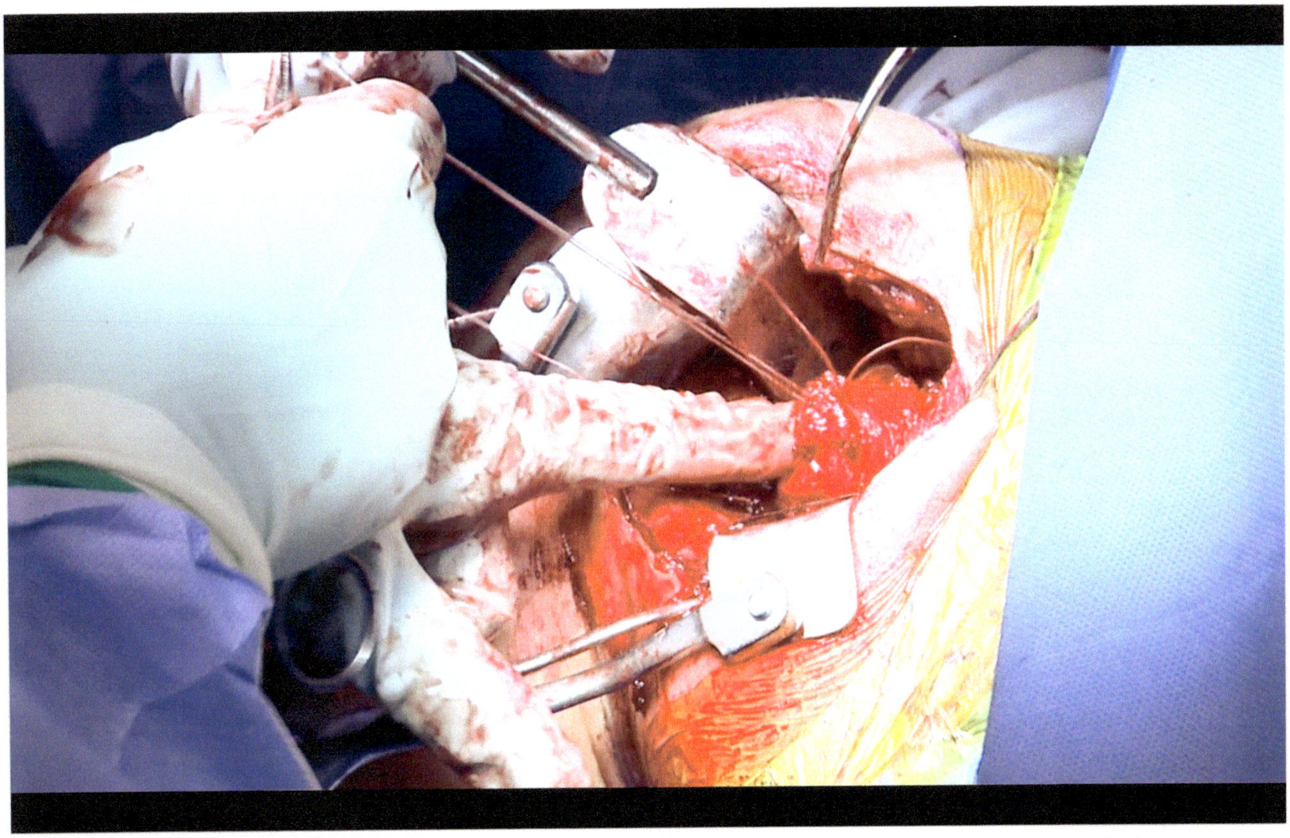

Fig. 29.3 Tenotomy of the subscapular tendon is performed near the tendon insertion site. It is then tagged with a no. 2 high-strength suture and retracted medially.

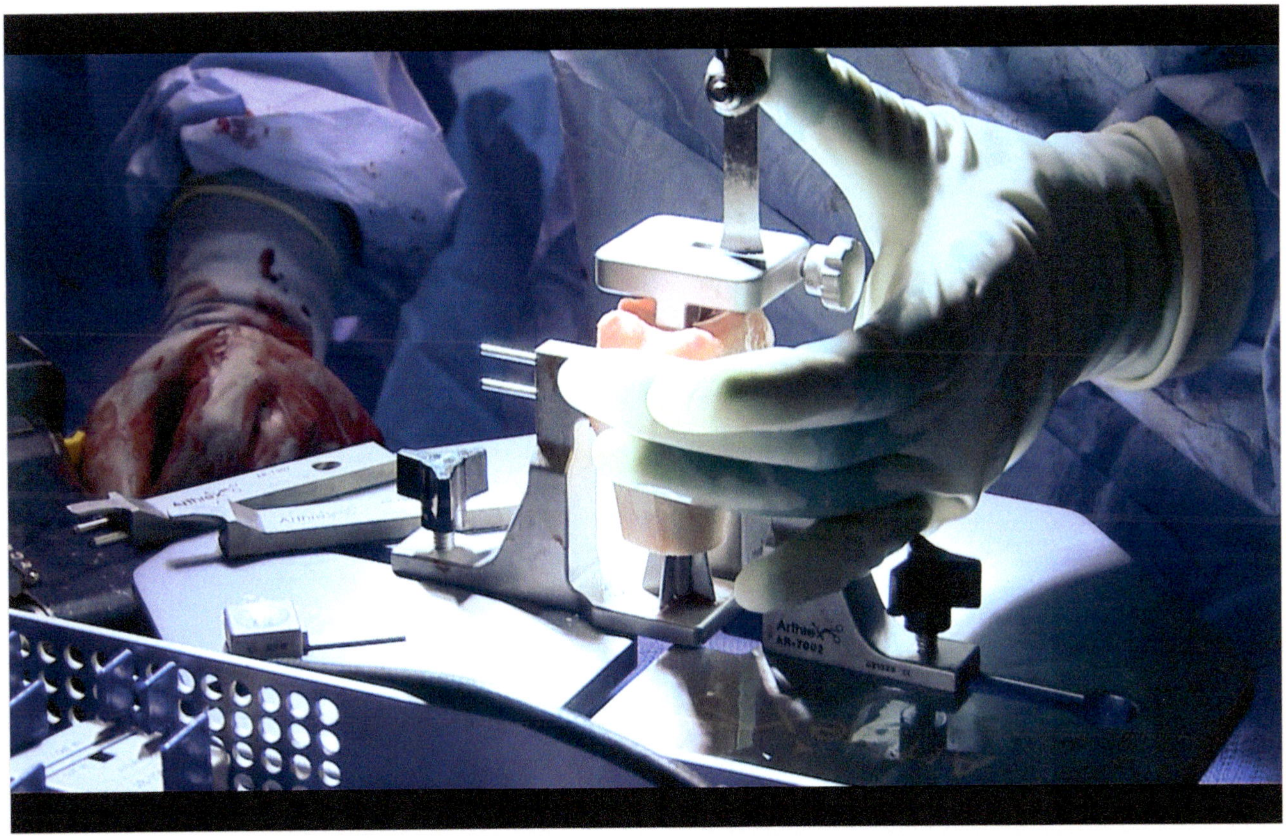

Fig. 29.4 Custom distal tibia allograft (DTA) cutting device (Arthrex) is used to perform necessary cuts of the DTA.

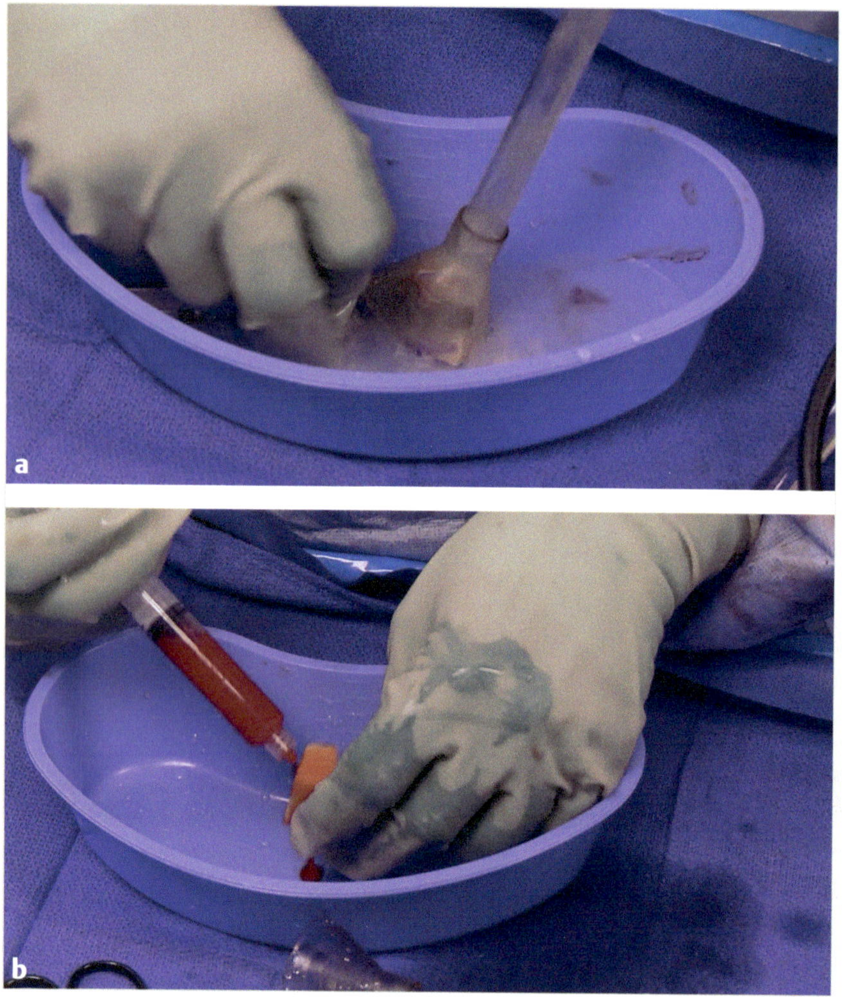

Fig. 29.5 **(a)** Pulsatile lavage of the distal tibia allograft (DTA) to remove marrow elements. **(b)** Graft is soaked in platelet-rich plasma to improve the potential for bony union.

ogous-conditioned plasma and platelet-rich plasma for application through use of a double-syringe system (Greyledge Technologies, Vail, CO; **Fig. 29.5b**). Before this, 60 cm^3 of peripheral blood is collected from the patient and submitted to centrifugation for approximately 10 minutes to heterogeneously divide the blood.

29.6.3 Graft Placement

Two small 1.6-mm Kirschner wires are placed in the graft bicortically from anterior to posterior in order to temporarily fixate it. If necessary, an additional K-wire can be used to improve fixation. The K-wires are measured and a cannulated drill is used over the first two K-wires through the previously drilled 4.0-mm holes, into the near cortex of the native glenoid, which will allow for lag screw compression of the graft to the glenoid. Following this, two 3.75-mm noncannulated fully threaded screws (typically 32–36 mm in length, determined by the K-wire measurement) with suture washers (Arthrex) are used to compress the graft into the anterior glenoid defect (**Fig. 29.6**). The sutures from the suture washer are used to repair the capsule that was sharply split or taken down. The tendon is repaired with multiple suture anchors (Arthrex) through a double-row technique when takedown is performed. The deltopectoral approach is closed in a standard fashion. **Table 29.1** summarizes the principal steps of the procedure.

29.7 Tips and Pearls/Expert Suggestions

To ensure the graft has the correct dimensions, we suggest the use of 3D CT to quantify the glenoid bone loss via the glenoid fossa circle method. All fibrotic tissue in the glenoid defect must be removed, as well as any graft or hardware from previous surgery in a revision setting. While exposing the capsule, every attempt should be made to preserve adequate tissue for repair of the capsular tissue to the DTA. A bleeding bone surface must be established in order to maximize healing potential. Special attention must be paid to the humeral head, as Hill–Sachs defects can lead to failure of the procedure; 3D CT can also be used to measure the glenoid track and assess the risk of engagement. During the preparation of the graft, precise cuts must be used to fashion the graft custom to the defect, ideally using a custom workstation in order to reduce the risk of errors or graft damage. It is also important that an assistant provides irrigation during cutting to minimize thermal damage to the graft bone and cartilage. Once the graft is prepared, we use pulsatile lavage and platelet-rich plasma to improve healing properties. Ensure the graft is flush and congruent with the anterior glenoid to allow for graft incorporation; this may take several attempts with intervening microadjustments.

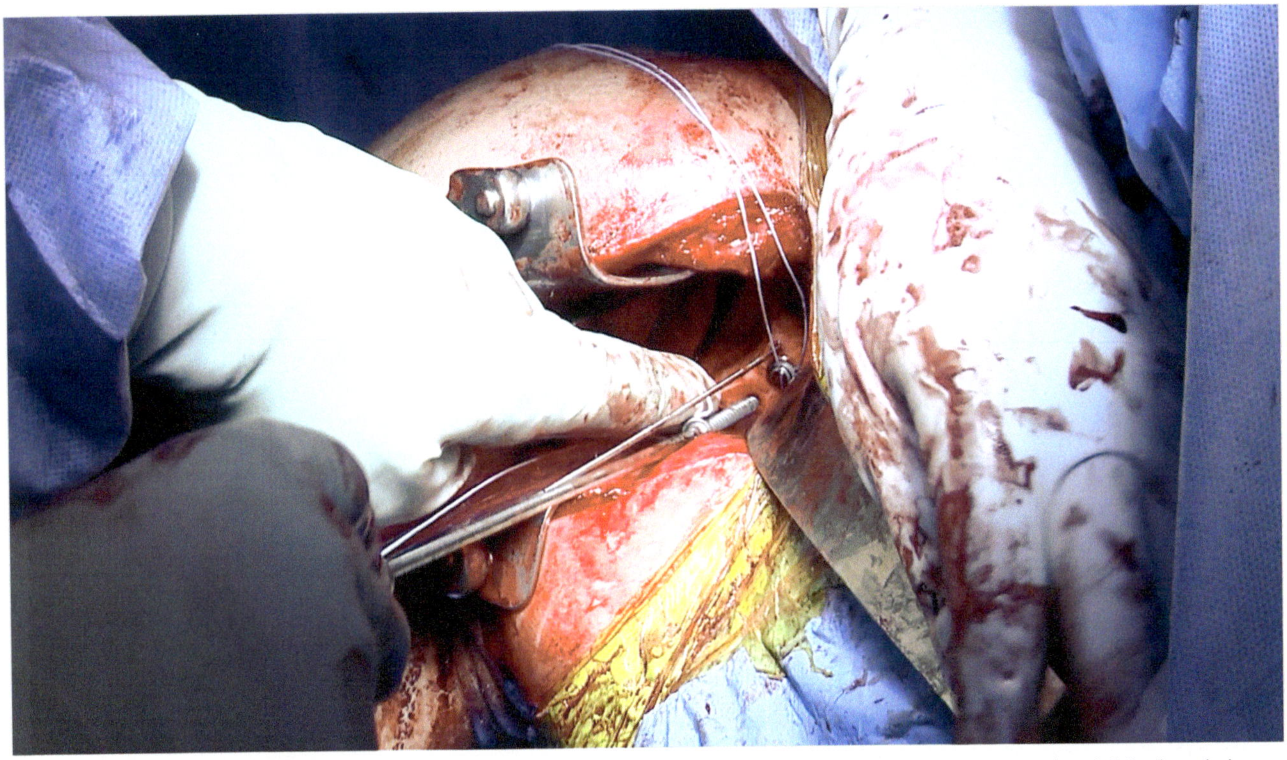

Fig. 29.6 Distal tibia allograft (DTA) graft fixation in correct position and orientation using two headless, noncannulated, fully threaded compression screws loaded with suture washers.

Table 29.1 Summary of the technique

Principal steps
1. Place the patient in the beach-chair position.
2. Use the deltopectoral approach.
3. Perform the subscapularis split in primary cases or subscapularis takedown in a revision setting.
4. Evaluate the glenoid and possible concomitant humeral defects.
5. Prepare the glenoid defect to a bony bleeding surface.
6. Prepare the DTA according to the glenoid defect.
7. Use platelet-rich plasma to improve healing potential.
8. Ensure the correct position of the graft into the glenoid defect.
9. Use screws with suture washers to perform a definitive fixation.
10. Close the medial aspect of the capsule using the loaded washer sutures.
11. Use anchors to repair the subscapularis when a takedown is performed.

29.8 What to Avoid

Whenever possible, a subscapularis tendon split is preferred to a subscapularis takedown; however, the subscapularis should not be split medial to the coracoid, as it puts the nerve to the subscapularis at risk. It is important to avoid placing excess medial retraction on the conjoined tendon, in order to protect the musculocutaneous nerve. Care should also be taken to avoid any damage to the axillary nerve during inferior dissection on the glenoid.

29.9 Complications

During the approach, damage to the cephalic vein can occur if it is not well identified and protected. In addition to the potential nerve injuries detailed earlier, traction injuries can also lead to neurologic complications. Inappropriate preparation of the glenoid defect can occur, leading to nonunion and failure. Damage to the graft can occur if prepared with an inappropriate device or without irrigation. When placed in an incorrect position or orientation, the graft will be unable to restore the anatomy and biomechanics of the shoulder. Allograft rejection and transmission of disease from the allograft are rare but potential complications.

29.10 Postoperative Care

Following the procedure, our postoperative protocol calls for the use an ultrasling for 4 to 6 weeks. In order to allow for better evaluation of the progression during the physiotherapy, we divide our protocol in phases.

29.10.1 Phase 1

This phase has a duration of 2 weeks and consists of aerobic exercises and passive shoulder range of motion. Aerobic exercises consist of stationary bike and walking on level surface, which are performed for 30 minutes. Passive range-of-motion exercises must be performed four times a week and progressed to the following limits: 120 degrees of forward flexion (FF),

120 degrees of motion in the scapular plane, 30 degrees of external rotation (ER) at side, and abduction (AB) to 90 degrees. We incentivize active wrist and elbow exercises; however, no biceps activation should be performed during this period.

29.10.2 Phase 2

This phase begins when the goals of the first phase are met, typically after 2 weeks. There is a progression in aerobic exercise duration to 45 to 60 minutes. Shoulder passive exercises also increase to 150 degrees of FF, 150 degrees of motion in the scapular plane, 45 degrees of ER at side, and AB of 90 degrees. We also encourage isometric exercises for extension, ER, internal rotation (IR), and AB. For patients who achieve rehabilitation goals without incident, the use of the sling is discontinued at 4 weeks postoperatively. Deltoid isometric exercises typically start at 4 weeks.

29.10.3 Phase 3

The third phase, usually from week 6 to 12, continues the incremental progression of passive range of motion to 160 degrees of FF, 160 degrees of motion in the scapular plane, 45 degrees of ER at side, and AB to 140 degrees. Passive range of motion is progressed to active-assisted, and ultimately, active range of motion. We also include more internal and external rotation exercises. Aerobic exercise intensity is increased. Treadmill with 7 degrees of inclination and stationary bike with progressed resistance are performed.

29.10.4 Phase 4

This phase consists of strength restoration, usually from week 12 to 16. For this phase, we use specific exercises including external and internal rotation at 90 degrees with cable, pushup, and plyometric exercises.

29.10.5 Phase 5

This phase marks the return to sports activities. The patient starts swimming, military press, and lat pull-down exercises. Throwing is progressed from short to long distances. The return to full sports activities is individualized to each patient according to patient confidence, progress during the physical therapy phases, and type of sport.

References

1. Bhatia S, Van Thiel GS, Gupta D, et al. Comparison of glenohumeral contact pressures and contact areas after glenoid reconstruction with. Latarjet or distal tibial osteochondral allografts. Am J Sports Med 2013;41(8):1900–1908
2. Gupta AK, Chalmers PN, Klosterman E, Harris JD, Provencher MT, Romeo AA. Arthroscopic distal tibial allograft augmentation for posterior shoulder instability with glenoid bone loss. Arthrosc Tech 2013;2(4):e405–e411
3. Frank RM, Romeo AA, Provencher MT. Glenoid reconstruction with distal tibia allograft for recurrent anterior shoulder instability. Orthopedics 2017;40(1):e199–e205
4. Provencher MT, Ghodadra N, LeClere L, Solomon DJ, Romeo AA. Anatomic osteochondral glenoid reconstruction for recurrent glenohumeral instability with glenoid deficiency using a distal tibia allograft. Arthroscopy 2009;25(4):446–452
5. Ferrari MB, Sanchez A, Sanchez G, Akamefula R, Kruckeberg BM, Provencher MT. Use of a cutting instrument for fresh osteochondral distal tibia allograft preparation: treatment of glenoid bone loss. Arthrosc Tech 2017;6(2):e363–e368
6. Sanchez A, Ferrari MB, Akamefula RA, Frank RM, Sanchez G, Provencher MT. anatomical glenoid reconstruction using fresh osteochondral distal tibia allograft after failed Latarjet procedure. Arthrosc Tech 2017;6(2):e477–e482

30 Partial Humeral Head Replacement: Allograft and Prosthetic

Daniel E. Davis and Joseph A. Abboud

Abstract

Full thickness osteochondral defects of the humeral head may occur most commonly as a result of avascular necrosis or glenohumeral dislocation. In the setting of defects comprising less than 40% of the articular surface, the lesion may be replaced with either allograft or prosthetic components. Allograft components have the benefit of replacing with a cartilaginous surface, but may resorb. Prosthetic components have the benefit of being more stable, but do have the downside of glenoid wear. This chapter will review the indications and techniques of each procedure.

Keywords: *humerus osteochondral defect, osteochondral allograft replacement, partial humerus arthroplasty, treatment of AVN, treatment of large humeral head defects*

30.1 Goals of Procedure

Cartilage defects involving a portion of the humeral head are a condition that may occur due to multiple causes, each of which poses a treatment challenge. A large portion of these osteochondral defects are caused by either avascular necrosis (AVN) or traumatic glenohumeral dislocation, both of which are relatively rare events.

AVN of the humeral head is the second most common site secondary to the femoral head. Frequently, this process is idiopathic, but may also be associated with steroid use, systemic lupus, chronic renal failure, or alcoholism.[1] In the presence of AVN, the subchondral bone of the humeral head becomes necrotic and loses the mechanical integrity to support the cartilaginous surface. The cartilage than collapses, leaving a lesion in the humeral head, which causes pain and dysfunction.[1]

Traumatic glenohumeral dislocations, a majority of which are anterior, may result in a defect in the posterosuperior humeral head known as a Hill–Sachs lesion. This lesion is caused when that area of the head traumatically contacts the anteroinferior glenoid edge after the dislocation.[2] A reverse Hill–Sachs lesion may occur through a similar mechanism in a posterior dislocation. In either event, a large enough defect can lead to recurrent instability by engaging with the glenoid edge and levering the head out of its articulation with the glenoid. While these lesions may not completely involve articulating cartilage of the joint surface, the presence of the defect leads to dysfunction through recurrent dislocation.

There is the possibility of limiting the pathology of these defects by replacing the defective surface of the humeral head with either osteochondral allograft or prosthetic replacement. The goal of either of these procedures is to reconstruct the native anatomy of the humeral head, while leaving the intact cartilage undisrupted.[3,4] Either reconstruction should fill the defect, be on the same level of the surrounding cartilage, and match the contour and radius of the surrounding head. While we recognize that other soft-tissue procedures can be performed for engaging Hill–Sachs lesions, this chapter will focus on partial arthroplasty with either allograft or prosthetic.

30.2 Advantages

Operative treatment options for partial surface humeral head lesions are limited and consist of either filling the defect or replacing the entire humeral head. There are multiple advantages involved in partially filling or replacing the defect rather than the whole cartilaginous surface. First, it allows the surgeon to maintain the normal anatomy of the humeral articular surface. When replacing the entire head, there is a risk of malalignment or incorrectly sizing the replacement. In a partial replacement, the natural inclination, version, and size are more easily maintained. Second, intact healthy cartilage is spared, allowing the patient to live with the greatest amount of their natural cartilage. Third, this minimalistic approach allows for greater reconstructive options in the future, which is ideal for younger patients. Finally, an advantage of an osteochondral allograft is the potential for bony healing and incorporation, but comes with the risk of not healing and resorption. A prosthetic partial replacement has the advantage of minimized wear and no risk of resorption with the risk of loss of fixation and loosening.

30.3 Indications

As mentioned earlier, the majority of indications for partial humeral head replacement are for osteonecrosis of the head and Hill–Sachs lesions. The size of the osteonecrotic lesion should be measured and be less than 40% of the entire surface area of the humeral head.[5] Hill–Sachs or reverse Hill–Sachs lesions are indicated for partial replacement if they are large enough to engage with the glenoid and create instability.

30.3.1 Contraindications

Partial humeral head replacement is contraindicated for lesions larger than 40% of the humeral articular surface. Lesions larger than this will create challenges with maintaining fixation and appropriately re-creating the articular surface anatomy. For these larger lesions, the humeral head should be resurfaced or replaced.[3,5] Additionally, global humeral arthritis as evidenced by joint space narrowing less than 4 mm, osteophyte formation, subchondral sclerosis, and subchondral cysts is contraindicated for partial resurfacing. If significant arthritic glenoid disease is present, partial replacement should be avoided as it will be difficult to eliminate pain. Finally, while age is not a strict contraindication, we usually only perform this procedure on patients younger than 60 years. In our experience, patients above this age have better clinical outcomes with lower chance of another operation with a full humeral head replacement and/or glenoid replacement if clinically indicated.

30.4 Preoperative Preparation/ Positioning

As with any orthopaedic evaluation, a thorough history and physical examination should be obtained. Focus should be on a history of steroid use for systemic disease or, otherwise, sickle cell anemia, alcohol use, and renal disease. Additionally, a history of dislocation events including number of dislocations and trauma should be focused on if concern is more for Hill–Sachs lesions. A standard shoulder examination including inspection, palpation, range of motion, and special examinations focusing on pain during midrange for AVN or apprehension and relocation tests for instability. Finally, imaging should be obtained to corroborate the history and findings of the physical examination. Standard X-rays are valuable to obtain information on the native alignment of the humerus, presence of arthritic changes, and initial evaluation of defect location. Advanced axial imaging is also needed to completely evaluate the location and size of the lesion. For AVN lesions, MRI is the best study to evaluate the lesion, its effect on the cartilage, and to determine the size relative to the head. For Hill–Sachs lesions, CT imaging is preferred for more detailed bony evaluation of the size and location of the lesion.

At our institution, the vast majority of these lesions will be treated through an anterior deltopectoral approach. For posteriorly oriented Hill–Sachs lesions, a posterior approach can also be utilized. The location of the lesion and the comfort of the surgeon with the approach will determine the preoperative positioning. For the deltopectoral approach, we use a beach-chair position with the patient's head elevated to approximately 30 degrees. If it is decided to perform a posterior approach, the patient is positioned in lateral decubitus with the operative arm draped free to allow free range of motion.

The choice of humeral head allograft versus prosthetic partial replacement should be made prior to the procedure; however, all options should be made available as backup for surgery. Indications for allograft are for the largest deepest lesions that are within the parameters of partial replacement. Additionally, allograft is reserved for younger, healthier patients with better bone stock for integration and also possesses a theoretical advantage of decreased glenoid wear. Partial replacement is generally reserved for the older end of the indicated population with the understood risk that there may be increased rate of glenoid wear.

30.5 Operative Techniques

As mentioned earlier, the vast majority of these cases will be performed anteriorly through a standard deltopectoral interval approach. Occasionally, a posterior Judet approach may be used for posteriorly based lesions (**Fig. 30.1**), but our preference is the anterior deltopectoral approach. The patient is positioned in the beach-chair position elevated at 30 degrees. Dissection is made through the internervous interval taking the cephalic vein laterally with the deltoid. A Cobb elevator is used to define the subdeltoid space first laterally, then superiorly deep and lateral to the coracoacromial ligament. Complete release of the subdeltoid space is mandatory to allow mobilization of the deltoid and improve visualization. A Brown deltoid retractor is placed laterally and a wide Richardson retractor medially. We like to avoid self-retaining retractors in open shoulder cases to limit constant stretch on the brachial plexus.

The subscapularis tendon is tagged with a suture and a blunt Hohmann is placed inferiorly to protect the axillary nerve. For partial resurfacing procedures, we prefer a subscapularis peel approach. We prefer a peel for management of our subscapularis to allow for full exposure and to not sacrifice any cartilage with the head that may occur with an osteotomy. When using the anterior approach for a posteriorly based lesion, wide and complete exposure is mandatory. For anteriorly based lesions, especially those more superior, a subscapularis sparing approach may be used through the rotator interval; however, this limits the ability to fully evaluate the entire humeral head as well as the glenoid. Before moving onto preparation of the lesion, the entirety of both articular surfaces should be evaluated to confirm stable, intact cartilage.

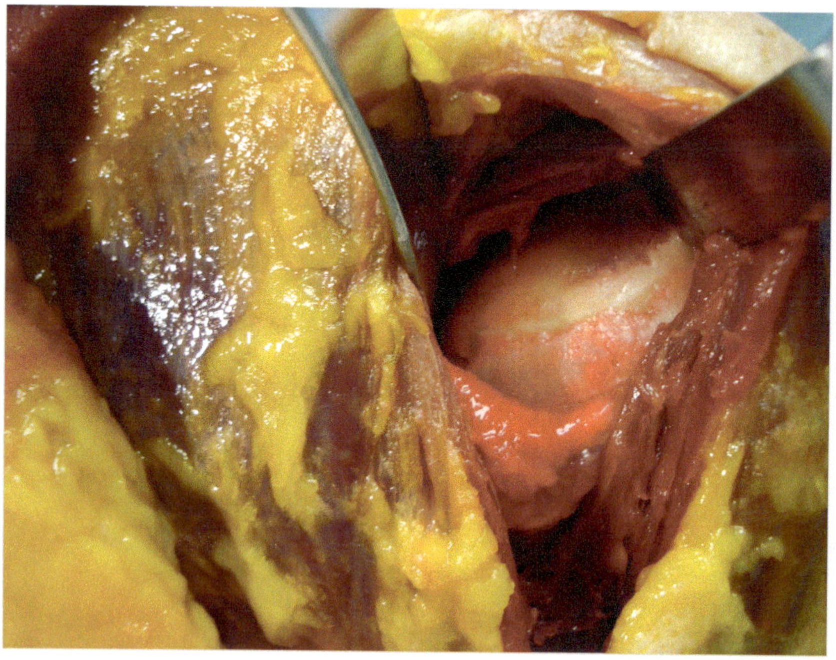

Fig. 30.1 An example of the posterior Judet approach is demonstrated in this cadaver case. After reflecting the deltoid, an internervous plane between the infraspinatus and teres minor is developed to expose the posterior humeral head. This can be used for posteriorly based lesions, which are determined too difficult to access through the more standard deltopectoral approach.

30.5.1 Allograft

If the choice is made to replace the defect with allograft, this can be done through either fresh bulk allograft or by filling the lesions with multiple plugs. We prefer to use a bulk matched allograft to fill the lesion and will highlight the steps later. Using the CT scan that was obtained preoperatively, the size of the humeral head is determined and sent to the tissue bank to obtain a size-matched humeral head. We prefer to use the Allograft OATS system from Arthrex, Inc. (Naples, FL), which is primarily designed for work in the knee, but may be transferred to the shoulder.

After the lesion is exposed adequately, a cannulated sizer is used to estimate the lesion diameter in order to obtain complete coverage of all affected cartilage. After the appropriate sizer is selected, the circumference of it is traced onto the humeral head surface to make sure the cylinder is perpendicular to the cartilaginous surface. A pin is then placed through the center of the cylinder, the cylinder is removed, and a mark is made with a pen at the 12 o'clock position of the traced circle. The donor-matched graft is then held near the recipient humeral head and the sizer is again used to mark a circumferential area in the corresponding area of the donor. A mark is also made in the 12 o'clock position on the donor (**Fig. 30.2**). Attention is turned back to the recipient humeral head and a cylindrical drill is used to score the cartilage around the lesion. A cannulated graduated drill of appropriate size is then used to drill out the lesion to a depth of approximately 6 to 8 mm, being sure to have bleeding subchondral bone (**Fig. 30.3**). The graft is then prepared on the provided workstation, which has a bushing and a cannulated sizer that are mounted over the graft to ensure drilling of the graft in the appropriate angle and direction. The graft cylinder is then drilled through the entirety of the patient head (**Fig. 30.4**). A depth measurement guide is then used to determine the depth of the drilled out lesion of the recipient and then the graft is trimmed accordingly. A dilator is used in the donor to extend the donor site by one-half of a millimeter and then the graft is delivered into the donor with a clear, graft delivery tube. Gentle taps are used to

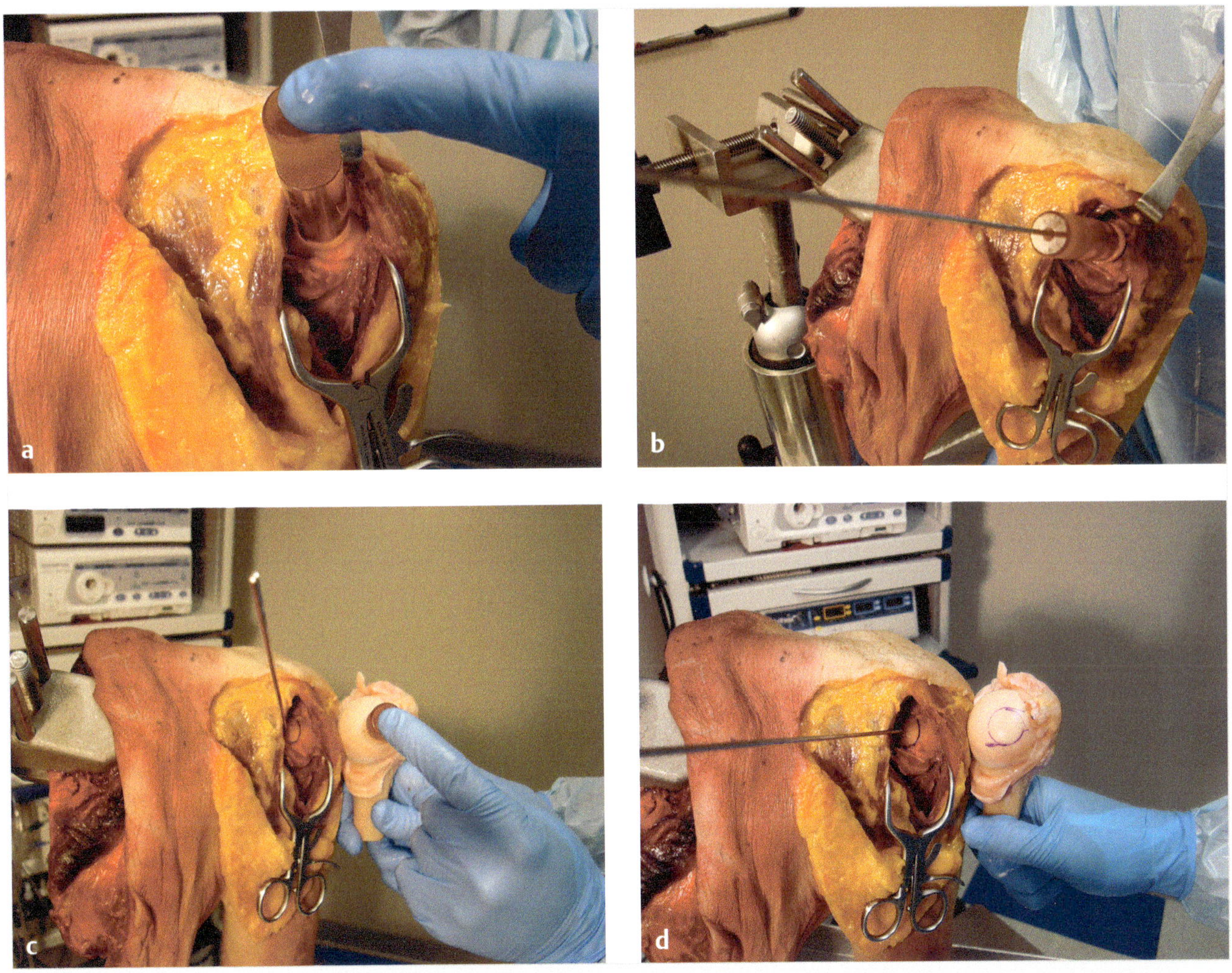

Fig. 30.2 A fresh bulk allograft system from Arthrex Inc. can be used to replace osteochondral defects in the humeral head. **(a)** The appropriately sized cylinder is used to define the size of the lesion that will be replaced. **(b)** A pin is placed through the cannulated cylinder to identify the exact center of the lesion. **(c)** The bulk graft is then held next to the patient to determine the exact spot from which to harvest the graft. **(d)** The graft is then marked out with the sizer cylinder and the polarity of the graft is marked along with the corresponding location in the patient.

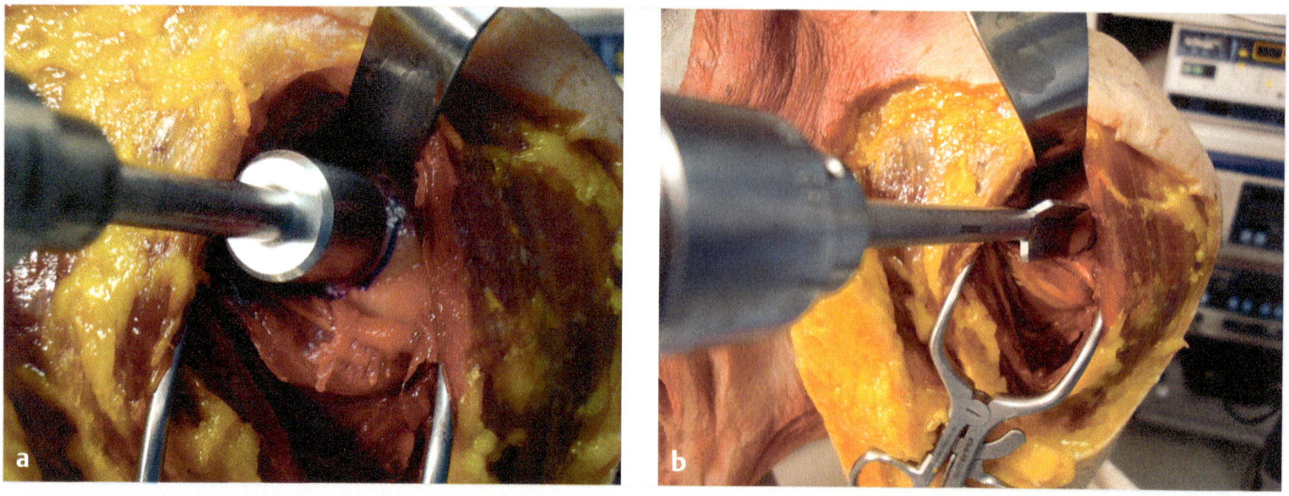

Fig. 30.3 Preparation of humeral defect. **(a)** A cannulated cylinder is used to score the edges of the lesion. **(b)** A graduated drill is then used to core out the lesion to bleeding subchondral bone.

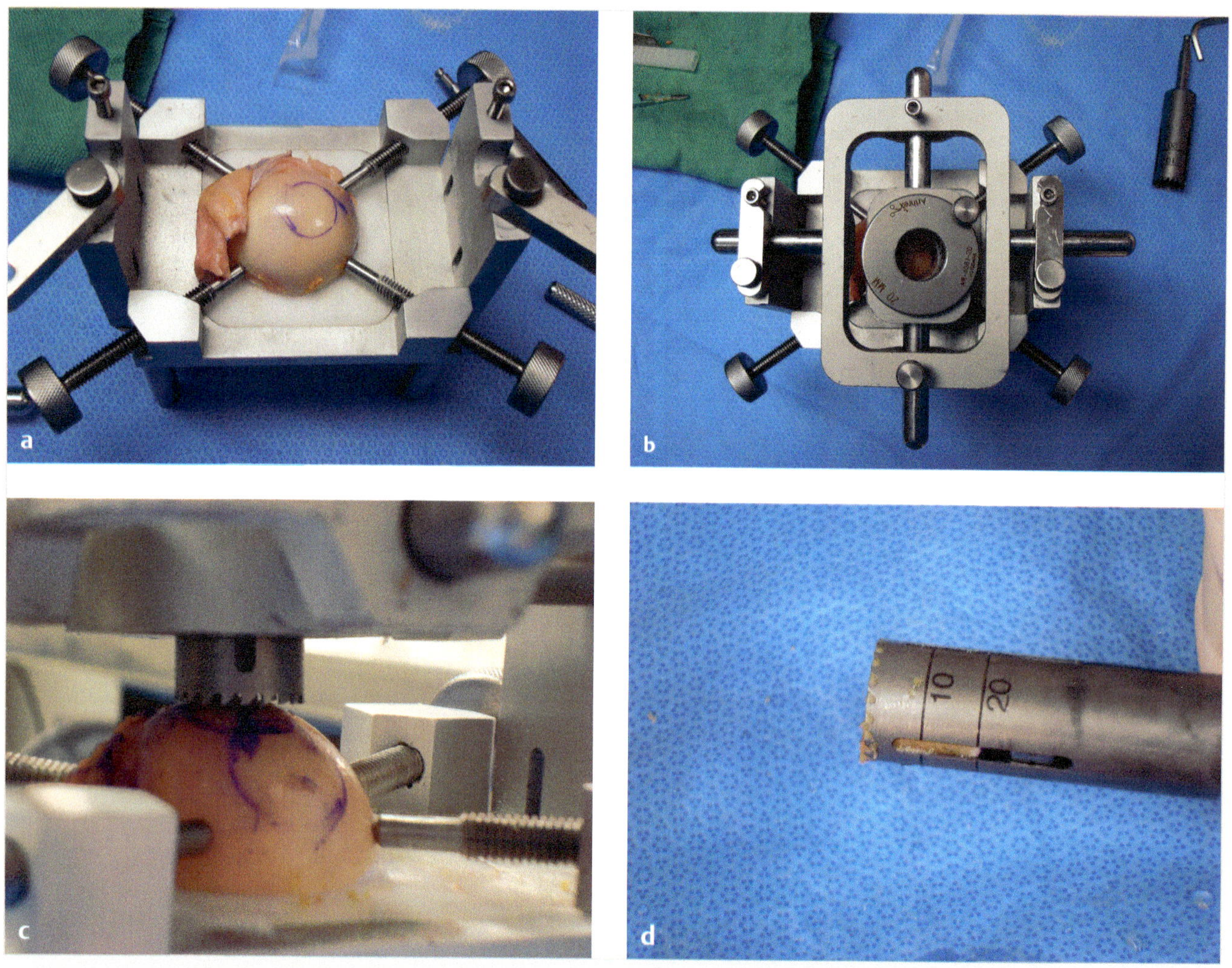

Fig. 30.4 **(a)** The workstation is built on the back table and the graft is mounted securely with four pins. **(b)** The bushing and cannulated sizer are then mounted over the graft to ensure drilling in the correct direction and position. **(c)** The graft is then drilled with the appropriate sized cannulated drill through the entirety of the graft. **(d)** The plug is then within the cannulated drill and should be carefully extracted.

seat the graft in place, making sure the marks at the 12 o'clock position are in line. Being flush with the adjacent graft is ideal, but we err on the side of a slight inset rather than leaving the cartilage proud (**Fig. 30.5**). In general, the interference fit of the bone is enough to firmly fix the graft. However, screw fixation may be added to provide extra security. A headless antegrade screw may be used, but we prefer a retrograde screw if necessary to avoid violating the donor cartilage.

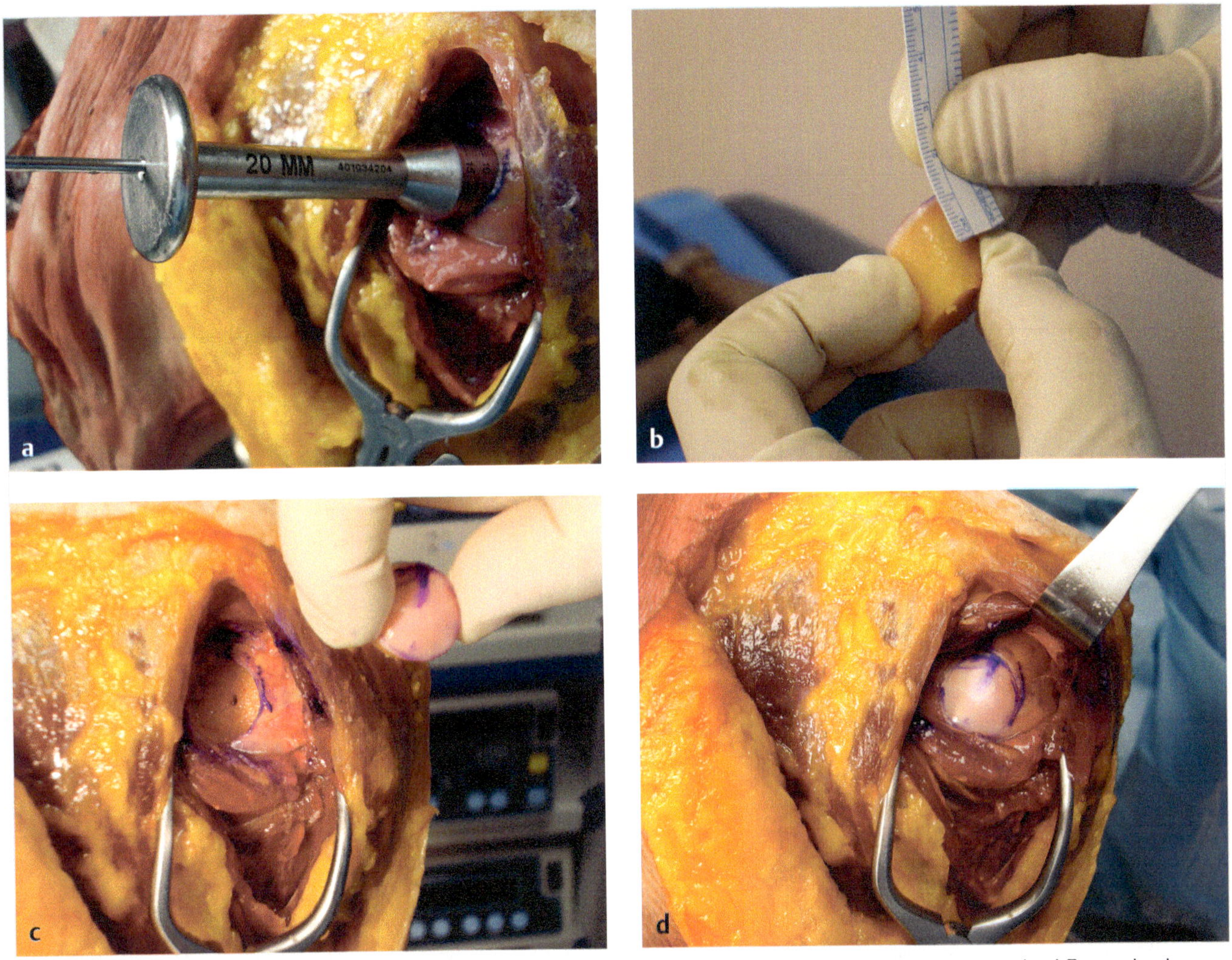

Fig. 30.5 **(a)** A sizer of the appropriate diameter is used to measure the size of the recipient site, being sure to note the different depths along the curvature of the head. **(b)** The graft plug is then measured and trimmed accordingly to the measurements. **(c)** The graft is then oriented to the lines that were drawn on the draft initially. **(d)** Tamps are used to insert the graft into the recipient site erring on the side of slightly countersunk.

30.5.2 Prosthetic Replacement

If the decision is made to replace the defect with a prosthetic, we prefer to use the HemiCap system made by Arthrosurface (Franklin, MA). After the lesion is exposed, the first step is placing the taper post, which will support the implant. A drill guide is placed over the lesion to place the starter pin (**Fig. 30.6**). The drill guide size should be selected so that it is just larger than the present defect. The goal is to remove the least amount of healthy cartilage while allowing to adequately fit an implant. The guide should also be centered over the defect and normal to the articular surface; the pin should then be placed through the guide. A stepped drill is then used until the step becomes flush to the articular surface and the hole is tapped. The hole is irrigated and a small amount of cement is placed prior to inserting the taper post with the provided driver until the line on the driver is equal to the articular surface. A trial cap is provided to then test the height of the taper post to the articular surface, the driver may be used to adjust as needed. Always remember, slightly countersunk is preferable to being proud.

After the taper post is in place, the surface must be prepared to accept the implant. A centering shaft is placed into the taper post and a contact probe is used to measure the articular offset at four points (superior, inferior, medial, and lateral) on the lesion. Four diameter sizes are available (25, 30, 35, and 40 mm). The appropriate diameter and offset is chosen. The appropriate diameter implant is selected, the cartilage is first prepared with a circle cutter, and the lesion is then reamed. The reamer will stop at the taper post. Be sure to start the reamer off the cartilage and then advance to avoid chipping intact cartilage. A trial implant is placed over the taper post to assess height and appropriate radius of curvature. Height can be adjusted by driving in or backing out the taper post. Radius can be adjusted with other implants. Once the appropriate size is chosen, the final implant is impacted onto the taper post (**Fig. 30.7**).

When using a subscapularis peel technique, we repair the tendon back to the lesser tuberosity. Two 1-mm Dacron tape sutures are woven through the tendon after being passed through drill holes in the lesser tuberosity and tied with the humerus in neutral rotation.

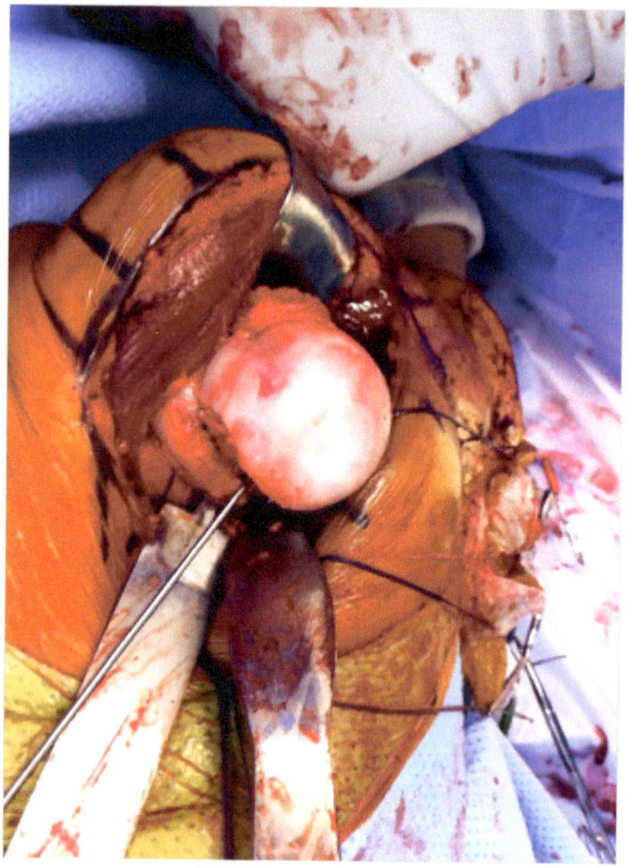

Fig. 30.6 After the sizing guide is used to determine the lesion size, a guide is used to insert a pin into the center of the lesion to assist with preparation of the site.

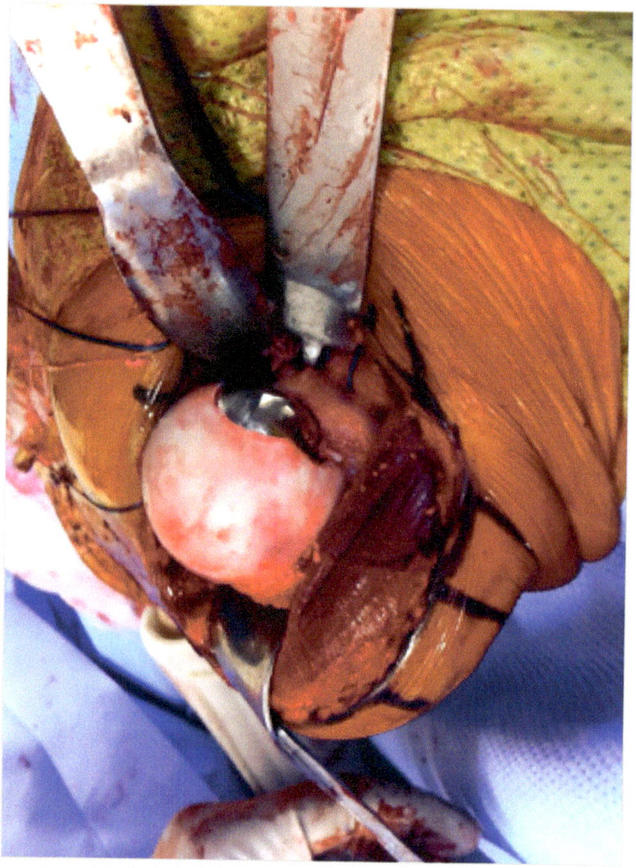

Fig. 30.7 The implant is seated into the prepared defect onto the taper post. Notice how the implant surface is slightly sunken compared to the articular surface, which is preferable to leaving the implant proud.

30.6 Tips and Pearls/Expert Suggestions

- Obtain a complete history and physical examination with appropriate imaging to fully diagnose and define the lesion to choose the appropriate treatment modality.
- Extensive preoperative counseling should be had with the patient that this may not be their last shoulder surgery as the graft may resorb, the implant may loosen, or cause significant glenoid disease requiring a total shoulder replacement.
- Preoperative planning must ensure the location of the lesion and the most appropriate approach to gain adequate exposure.
- Be sure to evaluate the remaining cartilaginous surfaces.
- Err on the side of countersinking the implant instead of leaving proud.
- Whenever reaming the cartilage, start the reamer on full speed first and then advance onto the cartilage.

30.7 What to Avoid

- Self-retaining retractors to avoid nerve injury: assistants using manual retractors will fatigue and need to reposition, which is of benefit to the nerves being retracted.
- Injury to intact cartilage: care must be taken on the approach compared to total joint arthroplasty as the majority of the cartilage is healthy in these cases.
- Overstuffing of the lesion: countersinking either the allograft or the prosthetic replacement is preferred to leaving proud to avoid damage to the intact glenoid cartilage.
- Damage to the rotator cuff insertion: more superior lesions are at a higher risk of injuring the attachment of the rotator cuff tendon; extra care should be taken for these lesions.

30.8 Complications/Bailout/Salvage

The complications associated with allograft replacement include errors during graft placement, such as incorrect sizing or rotation. These can be corrected by removing the graft with the supplied graft removal system. Care must be taken, however, not to fracture the graft or further compromise the host site. Additional complications include resorption of the graft, loosening of the graft, movement of the fixation device, or infection. Complications of the prosthetic replacement are similar and include loosening, glenoid wear, or infection.

Graft resorption or implant loosening should be treated on a case-by-case basis and dependent on the patient's symptoms and age. If the failure was within a year and the patient is symptomatic, it may be reasonable to perform a revision as long as the remaining, surrounding cartilage is intact. Movement of the fixation screw may require more immediate surgical intervention to avoid further, severe damage to the remaining articular surfaces. Progressive wear of the surrounding cartilage leading to advanced arthritis may be treated with a total shoulder arthroplasty as long as the rotator cuff is still intact and functioning. Infection should of course be treated on an urgent basis with removal of all foreign material along with thorough debridement. Further implants should not be replaced until all signs of infection have cleared.

If all else has failed, depending on the patient's age and activity level, there are multiple salvage options. Reverse total shoulder is an option for patients who have lost all rotator cuff integrity with relatively low demands for their shoulder. Range-of-motion limitations should be fully explained to the patient. If the patient is deemed too young for a reverse total shoulder, fusion of the glenohumeral joint may be performed until they have reached an age where conversion to a reverse total shoulder is a more reasonable option. Finally, in the setting of chronic, recurrent infections, resection arthroplasty may be necessary.

30.9 Postoperative Care

Depending on the patient's age and functional status, it is not unreasonable to perform these operations on an outpatient basis. A one-night stay may be more reasonable for pain control over the first night; however, with improved regional anesthesia, pain in the first postoperative day is not as common in our practice. To allow for appropriate healing of the subscapularis tendon, we limit range of motion to passive external rotation to 40 degrees and passive forward elevation to 140 degrees for the first 6 weeks postoperatively, during which time they also stay in a sling when not working on passive exercises. After those 6 weeks, the patient is allowed to come out of the sling and will undergo an additional 6 weeks of active and active assisted full range of motion and strengthening. At the 3-month mark, the patient may continue to work on range of motion and strength at home if they are progressing along a normal course. Postoperative X-rays are obtained at 2 weeks, 6 weeks, 3 months, 6 months, and 1 year to evaluate allograft integration and implant position.

References

1. Hasan SS, Romeo AA. Nontraumatic osteonecrosis of the humeral head. J Shoulder Elbow Surg 2002;11(3):281–298
2. Provencher MT, Frank RM, Leclere LE, et al. The Hill-Sachs lesion: diagnosis, classification, and management. J Am Acad Orthop Surg 2012;20(4):242–252
3. Uribe JW, Botto-van Bemden A. Partial humeral head resurfacing for osteonecrosis. J Shoulder Elbow Surg 2009;18(5):711–716
4. Armitage MS, Faber KJ, Drosdowech DS, Litchfield RB, Athwal GS. Humeral head bone defects: remplissage, allograft, and arthroplasty. Orthop Clin North Am 2010;41(3):417–425
5. Hattrup SJ. Indications, technique, and results of shoulder arthroplasty in osteonecrosis. Orthop Clin North Am 1998;29(3):445–451

31 Arthroscopic Posterior Stabilization

Fotios P. Tjoumakaris and James P. Bradley

Abstract
Arthroscopic posterior stabilization has evolved considerably over the past several years. Primary indication of this technique is in patients with recurrent posterior glenohumeral instability who have failed conservative management. Preoperative diagnostic imaging with MRA is often necessary to clearly delineate the pathology. Techniques of arthroscopic repair utilizing knotless fixation have allowed for anatomic repair without the risk of intra-articular knot abrasion. The risk of recurrence after arthroscopic plication is less than 10%, with the majority of patients returning to their preinjury level of function and athletic participation. Postoperative physical therapies utilizing developed protocols are key determinants to a successful outcome.

Keywords: *arthroscopic, posterior instability, posterior labral tear, recurrent posterior subluxation*

31.1 Goals of Procedure

The main purpose of arthroscopic posterior stabilization is to prevent recurrent macro (dislocation) or micro (recurrent posterior subluxation [RPS]) posterior instability of the glenohumeral joint. Traditional techniques focused on open capsular plication with labrum repair, bone block, or wedge osteotomy to prevent recurrent posterior instability. Evolving techniques have allowed for better access to the glenohumeral joint with an arthroscopic approach with accompanying superior clinical outcomes in recent years. The ultimate goal of arthroscopic management is to restore normal glenohumeral mechanics, prevent recurrent instability or subluxation, and allow for return to normal physiologic function of the joint and athletic participation. The arthroscopic method is also aimed at improving short-term range-of-motion goals and preventing disruption of the deltoid or scapular musculature, which can delay postoperative rehabilitation and may accompany an open technique.

31.2 Advantages

The arthroscopic approach to posterior stabilization has the advantage of treating a wide array of pathology. With open techniques, anterior pathology of the shoulder (labrum tearing, subscapularis disruption) in addition to superior pathology (supraspinatus, biceps tendon, and superior labrum tearing) is near impossible to address through the same exposure. The arthroscopic approach allows for clear visualization of the entire labrum, rotator cuff, and other pain-generating pathology around the glenohumeral joint, which also allows for adequate treatment. In addition, arthroscopic management of posterior instability allows for complete labrum repair, in addition to capsular plication in an "around the world" fashion. Recent studies evaluating postoperative outcomes of the arthroscopic approach have also surpassed those of open techniques, making the arthroscopic modality the current standard of care for the majority of patients.

31.3 Indications

Patients are candidates for arthroscopic posterior stabilization if they present with prior episodes of posterior dislocation or RPS of the glenohumeral joint that has not responded favorably to conservative management. Patients with macroinstability or joint dislocation may have accompanying osseous pathology (reverse Hill-Sachs lesion, reverse osseous Bankart lesion) that can accompany the soft-tissue pathology seen in patients with RPS (posterior labrum tear, Kim's lesion, capsular tearing, or patulous capsule). Patients who have suffered an initial posterior dislocation of the shoulder are initially closed reduced and assessed for instability. Once a pain-free shoulder with full range of motion is restored, patients are gradually returned to regular activity. If resultant instability or pain persists and physical therapy is not ameliorative, then the patient is counseled regarding surgical intervention. Patients with RPS may not report an initial traumatic event, however, and may have a more insidious course with deep-seated shoulder pain, reduced athletic participation (difficulty throwing a long ball or loss of velocity), and pain with cross-body and adducted shoulder movements. An initial course of physical therapy can be initiated in addition to a throwing regimen for overhead throwing athletes. If pain subsides, gradual return to play is begun and the patient can be assessed for recurrence of symptoms. If pain or subluxation returns, an MRA can be obtained to confirm the diagnosis. Once confirmed, the specific anatomical considerations can be evaluated and the patient can be counseled regarding the need for surgical intervention. Our primary indications for surgery are the following:

- History consistent with prior dislocation or RPS (as detailed earlier).
- Physical examination that is positive for any or all of the following:
  - Kim's test.
  - "Jerk" test.
  - Positive posterior load and shift test.
  - Pain with cross-body and adduction with reproduction of symptoms.
- Diagnostic imaging (MRA) demonstrating the following:
  - Patulous posterior capsule.
  - Posterior labral tear or concealed crack ("Kim's" lesion).
  - Reverse Hill-Sachs impaction fracture.
  - Relative increase in glenoid retroversion with hypoplastic labrum.
- Patients who failed conservative treatment with a stretching and strengthening rotator cuff rehabilitation program.

31.4 Contraindications

As arthroscopic techniques have evolved, so have the relative contraindications to an arthroscopic approach. Contraindications to arthroscopic surgery may include large glenoid (>25%) or reverse Hill-Sachs (>30%) lesions that may be better managed with an open bone grafting technique, capsular tearing with loss of capsular tissue (from prior surgery or thermal modification), excessive glenoid retroversion (type C glenoid), significant osteoarthritis or chondral erosion, neuromuscular abnormality resulting in motor deficit, and patients who have failed a prior arthroscopic procedure (relative contraindication). Any patient who is unable to comply with a postoperative regimen that consists of a brief period of immobilization followed by a structured therapy protocol is not a suitable candidate for surgical intervention.

31.5 Preoperative Preparation/ Positioning

31.5.1 Preoperative Preparation

Prior to surgery, the MRA is evaluated for degree of glenoid retroversion, significance of any osseous pathology, and the degree of labrum pathology (**Fig. 31.1**). Routine radiographs (anteroposterior [AP], scapular Y, and axillary views) are also typically obtained prior to MRA to exclude the presence of fracture, subluxation, or frank dislocation. Understanding the needs of each patient is critical to achieving success with this technique. For instance, patients who engage in high-risk contact sports are more likely to have significant labral pathology and require added capsular plication. Patients who are overhead throwing athletes will have difficulty returning to sports if excessive plication is performed causing a decrease in range of motion and capsular tightness. Patients are given information regarding the risks of surgery, which may include stiffness, infection, neurovascular injury, and recurrence of instability. On the date of the surgery, we routinely use an interscalene nerve block with general anesthesia for both intraoperative muscle relaxation and postoperative pain control.

31.5.2 Positioning

We prefer a lateral decubitus position, but recognize that a beach-chair position can be utilized for this technique. The lateral decubitus position offers excellent access to the posterior joint and capsule without the use of accessory traction by an assistant. A beanbag positioner is typically used with an axillary roll to protect the nonoperative extremity. The down leg is padded over the peroneal nerve, fibular head, and lateral malleolus. The operative arm is placed in 10 to 15 lb of balanced arm traction in 45 degrees of abduction and 20 degrees of forward flexion (**Fig. 31.2**). When the posterior, inferior aspect of the labrum is approached arthroscopically, forward flexion can be increased to gain better exposure. We will often angle the bed 45 degrees away from anesthesia and place the visualization tower across the surgical field and at eye level to the surgeon.

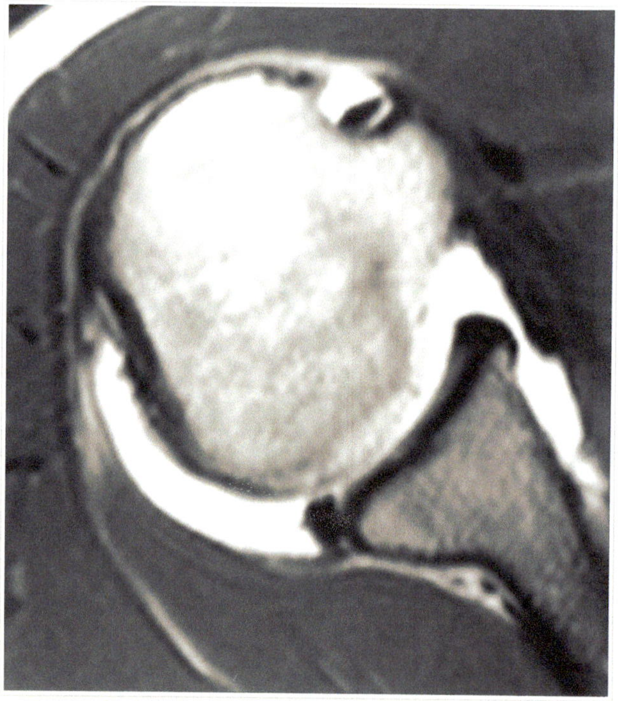

Fig. 31.1 Axial MRA demonstrating a crack/tear in the posterior labrum.

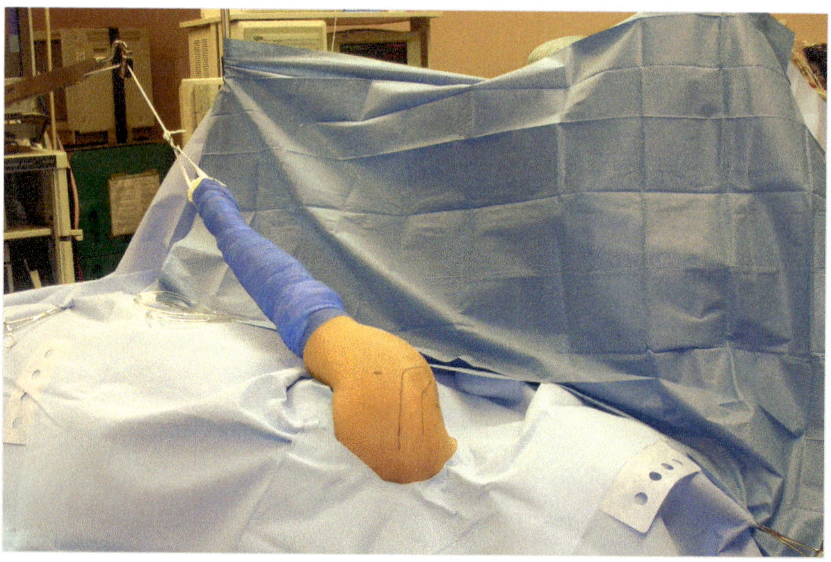

Fig. 31.2 Lateral decubitus positioning used for arthroscopic posterior stabilization.

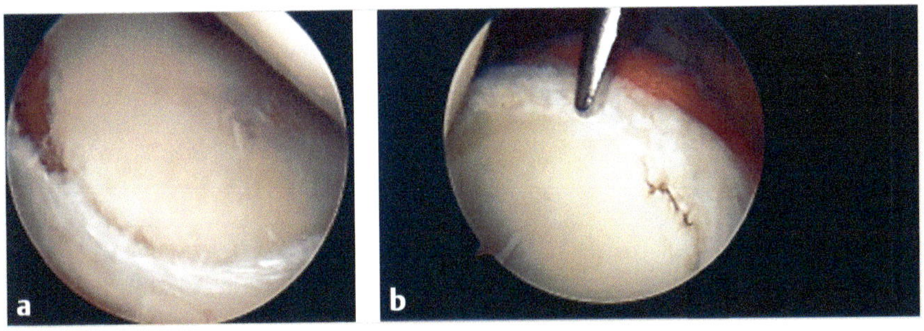

Fig. 31.3 (a) Arthroscopic view from the posterior portal demonstrating a superior and posterior labral tear in a right shoulder. (b) Arthroscopic view from the anterior portal looking posterior demonstrating the trajectory of the posterior portal that is adequate for placement of anchors tangential to the glenoid.

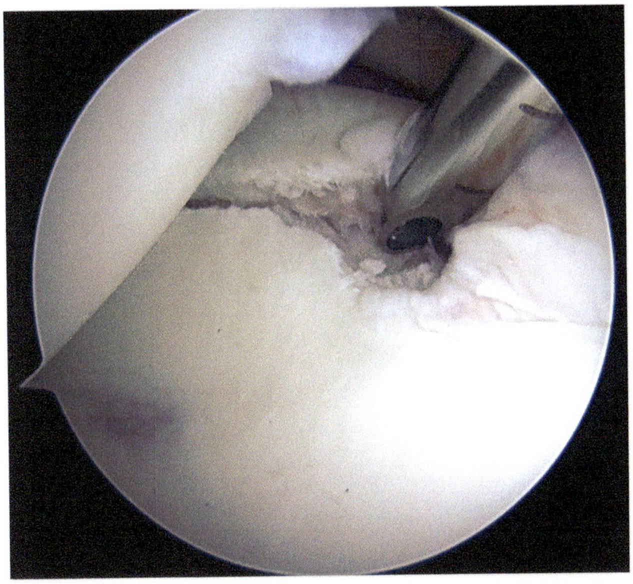

Fig. 31.4 A hooded burr or shaver can be used (as in this image) to debride the posterior glenoid in preparation for anchor placement.

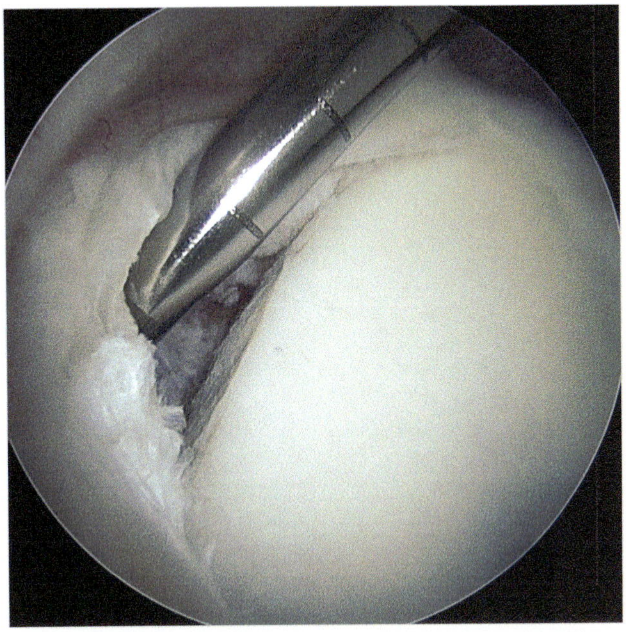

Fig. 31.5 Arthroscopic view from the posterior portal looking inferiorly along the glenoid after labrum mobilization and glenoid preparation are complete.

31.6 Operative Technique

31.6.1 Portal Placement

All bony landmarks are marked with a marking pen (the acromion, coracoid process, and acromioclavicular joint; **Fig. 31.2**). The anterior portal is typically placed in the rotator interval in a trajectory that is diagonal from the coracoid process to the anterolateral edge of the acromion. The posterior portal is created slightly lateral to a traditional posterior arthroscopy portal to allow tangential access to the posterior glenoid for anchor placement. The posterior portal is created first after insufflation of the joint with 30 mL of normal saline and the anterior portal is created using an "inside-out" technique. Once portals are created, a clear cannula is placed in the anterior portal using a traditional dilation technique. Either a 5.75- or 8.25-mm clear cannula (distally threaded) can be used for the anterior portal.

31.6.2 Diagnostic Arthroscopy

A 30-degree arthroscope placed through a posterior viewing portal is used to perform an initial diagnostic arthroscopy (**Fig. 31.3a, b**). The joint is checked for concomitant pathology such as superior labral tears, rotator cuff tears, and osteochondral injury. Debridement of the joint can be carried out with a 4.5-mm shaver through the anterior portal as needed. Following an initial diagnostic arthroscopy, the camera is placed into the anterior cannula and inflow is placed on the side port on the cannula. A switching stick is placed in the posterior portal and this portal is dilated to 8 mm. An 8.25-mm cannula (Arthrex, Naples, FL) is then placed in the posterior portal. The arthroscope can be switched to a 70-degree arthroscope, which allows better visualization of the posterior and inferior capsule and posteroinferior band of the inferior glenohumeral ligament.

31.6.3 Glenoid and Labrum Preparation

A meticulous glenoid preparation is critical to achieving success of the repair. An elevator is initially placed through the posterior portal and the labrum is sharply elevated off the glenoid. The labrum is mobilized as with anterior labral tears until the underside of the capsule edge of the glenoid rim is visualized. Care is taken during labral elevation and mobilization to not transect the labrum and adequate trajectory through the posterior portal is critical in achieving this mission. If the angle is difficult, the elevator can be brought in through the anterior portal and the labrum visualized posteriorly. Once adequate mobilization is achieved, a hooded burr is utilized to prepare the glenoid rim (**Fig. 31.4**). Great care should be used to ensure the labrum is protected during the bony debridement. A shaver is then utilized to remove any remaining soft-tissue debris from the glenoid rim, followed by rasping to create a fresh, bleeding surface conducive to soft-tissue healing (**Fig. 31.5**).

31.6.4 Suture Passing and Labral Repair

We have evolved our technique in recent years to a knotless anchor system (2.4-mm biocomposite short PushLock anchors [Arthrex] for patients with smaller glenoids [subequatorial width < 25 mm] or 2.9-mm short PushLock anchors for patients with normal or large glenoid widths) with 1.3-mm SutureTape (Arthrex) as our primary fixation method. Knotless fixation superior to the equator of the glenoid may minimize the risk of humeral head chondral injury as well as articular-sided rotator cuff knot abrasion. Furthermore, the SutureTape has a low profile, which allows it to lay flat against the labrum, minimizing tear-through and providing excellent reduction without humeral abrasion. The first step in labral repair is predicated on the surgeon understanding the patient-specific pathology and demands of the patient. Patients presenting with symptoms consistent with RPS and insidious shoulder pain without gross macroinstability may benefit from a primary labral repair without significant capsular plication/advancement (i.e., throwers). Patients with macroinstability or dislocation and who participate in high-demand contact sports capsule (e.g., offensive linemen) may require labral repair with plication of the posterior.

For the standard posterior labral repair, we prefer to place anchors from approximately the 6 o'clock to the 11 o'clock position on the glenoid. To achieve positioning of the inferior-most anchor, an accessory posterior portal may need to be created 45 degrees tangential to the glenoid. This portal is typically created slightly inferior and lateral to the posterior working portal. While viewing from the anterior portal, a spinal needle is used to localize the correct site of entry for the accessory posterior portal. Once the correct location and trajectory are identified for anchor placement, an accessory 5-mm cannula is introduced into the joint using the Seldinger technique. Great care should be taken to avoid damage to the axillary nerve on cannula introduction as it lies at risk in this area. The anchors are all placed from inferior to superior after suture passage.

A curved suture hook (Spectrum, Linvatec, Edison, NJ, or ReelPass Suture Lasso, Arthrex) loaded with a no. 0 monofilament suture is placed through the posterior working cannula while the arthroscope is placed in the anterior cannula. A bite of capsulolabral tissue is taken slightly inferior and lateral to the level of desired anchor location (to achieve capsular plication and advancement) and the suture is delivered through the labrum against the glenoid articular margin (**Fig. 31.6**). The monofilament suture is then shuttled through the posterior working cannula and a loop of SutureTape is placed in a knot of the monofilament suture. The goal is to create a "cinch" stitch akin to a luggage tag that will reduce the labrum and provide optimum suture security around the tissue. The loop of SutureTape is then shuttled back through the posterior working cannula and the tail ends of the suture are delivered through the loop created in the SutureTape. The two tails of the SutureTape are then pulled and the cinch stitch is reduced to the labrum. A knot pusher can be used to help reduce the knot to the labral tissue if needed when there is concern that the tissue is of poor quality. This creates 2.6 mm of SutureTape as the tape is essentially doubled over to create a stable fixation construct around the labrum and capsular complex. The SutureTape ends are then delivered through the accessory cannula for anchor placement. The drill guide is then placed through the accessory posterior cannula and a pilot hole drilled in the desired location. The suture ends are then shuttled through the eyelet of the knotless anchor and the anchor is then slid to the level of the glenoid and slight tension is applied to the limbs to reduce the labrum (**Fig. 31.7**). The anchor is then impacted into place within the pilot hole and the labrum and capsule are reduced to the glenoid margin. Additional anchors can be placed in an identical fashion as needed. Anchors in the 8 o'clock to 11 o'clock position are generally placed through the standard posterior portal, which provides a better angle of approach in this zone (**Fig. 31.8**).

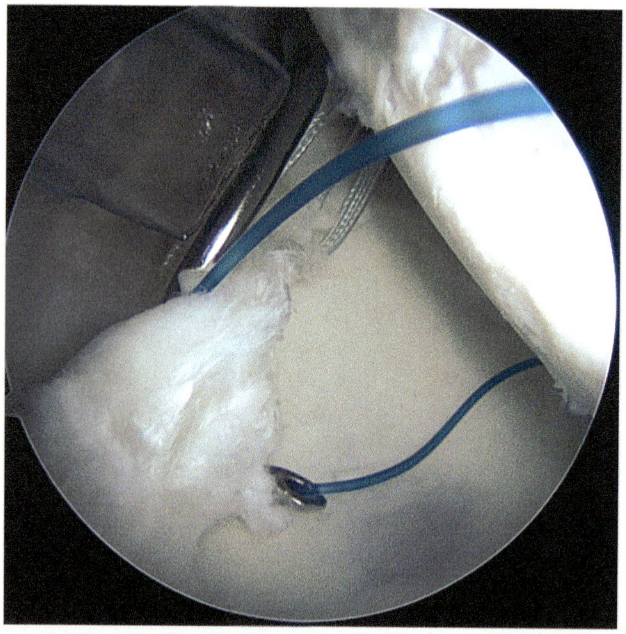

Fig. 31.6 A suture hook device is first used to shuttle a monofilament suture around the labrum for later suture tape passage.

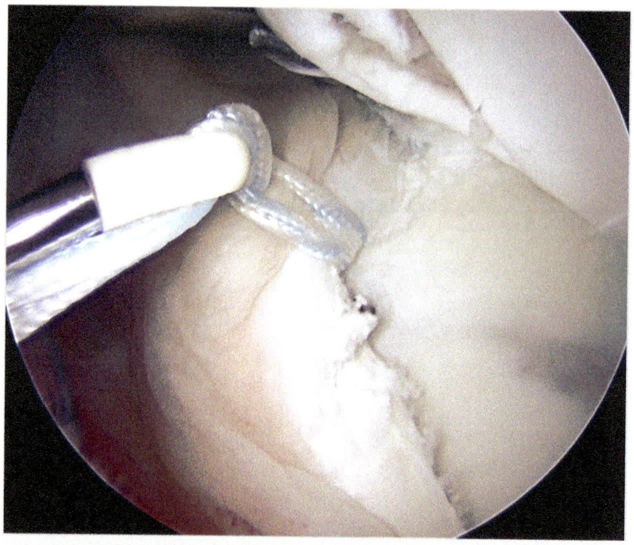

Fig. 31.7 A luggage tag or "cinch" stitch has been placed around the labrum and capsule and is delivered through the eyelet of the anchor for glenoid placement. Note the osteochondral injury present in this patient on the posterior aspect of the humeral head.

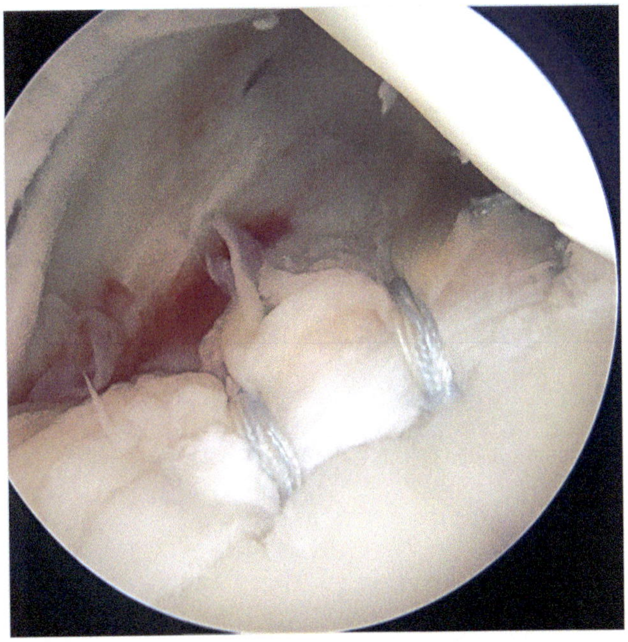

Fig. 31.8 Arthroscopic view from the posterior portal looking inferiorly at the completed labrum and capsular repair.

31.6.5 Posterior Portal Closure

The posterior portal is then closed using a no. 1 Polydioxanone (PDS) suture. The cannula is withdrawn to a level just external to the capsule. A suture passer is then used to pierce the capsule adjacent to the portal and the PDS suture is introduced into the joint. A penetrating suture grasper is then used to pierce the capsule on the opposite side of the portal and the suture is retrieved. A sliding Weston knot is then used to close down the capsule. Additional sutures can be placed in a wider fashion if additional plication is required based on the patient's predetermined needs from the preoperative plan.

31.7 Tips and Pearls/Expert Suggestions

- *Positioning:* The lateral decubitus position offers excellent exposure with minimal assistance to access the posterior joint capsule.
- *Portal placement*: Placement of the posterior portal slightly lateral to the standard portal allows for easier placement of the anchors when utilizing a single portal technique.
- *Anchor placement*: Anchors should be placed nearly perpendicular to the glenoid or at a tangent of 45 degrees to avoid chondral injury and "skiving."
- *Repair*: The repair should be tailored to the precise pathology of the patient as determined by history, examination, and diagnostic imaging. Knotless techniques can help avoid knot abrasion against the rotator cuff and scuffing against articular cartilage.

31.8 What to Avoid

- Avoid placement of anchors too close to one another as this could cause fragmentation of the glenoid bone and a "postage stamp"-style fracture.
- Avoid transecting the posterior labrum during labrum preparation. Use of a periosteal elevator should be done from the portal that allows for the most mobilization of tissue without iatrogenic injury.
- Avoid overtightening overhead throwing athletes as this could compromise their ability to return to play.

31.9 Complications/Bailout/Salvage

The most likely complication resulting from arthroscopic posterior stabilization is recurrent instability (<10%). The majority of patients, however, will achieve a successful outcome with proper technique and adherence to a strict protocol-driven rehabilitation program. Postoperative stiffness is relatively uncommon but can be encountered in patients who underwent concomitant posterior capsular plication. Early posterior capsular stretching can help avoid this complication and in those patients whose range of motion is not restored, posterior capsulotomy can be performed if deemed necessary. Transection of the labrum during preparation can occur and compromise the ability to achieve an anatomic repair. In instances where this occurs, the posterior capsule can be used utilizing an extracapsular technique to repair the capsule to the posterior glenoid margin.

31.10 Postoperative Care

Following surgery, patients are placed in a shoulder abduction sling to limit internal rotation. During the initial postoperative period, elbow and wrist active range-of-motion exercises are encouraged along with passive and active-assisted shoulder range of motion. Most patients are progressed to complete passive and active range of motion by postoperative weeks 8 to 12. Strengthening can begin at week 12, focusing on the periscapular musculature groups and the rotator cuff muscles. Throwers may begin a light toss program by week 16. Final return to play and competitive sports is typically achieved at 6 months, but may take up to a year for overhead throwing athletes to reach peak performance and throwing velocity. It is encouraged that patients have at least 80% of strength and near-normal range of motion prior to returning to full activities and athletics.

Suggested Readings

Arner JW, McClincy MP, Bradley JP. Arthroscopic stabilization of posterior shoulder instability is successful in American football players. Arthroscopy 2015;31(8):1466–1471

Bahk MS, Karzel RP, Snyder SJ. Arthroscopic posterior stabilization and anterior capsular plication for recurrent posterior glenohumeral instability. Arthroscopy 2010;26(9):1172–1180

Bradley JP, Baker CL III, Kline AJ, Armfield DR, Chhabra A. Arthroscopic capsulolabral reconstruction for posterior instability of the shoulder: a prospective study of 100 shoulders. Am J Sports Med 2006;34(7):1061–1071

Bradley JP, McClincy MP, Arner JW, Tejwani SG. Arthroscopic capsulolabral reconstruction for posterior instability of the shoulder: a prospective study of 200 shoulders. Am J Sports Med 2013;41(9):2005–2014

Bottoni CR, Franks BR, Moore JH, DeBerardino TM, Taylor DC, Arciero RA. Operative stabilization of posterior shoulder instability. Am J Sports Med 2005;33(7):996–1002

Goubier JN, Iserin A, Duranthon LD, Vandenbussche E, Augereau B. A 4-portal arthroscopic stabilization in posterior shoulder instability. J Shoulder Elbow Surg 2003;12(4):337–341

Kim SH, Ha KI, Park JH, et al. Arthroscopic posterior labral repair and capsular shift for traumatic unidirectional recurrent posterior subluxation of the shoulder. J Bone Joint Surg Am 2003;85-A(8):1479–1487

Kim SH, Park JS, Jeong WK, Shin SK. The Kim test: a novel test for posteroinferior labral lesion of the shoulder: a comparison to the jerk test. Am J Sports Med 2005;33(8): 1188–1192

Lenart BA, Sherman SL, Mall NA, Gochanour E, Twigg SL, Nicholson GP. Arthroscopic repair for posterior shoulder instability. Arthroscopy 2012;28(10):1337–1343

Pennington WT, Sytsma MA, Gibbons DJ, et al. Arthroscopic posterior labral repair in athletes: outcome analysis at 2-year follow-up. Arthroscopy 2010;26(9):1162–1171

owski CA, Chhabra A, Baker CL III, Tejwani SG, Bradley JP. Arthroscopic capsulolabral repair for posterior shoulder instability in throwing athletes compared with nonthrowing athletes. Am J Sports Med 2008;36(4):693–699

Savoie FH III, Holt MS, Field LD, Ramsey JR. Arthroscopic management of posterior instability: evolution of technique and results. Arthroscopy 2008;24(4):389–396

Tjoumakaris FP, Bradley JP. The rationale for an arthroscopic approach to shoulder stabilization. Arthroscopy 2011;27(10):1422–1433

Walch G, Badet R, Boulahia A, Khoury A. Morphologic study of the glenoid in primary glenohumeral osteoarthritis. J Arthroplasty 1999;14(6):756–760

Williams RJ III, Strickland S, Cohen M, Altchek DW, Warren RF. Arthroscopic repair for traumatic posterior shoulder instability. Am J Sports Med 2003;31(2):203–209

Wooten CJ, Krych AJ, Schleck CD, Hudgens JL, May JH, Dahm DL. Arthroscopic capsulolabral reconstruction for posterior shoulder instability in patients 18 years old or younger. J Pediatr Orthop 2015;35(5):462–466

32 Open Posterior Stabilization

Joo Han Oh

Abstract

Posterior shoulder instability is mostly caused by acute traumatic events; it is rare and also challenging to treat. Patients with posterior instability have vague symptoms that make surgical decisions more difficult. Therefore, detailed history taking and thorough physical examination are crucial for proper patient selection and better outcomes. Despite rapid advances in arthroscopic treatment for posterior instability, there is still need for open surgery for challenging cases. If there is significant posterior capsular redundancy, open posterior capsulorrhaphy should be done. Since up to 40% of patients with posterior instability have concomitant posterior labral lesions, these can be repaired simultaneously with open posterior capsulorrhaphy. In the case of significant bone loss, dysplasia, or glenoid retroversion, bone graft on the posterior rim or wedged open osteotomy is required. With advances in surgical techniques and skills, numerous studies have reported good to excellent outcomes with open posterior capsulorrhaphy. However, most are level IV studies that are difficult to interpret. In terms of bony procedures, debate is ongoing regarding outcomes, since some studies reported complication rates as high as 36%. To ensure better outcomes, care must be taken to select the proper patients for surgery. As not every case can be treated by arthroscopic posterior stabilization, knowledge of open posterior stabilization would help the surgeon to plan and treat patients with challenging cases.

Keywords: *posterior instability, open posterior stabilization, posterior capsulorrhaphy, reverse Bankart repair, posterior bone block, wedged open osteotomy*

32.1 Introduction

Posterior shoulder instability, first described in 1838 in a patient who had an epileptic seizure, is rare but challenging to treat, and even difficult to diagnose due to vague symptoms.[1–4] It is caused by an acute traumatic event, repetitive microtrauma, or atraumatic causes in only 2 to 5% of all cases.[5–8] Among individuals with posterior instability, up to 40% have concomitant posterior labral lesions.[9]

With rapid advances in arthroscopy, many studies have reported high satisfaction rates and low recurrence rates.[10–12] However, open surgery is still needed for revision, significant capsular insufficiency, poor-quality tissue, significant bone loss on glenoid, glenoid dysplasia, or retroverted glenoid.[9]

32.2 Patient History and Physical Examination

As the symptoms are not always obvious, detailed history taking is important. Patients may have weakness or pain in their shoulder, and sometimes complain of difficulty performing pushups. The most important thing to ask is whether the patient's main symptom is pain or instability. Patients who complain of pain usually describe it as a deep, posterior shoulder pain.[2,13] The severity and frequency of the pain should also be determined. In addition, since most patients have had traumatic events, determining the details including the position of the arm at the time of injury is important.[14,15] Inquiring as to the number of prior dislocations or subluxations, the first and most recent episodes, and self-reduction or reduction by a medical professional may help the surgeon decide how to treat the patient. If the patient had prior surgeries, obtaining information about the procedures could aid in deciding the next step. In addition, chronicity, general laxity, family history of disease, and history of voluntarily reproduced instability should be determined, since those cases may have more difficulty achieving good outcomes. Finally, the surgeon should acquire the information about sports or work activity levels.

Range of motion (ROM) and pain location should be evaluated. Patients may have full ROM, but comparison with the contralateral shoulder should be assessed. Focal tenderness in the posterior glenohumeral joint area should be determined. Provocative tests, including the posterior stress test, jerk test, load and shift test, and Kim's tests may help with diagnosing posterior instability.[7,16] In addition, a positive sulcus test in 30 degrees of external rotation while applying longitudinal traction suggests that the patient may have multidirectional instability and may need rotator interval closure.[17] Finally, it is crucial to determine whether the patient has general laxity. Patients with general laxity may have positive results in three of the following five tests: ability to perform thumb approximation to the volar surface of the forearm; ability to place the palm of the hand flat on the floor with the knees straight or show hyperextension of the second metacarpophalangeal joint greater than 90 degrees; ability to hyperextend the elbow over 10 degrees, or show genu recurvatum/hyperextension of the knee over 10 degrees.[18]

32.3 Imaging Evaluation

32.3.1 Plain Radiographs

Standard X-rays including true anteroposterior (AP) view, "Y" view, and an axillary view provide critical information. Among the plain X-rays, the axillary view (**Fig. 32.1a**) is the most informative for evaluating the relationship between the humeral head and glenoid. By evaluating X-rays, the surgeon can assess whether the patient has bony lesions such as a reverse Hill–Sachs lesion, reverse Bankart lesion, glenoid retroversion, or glenoid dysplasia.

32.3.2 Computed Tomography or CT Arthrography

CT with 3D images also help with planning by giving more detailed information of bone loss. The author calculates the percentage of glenoids remaining in patients with bone loss and glenoid version by use of CT (**Fig. 32.1b**). Moreover, 3D images

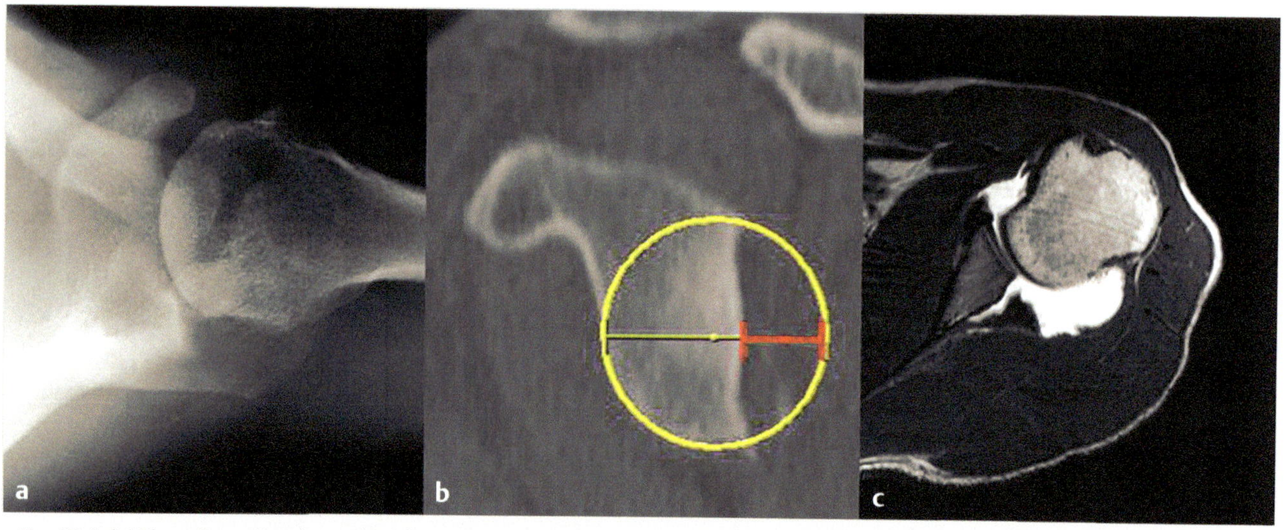

Fig. 32.1 (a) The axillary view shows the relationship between the humeral head and the glenoid. (b) The percentage of glenoids remaining in patients with bone loss can be calculated by CT. (c) MR images facilitate evaluation of soft tissues of the shoulder including the labrum, capsule, rotator cuff muscles, and biceps.

provide considerable information for planning if the patient needs a bone graft. CT arthrography is useful to evaluate any soft-tissue lesions as well as bone loss, such as a reverse Bankart lesion, capsular redundancy, or any concomitant anterior lesion of the glenoid.

32.3.3 Magnetic Resonance Imaging or MR Arthrography

MRI or MRA (**Fig. 32.1c**) may help with evaluation of soft tissues of the shoulder including the labrum, capsule, rotator cuff muscles, and biceps. Furthermore, the existence of any bony edema, hematoma, or swelling may help distinguish between acute traumatic or chronic causes of posterior instability.

32.4 Operative Management: Overview

Numerous studies have reported various surgical techniques for posterior instability.[2,6,9,15,19–21] However, possibly due to vague symptoms that cause difficulty in decision-making regarding the cause of shoulder pain, the outcomes have not been very satisfactory, compared to those in anterior instability.[20,22]

One solution for posterior capsular redundancy, which is the most common reason for posterior instability, is capsular plication or shift.[9] This can be done by using arthroscopy only, but if significant capsular redundancy is found, treatment should be performed with open capsular shift. If the patient has a reverse Bankart lesion, it should be repaired. In addition, sometimes bone graft or posterior opening wedge osteotomy is needed to treat a large bone defect or excessive glenoid retroversion in an open posterior stabilization procedure.[20,23–25] However, with open surgery, it is impossible to assess or treat other concomitant pathology such as a Bankart lesion, which requires arthroscopy before open surgery.

32.5 Operative Management: Technique

32.5.1 Patient Positioning

Under general anesthesia, the patient is positioned in a lateral decubitus position with a beanbag or anterior and posterior body support. Every protruding area of the patient that is in direct contact with the bed should be protected with padding. To prevent common peroneal nerve palsy, padding under the distal thigh is necessary. In addition, one pad should be placed below the axilla to prevent axillary nerve palsy. With slight flexion of the knee, stretching of the neurovascular system of the lower leg can be avoided. Draping should be done without causing any limitation of motion of the upper arm. Putting a pillow between the anterior chest and the arm with slight abduction can help stabilize the arm during surgery (**Fig. 32.2**).

- Due to difficulty in observing the anterior glenoid in an open procedure, using a mechanical arm holder at the opposite side of the operating table is helpful for arthroscopic evaluation to explore any combined lesions and treat a Bankart lesion or perform rotator interval closure.

32.5.2 Surgical Approach

Among the various surgical approaches, the author prefers the vertical approach. It is the most cosmetic and has the advantage of exposing the glenohumeral joint without detaching the posterior deltoid. However, careful dissection should be done to avoid injury to the axillary nerve while splitting the distal area.

From the scapular spine at the same level of the acromioclavicular joint anteriorly, the incision should be made distally in the direction of the axillary fold. After dissecting subcutaneous tissues, the deltoid is exposed. By blunt longitudinal dissection through the posterior deltoid fibers above the posterior glenohumeral joint line, beginning from the scapular spine to approximately 4 to 5 cm distally, the infraspinatus and teres minor are exposed (**Fig. 32.3a**). After identifying the interval between the infraspinatus and teres minor, continue dissection on the fat stripe over the raphe separating the two heads of the infraspinatus (**Fig. 32.3b**). Usually, the raphe of the infraspinatus lies on the equator of the glenohumeral joint. Care should be taken to avoid confusing the raphe with the interval between the infraspinatus and teres minor, which lies below the equator of the glenohumeral joint. Splitting the infraspinatus has several advantages, such as obtaining good exposure to the posterior capsule, labrum, and glenoid, or preserving the insertion of the infraspinatus to the humerus. Careful separation of infraspinatus from the posterior capsule is needed due to the axillary nerve passing inferiorly and the suprascapular nerve passing around 15 mm medial to the line of the posterior glenoid rim (**Fig. 32.3c**).

- Careful dissection is needed while splitting the distal part of the deltoid to avoid axillary nerve injury.
- If the surgeon does not want to dissect the deltoid, the infraspinatus and teres minor can be exposed by abducting the arm to 90 degrees and retracting the deltoid upward in the direction of the patient's head. At this point, care should be taken at the inferior border of the teres minor to prevent injury to the axillary nerve or posterior humeral circumflex vessels (**Fig. 32.4**).
- When the interval between infraspinatus and teres minor is difficult to determine, try to dissect along a muscular section instead of at the humeral insertion site of two muscles.
- Try to use a blunt elevator while dissecting infraspinatus from posterior capsule to avoid any damage to the suprascapular nerve medially.
- By rotating the arm slightly externally, relaxation of the axillary nerve can be achieved to prevent any damage, while dissection and rotator interval dissection can also be facilitated if needed.

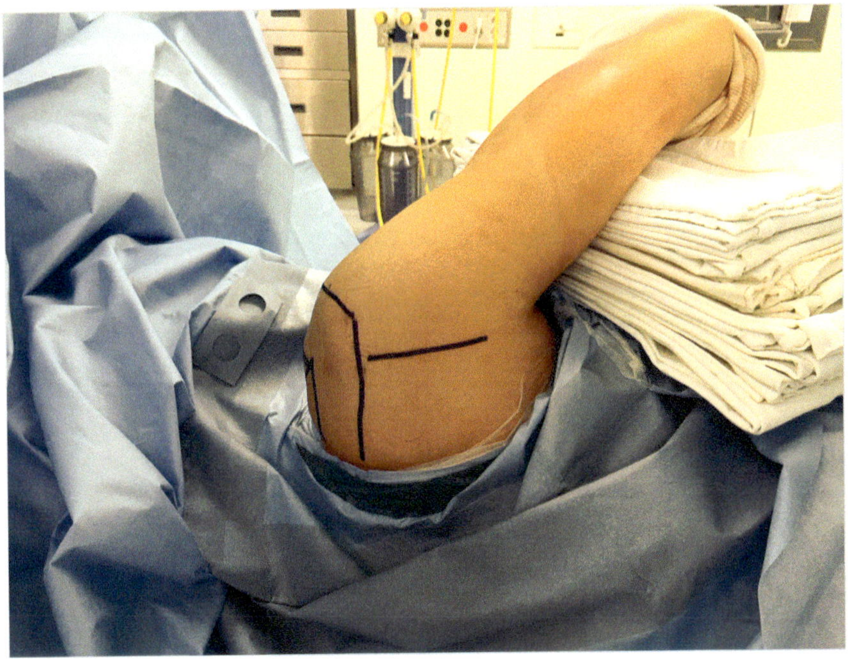

Fig. 32.2 Abduction of the shoulder helps with superior retraction of the posterior deltoid. The arm is in the lateral decubitus position with 30 degrees of abduction.

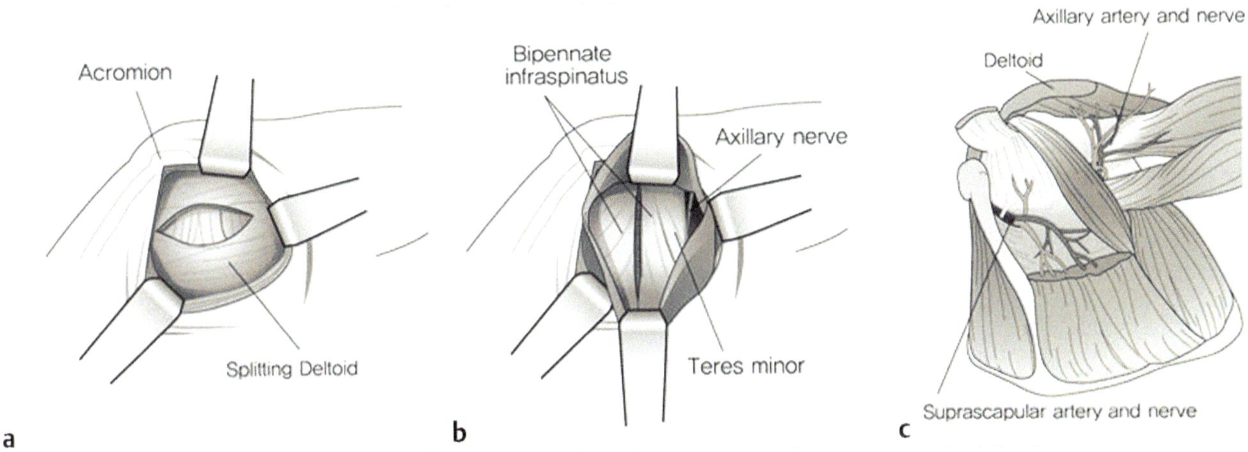

Fig. 32.3 (a) After longitudinal splitting of posterior deltoid fibers, the infraspinatus and teres minor are exposed. (b) The fat stripe over the raphe separating the two heads of the infraspinatus is shown and the axillary nerve is located below the teres minor. (c) The suprascapular nerve passes approximately 15 mm medial to the posterior glenoid rim and the axillary nerve passes inferior to the teres minor.

32.5.3 Posterior Capsulorrhaphy

After exposing the posterior capsule sufficiently, a transverse incision is made above the equator of the glenohumeral joint from 5 mm lateral to the glenoid rim to 5 mm medial to the lateral humeral capsular attachment. Additional incision should be made vertically at the same level of the medial tip of the transverse incision (**Fig. 32.5a**). Traction sutures are necessary to mobilize superior and inferior capsules with ease (**Fig. 32.5b**). Extra care is required while mobilizing the posterior capsule, since its thickness is less than half that of the anterior capsule and is thinner in patients with posterior instability.[26,27] The superomedial site of the inferior flap of the capsule should be advanced in a superior direction, while the inferomedial site of the superior flap of the capsule should be advanced in an inferior direction. After passing three to four nonabsorbable sutures from bottom to top of the labrum, the inferior flap is first penetrated and sutured with a horizontal mattress suture from inferior to superior, since the inferior flap is usually larger than the superior flap and more redundant (**Fig. 32.5c**). By using sutured thread, the superior flap is also penetrated and sutured above the inferior flap, making an overlap with horizontal mattress sutures (**Fig. 32.5d**). Additional side-to-side sutures are needed to close the interval between the superior and inferior leaflets.

If a reverse Bankart lesion is present, medial-based capsular shift is preferred by making a vertical incision at the level of the medial tip of the transverse incision. Repair of reverse Bankart lesion and capsulorrhaphy is discussed in the preceding section.

After the operation, the incised site of the muscle should be returned to normal position with absorbable suture. A drain to evacuate hematoma is inserted, and subcutaneous tissue and skin are sutured.

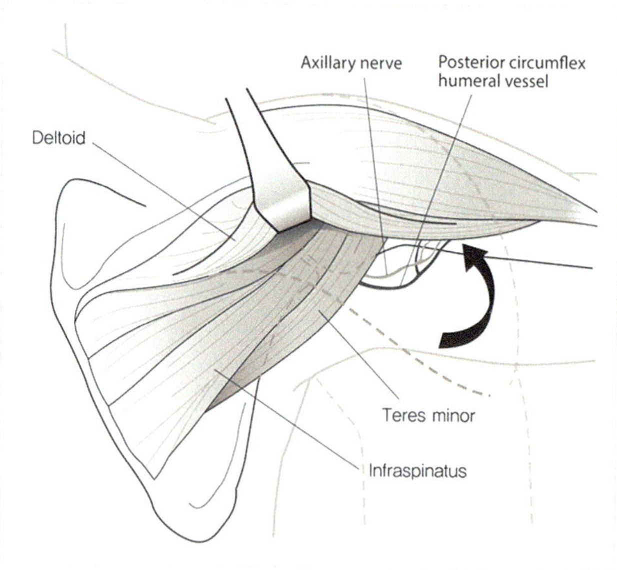

Fig. 32.4 By retracting the deltoid superiorly, the infraspinatus and teres minor can be exposed. The arm needs to be in 90 degrees of abduction to facilitate exposure.

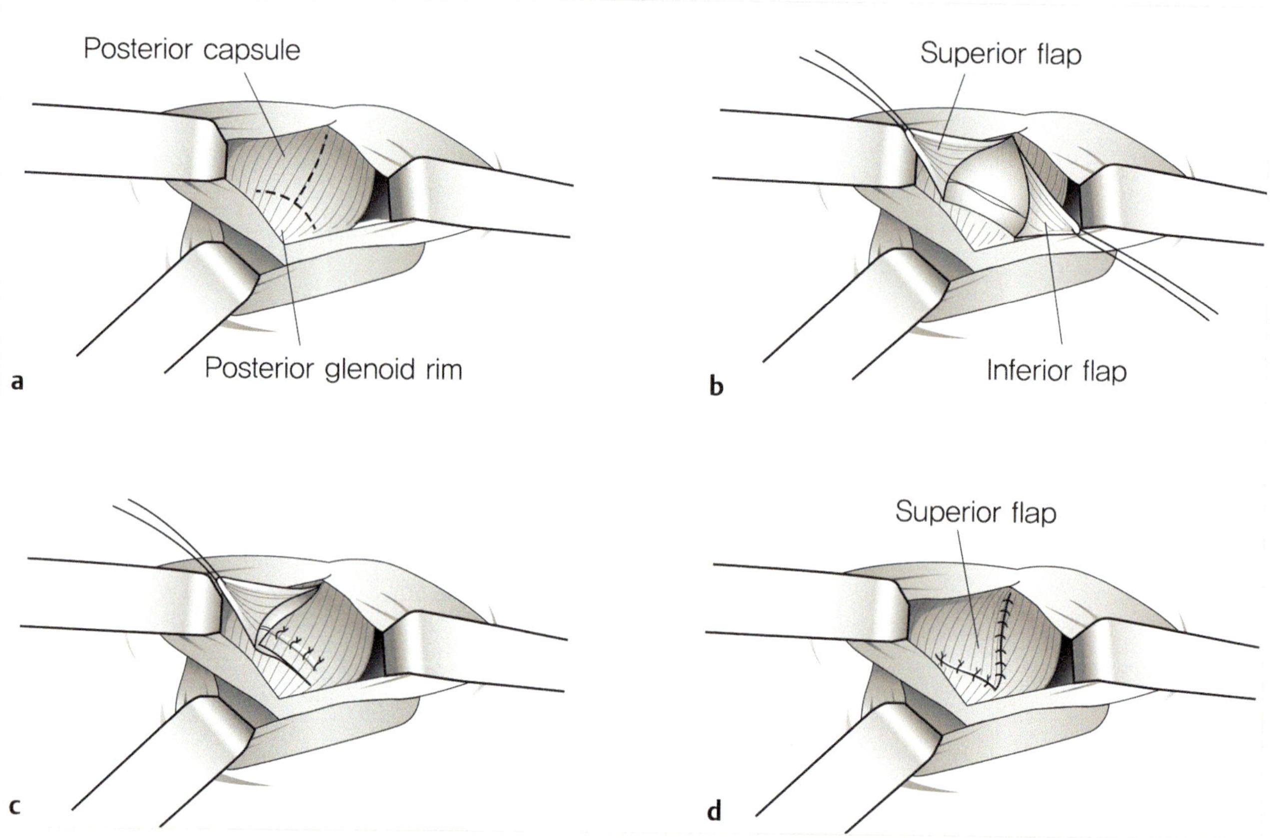

Fig. 32.5 Illustration of the sequence of procedures. **(a)** Capsulotomy is done in a T shape. **(b)** Traction sutures help with mobilizing superior and inferior flaps of the capsule. **(c)** The inferior flap is advanced superiorly first with fixation on the glenoid. **(d)** The superior flap is advanced inferiorly and overlaps the inferior flap.

- The arthrotomy should be done after full visualization of the posterior capsule is achieved.
- Excessive external rotation during capsulorrhaphy results in limitation of internal rotation after surgery. Therefore, 30 degrees of abduction in the scapular plane and neutral rotation seems to give appropriate capsular tension.

32.5.4 Posterior Labral Repair

After exposing the posterior capsule as previously described, horizontal capsulotomy is performed. If posterior capsular redundancy exists, the author usually performs a glenoid-based T-cut capsulotomy. The joint can be well exposed by using a humeral head retractor. For the reverse Bankart lesion, the capsulolabral tissue should be mobilized first and detached from the glenoid rim. After preparing the glenoid rim down to bleeding bone with a rasp and power burr, three to four suture anchors are inserted just at the edge of the articular surface and the labrum is reattached to the posterior glenoid (**Fig. 32.6**). Closure of horizontal capsulotomy site is done by side-to-side suture. If posterior capsular redundancy is also presented, the author uses the same procedure noted earlier.

- In the case of reverse Bankart repair, humeral-based capsulotomy has the advantage of preventing injury of the labrum while making a vertical incision on the capsule. However, the author performs glenoid-based capsulotomy since it seems to facilitate procedures on both the labrum and the capsule.
- To prevent any knot-induced complications in the repaired posterior labrum, the author tries to place suture knots away from the joint surface or use knotless suture anchors.

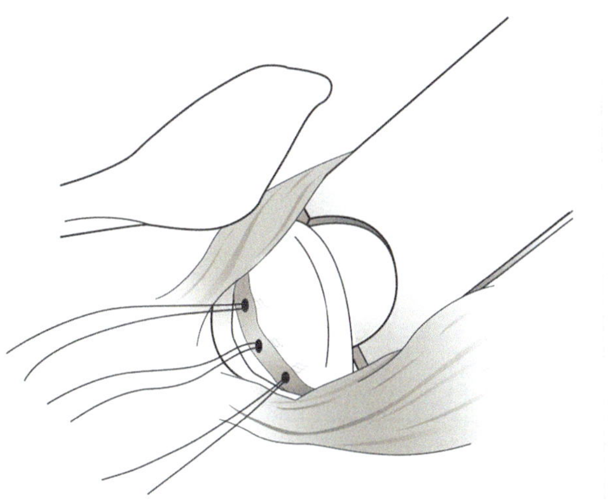

Fig. 32.6 Glenoid exposure is facilitated by using a humeral head retractor. After preparing the posterior glenoid, three to four anchors are inserted for a reverse Bankart repair.

32.5.5 Posterior Bone Block

Posterior bone block is used to restore an anatomic glenoid arc. If the patient has glenoid dysplasia or more than 25% posterior glenoid wear, a posterior bone graft can solve the instability. In addition, this can be done for revision surgery if there is insufficient soft tissue to be repaired. Harvesting for the bone graft can be done by making another incision at the level of iliac crest or scapular spine. Usually the author prefers harvesting from scapular spine to decrease morbidity. However, if considerable bone block is required, the author prefers using bone graft from posterior iliac crest. For harvesting bone, saws, osteotomes (curved or straight), and 4.0-mm cannulated screws should be prepared.

The approach to the posterior capsule is the same as previously described. As shown in **Fig. 32.7a**, the bone is harvested from the midportion of the scapular spine. The author usually takes a 3-cm length of bone. For patients without any labral lesion, the author fixes the graft at the extra-articular site. First, the posteroinferior quadrant of the glenoid rim is decorticated using rasp and power burr to make a bleeding bone bed. Then, the cancellous side of the harvested bone is placed extra-articularly to the prepared site. The goal of placing a graft at the site of defect is to augment the contour of glenoid arc rather than create "a blocking effect." Care should be taken to avoid placing the graft beyond the glenoid rim. If no advancement beyond the glenoid rim is confirmed, then graft fixation is done with two 4.0-mm cannulated screws. Again, the surgeon should be certain there is no advancement of bone graft beyond the fixation. If there is, it should be reduced by using a power burr to follow the contour of the posterior glenoid. Bone graft should be placed approximately 5 mm lateral to the posterior labrum and approximately 10 mm posterior to the posterior rim of the glenoid (**Fig. 32.7b**).[23]

- When harvesting bone from scapular spine, as the width increases at the base of the scapular spine, the author cuts the bone at the base to obtain around 2 cm in width.
- The bone graft can be located after repairing any concomitant labral lesion. If any capsular redundancy exists, humeral-based capsulorrhaphy can be done.

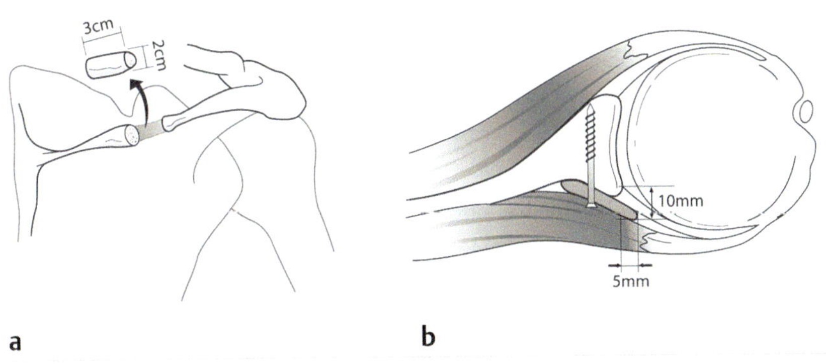

Fig. 32.7 (a) Harvesting bone graft from midportion of the scapular spine is shown. (b) Approximately 5 mm lateral and 10 mm posterior to the glenoid rim seem adequate for graft fixation.

- Using Kirschner's wire temporarily can help with confirming the absence of extension beyond the posterior glenoid rim before fixation.

32.5.6 Posterior Opening Wedge Glenoid Osteotomy

The ideal correction angle to achieve 5 degrees of glenoid retroversion or neutral version is calculated by preoperative CT. The approach to the posterior capsule is the same as previously described. The procedure for harvesting bone graft was also discussed previously; the author harvests before the osteotomy procedure for opening wedge glenoid osteotomy. Capsulotomy is done from superior to inferior at the midlevel of the capsule. After evaluation of joint pathologies, exposure of the posteromedial glenoid neck should be done with extreme care to avoid injury to the suprascapular nerve, which is located 15 mm medial to the posterior glenoid rim. Then a flat osteotome is placed 10 mm medial to the posterior glenoid rim and a cut is made parallel to the glenoid surface. The most important thing at this point is not to breach the anterior glenoid cortex to maintain stability of the osteotomy. Harvested wedged bone graft from scapular spine is inserted at the osteotomy site to the desired degree of correction. Usually, internal fixation for stabilization of bone graft is not needed (**Fig. 32.8**). If capsular redundancy exists, capsulorrhaphy can be done as described previously.

- Portable X-ray equipment can facilitate maintaining the anterior cortical hinge.

32.6 Postoperative Care

An external rotation brace is used to maintain 30 degrees of abduction and neutral rotation for 4 to 6 weeks postoperatively. In the case of revision or in patients with ligament laxity or a thin posterior capsule, the brace is applied for 6 weeks. To reduce any tension on the repaired site, the brace should be placed so that the patient's elbow is slightly posterior to the body. During the brace-wearing period, passive and active shoulder motions were restricted.

After discontinuation of the brace, the patients are permitted active-assisted forward flexion, and external rotation stretching exercises. Care should be taken to avoid concomitant internal rotation and flexion at this time. At 2 to 3 months after gaining full ROM, strengthening exercise is taught. Most of the patients are able to return to sports at 6 months postoperatively.

32.7 Complications

Recurrence is the most common complication due to new injury or the failure of the stabilization procedure, occurring in 7 to 23%.[6,28,29] This can be due to poor tissue quality in the posterior capsule or inadequate surgical skill. To reduce failure rates, strict management and education of the patient to maintain use of the brace and to exercise in a correct manner are important.

Another common complication is stiffness, which causes limitation of forward flexion and internal rotation.[28] This occurs in 4 to 36%,[28–30] usually due to excessive tightening of the posterior capsule, and can result in early osteoarthritis.[31] In addition, excessive tightness can result in subcoracoid impingement of the subscapularis due to anterior shift of the humeral head.[32]

Axillary or suprascapular nerves can be damaged. Usually, the axillary nerve is injured while incising vertically on the posterior capsule to make an inferior flap. Therefore, full exposure of the posterior capsule, especially at the inferior area, should be achieved to prevent iatrogenic axillary nerve injury. The suprascapular nerve runs approximately 15 mm medial to the glenoid rim. Thus, it is important not to invade more than 15 mm medial to the posterior glenoid while dissecting or splitting the infraspinatus.[33]

32.8 Outcomes

Although outcomes of surgical treatment for posterior stabilization have improved due to proper patient selection and advanced surgical technique, conservative treatment such as strengthening rotator cuff, deltoid, and scapular muscles should be applied first. The author performs surgical reconstruction in patients who have persistent symptoms after physical therapy.

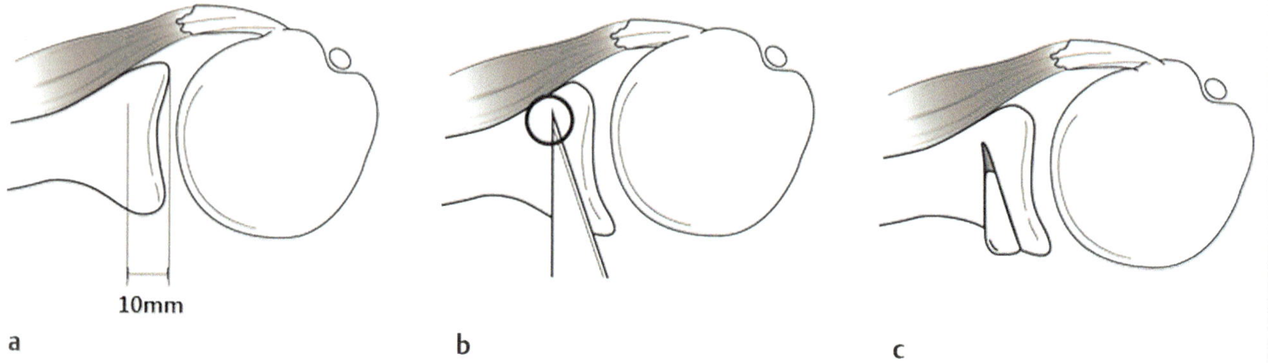

Fig. 32.8 **(a)** The osteotomy of glenoid can be done at 10 mm medial to the glenoid rim. **(b)** It is crucial to avoid breaking the anterior cortex during osteotomy. The *circle* denotes the importance of not breaching the anterior glenoid cortex. **(c)** A wedge of the bone graft is inserted with no need for additional fixation.

However, in terms of outcomes of surgical treatment, there are still controversies due to different interpretations of the results.

Fronek et al showed a 91% success rate in 24 patients who had posterior capsulorrhaphy for isolated posterior subluxation.[6] This result is consistent with that in a study by Wolf et al. In their study, 84% of patients showed successful outcomes, and 74% were able to return to sports at the prior level; recurrent postoperative instability was observed in 19%.[21] Furthermore, the outcome with a longer term of follow-up was reported by Pollock et al[34] and Bigliani et al,[28] who reported an 83% satisfaction rate at an average of 5 years postoperatively. Moreover, a systematic review comparing open versus arthroscopic posterior stabilization showed no statistical difference in clinical outcomes.[35]

In terms of bony procedures such as bone graft or posterior opening wedge osteotomy, the outcomes are unclear. Early studies reported unsatisfactory results with a posterior bone block. In the study by Ahlgren et al, recurrent posterior instability occurred in three of five patients treated with posterior bone block.[36] Additional studies, including a long-term follow-up study by Meuffels et al, reported a complication rate as high as 36%, including residual instability or osteoarthritic change.[19,20] In a biomechanical study, Wellmann et al stressed that a posterior bone block may overconstrain the posterior shoulder and may not gain adequate inferior instability compared with arthroscopic repair techniques.[37] However, another study by Servien et al reported that all patients who had bone-block procedures showed good to excellent satisfaction, with a mean Constant score of 93.3 points (range: 80–103 points).[23]

For posterior opening wedge osteotomy, a few studies showed good results, but other studies addressed its high complication rates and recurrence.[24,25,38,39] In the study by Norwood et al, three patients (16%) had posterior instability after surgery, while four patients (21%) showed new anterior instability.[38] Furthermore, another study by Gerber et al reported that posterior glenoplasty was shown to thrust the humeral head forward and subsequently cause impingement of the anterior cuff between the coracoid process and the humeral head.[31]

32.9 Conclusion

Compared with procedures for anterior instability, treatment for posterior instability is still challenging due to difficulty with diagnosis and surgery. Detailed history taking, thorough physical examination, and radiologic evaluation are critical to appropriately identify patients who require surgery. With advanced treatment skills, most cases can be treated with arthroscopy. However, arthroscopy cannot be used for revisions, significant capsular redundancy, glenoid hypoplasia, excessive glenoid retroversion, or posterior glenoid bone loss. Although few data have been reported on outcomes for open posterior stabilization, this may be the final option to achieve a better result in challenging cases.

32.10 Acknowledgments

The author would like to acknowledge Sung-Min Rhee for his assistance in the preparation of this manuscript and illustrations.

References

1. Hawkins RJ. Unrecognized dislocations of the shoulder. Instr Course Lect 1985;34:258–263
2. Provencher MT, Bell SJ, Menzel KA, Mologne TS. Arthroscopic treatment of posterior shoulder instability: results in 33 patients. Am J Sports Med 2005;33(10):1463–1471
3. Rouleau DM, Hebert-Davies J, Robinson CM. Acute traumatic posterior shoulder dislocation. J Am Acad Orthop Surg 2014;22(3):145–152
4. Kowalsky MS, Levine WN. Traumatic posterior glenohumeral dislocation: classification, pathoanatomy, diagnosis, and treatment. Orthop Clin North Am 2008;39(4):519–533, viii
5. Hawkins RJ, Belle RM. Posterior instability of the shoulder. Instr Course Lect 1989;38:211–215
6. Fronek J, Warren RF, Bowen M. Posterior subluxation of the glenohumeral joint. J Bone Joint Surg Am 1989;71(2):205–216
7. Hawkins RJ, Koppert G, Johnston G. Recurrent posterior instability (subluxation) of the shoulder. J Bone Joint Surg Am 1984;66(2):169–174
8. Robinson CM, Aderinto J. Recurrent posterior shoulder instability. J Bone Joint Surg Am 2005;87(4):883–892
9. Antosh IJ, Tokish JM, Owens BD. Posterior shoulder instability: current surgical management. Sports Health 2016;8(6): 520-526
10. DeLong JM, Bradley JP. Posterior shoulder instability in the athletic population: Variations in assessment, clinical outcomes, and return to sport. World J Orthop 2015;6(11):927–934
11. DeLong JM, Jiang K, Bradley JP. Posterior instability of the shoulder: a systematic review and meta-analysis of clinical outcomes. Am J Sports Med 2015;43(7):1805–1817
12. Lenart BA, Sherman SL, Mall NA, Gochanour E, Twigg SL, Nicholson GP. Arthroscopic repair for posterior shoulder instability. Arthroscopy 2012;28(10):1337–1343
13. Yeargan SA III, Briggs KK, Horan MP, Black AK, Hawkins RJ. Determinants of patient satisfaction following surgery for multidirectional instability. Orthopedics 2008;31(7):647
14. Robinson CM, Seah M, Akhtar MA. The epidemiology, risk of recurrence, and functional outcome after an acute traumatic posterior dislocation of the shoulder. J Bone Joint Surg Am 2011;93(17):1605–1613
15. Antoniou J, Duckworth DT, Harryman DT II. Capsulolabral augmentation for the management of posteroinferior instability of the shoulder. J Bone Joint Surg Am 2000;82(9):1220–1230
16. Kim SH, Park JS, Jeong WK, Shin SK. The Kim test: a novel test for posteroinferior labral lesion of the shoulder: a comparison to the jerk test. Am J Sports Med 2005;33(8): 1188–1192
17. Tzannes A, Murrell GA. Clinical examination of the unstable shoulder. Sports Med 2002;32(7):447–457
18. Beighton P, Solomon L, Soskolne CL. Articular mobility in an African population. Ann Rheum Dis 1973;32(5):413–418
19. Schwartz DG, Goebel S, Piper K, Kordasiewicz B, Boyle S, Lafosse L. Arthroscopic posterior bone block augmentation in posterior shoulder instability. J Shoulder Elbow Surg 2013;22(8):1092–1101

20. Meuffels DE, Schuit H, van Biezen FC, Reijman M, Verhaar JA. The posterior bone block procedure in posterior shoulder instability: a long-term follow-up study. J Bone Joint Surg Br 2010;92(5):651–655
21. Wolf BR, Strickland S, Williams RJ, Allen AA, Altchek DW, Warren RF. Open posterior stabilization for recurrent posterior glenohumeral instability. J Shoulder Elbow Surg 2005;14(2):157–164
22. Tibone JE, Bradley JP. The treatment of posterior subluxation in athletes. Clin Orthop Relat Res 1993(291):124–137
23. Servien E, Walch G, Cortes ZE, Edwards TB, O'Connor DP. Posterior bone block procedure for posterior shoulder instability. Knee Surg Sports Traumatol Arthrosc 2007;15(9):1130–1136
24. Metcalf MH, Duckworth DG, Lee SB, et al. Posteroinferior glenoplasty can change glenoid shape and increase the mechanical stability of the shoulder. J Shoulder Elbow Surg 1999;8(3):205–213
25. Bessems JH, Vegter J. Glenoplasty for recurrent posterior shoulder instability. Good results in 13 cases followed for 1-16 years. Acta Orthop Scand 1995;66(6):535–537
26. Bottoni CR, Franks BR, Moore JH, DeBerardino TM, Taylor DC, Arciero RA. Operative stabilization of posterior shoulder instability. Am J Sports Med 2005;33(7):996–1002
27. Shin RD, Polatsch DB, Rokito AS, Zuckerman JD. Posterior capsulorrhaphy for treatment of recurrent posterior glenohumeral instability. Bull Hosp Jt Dis 2005;63(1–2):9–12
28. Bigliani LU, Pollock RG, McIlveen SJ, Endrizzi DP, Flatow EL. Shift of the posteroinferior aspect of the capsule for recurrent posterior glenohumeral instability. J Bone Joint Surg Am 1995;77(7):1011–1020
29. Fuchs B, Jost B, Gerber C. Posterior-inferior capsular shift for the treatment of recurrent, voluntary posterior subluxation of the shoulder. J Bone Joint Surg Am 2000;82(1):16–25
30. Misamore GW, Facibene WA. Posterior capsulorrhaphy for the treatment of traumatic recurrent posterior subluxations of the shoulder in athletes. J Shoulder Elbow Surg 2000;9(5):403–408
31. Gerber C, Ganz R, Vinh TS. Glenoplasty for recurrent posterior shoulder instability. An anatomic reappraisal. Clin Orthop Relat Res 1987(216):70–79
32. Harryman DT II, Sidles JA, Clark JM, McQuade KJ, Gibb TD, Matsen FA III. Translation of the humeral head on the glenoid with passive glenohumeral motion. J Bone Joint Surg Am 1990;72(9):1334–1343
33. Shaffer BS, Conway J, Jobe FW, Kvitne RS, Tibone JE. Infraspinatus muscle-splitting incision in posterior shoulder surgery. An anatomic and electromyographic study. Am J Sports Med 1994;22(1):113–120
34. Pollock RG, Bigliani LU. Recurrent posterior shoulder instability. Diagnosis and treatment. Clin Orthop Relat Res 1993(291):85–96
35. Kakar S, Voloshin I, Kaye EK, et al. Posterior shoulder instability: comprehensive analysis of open and arthroscopic approaches. Am J Orthop 2007;36(12):655–659
36. Ahlgren SA, Hedlund T, Nistor L. Idiopathic posterior instability of the shoulder joint. Results of operation with posterior bone graft. Acta Orthop Scand 1978;49(6):600–603
37. Wellmann M, Bobrowitsch E, Khan N, et al. Biomechanical effectiveness of an arthroscopic posterior Bankart repair versus an open bone block procedure for posterior shoulder instability. Am J Sports Med 2011;39(4):796–803
38. Norwood LA, Terry GC. Shoulder posterior subluxation. Am J Sports Med 1984;12(1):25–30
39. Scott DJ Jr. Treatment of recurrent posterior dislocations of the shoulder by glenoplasty. Report of three cases. J Bone Joint Surg Am 1967;49(3):471–476

33 Arthroscopic Posterior HAGL Repair

Zachary J. Finley, Michael O'Brien, and Felix H. Savoie

Abstract
Reverse humeral avulsion of the glenohumeral ligament (RHAGL), or posterior HAGL, is an uncommon but traumatic cause of posterior shoulder instability. HAGL/RHAGL lesions are defined as a disruption of the inferior glenohumeral ligament complex from the humerus, and in rare cases avulsion from both the humerus and the glenoid. The goal of arthroscopic posterior HAGL repair is to restore anatomy and regain stability of the joint.

Keywords: *instability, shoulder, RHAGL*

33.1 Goals of Procedure

The goals of the procedure are to identify the injury to the posterior capsule of the shoulder and repair the capsule to the site of the avulsion from the humerus without compromising the posterior rotator cuff muscle and tendon.

33.2 Advantages

Open, mini-open, and arthroscopic repair techniques of HAGL/RHAGL lesions have all obtained successful outcomes.[1–5] All have proven to be successful with few failures in a recent review[3]; however, arthroscopic treatment provides easier identification of the lesion, minimal damage to the surrounding soft tissues, maximum visualization, less postoperative pain, and improved rehabilitation. Unless other pathology in the shoulder dictates an open approach, we recommend an all-arthroscopic technique for these repairs.

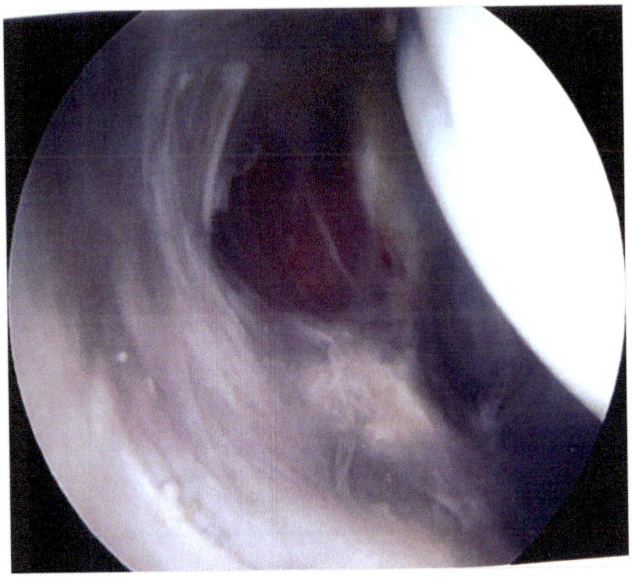

Fig. 33.1 A humeral avulsion of the glenohumeral ligament (HAGL) lesion with subscapularis muscle fibers seen beneath the anterior capsule. This lesion extended inferiorly and then posteriorly to make this both an HAGL and a reverse HAGL.

33.3 Indications

All indications and contraindications are considered relative and are dictated by the patient's pathology and level of disability. As with all instability complaints, the patient's level of dysfunction dictates the need for operative intervention. Pain and disability are the most important factors to consider when they interfere with normal or desired activity. The majority of patients will present with a traumatic dislocation event, often occurring during a sporting activity. If at all possible, it is important to determine the position of the arm at the time of injury. The most common position of the arm in the setting of RHAGL lesions is abducted and internally rotated at the time of injury. Other signs and symptoms include recurrent dislocations, general sense of "looseness" of the shoulder, shoulder pain, and intermittent popping/catching.[6,7]

Current thinking may suggest initial nonoperative treatment for traumatic posterior instability focusing on scapular stabilization and rotator cuff strengthening; however, nonoperative management was once the mainstay for treatment after anterior dislocation, and investigations have since shown a lower recurrence of anterior instability after early arthroscopic stabilization in young athletes.[8–10] Because of this, we advise that young, active patients, especially athletes, undergo surgical correction.

33.4 Contraindications

Contraindications are the presence of an active infection or lack of surgical skill for the appropriate technique.

33.5 Preoperative Preparation/Positioning

A thorough physical examination should be performed on each patient, including comparison to the contralateral shoulder. Great care should be taken to assess for differences in active and passive range of motion as well as strength between the two sides. Extra focus should be placed on the evaluation of the infraspinatus muscle in the presence of RHAGL lesions. While none are specific for HAGL/RHAGL lesions, tests for instability should be performed, including apprehension, posterior jerk, sulcus, and a load and shift. In patients without concomitant labral pathology, one will not feel the usual "grind" during subluxation, as it feels more like an elastic-type shift without the crepitation as the lateral attachment separates from the humerus. Performing a thorough physical examination will also help eliminate or confirm other pathology, which is important as RHAGL lesions have a high incidence of concomitant injuries.[7,11,12]

Standard radiographs are rarely useful to specifically diagnose HAGL/RHAGL lesions except in the setting of a bony HAGL. MRI or an MR arthrogram is the mainstay of diagnosis. The IGHL complex is best viewed on coronal oblique or sagittal oblique images on a T2-weighted MRI. In a normal shoulder, the IGHL complex forms a "**U** shape" at the inferior margin of the joint. In the presence of an RHAGL lesion, this is changed to a backward **J** shape as a result of the deficient capsule. Additionally, the use of an MR arthrogram can confirm the presence of an HAGL lesion. The axillary pouch of the IGHL drops inferiorly and extravasation of contrast media can be seen to cross the humeral attachment. While MRI is a helpful diagnostic tool, it has been shown to miss the diagnosis of an HAGL/RHAGL lesion in up to 50% of cases based on imaging alone. Conflicting pathology on MRI may distract from the HAGL diagnosis.

The arthroscopic repair of an RHAGL lesion can be performed in both the lateral decubitus and the beach-chair positions; however, we recommend the lateral position as it provides increased access and viewing of the inferior glenohumeral joint as compared to the beach-chair position. We perform most procedures for instability in the lateral decubitus position.

After successful induction of anesthesia, the patient is placed in the lateral decubitus position with the operative shoulder rolled posteriorly 30 to 45 degrees. An examination under anesthesia is performed to confirm preoperative clinical findings. Standard draping is applied and the arm is suspended (abducted 45–50 degrees, forward flexed 15–20 degrees) and attached to approximately 5 to 15 lb of weight (depending on the patient size).

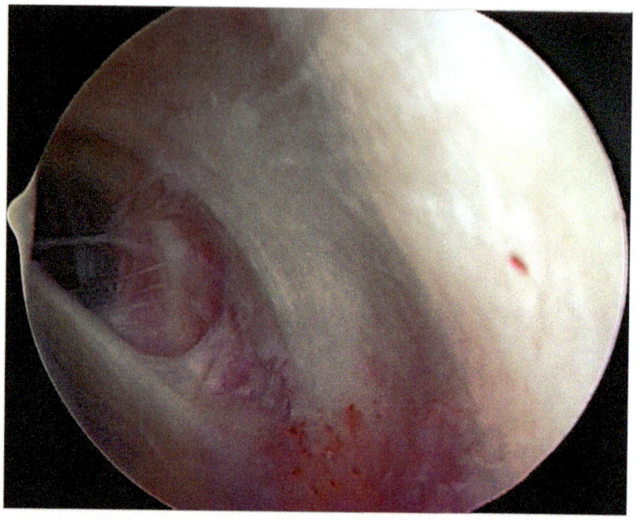

Fig. 33.2 Reverse humeral avulsion of the glenohumeral ligament (RHAGL) lesion with infraspinatus muscle fibers able to be visualized through the posteroinferior capsule.

33.6 Operative Technique

A standard posterior viewing portal is then established at the equator of the joint through the soft spot between the upper and lower infraspinatus muscle belly (see **Video 33.1**). This portal should be in line with the glenoid so as to be able to access the lateral capsule for HAGL repair. A diagnostic arthroscopy is performed using a 30-degree arthroscope. We suggest diagnostic arthroscopy be performed not only from the posterior portal but also, once completed, from the anterior portal to fully assess the shoulder joint. As outlined earlier, HAGL/RHAGL lesions are most commonly associated with other shoulder pathologies. When an HAGL/RHAGL lesion is suspected preoperatively, extra care should be taken when looking at the axillary recess in the inferior portion of the joint. Both the origins and insertion of the entire IGHL complex should be assessed on the glenoid as well as the humeral side. Internal and external rotations of the arm aid in visualization of these areas; external rotation will tighten the intact anterior band and internal rotation will tighten the intact posterior band. It is recommended that the lateral capsular insertion be visualized for all patients undergoing arthroscopic surgery for instability. An RHAGL lesion can often be identified by the visualization of muscle fibers in the posterior inferior capsule, which correspond to the underlying infraspinatus muscle fibers (**Fig. 33.2**).

33.7 Portals Needed (in the Order They Should Be Established)

1. *Standard posterior portal.* "Soft point" portal found approximately 2 cm inferior and 2 cm medial to the posterolateral corner of the acromion. This portal is used for instrumentation.
2. *Midanterior portal.* Outside-in technique with an 18-gauge spinal needle just above the subscapularis; this portal is used for suture positioning.
3. *Anterior superior portal.* This portal is established just off the anterior lateral corner of the acromion and enters the joint just anterior to the supraspinatus tendon used for viewing. If necessary, a 70-degree arthroscope can be used to facilitate a more complete view of the inferior extent of the RHAGL.
4. *Posteroinferior portal* (the 7 o'clock position portal). This portal is established outside-to-in with an 18-gauge spinal needle 2 cm inferior to the posterior viewing portal, and rarely used for RHAGL lesions; one must be careful not to get too close to the quadrangular space when using this portal.

33.7.1 Steps

1. Establish the portals as listed earlier.
2. Place the arthroscope in the superior viewing portal to obtain visualization of the lesion. A slight anteriorly directed force on the humeral head will move the humerus forward, creating more room for instrumentation.
3. The lesion should be completely evaluated for the extent of injury at this time. If there are any adhesions between the capsule and the overlying infraspinatus muscle, they can be released at this time. Once released, the posterior capsule can be properly tensioned to the posterior humeral neck.
4. The capsule usually attaches lateral to the normal bare spot on the humerus. One can use the shaver to prepare the bed for reinsertion. We do not usually abrade the bare spot in RHAGL repairs, and try not to damage the intact infraspinatus tendon.
5. A double- or triple-loaded vented suture anchor is then placed into the humerus at the 3 to 9 o'clock position (**Fig. 33.3**). The sutures are then retrieved out of the anterior portal for ease of suture management during repair.
6. A small, sharp 30-degree retrograde suture retriever is used via the posterior portal to pass the sutures in sequence from inferior to superior. It helps to have an assistant push the humeral head anteriorly during suture passage, creating more "room" and separating the capsule from the overlying muscle. We use mattress configuration, retrieve and tie the most inferior set first, and then judge the restoration of normal anatomy. The

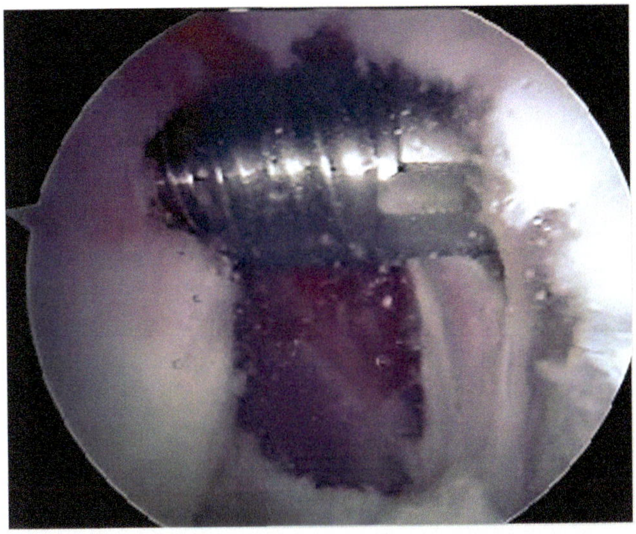

Fig. 33.3 A tap/awl is used to create a tunnel for the first suture anchor to be placed into the right humerus at the 4 o'clock position.

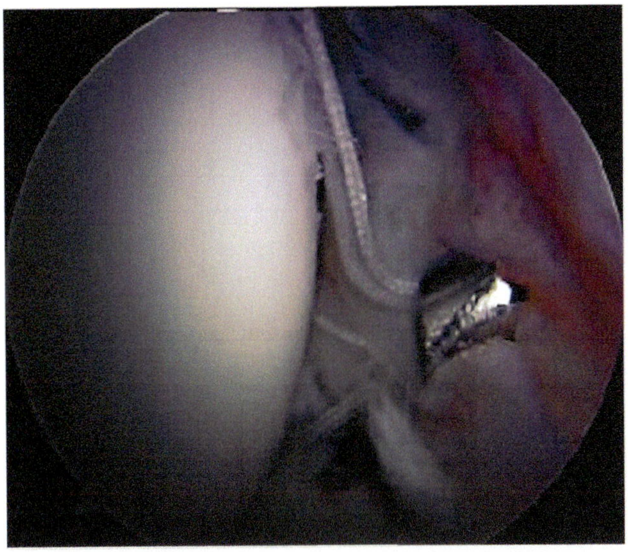

Fig. 33.4 In this right shoulder, the sutures are being prepared for retrieval in posterior reverse humeral avulsion of the glenohumeral ligament repair.

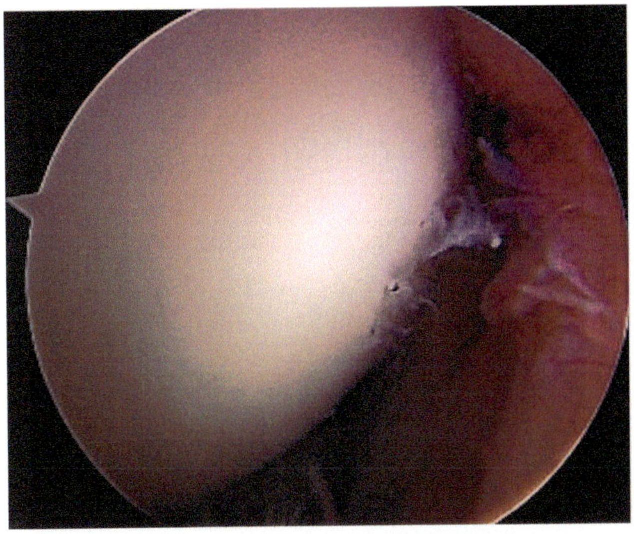

Fig. 33.5 In this right shoulder, the repaired reverse humeral avulsion of the glenohumeral ligament (above) and posterior labral repair (bottom center) can be seen to have restored the posterior capsule tension.

second and third sets are sequentially retrieved and properly tensioned to complete the repair (**Fig. 33.4**).

7. Once all the sutures are tied, the repair is reassessed regarding the need for an additional anchor and sutures to complete the repair. This is usually needed when the RHAGL extends across the inferior humerus and the lower anchor is placed more closely to the 6 o'clock position. The second anchor is placed more superiorly on the humerus and the sutures are retrieved and tied by repeating the same steps as detailed earlier (**Fig. 33.5**).
8. On occasion, the RHAGL may extend across the entire inferior humerus and include the attachment of the anterior band of the IGHL complex. In these cases, we use a small all-suture anchor placed near the 6 o'clock position and accessed by internally rotating the humerus to bring that spot into view. Once the anchor is placed, the sutures are retrieved as previously described using a more angled (60-degree or sixter type retrograde retriever) and this portion is repaired first. The rest of the RHAGL can be repaired as detailed earlier.

33.8 Tips and Pearls/Expert Suggestions

We believe that the following are key to successful treatment of RHAGL lesions:

- Look for the lesion during diagnostic arthroscopy.
- Set up the portals correctly to make the repair as easy as possible. Have a 70-degree arthroscope available to assist with complete visualization.
- If there is concomitant labral pathology, repair the labrum first though the RHAGL lesion. The defect provides easier access for instrumentation and also prevents having to penetrate the repaired capsule to repair the labrum.
- Recognize that while this repair may be technically demanding, conceptually this repair is very similar to, and requires many of the same skills as, other more common arthroscopic shoulder repairs. The technical difficulty comes from working in the posterior portion of the glenohumeral joint and tying sutures blindly within the subacromial space while viewing from within the joint.[3]

Key points for the repair include the following:

- Viewing through an anterosuperior portal.
- Carefully and bluntly releasing the posterior capsular tissue from the overlying rotator cuff muscular tissue in order to identify the native position of the tissue.
- Using multiple mattress stitches to reapproximate the posterior capsule and the posterior band of the IGHL back to the native footprint on the humeral head.
- Tying sutures blindly within the joint while viewing the two layers of the repair from within the glenohumeral joint.

- Finally, if some of the infraspinatus insertion is involved, one should be comfortable retrieving and tying the sutures from the subacromial area while visualizing from within the joint to confirm repair.

33.9 What to Avoid

The primary issue with RHAGL lesions is failure to look for the lesion. RHAGL lesions are actually more common than HAGL lesions, as the pathology of posterior instability is more variable. The second problem is using a too inferior posterior portal and violating the quadrangular space and the axillary nerve. Finally, when the entire inferior capsule is involved, a too large bite of the capsule may endanger the axillary nerve.

33.10 Complications/Bailout/ Salvage

In cases of insufficient capsule, the tendon of the infraspinatus may be used to reinforce the capsule. An open posterior T capsular shift may also be effective.

33.11 Postoperative Care

Postoperatively, the arm is placed into an abduction sling. The patient should remain in the sling for 6 weeks. In weeks 0 to 6, the patient may work on scapular retraction while in the sling. Passive motion and further scapular stabilization exercises can be started at week 6. At week 8, active-assisted exercises can begin. The patient is limited in internal rotation to protect repairs. At 12 weeks, the patient may begin active exercises and strengthening of the shoulder. If the patient is a throwing athlete, an interval throwing program can be initiated at 16 weeks postoperatively. The patients should expect strength and range of motion to improve for up to 1 year. It is reasonable for both physician and patient to expect some mild but clinically insignificant losses in range of motion, particularly in internal rotation for the posterior repair.

References

1. Bach BR, Warren RF, Fronek J. Disruption of the lateral capsule of the shoulder. A cause of recurrent dislocation. J Bone Joint Surg Br 1988;70(2):274–276
2. Wolf EM, Cheng JC, Dickson K. Humeral avulsion of glenohumeral ligaments as a cause of anterior shoulder instability. Arthroscopy 1995;11(5):600–607
3. Longo UG, Rizzello G, Ciuffreda M, et al. Humeral avulsion of the glenohumeral ligaments: a systematic review. Arthroscopy 2016;32(9):1868–1876
4. Warner JJ, Beim GM. Combined Bankart and HAGL lesion associated with anterior shoulder instability. Arthroscopy 1997;13(6):749–752
5. Arciero RA, Mazzocca AD. Mini-open repair technique of HAGL (humeral avulsion of the glenohumeral ligament) lesion. Arthroscopy 2005;21(9):1152
6. Field LD, Bokor DJ, Savoie FH III. Humeral and glenoid detachment of the anterior inferior glenohumeral ligament: a cause of anterior shoulder instability. J Shoulder Elbow Surg 1997;6(1):6–10
7. Chhabra A, Diduch DR, Anderson M. Arthroscopic repair of a posterior humeral avulsion of the inferior glenohumeral ligament (HAGL) lesion. Arthroscopy 2004;20(Suppl 2):73–76
8. Abrams JS. Arthroscopic repair of posterior instability and reverse humeral glenohumeral ligament avulsion lesions. Orthop Clin North Am 2003;34(4):475–483
9. DeBerardino TM, Arciero RA, Taylor DC, Uhorchak JM. Prospective evaluation of arthroscopic stabilization of acute, initial anterior shoulder dislocations in young athletes. Two- to five-year follow-up. Am J Sports Med 2001;29(5):586–592
10. Brown T, Barton RS, Savoie FH III. Reverse humeral avulsion glenohumeral ligament and infraspinatus rupture with arthroscopic repair: a case report. Am J Sports Med 2007;35(12):2135–2139
11. Bankart ASB. Recurrent or habitual dislocation of the shoulder-joint. BMJ 1923;2(3285):1132–1133
12. Stoller DW, Wolf EM. The shoulder. In: Stoller DW, ed.Magnetic Resonance Imaging in Orthopaedics and Sports Medicine. 2nd ed. Philadelphia, PA: JB Lippincott;1997:597–748

34 Modified McLaughlin for Posterior Dislocation

Michael Angeline

Abstract

For patients with recurrent instability after an acute posterior shoulder dislocation, operative stabilization with a modified McLaughlin procedure using the middle glenohumeral ligament can treat humeral head defects less than 40%.

Keywords: *posterior shoulder instability, reverse Hill–Sachs lesion, arthroscopic stabilization, arthroscopic McLaughlin procedure, posterior shoulder dislocation*

34.1 Goals of Procedure

Locked posterior shoulder dislocations are uncommon and often misdiagnosed. Overall, posterior shoulder instability accounts for approximately 3% of all shoulder dislocations with a reported prevalence of 1.1 per 100,000 per year.[1] The general causes include epileptic seizures, high-energy trauma, electric shock, or electroconvulsive therapy. In the case of involuntary muscle contraction, the strong internal rotators of the shoulder such as the latissimus dorsi, pectoralis major, subscapularis, and teres major overpower the weak external rotators and drive the humeral head posteriorly.

During a posterior dislocation event, the shoulder is typically axially loaded with the arm in a forward elevated, adducted, and internally rotated position. As the humeral head impacts on the posterior aspect of the glenoid, an osteochondral impression fracture (also termed encoche fracture or reverse Hill–Sachs lesion) is produced.[2] If the shoulder is not reduced acutely, the impression fracture can enlarge due to the grinding effects of rotational shoulder movements. A secondary deformity within the humeral head articular cartilage may also develop with prolonged dislocation. Additionally during the acute dislocation event, an injury may also occur within the posterior stabilizers of the shoulder including capsulolabral tears/avulsions, glenoid rim fractures, or rotator cuff tears.

After sustaining a posterior dislocation, patients will present with their arm held in an adducted/internally rotated position. The patient will complain of loss of motion, particularly external rotation; on examination, there may be a prominence of the coracoid process anteriorly limited to no external rotation due to the humeral head being fixed on the posterior glenoid rim. Initial radiographic evaluation includes a true anteroposterior (AP) view of the shoulder, scapular Y view, and an axillary view. If the patient's pain and limited abduction do not allow for a standard axillary lateral, a modified axillary view, apical oblique view, or a Velpeau view may need to be considered. An axillary view is essential for the diagnosis of a posterior dislocation, as the standard AP view may appear normal (**Fig. 34.1**). A CT scan of the shoulder with glenoid subtraction and 3D reconstruction of the humeral head is also helpful to evaluate the size and location of the humeral head defect. The CT scan is also useful in detecting any potential occult anatomical/surgical neck fractures of the humerus. An MRI should also be considered to evaluate for possible rotator cuff tears and/or injury to the ligamentous soft-tissue restraints of the posterior shoulder.

When evaluating treatment options for a posterior dislocation of the shoulder, the clinician should consider the age/demands of the patient, the size of the humeral head defect, associated pathology, and the duration of the dislocation.[3] Nonoperative treatment can be considered for elderly patients with low demands, patients with multiple medical comorbidities, or

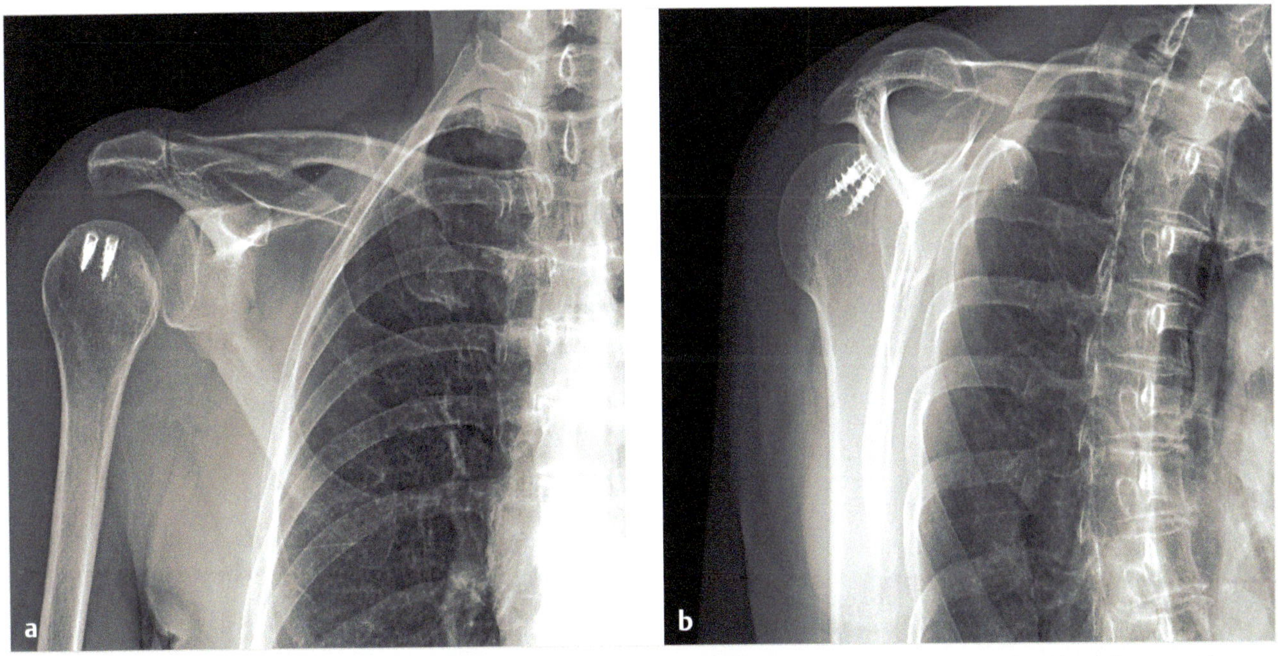

Fig. 34.1 Conventional radiographs showing **(a)** anteroposterior and **(b)** lateral scapular Y views of a posterior shoulder dislocation. The metal anchors noted are from a prior rotator cuff repair.

patients with unstable epilepsy. For acute shoulder dislocations, one that has occurred within 3 weeks of the traumatic event, a closed reduction can usually be successfully performed in patients with smaller humeral head defects. If the dislocation has been present for greater than 3 weeks, a successful closed reduction may be more difficult to perform and a potential open/arthroscopically assisted reduction may need to be considered. Overall, the degree of posterior shoulder instability after a successful reduction is determined by the size of the anterior humeral defect and the associated capsulolabral injury.

If the shoulder is stable after a successful closed reduction, continued closed treatment in an abduction sling in neutral rotation for 6 weeks can be considered. If, however, the shoulder is unstable after a successful closed reduction, the clinician should assess and quantify the relevant bony lesion of the humeral head.[3] In cases without a significant reverse Hill-Sachs lesion, isolated treatment of the posterior labral pathology can be performed for the unstable shoulder. For patients with associated fractures of either the surgical neck or greater tuberosity, these fractures should be considered separately and addressed directly. When the bone defect of the Hill–Sachs lesion is greater than 45%, biologic reconstruction techniques utilizing an allograft to fill the segmental defect and restore the sphericity of the humeral head should be considered for young/active patients. Elderly or low-demand patients with these large humeral head defects (> 45%) may be ideal candidates for a primary joint replacement. In patients with humeral head defects less than 40% and instability after a posterior shoulder dislocation, operative stabilization with a McLaughlin or modified McLaughlin is considered the gold standard. Disimpaction bone grafting or autologous bone graft procedures such as osteochondral transplantation can be considered in addition to the soft tissue–based stabilization of the humeral defect for lesions measuring 20 to 40%.

34.2 Advantages

In a small case series, McLaughlin outlined his original technique for treating chronic locked posterior dislocations by a split in the subscapularis tendon close to its insertion with subsequent open reduction and filling the tendon into the reverse Hill–Sachs lesion.[4] The subscapularis tendon was then secured to the humerus through transosseous tunnels. Neer subsequently modified this technique with an osteotomy of the lesser tuberosity and transfer of the subscapularis-tendon-bone unit into the reverse Hill–Sachs lesion.[3] As a consequence of these nonanatomic techniques, there is a significant loss in internal rotation motion and strength. Additionally, the shoulder anatomy is distorted, which can complicate any future arthroplasty-based procedures. Less invasive arthroscopic modifications have been more recently described in which the attachment of the subscapularis tendon to the lesser tuberosity is maintained while insetting it into the bony defect.[1] This converts the reverse Hill–Sachs lesion into an extra-articular defect. While this modification is less invasive, it can still lead to deficits with internal rotation and alters the direction of force transmission/working length of the subscapularis tendon. A subsequent modification of this arthroscopic technique initially described by Duey et al utilizes the middle glenohumeral ligament (MGHL) instead of the subscapularis at the lesser tuberosity to fill the reverse Hill–Sachs lesion.[1] While the use of the MGHL may still result in a slight loss of internal rotation, the anatomy, force vector, and function of the subscapularis are not altered. This chapter will highlight the modified McLaughlin procedure with the use of the MGHL to treat instability after a posterior shoulder dislocation.

34.3 Indications

As previously noted, reverse Hill–Sachs lesions are common after a posterior shoulder dislocation and the location/size remain the most important factors in determining treatment options. The modified McLaughlin procedure can be utilized to treat humeral defects measuring 20 to 40%. It is important to note, however, that these nonanatomic techniques are less successful when the humeral defect occupies 33 to 50% of the articular surface.[3] In cases with larger lesions, the soft tissue–based modified McLaughlin procedure can be combined with an osteochondral transplantation. For lesions greater than 45%, allograft- or arthroplasty-based procedures may need to be considered.

34.4 Contraindications

The main contraindication for the use of an isolated modified McLaughlin procedure to treat recurrent instability after a posterior shoulder dislocation is a larger reverse Hill–Sachs lesion, greater than 45%. A relative contraindication for the use of the MGHL is mainly related to certain anatomical variations in which the ligament does not have a normal size or consistency. In these cases, the subscapularis tendon can be utilized instead and inset into the humeral head defect arthroscopically. Nonoperative treatment should be considered for elderly patients with low demands and patients with unstable epilepsy or multiple medical comorbidities/advanced dementia.

34.5 Preoperative Preparation/ Positioning

Most posterior shoulder dislocations are missed in up to 79% of cases and as a result a high index of suspicion along with proper radiographs are required for the proper diagnosis.[5] Standard radiographs are obtained including a true AP view of the shoulder, an axillary view, and a lateral scapular view. The axillary radiograph is essential to evaluate for a posterior dislocation. If the patient's pain or limited abduction does not allow for a standard axillary view, a modified axillary lateral, apical oblique, or Velpeau view can be considered. Additionally, a CT scan of the shoulder with 3D reconstructions of the humeral head along with an MRI (**Fig. 34.2**) of the shoulder can be utilized to evaluate the size of the humeral head defect and assess for potential rotator cuff and/or labral pathology. The size of the reverse Hill–Sachs lesion, associated pathology, and the duration of the dislocation are the most important factors in determining the treatment for a posterior shoulder dislocation.

Once the patient has been diagnosed with a locked posterior dislocation and assessed to be an optimal surgical candidate, a reduction of the shoulder should be performed. A posterior dislocation of the shoulder should be reduced in the operating room under general anesthesia with a regional brachial plexus

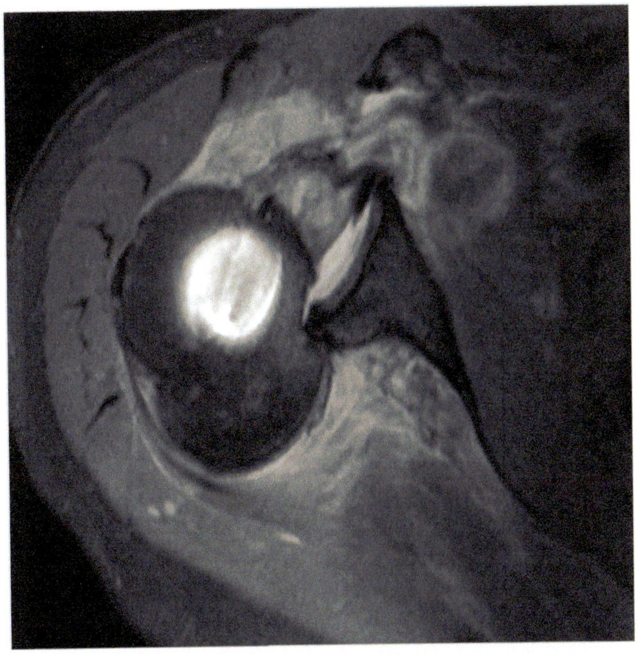

Fig. 34.2 Axial MRI view of a locked posterior dislocation of the shoulder with an impression fracture of the humeral head.

block, as a full assessment of stability is difficult to perform in a conscious, sedated patient. For the initial closed reduction, the patient is positioned supine on the operating table and image intensification is utilized to confirm the reduction. The reduction maneuver is performed with initial gentle traction applied to the affected arm while it is in a flexed, adducted, and internally rotated position. While the traction is being applied, pressure is placed on the posterior humeral head to guide it out of the engaged position along with slow sustained external rotation. For dislocations that have been present for greater than 3 weeks or if there is a larger reverse Hill–Sachs lesion present (>25%), a closed reduction may be more difficult and subsequent open or arthroscopically assisted reduction may be required. If an open reduction is performed, the patient is placed in the beach-chair position. A standard deltopectoral approach is utilized and the biceps tendon is used as a reference point to find the lesser tuberosity and rotator interval. The rotator interval is then opened and a small Darrach-type retractor is inserted to dislodge the humeral head from the posterior glenoid, followed by distraction, external rotation, and pressure applied posteriorly on the humeral head. An arthroscopically assisted reduction can also be performed utilizing trocars through the working portals to assist in the reduction.

If the reduction is successful, shoulder stability is then assessed by bringing the arm into forward flexion, adduction, and internal rotation. In the setting of an unstable shoulder after a closed/open reduction, adjunctive stabilization procedures are required to restore function and prevent recurrent instability. As noted previously, the size of the bone defect within the reverse Hill–Sachs lesion determines the treatment options. For unstable shoulders with humeral lesions measuring less than 40%, a modified McLaughlin procedure utilizing the MGHL can be performed. It is additionally important to note that associated posterior labral pathology and associated rotator cuff pathology should be concomitantly addressed.

34.6 Operative Technique

To perform the modified McLaughlin procedure utilizing the MGHL, the patient is placed in the beach-chair position. The operative extremity is prepped and draped in the usual sterile fashion. A pneumatic arm-positioning device is utilized to allow for stable positioning of the operative extremity. An examination under anesthesia is not performed as stability was already assessed after the closed reduction. A standard posterior portal is made and the 30-degree arthroscope is then inserted. Portals are then created first anteriorly and second anterosuperolaterally with cannulas subsequently placed in each portal. The anterior portal is the working portal and a larger diameter cannula, typically 8.0 mm, is utilized. The outflow is attached to the anterior cannula. For the anterosuperolateral portal, a smaller diameter cannula, typically 5.5 mm, is utilized. This portal is through the rotator interval and additionally serves as a viewing portal. A diagnostic arthroscopy is then performed with evaluation of the reverse Hill–Sachs lesion and any associated rotator cuff or biceps labral complex pathology. If the patient has any tearing in the biceps tendon greater than 50% of the total tendon integrity or tearing in the superior labrum, the long head of the biceps tendon is tenotomized for later tenodesis, which can be performed arthroscopically or open. The rotator cuff pathology is addressed after performing the modified McLaughlin procedure. After completion of viewing posteriorly, the arthroscope is then switched into the anterosuperolateral portal. The posterior capsulolabral complex and glenoid are then evaluated for possible pathology. If posterior labral pathology is present, this must be addressed along with the reverse Hill–Sachs lesion.

To repair the posterior capsulolabral complex, the arthroscope is maintained in the anterosuperolateral portal and a second 8.0-mm cannula is placed in the posterior portal over a switching stick. The posterior glenoid and labrum are then prepared with a combination of an arthroscopic shaver, periosteal elevator, and radiofrequency ablation device via the anterior portal. A bleeding bony bed is created on the posterior glenoid rim in order to optimize the healing surface for the capsulolabral repair. In order to increase accesses/visualization of the posterior shoulder, the arm is positioned in 45 degrees of forward flexion and limited elbow flexion. An assistant can additionally apply a distracting lateral-based force on the axilla, which increases the access to the inferior glenoid. Once the posterior labrum and associated capsular complex have been mobilized, an anchor is placed at the most inferior aspect of the tear. If a standard 2.9-mm double-loaded anchor is utilized, a separate percutaneous posterolateral portal is made just distal to the posterolateral border of the acromion. A spinal needle is utilized as an initial guide for the angle of approach, and the drill guide for the anchor is placed through the infraspinatus tendon near the muscle–tendon junction in an effort to minimize trauma to the tendon unit. Anchors are then placed sequentially along the glenoid rim and the sutures are shuttled through the capsulolabral complex via the posterior portal with a 45-degree Ideal (Depuy Mitek, Raynham, MA) in the opposite direction of the operative extremity. For a right operative shoulder, a left 45-degree Ideal is utilized and vice versa for a left operative shoulder. The sutures are sequentially passed in a horizontal mattress configuration through the capsulolabral complex for later repair but not tied. More recently, we have utilized an all-suture double-loaded anchor, Iconix 2.3 mm (Stryker, Mahwah, NJ), with a curved 25-degree guide system. This allows for placement of the anchors via the anterior portal and obviates the need for a separate posterolateral portal (**Fig. 34.3**).

After completion of suture passage, attention is then turned to the reverse Hill–Sachs lesion. The 30-degree arthroscope is exchanged for a 70-degree arthroscope, which is then placed into the posterior portal through the cannula. The 5.5-mm cannula is then placed back into the anterosuperolateral portal and the arm is repositioned in 45 degrees of forward flexion, 90 degrees of elbow flexion, 15 to 30 degrees of arm abduction, and maximal internal rotation. The bed of the reverse Hill–Sachs lesion is then debrided down to a bleeding base with an arthroscopic burr and ring curette via the anterosuperolateral portal (**Fig. 34.4**). A periosteal elevator is then utilized via the anterior and anterosuperolateral portals to free the underlying capsule and MGHL off the undersurface of the subscapularis (**Fig. 34.5**). Once the reverse Hill–Sachs lesion and MGHL complex have been prepared, a double-loaded 5.5-mm Healix

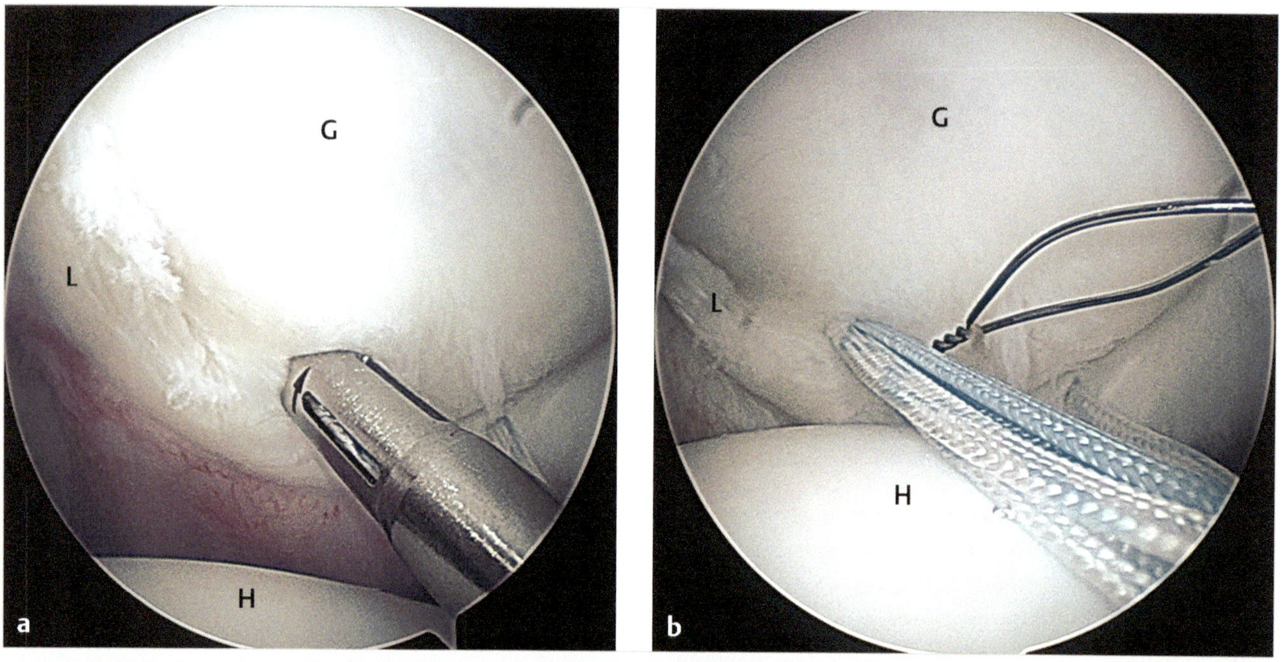

Fig. 34.3 View from the anterosuperolateral portal showing the **(a)** placement of an all-suture anchor within the posterior glenoid via a curved guide system and **(b)** suture shuttling with a 45-degree Ideal placed in the posterior portal. G, glenoid; H, humeral head; L, labrum.

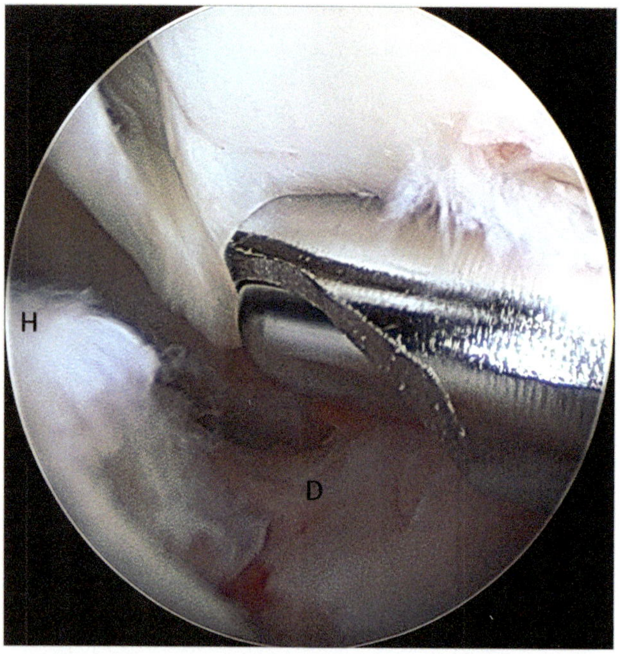

Fig. 34.4 View from the anterosuperolateral portal showing preparation of the reverse Hill–Sachs lesion with an arthroscopic shaver. D, reverse Hill–Sachs lesion; H, humeral head.

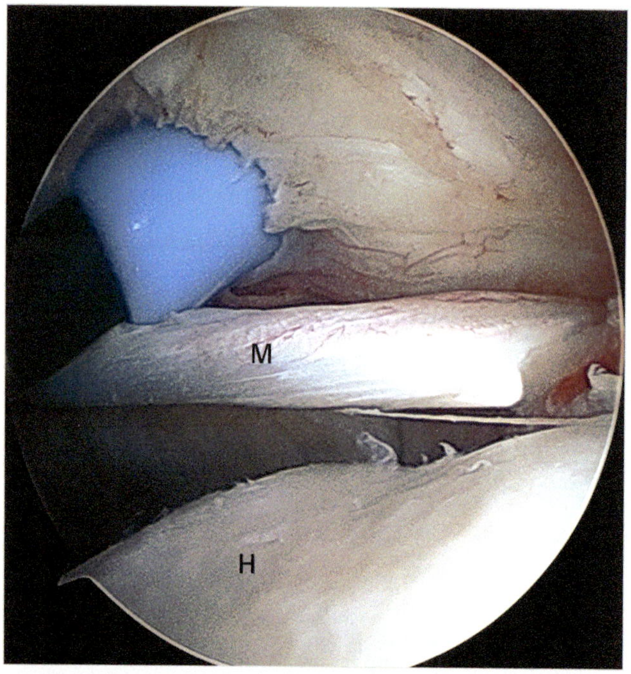

Fig. 34.5 View from the posterior portal showing the middle glenohumeral ligament (MGHL) once it has been elevated off the undersurface of the subscapularis. H, humeral head; M, MGHL.

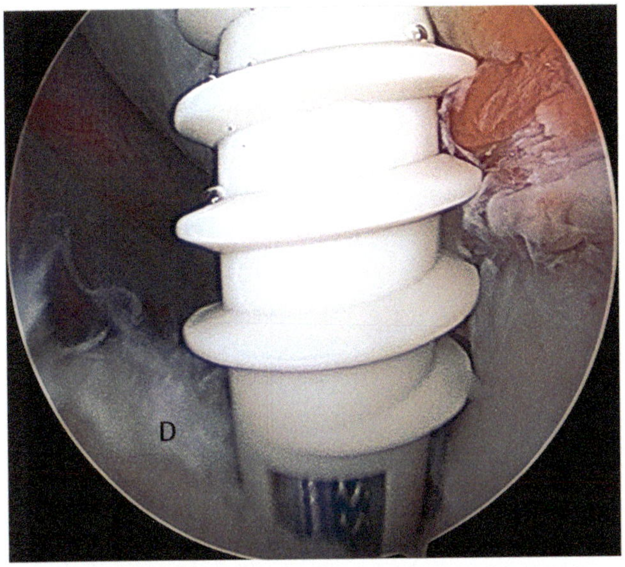

Fig. 34.6 View from the anterosuperolateral portal showing the placement of a double-loaded 5.5-mmHealix anchor (DePuy Mitek) into the superior aspect of the reverse Hill–Sachs lesion. D, reverse Hill–Sachs lesion.

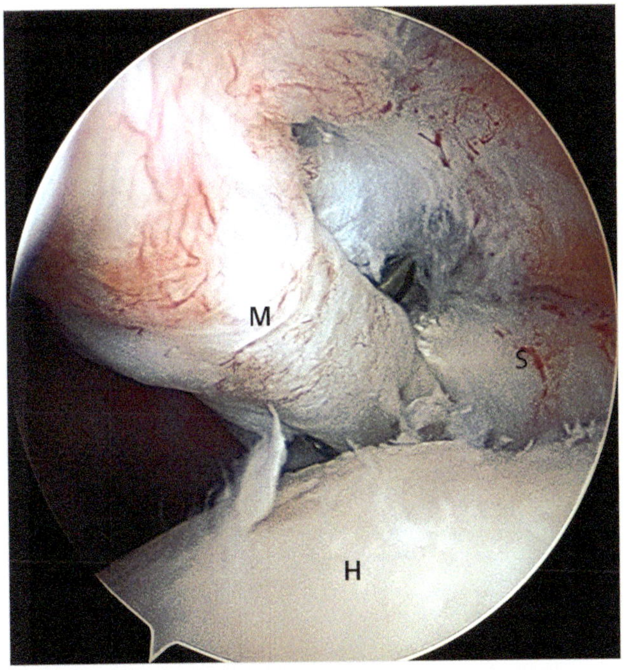

Fig. 34.8 View from the posterior portal showing the placement of the middle glenohumeral ligament (MGHL) and underlying capsule into the reverse Hill–Sachs lesion. H, humeral head; M, MGHL; S, subscapularis.

anchor (DePuy Mitek) is placed into the superior aspect of the lesion (**Fig. 34.6**). Depending on the angle of approach, the anchor can be placed via the anterior portal or percutaneously via an anterosuperolateral stab incision. The sutures are then passed through the MGHL in a modified Mason–Allen configuration with either an Expressew III (DePuy Mitek) or a right/left 45-degree Ideal via the anterior portal. Provisionally, the sutures are docked out through the anterosuperolateral por-

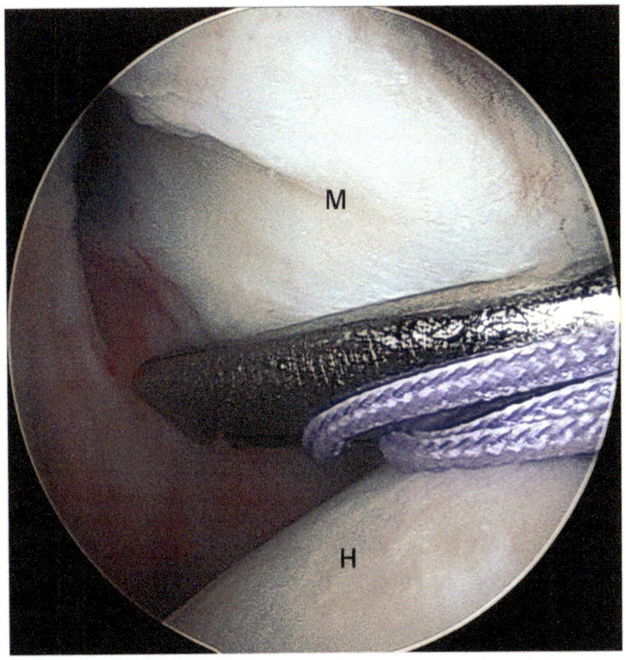

Fig. 34.7 View from the posterior portal showing the passage of sutures through the middle glenohumeral ligament (MGHL) with an Expressew III (DePuy Mitek). H, humeral head; M, MGHL.

tal (**Fig. 34.7**). For larger bone defects, additional anchors may be necessary.

Once all sutures have been passed through the MGHL, the arm is repositioned in 45 degrees of forward flexion, limited abduction, and limited elbow flexion. The arthroscope is switched back into the anterosuperolateral portal and the previously passed sutures through the posterior capsulolabral complex are tied down. After the posterior capsulolabral complex has been repaired, the arthroscope is switched back into the posterior portal and the arm is repositioned in limited forward flexion, limited abduction/rotation, and 90-degree elbow flexion.

The previously passed sutures through the MGHL are then tied via the anterior portal insetting the MGHL and underlying capsule into the reverse Hill–Sachs lesion (**Fig. 34.8**). If present, any subsequent rotator cuff and biceps pathology is then addressed.

34.7 Tips and Pearls/Expert Suggestions

In an effort to help optimize the success and technical efficiency of the modified McLaughlin procedure, some tips/suggestions are noted:

- Utilize the 70-degree arthroscope via the posterior portal when addressing the reverse Hill–Sachs lesion. Additionally, the arm should be positioned in 45 degrees of forward flexion, 90 degrees of elbow flexion, and 15 to 30 degrees of arm abduction with maximal internal rotation. A posteriorly directed force on the proximal humerus with a combined anteriorly directed force on the distal humerus could also increase the visualization of the lesser tuberosity if required.

- The anterosuperolateral portal is established 5 to 10 mm distal to the anterolateral border of the acromion and enters the glenohumeral joint through the rotator interval. The angle of approach is typically 5 to 10 degrees and a spinal needle should be utilized first to define this angle. The anterosuperolateral portal is utilized for viewing if performing a posterior labral repair and for suture shuttling during the modified McLaughlin procedure.
- Anchors should be placed percutaneously in the reverse Hill–Sachs lesion with the use of a spinal needle first to localize the angle of approach. This enables independent placement if multiple anchors are required and also assists in suture management. Due to the bony architecture of the reverse Hill–Sachs lesion, a 5.5-mm anchor is preferred over the smaller 4.75-mm anchors.
- If more than one anchor is required for the filling of the MGHL into the reverse Hill–Sachs lesion, the sutures from the more inferior anchor should be shuttled retrograde, while the sutures from the more superior anchor should be shuttled antegrade. Additionally, all anchors and sutures should be shuttled first prior to knot tying. The previously passed sutures can be docked out through the posterior portal prior to tying.
- When combining a posterior labral repair with the modified McLaughlin procedure, all anchors and sutures should be passed on both the glenoid and the humeral sides prior to knot tying. Once all sutures have been passed, the posterior labral sutures should be tied down and then the humeral-based sutures.

34.8 What to Avoid

Any soft tissue–based stabilization of a reverse Hill–Sachs lesion should be avoided if the size of the osteochondral defect is larger than 40% of the articular surface. With these larger lesions, the modified McLaughlin procedure can be combined with an osteochondral transplantation. If the lesion is greater than 45%, an isolated allograft- or arthroplasty-based procedure should be considered.

34.9 Complications/Bailout/Salvage

The MGHL functions to resist anterior and posterior translation in the midrange of shoulder abduction and external rotation. It typically arises from the labrum just below the superior glenohumeral ligament or from the adjacent neck of the glenoid and inserts onto the humerus just medial to the lesser tuberosity. Unfortunately, the MGHL has the greatest variation in size of all the glenohumeral ligaments and may be absent more often than the other ligaments. The most common variant of the MGHL is a well-formed and distinct structure that has a flat/broad appearance. Another variant of the MGHL exists with a cordlike appearance and insertion onto the base of the biceps anchor. In the cases where the MGHL is deficient or poorly defined, a portion of the subscapularis should be inset into the reverse Hill–Sachs lesion utilizing the same outlined technique.

34.10 Postoperative Care

All patients are immobilized in an abduction sling in the neutral position for 6 weeks. It is important to avoid an internally rotated position of the arm after surgical intervention, as this will place stress on the repair. Table slides are initiated at the 2-week mark from the date of surgery. After 6 weeks, patients are allowed to come out of the sling, and a progressive self-directed home-based therapy program is initiated. No formalized physical therapy is initiated. Patients progress with an active and active-assisted motion protocol focusing mainly on forward flexion and an initial limitation of external rotation to 30 degrees. Once patients are able to achieve 90 to 95% of their motion, a functional strengthening program is initiated. A complete return to full activity without limitation is delayed up until the 6- to 9-month mark from the date of surgery depending on the patient's tissue quality and the strength of the repair.

References

1. Duey RE, Burkhart SS. Arthroscopic treatment of a reverse Hill-Sachs lesion. Arthrosc Tech 2013;2(2):e155–e159
2. Robinson CM, Aderinto J. Posterior shoulder dislocations and fracture-dislocations. J Bone Joint Surg Am 2005;87(3):639–650
3. Paul J, Buchmann S, Beitzel K, Solovyova O, Imhoff AB. Posterior shoulder dislocation: systematic review and treatment algorithm. Arthroscopy 2011;27(11):1562–1572
4. McLaughlin HL. Posterior dislocation of the shoulder. J Bone Joint Surg Am 1952;24 A(3):584–590
5. Spencer EE Jr, Brems JJ. A simple technique for management of locked posterior shoulder dislocations: report of two cases. J Shoulder Elbow Surg 2005;14(6):650–652

35 Latissimus Dorsi Tendon Transfer

Brendan M. Patterson and Jay D. Keener

Abstract

Patients with irreparable rotator cuff tears remain a significant clinical challenge. The latissimus dorsi tendon transfer is a viable option for patients with irreparable posterosuperior rotator cuff tears. Ideally indicated patients are those considered to young for reverse shoulder arthroplasty and without evidence of advanced cuff tear arthropathy or fixed proximal humeral migration. A functional deltoid and intact subscapularis are required as well. The surgical technique has multiple options. We describe a single posterior incision technique facilitated by arm positioning. Care is taken to protect surrounding neurovascular structures. Final placement of the transferred tendon can be modified based on the presence of external rotation lag signs. Careful protection of the repair is required for 6-12 weeks with a graduated progressive rehabilitation program. Final recovery can take 8-9 months. The results of latissimus dorsi tendon transfer have been shown to be reliable for pain relief and inconsistent for functional recovery. The functional results are better in shoulders with an intact teres minor. Successful early results in patients following latissimus dorsi tendon transfer have been shown to be durable long term.

Keywords: *latissimus dorsi transfer, irreparable rotator cuff tear, shoulder reconstruction*

35.1 Goals of Procedure

The goals of the latissimus dorsi tendon transfer are to improve function and decrease pain for patients with shoulder dysfunction caused by irreparable posterosuperior rotator cuff tears. Latissimus dorsi tendon transfer achieves improved shoulder function in the setting of irreparable cuff tears by helping restore the force couples of the shoulder originally described by Burkhart.[1] Transfer of the latissimus dorsi tendon to the greater tuberosity imparts external rotation and head depressor moments to the proximal humerus allowing for improved balance between the anterior and posterior force couples.

35.2 Advantages

Surgical options for the treatment of symptomatic irreparable rotator cuff tears in younger more active patients are limited. Many older patients with irreparable rotator cuff tears having failed nonoperative management would be served well with a reverse shoulder arthroplasty or in some cases an arthroscopic debridement and biceps tenodesis or tenotomy. The latissimus dorsi tendon transfer provides a durable nonarthroplasty treatment option for younger patients with shoulder pain and dysfunction secondary to irreparable posterosuperior rotator cuff tears.

Improvements in range of motion, strength, and pain scores have been demonstrated at both short-term and long-term follow-up.[2,3] Gerber et al reported durable improvements in forward elevation, abduction, external rotation, pain scores, strength, and Constant scores for patients with a minimum of 10 years of postoperative follow-up after latissimus dorsi tendon transfer for irreparable rotator cuff tears.[3] Warner and Parsons described less favorable results particularly for patients undergoing latissimus dorsi tendon transfer in setting of a failed rotator cuff repair.[4] Although the published success rates and functional outcome improvements vary to some degree, the latissimus dorsi tendon transfer has a proven clinical track record for the management of irreparable rotator cuff tears in properly indicated patients. Of note, currently it remains controversial if this transfer has primarily a tenodesis effect or if active recruitment is consistently achievable.[5] Maintenance of at least partial teres minor function has been linked to better outcomes after latissimus dorsi tendon transfer.[6]

35.3 Indications

The latissimus dorsi tendon transfer is indicated for younger (60 years and younger) and/or active patients with massive irreparable posterosuperior rotator cuff tears with continued pain and shoulder dysfunction despite nonoperative treatment. This procedure is also indicated for failed rotator cuff repair or failed debridement of irreparable rotator cuff tears. More refined indications for latissimus dorsi tendon transfer also include absence of significant glenohumeral arthritis, an intact subscapularis tendon, and maintenance of active overhead elevation. Additionally, significant patient compliance is needed to commit to the extended period of recovery and rehabilitation.

35.4 Contraindications

Latissimus dorsi tendon transfer is contraindicated for patients with advanced rotator cuff arthropathy defined as glenohumeral arthritis and/or advanced fixed proximal humeral migration. Success is predicated on the presence of healthy deltoid and periscapular muscles. Proximal humeral escape is an absolute contraindication to this procedure. Given the importance of the subscapularis for preserving the rotator cuff force couple, this tendon must be intact or repairable with minimal muscle atrophy. While the clinical results of latissimus dorsi tendon transfer are somewhat variable, there is evidence that patients with poor subscapularis function have decreased outcomes following latissimus dorsi tendon transfer.[2,3] It is also important to consider that patients with pseudoparalysis are less likely to demonstrate satisfactory improvement after latissimus dorsi tendon transfer.[7] Patients who are unable or unwilling to adhere to the required postoperative restrictions and prolonged rehabilitation protocol are poor candidates for this procedure. Furthermore, expectations to return to occupations with excessive overhead motion or heavy manual labor are not realistic given the modest gains in function realized following this procedure.

35.5 Preoperative Preparation/ Positioning

35.5.1 Initial Evaluation

A complete history and physical examination is required prior to consideration of latissimus dorsi tendon transfer. The history will help further characterize the duration and severity of symptoms and reveal the patient's expectations in regard to postoperative functional goals. Prior surgeries should be noted, especially those that may affect deltoid function such as open cuff repair. A careful review of occupational and recreational demands is warranted.

Inspection is initially performed to assess for muscle atrophy, integrity of the deltoid, and scapular posture. The physical examination should include a focused and complete assessment of range of motion and strength of the shoulder. The patient should have good passive range of motion (PROM) of the shoulder. Active range of motion (AROM) should assess elevation, external rotation in both adduction and abduction, and internal rotation with additional attention on scapular control. Strength testing in scapular plane elevation and external rotation is performed. Assessment of teres minor function is relevant given the known benefit of teres minor integrity on the clinical results of latissimus dorsi tendon transfer.[6] The presence of severe external rotation lag signs is important in potential latissimus dorsi tendon transfer candidates as these may influence the chosen insertion point of the tendon transfer. Subscapularis testing with belly-press or bear-hug test can be performed to determine the presence of subscapularis dysfunction. An upper quarter screen is important to rule out cervical radiculopathy.

35.5.2 Imaging

Preoperative imaging should include a full shoulder series: anteroposterior (AP), true AP, scapular Y, and axillary radiographs. The true AP and axillary views can be used to assess for glenohumeral joint space narrowing or other signs of arthritis. Severe or fixed proximal humeral head migration should be noted and caution is noted in cases with complete loss of the acromiohumeral interval with signs of chronic wear of the humeral head against the acromion. In the setting of a massive irreparable rotator cuff tear, an MRI, ultrasound, or CT arthrography of the shoulder can be used to assess for tear size, tendon retraction, and muscular fatty infiltration and atrophy.

35.5.3 Positioning

Lateral decubitus with the operative extremity prepped free is the preferred position for a single-incision technique. Alternatively, beach-chair positioning can be performed. There are many described techniques for latissimus dorsi tendon transfer including isolated or combined posterior, anterior, deltoid split, and axillary approaches with harvesting of the latissimus dorsi tendon in isolation or combined with the teres major that can be accomplished in either the lateral decubitus or the beach-chair position.

35.6 Operative Technique

35.6.1 Preferred Technique

We prefer a single-incision posterior approach similar to the approach described by Habermeyer et al.[8] A longitudinal incision (10–12 cm) is made just medial to the posterior axillary fold from the posterolateral acromion inferiorly (**Fig. 35.1**). The subcutaneous tissue is then dissected down to the level of the muscular fascia. The deltoid is identified and retracted superiorly, and the subdeltoid fascia is opened and the deltoid is swept off of the posterior cuff muscles. After the deltoid is reflected, the teres minor and infraspinatus can be visualized. The approach continues inferiorly and deep to the teres major, identifying the latissimus dorsi muscle and tendon. The fatty tissue inferior to the teres minor is not dissected facilitating easier identification of the teres major and latissimus dorsi tendons as well as minimizing bleeding (**Fig. 35.2**).

The operative extremity is then abducted and maximally internally rotated (**Fig. 35.3**). Any fascial adhesions connecting the latissimus dorsi to the long head of the triceps are dissected and released. The teres major and latissimus dorsi tendons are traced to their humeral attachments, and all soft tissues are cleared off the tendons with a sponge directly toward their humeral insertions. The latissimus dorsi tendon is separated from

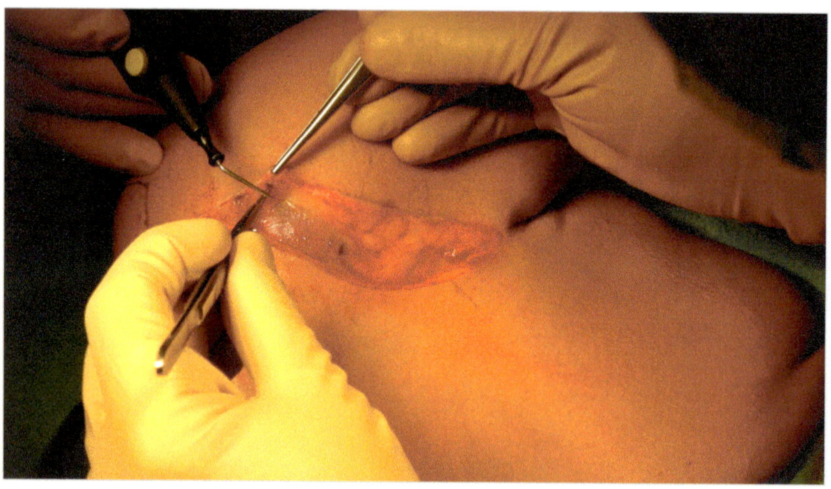

Fig. 35.1 A longitudinal incision is made from the posterolateral acromion directed just medial to the posterior axial fold.

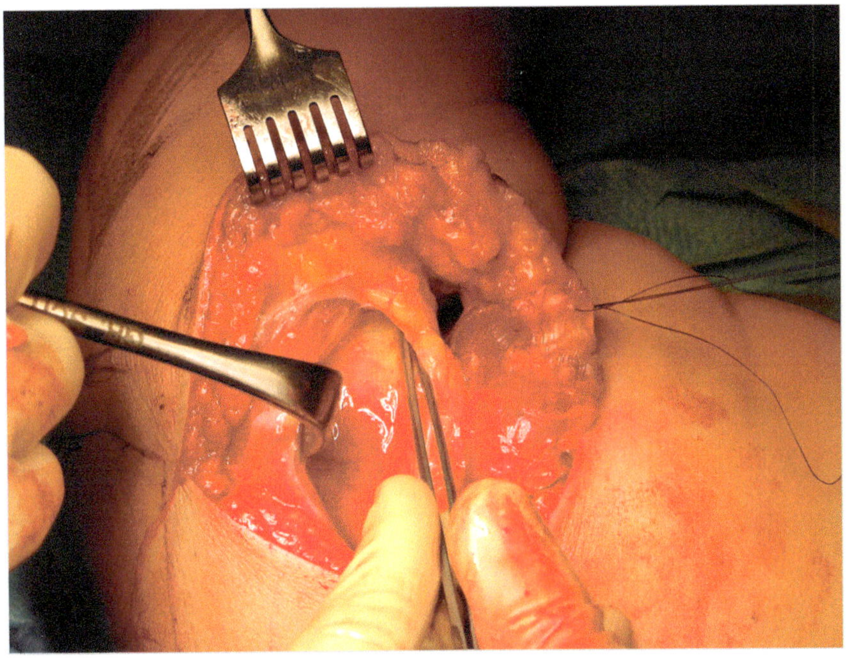

Fig. 35.2 The deltoid is retracted superiorly with the fatty tissue inferior to the teres minor left in continuity with the teres minor.

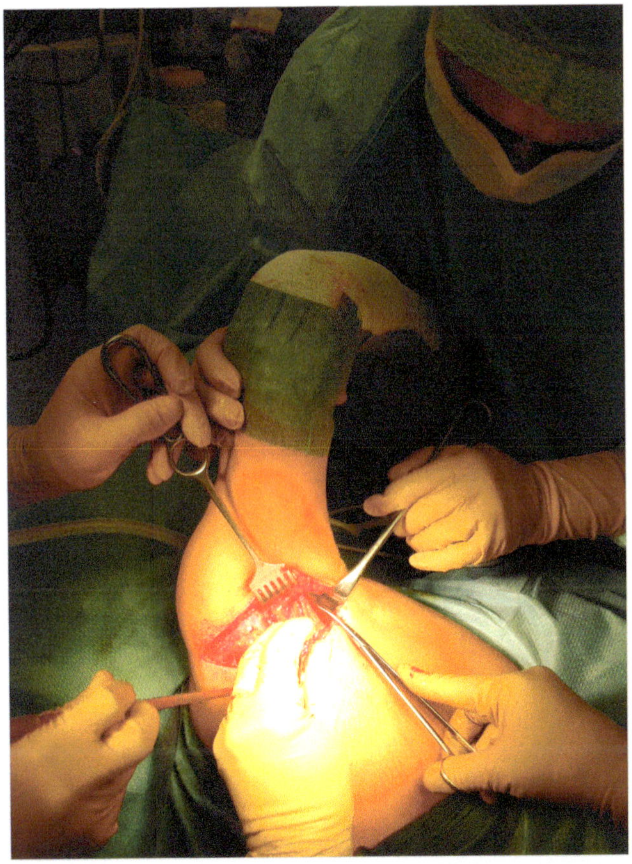

Fig. 35.3 Maximal abduction and internal rotation are demonstrated, which facilitate exposure of the latissimus dorsi and teres major tendons.

the teres major tendon and then released from the humeral insertion maximizing tendon length for harvest (**Fig. 35.4**). The latissimus dorsi tendon is deep to the teres major from the posterior approach. Alternatively, both the teres major and the latissimus dorsi can be harvested together. Care should be taken to protect the surrounding neurovascular structures, in particular the radial nerve directly anterior to the tendon and 2.3 to 2.9 cm medial to the boney insertion (**Fig. 35.5**).[9] Each side and the end of the tendon are reinforced with a running locked no. 2 caliber braided suture and the corners of the tendon are tagged for control (**Fig. 35.6**).

The tendon is then mobilized with blunt dissection and Metzenbaum scissors circumferentially. Care should be taken to preserve the neurovascular bundle on the anteromedial surface of the muscle belly. The latissimus dorsi is innervated by the thoracodorsal nerve which inserts 13.1 cm (11.0–15.3 cm) inferior to the humeral insertion (**Fig. 35.7**).[10] With the tendon harvested and freed from adhesions, the arm is then abducted and externally rotated to bring the posterior cuff humeral insertions into view.

With the arm held in this position, Bankart retractors are placed along the anterior aspect of the greater tuberosity to retract the deltoid (**Fig. 35.8**). Any remaining intact rotator cuff tendon should be preserved while all residual soft tissue is freed from the greater tuberosity. The greater tuberosity should then be gently decorticated to further promote tendon to bone healing.

Three humeral suture anchors double loaded with high tensile braided sutures are then placed at the planned transfer site on the greater tuberosity (**Fig. 35.9**). A commonly chosen insertion site for the tendon transfer is the superior aspect of the anterior greater tuberosity posterior to the biceps groove, which is now oriented horizontally with the shoulder in abduction and external rotation. Alternatively, the tendon can be attached more laterally and inferiorly on the greater tuberosity to facilitate external rotation control.

A combination of the horizontal mattress and the Mason–Allen suture technique is used to secure the tendon to the greater tuberosity. Horizontal mattress sutures are placed superiorly and tied first followed by the Mason–Allen sutures to allow appropriate compression of the tendon down to the greater tuberosity (**Figs. 35.10, 35.11**). If there is any residual infraspinatus or teres minor tendon present, we recommend a side-to-side repair to the medial aspect of the latissimus dorsi tendon with no.

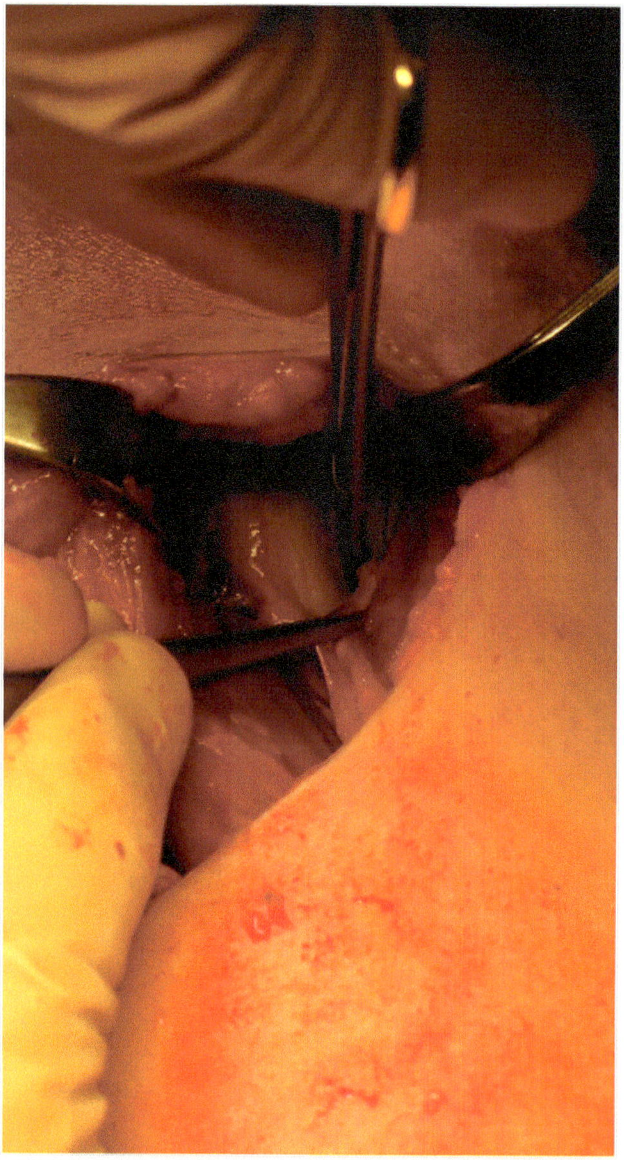

Fig. 35.4 Tendon length is maximized prior to release of the latissimus dorsi tendon from the humeral insertion.

2 braided nonabsorbable sutures. The arm is then taken through a range of motion to confirm appropriate excursion of the muscle and tendon unit in both external and internal rotations.

35.7 Tips and Pearls/Expert Suggestions

Visualization of the latissimus dorsi tendon insertion can be difficult from the posterior approach, especially in larger patients. Superficial dissection should be inferior to the fat pad of the quadrangular space. Fascial connections to the long head of the triceps must be released. The lateral head of the triceps must be retracted superiorly. Identify the teres major tendon initially and then work toward the deeper latissimus dorsi with the arm in abduction and maximal internal rotation. The use of sponge peanuts will facilitate separation of the teres major and latissimus dorsi tendons.

If delineation of the latissimus dorsi tendon from the teres major tendons is difficult, harvest both tendons for transfer. Maximizing length of the latissimus dorsi tendon is also important, and one should attempt to release the tendon sharply directly off the bone. This is more difficult at the superior

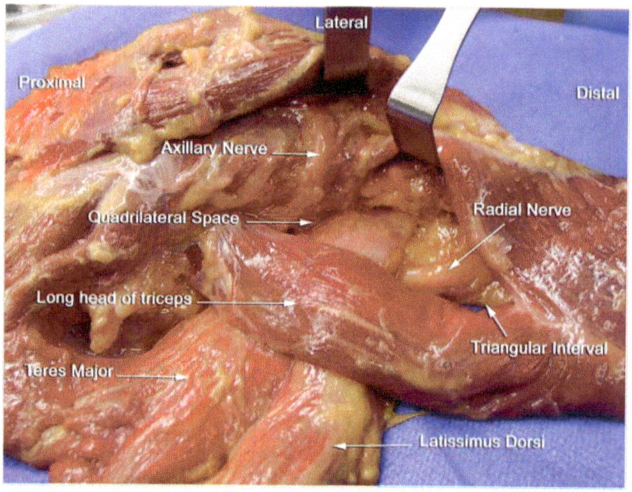

Fig. 35.5 Cadaveric dissection demonstrating the key anatomic structures involved in the posterior single-incision approach.[9]

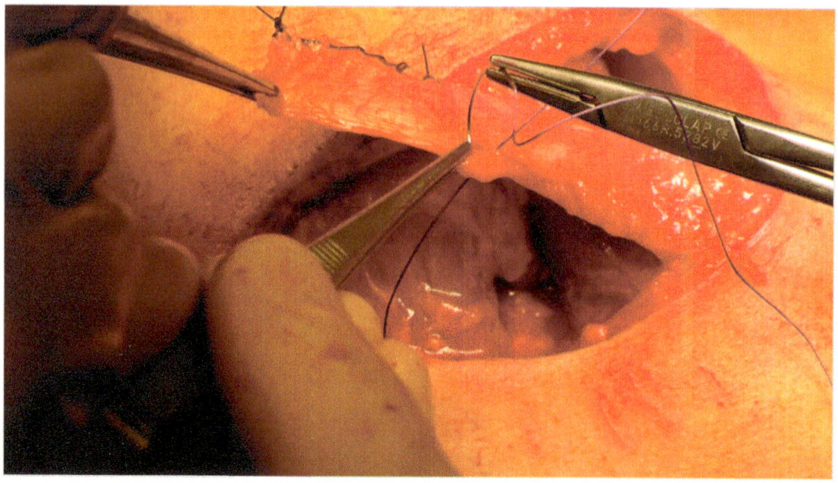

Fig. 35.6 Locked no. 2 caliber braided sutures are used to reinforce the tendon and aid in tendon control.

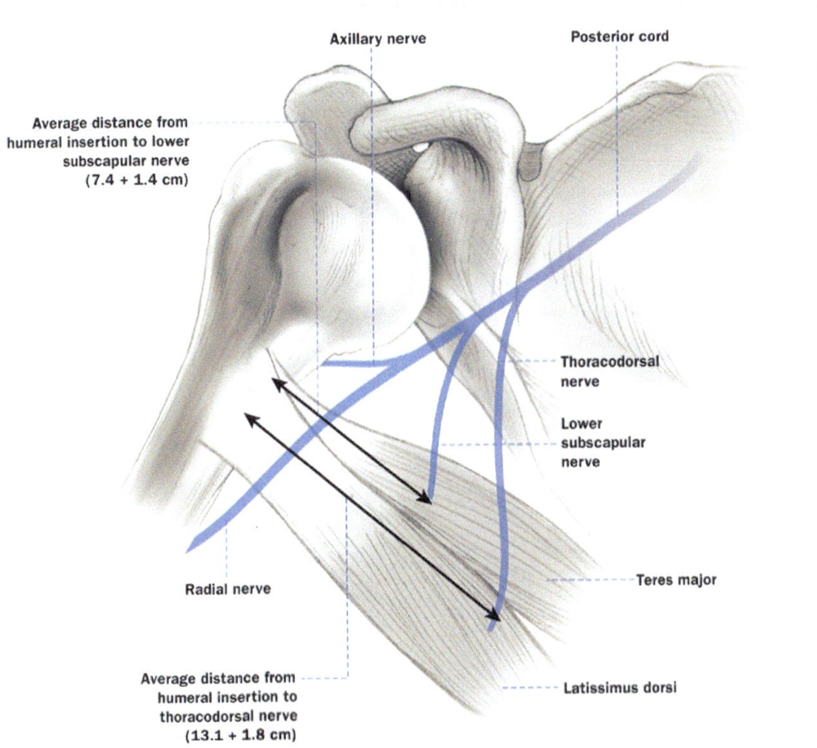

Fig. 35.7 The thoracodorsal nerve innervates the latissimus dorsi and inserts an average of 13.1 cm inferior to the humeral insertion.[10]

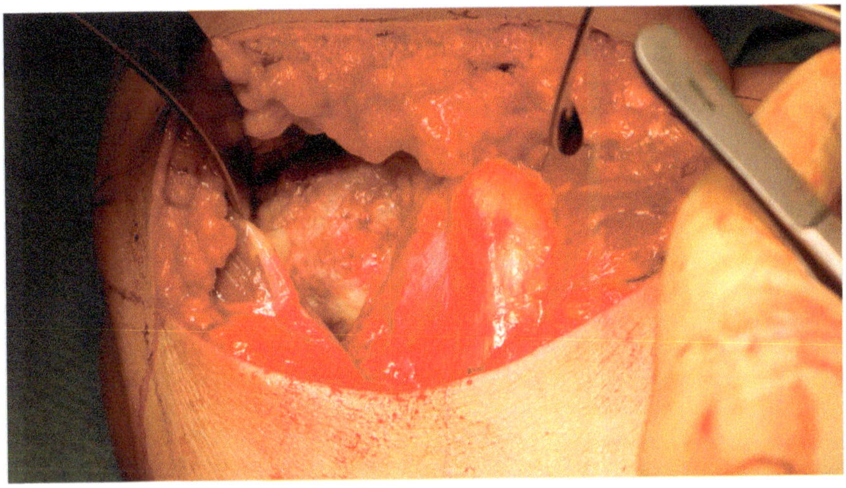

Fig. 35.8 The deltoid is retracted by Bankart retractors placed along the anterior aspect of the greater tuberosity.

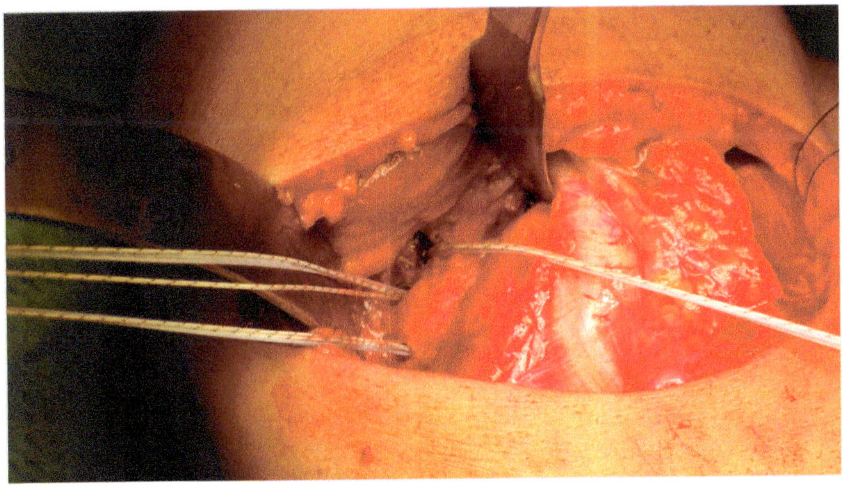

Fig. 35.9 Double-loaded suture anchors are evenly spaced at the greater tuberosity.

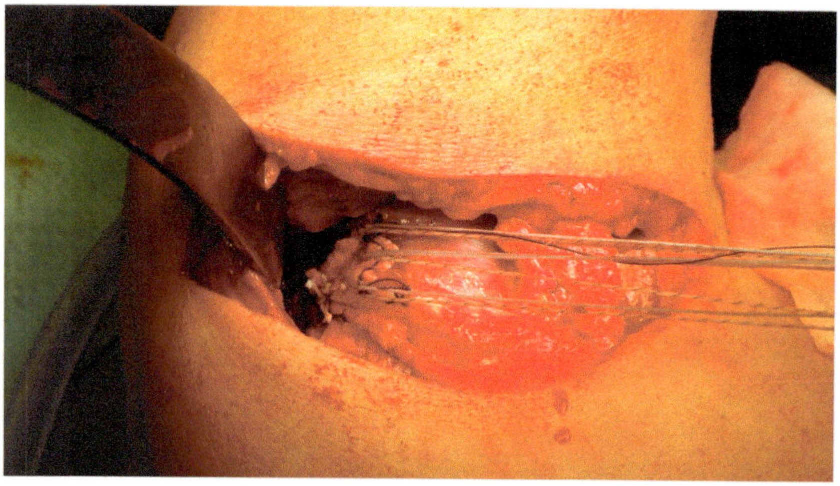

Fig. 35.10 Sutures from the previously placed suture anchors are used to repair the tendon with a combination of the horizontal mattress and the Mason–Allen suture technique.

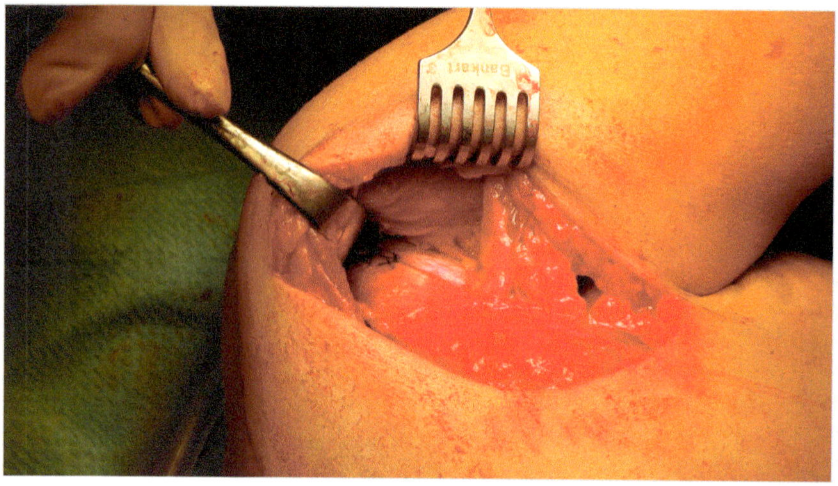

Fig. 35.11 Final repair construct is demonstrated with the latissimus dorsi tendon transferred to the greater tuberosity.

aspect of the insertion. Following tendon harvest, reinforcement of the thin latissimus dorsi tendon edges with suture will help minimize pullout of the repair sutures.

Abduction with maximal external rotation will facilitate proper visualization of the anterior and superior aspects of the greater tuberosity for tendon attachment. It is very helpful to use spiked glenoid retractors over the top of the humeral head to facilitate exposure. The tendon should be attached superior and anterior for standard transfers. If severe external rotation lag signs are present, we prefer to transfer the tendon a couple of centimeters more inferior and lateral adjacent to the teres minor attachment.

35.8 What to Avoid

Avoid dissection within the quadrangular space (identified by fatty tissue) below the teres minor to protect the axillary nerve. The tendon should be released directly off the bone. Sharp tendon release too medial will shorten the tendon and place the radial nerve at greater risk of injury. Careful dissection of adhesions along the anterior surface of the latissimus dorsi is important inferiorly to avoid injury to the thoracodorsal nerve.

35.9 Complications/Bailout/Salvage

If visualization of the latissimus dorsi tendon insertion is difficult from the posterior approach, a limited deltopectoral approach can be performed. The upper border of the pectoralis major tendon is released exposing the latissimus dorsi and teres major, which can be directly released from their humeral insertions. If preferred, the tendon(s) can be harvested with a small fleck of bone, which has been shown to result in a higher rate of healing.[11]

Full mobilization of the latissimus dorsi muscle may require extension of the skin incision inferiorly along the posterior axillary line. Occasionally, the length of the transferred tendon is not adequate to reach the desired transferred point on the greater tuberosity. If needed, an allograft (Achilles tendon preferred) can be sewn into the latissimus dorsi and attached to the humerus.

If the proper insertion point on the superior aspect of the anterior greater tuberosity cannot be visualized, a secondary lateral incision with a deltoid split can be performed for proper tendon site attachment. This approach can also be used to repair the upper subscapularis if needed.

35.10 Postoperative Care

The shoulder should be immobilized in a gunslinger brace with the shoulder in a position of approximately 20 to 30 degrees of abduction, 20 degrees of flexion, and 20 to 30 degrees of external rotation to minimize repair tension. At 1 week post-op, PROM is initiated into flexion and external rotation as tolerated. Internal rotation past the midline, combined adduction and extension motions, and AROM are prohibited for 6 weeks. The brace can be removed for elbow range of motion. At 6 weeks post-op, patients are transitioned to a sling with an abduction pillow. PROM exercises are continued avoiding internal rotation behind the back. Active-assisted range of motion (AAROM) elevation with pulleys is permitted. At 12 weeks post-op, the sling is discontinued. Full passive stretching is allowed as well as a full AAROM/AROM progression. Scapular control exercises are initiated and gentle shoulder isometrics are permitted. At 16 weeks, formal isotonic shoulder strengthening exercises are performed to include the rotator cuff, deltoid, and scapular stabilizers.

During the strengthening phase, external rotation AROM is initially performed without weight while facilitating recruitment of the latissimus dorsi tendon transfer. This is achieved by stabilizing the humerus in mid elevation and adducting against resistance while actively externally rotating the shoulder. As control improves, resistance to external rotation is progressed. Biofeedback devices can be used to facilitate active recruitment of the latissimus dorsi muscle. Generally, full strengthening of the shoulder is not complete until 8 to 9 months following surgery.

References

1. Burkhart SS. Arthroscopic treatment of massive rotator cuff tears. Clinical results and biomechanical rationale. Clin Orthop Relat Res 1991;(267):45–56
2. Gerber C, Maquieira G, Espinosa N. Latissimus dorsi transfer for the treatment of irreparable rotator cuff tears. J Bone Joint Surg Am 2006;88(1):113–120
3. Gerber C, Rahm SA, Catanzaro S, Farshad M, Moor BK. Latissimus dorsi tendon transfer for treatment of irreparable posterosuperior rotator cuff tears: long-term results at a minimum follow-up of ten years. J Bone Joint Surg Am 2013;95(21):1920–1926
4. Warner JJ, Parsons IM IV. Latissimus dorsi tendon transfer: a comparative analysis of primary and salvage reconstruction of massive, irreparable rotator cuff tears. J Shoulder Elbow Surg 2001;10(6):514–521
5. Iannotti JP, Hennigan S, Herzog R, et al. Latissimus dorsi tendon transfer for irreparable posterosuperior rotator cuff tears. Factors affecting outcome. J Bone Joint Surg Am 2006;88(2):342–348
6. Costouros JG, Espinosa N, Schmid MR, Gerber C. Teres minor integrity predicts outcome of latissimus dorsi tendon transfer for irreparable rotator cuff tears. J Shoulder Elbow Surg 2007;16(6):727–734
7. Namdari S, Voleti P, Baldwin K, Glaser D, Huffman GR. Latissimus dorsi tendon transfer for irreparable rotator cuff tears: a systematic review. J Bone Joint Surg Am 2012;94(10):891–898
8. Habermeyer P, Magosch P, Rudolph T, Lichtenberg S, Liem D. Transfer of the tendon of latissimus dorsi for the treatment of massive tears of the rotator cuff: a new single-incision technique. J Bone Joint Surg Br 2006;88(2):208–212
9. Pearle AD, Kelly BT, Voos JE, Chehab EL, Warren RF. Surgical technique and anatomic study of latissimus dorsi and teres major transfers. J Bone Joint Surg Am 2006;88(7):1524–1531
10. Pearle AD, Voos JE, Kelly BT, Chehab EL, Warren RF. Surgical technique and anatomic study of latissimus dorsi and teres major transfers. Surgical technique. J Bone Joint Surg Am 2007;89(Suppl 2, Pt 2):284–296
11. Moursy M, Forstner R, Koller H, Resch H, Tauber M. Latissimus dorsi tendon transfer for irreparable rotator cuff tears: a modified technique to improve tendon transfer integrity. J Bone Joint Surg Am 2009;91(8):1924–1931

36 Lower Trapezius Transfer

William R. Aibinder and Bassem T. Elhassan

Abstract

The lower trapezius tendon transfer aims to restore shoulder flexion and external rotation in patients with either paralysis or irreparable rotator cuff tears. This particular transfer utilizes a more direct line of pull to restore external rotation compared to the traditional latissimus dorsi transfer. The procedure can be performed via an open technique or an arthroscopically assisted technique. Appropriate tensioning of the tendon transfer in external rotation is crucial to a satisfactory outcome. Additionally, careful patient selection can prevent deleterious results, as compliance with a rehabilitation protocol is imperative.

Keywords: *lower trapezius tendon transfer, shoulder paralysis, irreparable rotator cuff tear*

36.1 Goals of Procedure

- To eliminate pain and restore function, particularly shoulder flexion and external rotation, in patients with either massive rotator cuff tears not amenable to repair or shoulder paralysis, such as after brachial plexus injury.

36.2 Advantages

The lower trapezius transfer is a simple procedure. In restoration of shoulder function, the lower trapezius provides a more direct line of pull for external rotation compared to the traditional latissimus dorsi transfer.[1,2] Additionally, the lower trapezius muscle is able to the stabilize the humeral head, even in the absence of subscapularis or deltoid function.[2] The lower trapezius tendon transfer can be performed as a single-tendon transfer or in combination with other tendon transfers to restore multiple planes of motion.

36.3 Indications

- Paralytic shoulders that lack active external rotation.
- Massive posterosuperior rotator cuff tears not amenable to repair or after failure of previous attempts at repair/reconstruction.

36.4 Contraindications

- Paralysis of the trapezius muscle, such as after spinal accessory nerve transfer.
- Active soft-tissue infections with or without associated open wounds.
- Advanced degenerative joint disease affecting the glenohumeral articulation.
- Inability to comply with the postoperative bracing and physical therapy protocol.

36.5 Preoperative Preparation/ Positioning

- Preoperative trapezius function must be assessed clinically by a shoulder shrug with evidence of muscle activation.
- When approaching a massive posterosuperior rotator cuff, an Achilles tendon allograft should be available.
- The patient is positioned laterally with the affected side up. A dynamic arm holder (SPIDER2; Smith & Nephew, Andover, MA) is utilized to position and stabilize the shoulder during the procedure and allow the assistant to retract.
- The operative extremity, and posterior and anterior thorax are prepped and draped passed midline.

36.6 Operative Technique

Anatomic landmarks are drawn on the patient including the scapula and scapular spine to identify the direction and location of the trapezius muscle fibers (**Fig. 36.1**). An incision is made 2 cm medial to the medial aspect of the scapular spine and extending distally approximately 5 to 7 cm. The lower and middle trapezius muscle bellies are then separated by identifying the triangular-shaped tendon insertion on the medial scapular spine of the lower trapezius and dissecting along the superior border. The spinal accessory nerve is identified and protected. It can usually be visualized two fingerbreadths medial to the medial border of the scapula on the undersurface of the muscle. Occasionally, a nerve stimulator is required. The insertion is

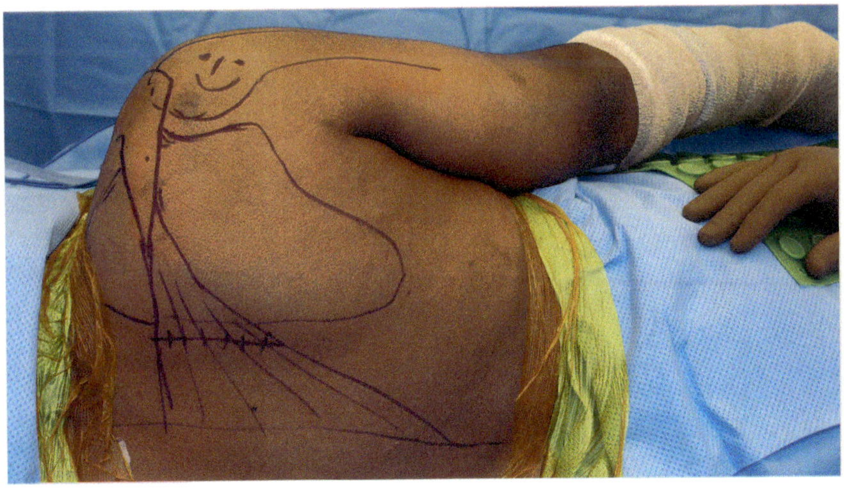

Fig. 36.1 A patient in the lateral decubitus position with the arm draped free and exposed passed midline. All anatomic landmarks are drawn including the humeral head, scapula, spinous processes, as well as the orientation and fibers of the trapezius muscle.

detached and the tendon is secured with a no. 2 nonabsorbable suture (ORTHOCORD; DePuy Synthes, Warsaw, IN) in a Krackow technique (**Fig. 36.2**). The tendon is then placed in the wound and the tendon transfer site is prepared.

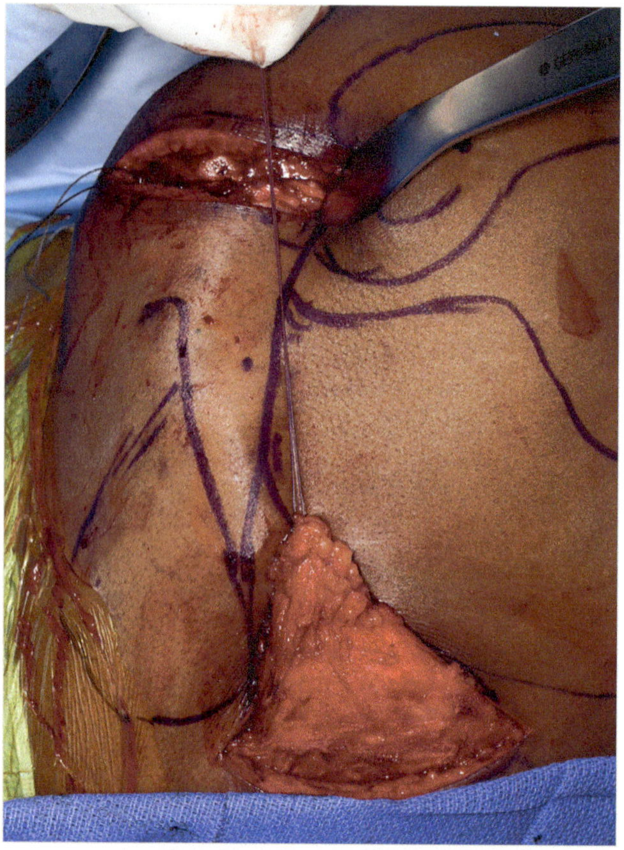

Fig. 36.2 The triangular-shaped lower trapezius tendon following harvest, secured with a Krackow suture.

36.6.1 Paralytic Shoulder

In paralytic shoulders, the infraspinatus tendon is usually intact and its attachment is preserved. A vertical incision is placed just posterior to the lateral end of the acromion over the insertion of the infraspinatus. The posterior deltoid is detached. The infraspinatus tendon is identified and dissected to expose its full extent, which is usually 3 to 4 cm longer than the visible portion. A portion of the superficial muscle should be peeled back to allow visualization of the entire tendinous portion. A Krackow suture is placed in the visible infraspinatus tendon with a no. 2 nonabsorbable suture. A subcutaneous tunnel is created between the medial and lateral wounds and the suture in the lower trapezius tendon is pulled into the medial wound. To relieve tension, finger dissection may be needed to provide length to the tendon. Occasionally, the length is not sufficient to attach the tendons without tension. Therefore, an Achilles tendon allograft should be available. The broad proximal end is secured to the trapezius tendon with multiple sutures, while the distal end is prepared with a Krackow suture, which is used to pull the allograft into the lateral wound. The allograft is sized appropriately, and a free needle can be used to secure the distal end to the intact infraspinatus tendon. The transfer should be performed in maximal external rotation. The end of the Krackow suture in each tendon is then sewn into the other tendon to create a stout repair. TenoGlide (Integra LifeSciences Corporation, Plainsboro, NJ) is routinely placed around the repair to prevent adhesions and maximize the gliding of the tendon transfer.

36.6.2 Massive Posterosuperior Rotator Cuff Tear

When approaching a massive rotator cuff tear, the infraspinatus tendon must always be augmented. The lateral approach involves an incision placed over the lateral edge of the acromion and an osteotomy is performed so that at least 5 mm of lateral acromion is preserved (**Fig. 36.3**). Excellent visualization of the rotator cuff tear is achieved, allowing for the supraspinatus

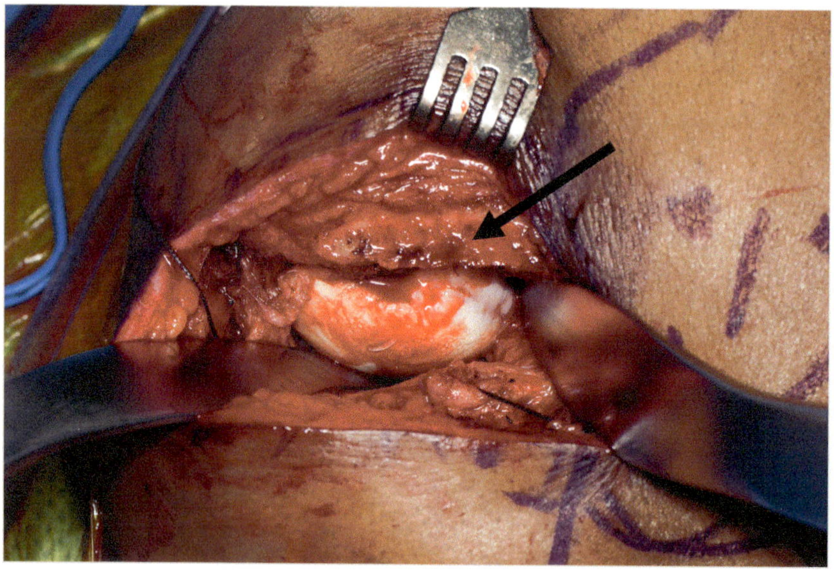

Fig. 36.3 Exposure of the humeral head following an osteotomy of the lateral acromion (*black arrow*). Note the deltoid musculature still attached to the acromion. Note the bare humeral head with a massive posterosuperior rotator cuff tear.

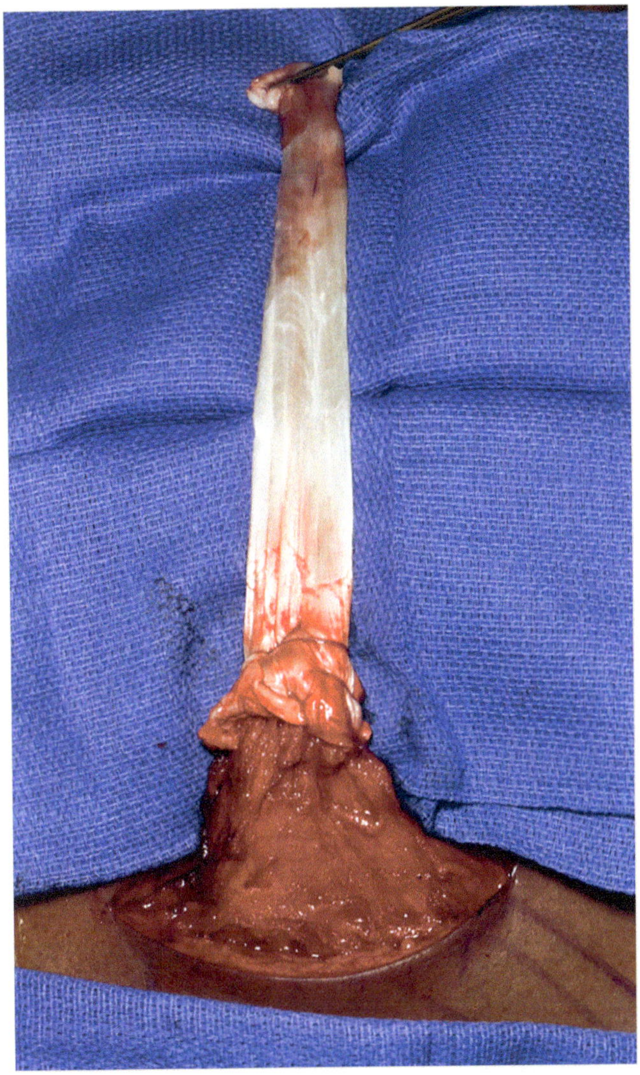

Fig. 36.4 The broad proximal end of the Achilles tendon allograft is secured to the lower trapezius tendon with multiple sutures.

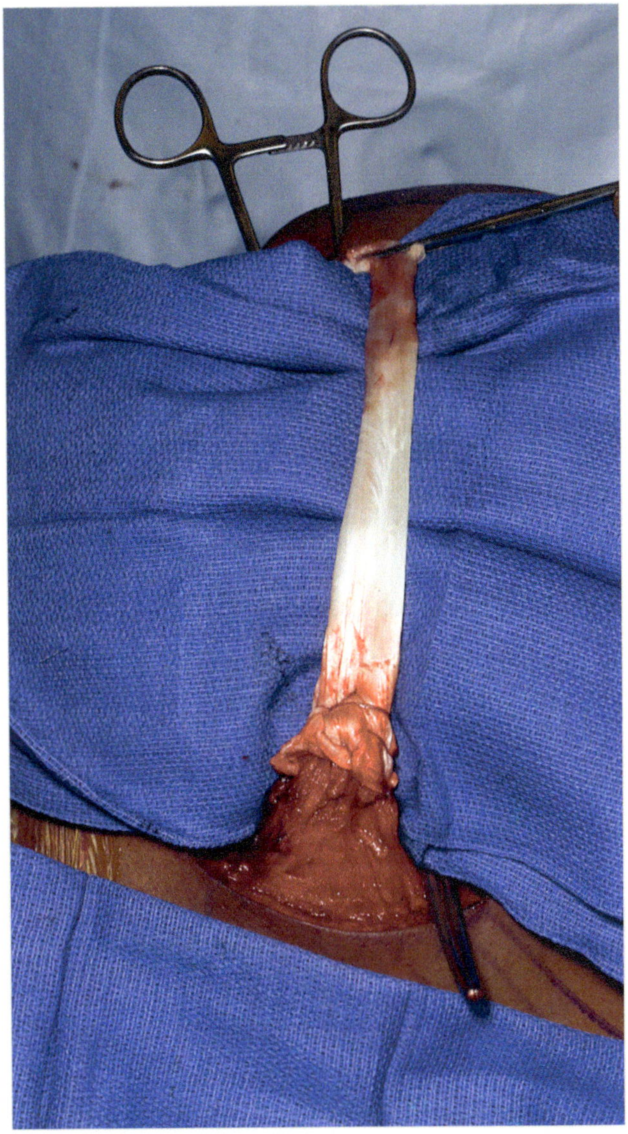

Fig. 36.5 A large curve clamp is passed between the medial and lateral incisions via a subcutaneous tunnel.

and infraspinatus footprint to be identified and debrided. Multiple transosseous sutures or suture anchors are then placed at the footprint.

Meanwhile, an Achilles tendon allograft is prepared with a Krackow suture utilizing a no. 2 nonabsorbable suture. The proximal end of the graft is then laid on the harvested lower trapezius tendon and secured (**Fig. 36.4**). A subcutaneous tunnel is then created between the medial and lateral incisions in a similar fashion to that described earlier, allowing the allograft to be passed into the lateral wound (**Fig. 36.5**). The shoulder is then placed in maximum external rotation and the allograft is appropriately tensioned using the attached sutures. Then, a free needle is used to pass the sutures from the anchors or transosseous position into the distal end of the allograft. Any remaining rotator cuff tissue is sewn into the allograft to improve on the robustness of the transfer.

The acromial osteotomy is then repaired with transosseous strong no. 2 nonabsorbable suture.

36.6.3 Arthroscopically Assisted Technique

An arthroscopically assisted technique may be performed for massive rotator cuff tears.[3] Although this can be performed in the lateral decubitus position, the senior author (BTE) prefers the beach-chair position with a McConnell headpiece and an open back so that the posterior aspect can be draped passed midline (**Fig. 36.6**). Harvest of the lower trapezius transfer is performed as described earlier. The Achilles tendon allograft is prepared in a similar fashion.

A shoulder arthroscopy is performed using a posterior viewing portal that is placed more proximal and lateral than usual. An anterolateral and direct lateral portal are established. The supraspinatus and infraspinatus footprints are identified and prepared with an arthroscopic burr.

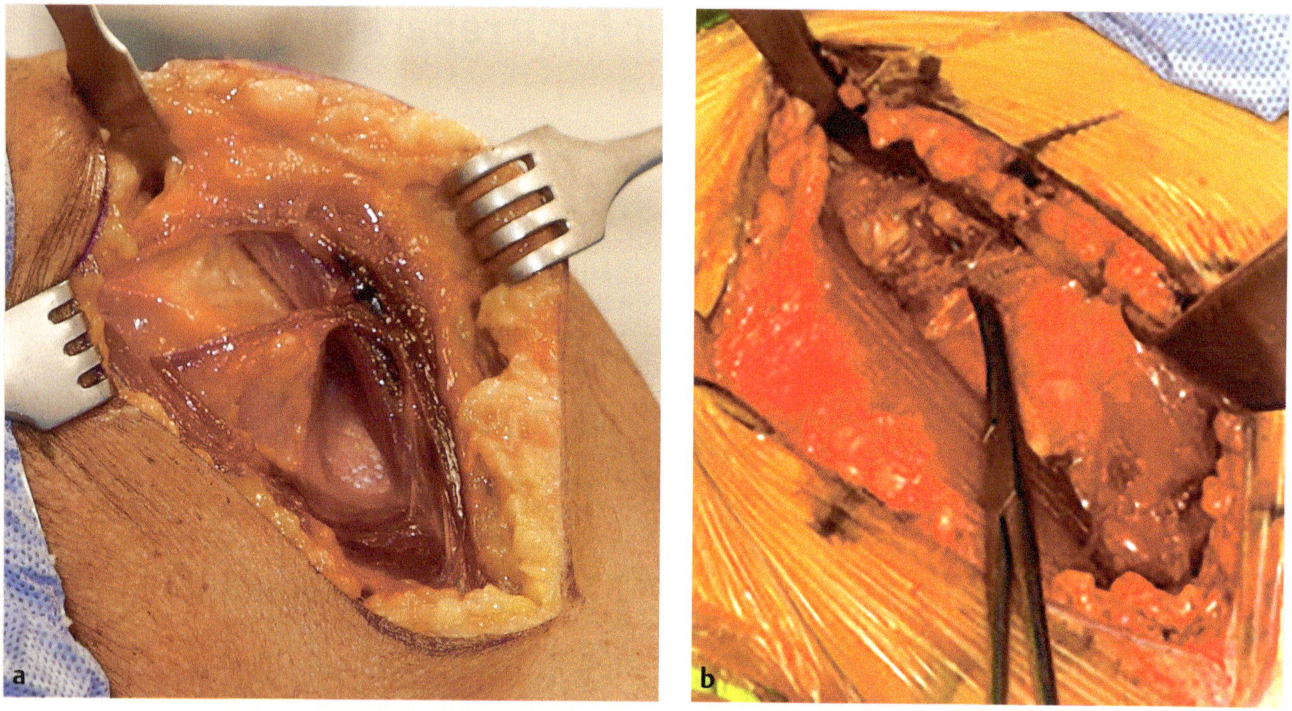

Fig. 37.1 “French vessels” traversing the proximal aspect of the deltopectoral interval.

- Beneath the clavipectoral fascia, the conjoint group is readily visualized and the large subscapularis tear will be identified. Preservation of the frequently intact inferior subscapularis is critical.
- Care must also be taken to identify the long head of the biceps tendon, which may have subluxed from the intertubercular groove. This may be released and tagged for later tenodesis.
- The pectoralis major is then identified and any adhesions around its posterior margin are released. The sternal head of the pectoralis major is isolated by exploiting the natural raphe between the clavicular and sternal heads and bluntly extending it from medial to lateral (**Fig. 37.2**). It is important to avoid dissecting this interval more than 8 cm from the lateral border of the muscle, as this could disrupt the lateral pectoral nerve. The arm is then positioned in forward flexion and internal rotation.
- A plane is then carefully developed between the conjoint group and the pectoralis minor as well as beneath the conjoint muscle/tendon group itself. Care is taken to ensure that the brachial plexus, which sits posteromedially, is protected. This step is completed prior to harvesting to ensure the volume of muscle harvested will pass through this interval.
- Laterally, the fibers of the sternal head are released from their insertion, which lies posterior to the fibers of the clavicular head with the knowledge of the size of the aperture in the retrocoracoid space (**Fig. 37.3**). The released sternal head is then tubularized with no. 2 FiberWire sutures passed in a running Kessler fashion (**Fig. 37.4**).
- The transferred sternal head is then passed posterior to the clavicular head and through the space developed under the conjoint group (**Fig. 37.5**).
- Four no. 5 FiberWire sutures are passed through the sternal head tendon in a Mason–Allen fashion.
- The lesser tuberosity is then prepared by removing soft tissue and decorticating the bone at the planned insertion site of the muscle/tendon transfer.

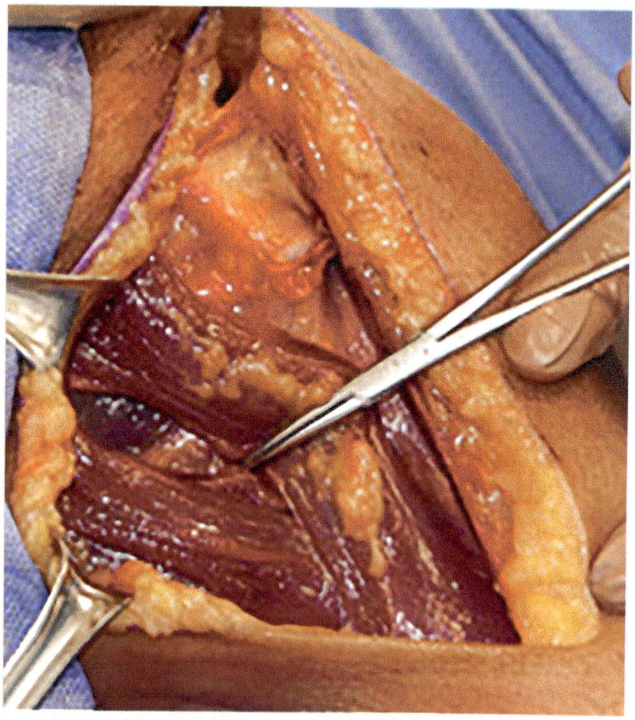

Fig. 37.2 Isolating the sternal head of pectoralis major.

- The sutures of the sternal head are then passed transosseously through the lesser tuberosity (**Fig. 37.6**). Note that the location at which the sutures are passed is carefully chosen to ensure that the transferred sternal head is appropriately tensioned. After transosseous passage of the sutures, they are passed through and tied over a button to prevent the sutures from pulling through the bone. Typically, the sutures are tied from inferior to superior to ensure optimal tensioning (**Fig. 37.7**).

- The arm is then put through a range of motion, paying attention to the degree of external rotation at which the transferred tendon begins to tension.
- The surgical site is copiously irrigated and closed in layered fashion.

37.7.2 Postoperative Physical Therapy Protocol

- Postoperatively, patients are immobilized for a period of 8 weeks, with no active or passive range of motion of the shoulder allowed over the first 4 weeks.
- Elbow, wrist, and hand range of motion is allowed beginning at week 2.
- After week 4, pendulum exercises begin.

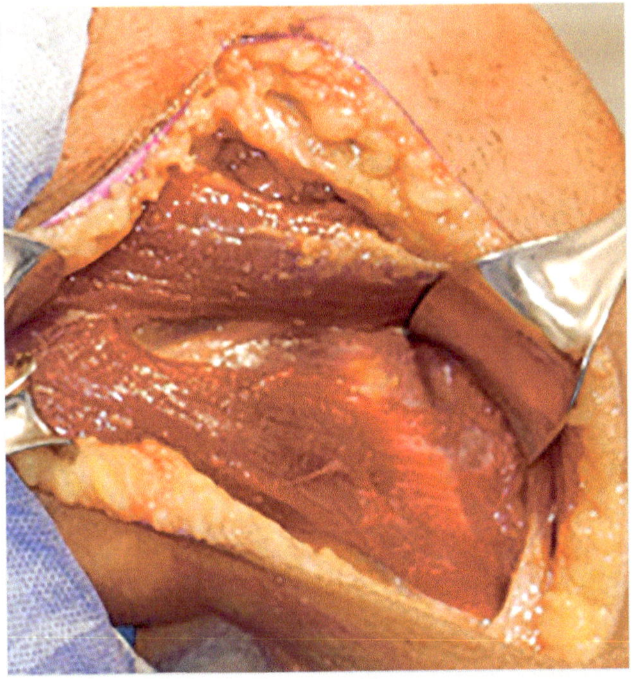

Fig. 37.3 Releasing the fibers of the sternal head, which lie posterior to the clavicular head.

- At week 6, passive supine forward flexion is initiated with a physical therapist. At 8 weeks, active-assisted range of motion is initiated.
- External rotation is limited to 10 degrees for the first 2 weeks and is advanced 10 degrees over the following 2 weeks. Thereafter, passive external rotation is increased 5 degrees per week to a maximum, terminal stop, of 45 degrees of external rotation.
- Beginning at weeks 16 to 18 and once the patient has regained greater than 90 degrees of forward elevation and 30 degrees of external rotation, strengthening exercises are initiated.

37.7.3 Follow-up and Monitoring

- Patients are seen at regular intervals postoperatively to ensure that the surgical site heals appropriately, and that physical therapy is progressing as expected.
- At 6 weeks, pain should have resolved and lingering pain or increased pain, for example, following a session of physical therapy, should raise concern for failure of tendon transfer and may warrant further investigation.

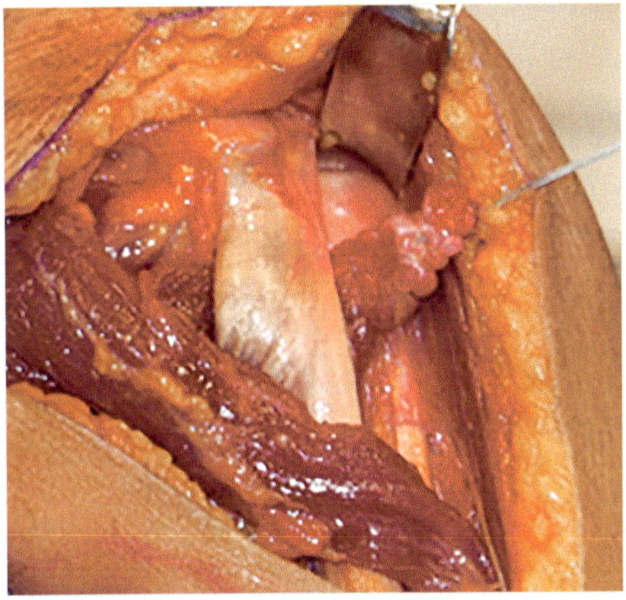

Fig. 37.5 Passing the harvested tendon under the conjoint group.

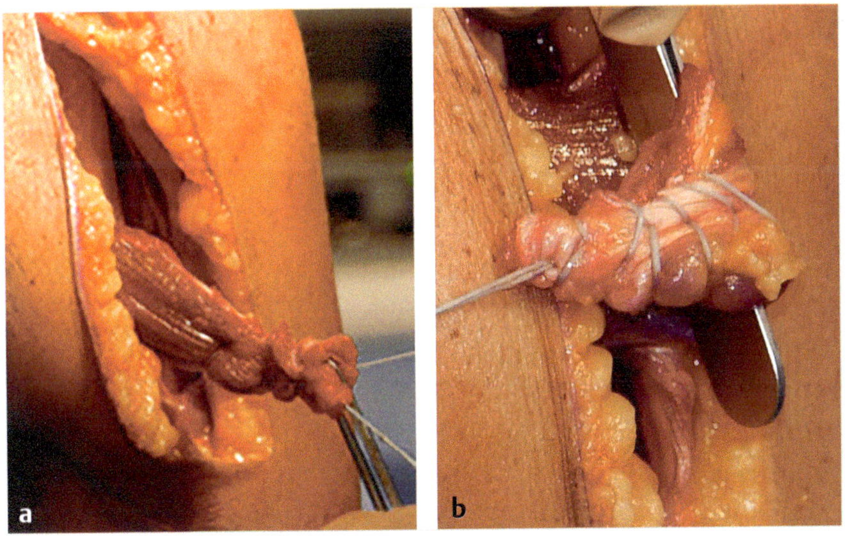

Fig. 37.4 Tubularizing the harvested tendon of the sternal head.

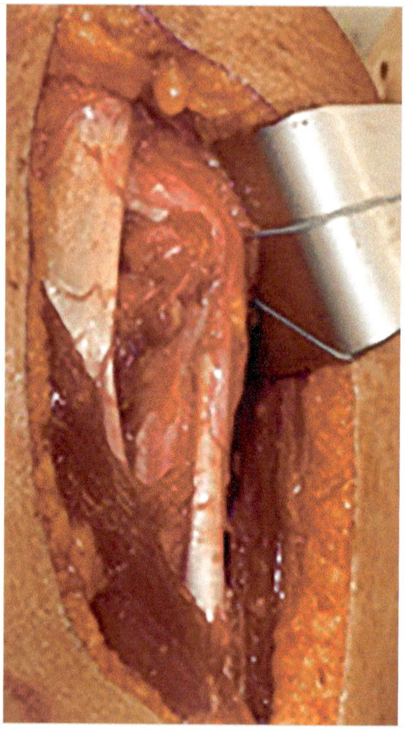

Fig. 37.6 Transosseous passage of the sternal head FiberWire sutures.

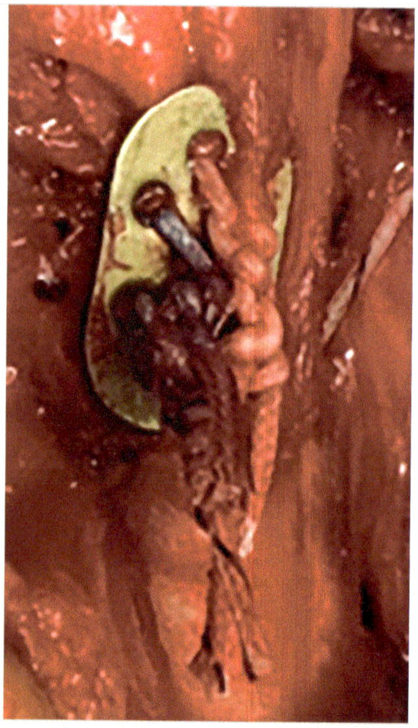

Fig. 37.7 Transosseous FiberWire sutures secured over a button.

- Some patients may be delayed in recovering their range of motion and may be best served by delaying the initiation of the strengthening phase of their rehabilitation.

37.8 Tips, Pearls, and Lessons Learned

The muscle belly of the subscapularis is anatomically positioned posterior, relative to the humeral head. Therefore, the subscapularis stabilizes the humeral head by pulling it posteriorly and inferiorly when the arm is abducted.[10] To best re-create this vector of pull, the sternal head of pectoralis major is routed under the clavicular head and then passed under the conjoined tendon. Both of these aspects of the transfer bring its line of action closer to that of the subscapularis, thereby restabilizing the humeral head. Additionally, when mobilizing the sternal head of the pectoralis major, it is important to avoid dissecting more than 8 cm medial to its insertion, as this could disrupt the lateral pectoral nerve and denervate the clavicular head of pectoralis major.[3,11]

37.9 Pitfalls

37.9.1 Intraoperative

- A considerable amount of scar tissue is frequently encountered. It is important to carefully identify and protect the axillary and musculocutaneous nerves.
- The sternal head of the pectoralis major must be adequately released from the clavicular head and any posterior adhesions must be released for sufficient excursion to enable transfer of the tendon to the appropriate position on the humeral head.
- Care should be taken to avoid disrupting the lateral pectoral nerve when mobilizing the sternal head of pectoralis major.

37.9.2 Late Postoperative

- Adhering to the aforementioned postoperative restrictions, particularly with respect to passive external rotation, as well as the physical therapy protocols is vitally important for a successful outcome. Early aggressive physical therapy may result in failure of fixation of the transferred pectoralis major tendon.

References

1. Rockwood CA Jr, Williams GR Jr, Burkhead WZ Jr. Débridement of degenerative, irreparable lesions of the rotator cuff. J Bone Joint Surg Am 1995;77(6):857–866
2. Burkhart SS. Arthroscopic debridement and decompression for selected rotator cuff tears. Clinical results, pathomechanics, and patient selection based on biomechanical parameters. Orthop Clin North Am 1993;24(1):111–123
3. Resch H, Povacz P, Ritter E, Matschi W. Transfer of the pectoralis major muscle for the treatment of irreparable rupture of the subscapularis tendon. J Bone Joint Surg Am 2000;82(3):372–382
4. Galatz LM, Connor PM, Calfee RP, Hsu JC, Yamaguchi K. Pectoralis major transfer for anterior-superior subluxation in massive rotator cuff insufficiency. J Shoulder Elbow Surg 2003;12(1):1–5

5. Jost B, Puskas GJ, Lustenberger A, Gerber C. Outcome of pectoralis major transfer for the treatment of irreparable subscapularis tears. J Bone Joint Surg Am 2003;85-A(10):1944–1951
6. Jennings GJ, Keereweer S, Buijze GA, De Beer J, DuToit D. Transfer of segmentally split pectoralis major for the treatment of irreparable rupture of the subscapularis tendon. J Shoulder Elbow Surg 2007;16(6):837–842
7. Elhassan B, Ozbaydar M, Massimini D, Diller D, Higgins L, Warner JJ. Transfer of pectoralis major for the treatment of irreparable tears of subscapularis: does it work? J Bone Joint Surg Br 2008;90(8):1059–1065
8 Gavriilidis I, Kircher J, Magosch P, Lichtenberg S, Habermeyer P. Pectoralis major transfer for the treatment of irreparable anterosuperior rotator cuff tears. Int Orthop 2010;34(5):689–694
9. Shin JJ, Saccomanno MF, Cole BJ, Romeo AA, Nicholson GP, Verma NN. Pectoralis major transfer for treatment of irreparable subscapularis tear: a systematic review. Knee Surg Sports Traumatol Arthrosc 2016;24(6):1951–1960
10. Warner JJ. Management of massive irreparable rotator cuff tears: the role of tendon transfer. Instr Course Lect 2001;50:63–71
11. Klepps SJ, Goldfarb C, Flatow E, Galatz LM, Yamaguchi K. Anatomic evaluation of the subcoracoid pectoralis major transfer in human cadavers. J Shoulder Elbow Surg 2001;10(5):453–459

Part III

Arthritis/Arthroplasty

38 Comprehensive Arthroscopic Management Procedure for the Treatment of Glenohumeral Osteoarthritis

Sandeep Mannava, Salvatore J. Frangiamore, Erik M. Fritz, Justin J. Mitchell, and Peter J. Millett

Abstract

The goal of arthroscopic management of shoulder arthritis is to address the multiple generators of pain associated with the degenerative shoulder joint. This is accomplished primarily with glenohumeral debridement, lysis of adhesion, osteoplasty, neurolysis, capsular release, and microfracture if indicated. This multimodal approach to anatomic pain generators results in restoration of motion and reduction of pain for the patient with good two-year survival and improvement in outcome scores. Appropriate patient selection is important to successful outcomes as the comprehensive arthroscopic management procedure is best suited to younger patients or more active older patients desiring joint preservation.

Keywords: *arthroscopy, arthritis, shoulder*

38.1 Goals of Procedure

Glenohumeral osteoarthritis (GHOA) is a debilitating condition that can lead to shoulder pain, loss of function, and decreased quality of life.[1] Cadaveric studies have demonstrated that the disease prevalence may be as high as 20 to 30% in patients older than 60 years.[2] When nonoperative treatment fails, many patients seek surgical options for palliation of their pain and to improve their function.

Traditionally, surgical treatment for shoulder osteoarthritis with an intact rotator cuff is prosthetic joint replacement with either total shoulder arthroplasty (TSA) or hemiarthroplasty (HA). Arthroplasty options in this setting have the benefits of pain relief and functional improvements with good to excellent patient-reported outcomes, predictability, and durability.[3] In recent years, the number of TSAs performed has increased. In 2008, approximately 27,000 TSAs and 20,000 HAs were performed.[4] This increased to 30,000 TSAs and 15,000 HAs in 2011.[5] However, there remains a subset of patients with symptomatic GHOA in which shoulder arthroplasty may not be ideal or desirable. This is especially true in relatively young and active patients, manual laborers, or those with high demands for the upper extremity.[6,7] This patient population may benefit from arthroscopic and minimally invasive treatments for shoulder osteoarthritis in an attempt to relieve pain, restore function, and preserve the native anatomy.[8]

This chapter presents the Comprehensive Arthroscopic Management (CAM) procedure, which was developed as a minimally invasive surgical intervention to address shoulder osteoarthritis arthroscopically. This is a joint-preserving procedure that attempts to surgically address the pain generators in GHOA, thereby decreasing patient pain and improving quality of life. Ultimately, the procedure strives to avoid or delay shoulder arthroplasty without compromising the local bony or soft-tissue anatomy in the event that an arthroplasty becomes necessary at a later time.

38.2 Advantages

The CAM procedure aims to address known pain generators about the shoulder with minimally invasive surgical techniques. The components of the CAM procedure include arthroscopic glenohumeral joint debridement, loose body removal, chondroplasty, synovectomy, inferior humeral osteoplasty, axillary nerve neurolysis, and capsular release when indicated. Subcoracoid decompression, subacromial decompression, and biceps tenodesis are also frequently performed when indicated.

38.3 Indications

Indications for the CAM procedure include patients with advanced symptomatic GHOA who are young, active, or desire joint-preserving treatment. Patients with osteoarthritic changes on either the humeral or the glenoid surface and who have failed an extensive course of nonsurgical management including activity modification, anti-inflammatory medications, physical therapy, viscosupplementation, or corticosteroid injections are good candidates for the CAM procedure (**Table 38.1**).

38.4 Contraindications

Patients should not undergo CAM procedure if they are found to have mild or early-stage osteoarthritis or have not attempted conservative measures. Additional contraindications include severely incongruous joint space and severe deformity. Relative contraindications include less than 2 mm of glenohumeral joint space, acetabulization of the acromion, and significant superior

Table 38.1 Indications and contraindications for CAM procedure.

Indications	Contraindications
Advanced symptomatic GHOA	*Absolute*
Young	Mild GHOA
Active	Have not attempted conservative treatment
Desire joint preservation	Incongruous joint space and severe deformity
Failed nonsurgical management	
	Relative
	<2 mm GH joint space
	Severely limited GH PROM (especially IR)
	Large osteophytes
	Bipolar chondral lesions
	Low critical shoulder angle
	Kellgren–Lawrence grade III or IV arthritis
	Walch type B2 or C glenoid changes

Abbreviations: GH, glenohumeral; GHOA, glenohumeral osteoarthritis; GH, glenohumeral; IR, internal rotation; PROM, passive range of motion.

humeral head migration.[9] Other factors that are often present and may lead to slightly inferior outcomes are severely limited passive glenohumeral motion (especially internal rotation), large osteophytes, bipolar chondral lesions, low critical shoulder angle, Kellgren–Lawrence grade III or IV arthritis, and Walch type B2 or C glenoid changes (**Table 38.1**).[10–12] However, the CAM procedure does seek to arthroscopically address some of these clinical, physical examination, and radiographic findings.

38.5 Operating Room Setup, Preoperative Preparation, and Patient Positioning

An interscalene nerve block is used for postoperative analgesia. After induction of general anesthesia, the patient is positioned in the beach-chair position (Tenet T-Max Beach Chair and Spider arm positioner; Smith & Nephew, Memphis, TN; **Fig. 38.1**). The surgeon then performs an examination of the surgical and contralateral shoulders; in particular, the range of motion (ROM) is assessed for deficits. Capsular contractures resulting in an ROM deficit, which are noted on the examination under anesthesia, of more than 15 degrees in any plane are consistent with capsular contracture and may warrant the addition of a capsular release to the procedure. Loss of shoulder abduction is consistent with the inferior humeral osteophyte (known as the "goat's beard"; **Fig. 38.2**) and resection/osteoplasty of this region improves movement in this plane of motion (**Fig. 38.2**).[13]

A dynamic fluoroscopic examination is then undertaken using intraoperative fluoroscopy. Prior to sterile preparation, the surgeon should ensure that the humeral head osteophyte can be completely visualized utilizing fluoroscopy of the shoulder in both internal and external rotations of the humerus (**Fig. 38.1**). Standard preparation and draping are performed, to include sterile draping of the C arm, such that adequacy of osteophyte resection can later be radiographically confirmed (**Fig. 38.1**).

38.6 Operative Technique

Standard arthroscopic portals are placed, including a posterior viewing portal (~2 cm inferior and 2 cm medial to the posterolateral corner of the acromion) and an anterosuperior working portal through the rotator interval. The procedure is performed with visualization using a standard 30-degree arthroscope. We avoid entry into the subacromial or subcoracoid spaces and do not release the capsule until after the inferior humeral head osteophyte is resected to avoid fluid extravasation. Similarly, the axillary nerve neurolysis and capsular releases (**Fig. 38.3**) are performed prior to entry into the subacromial space to avoid excessive extravasation, as this

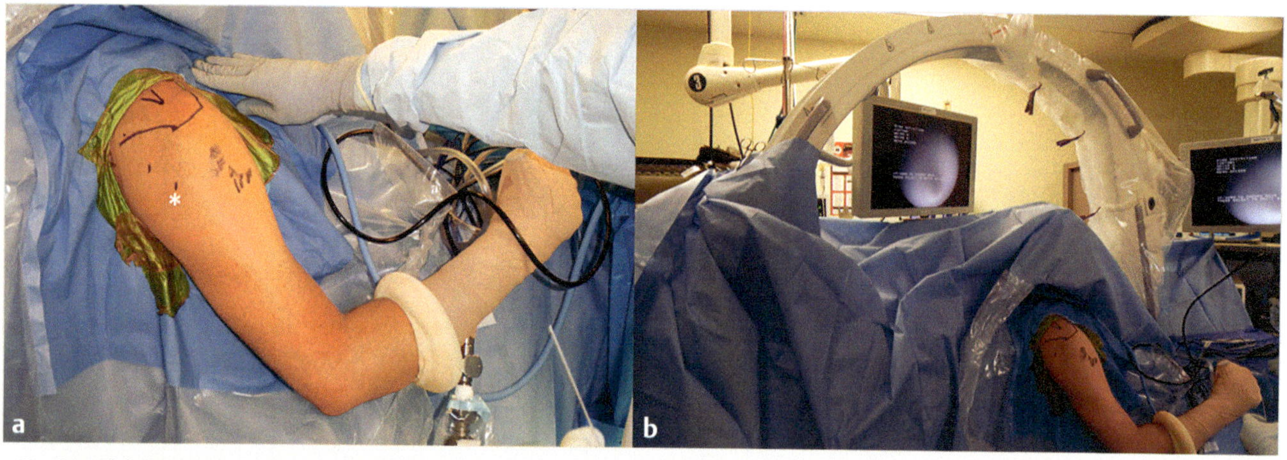

Fig. 38.1 (a) Patient prepped and draped in the beach-chair position (*, accessory posterior inferolateral portal at the 7 o'clock position). (b) C-arm draped along with patient to permit intraoperative confirmation of osteophyte resection.

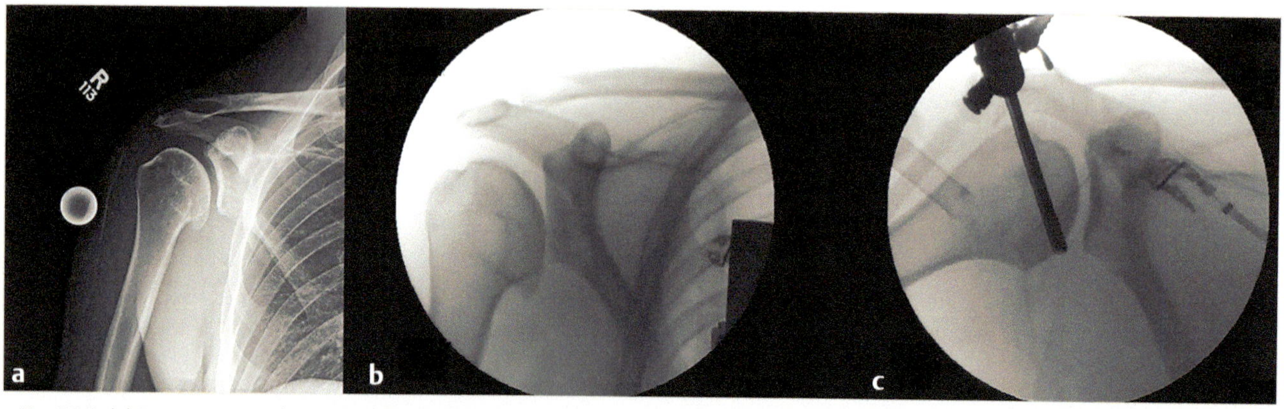

Fig. 38.2 (a) Preoperative radiograph demonstrating "goat's beard" deformity. (b) Intraoperative fluoroscopy visualizing the "goat's beard." (c) Fluoroscopy confirming complete resection of the "goat's beard."

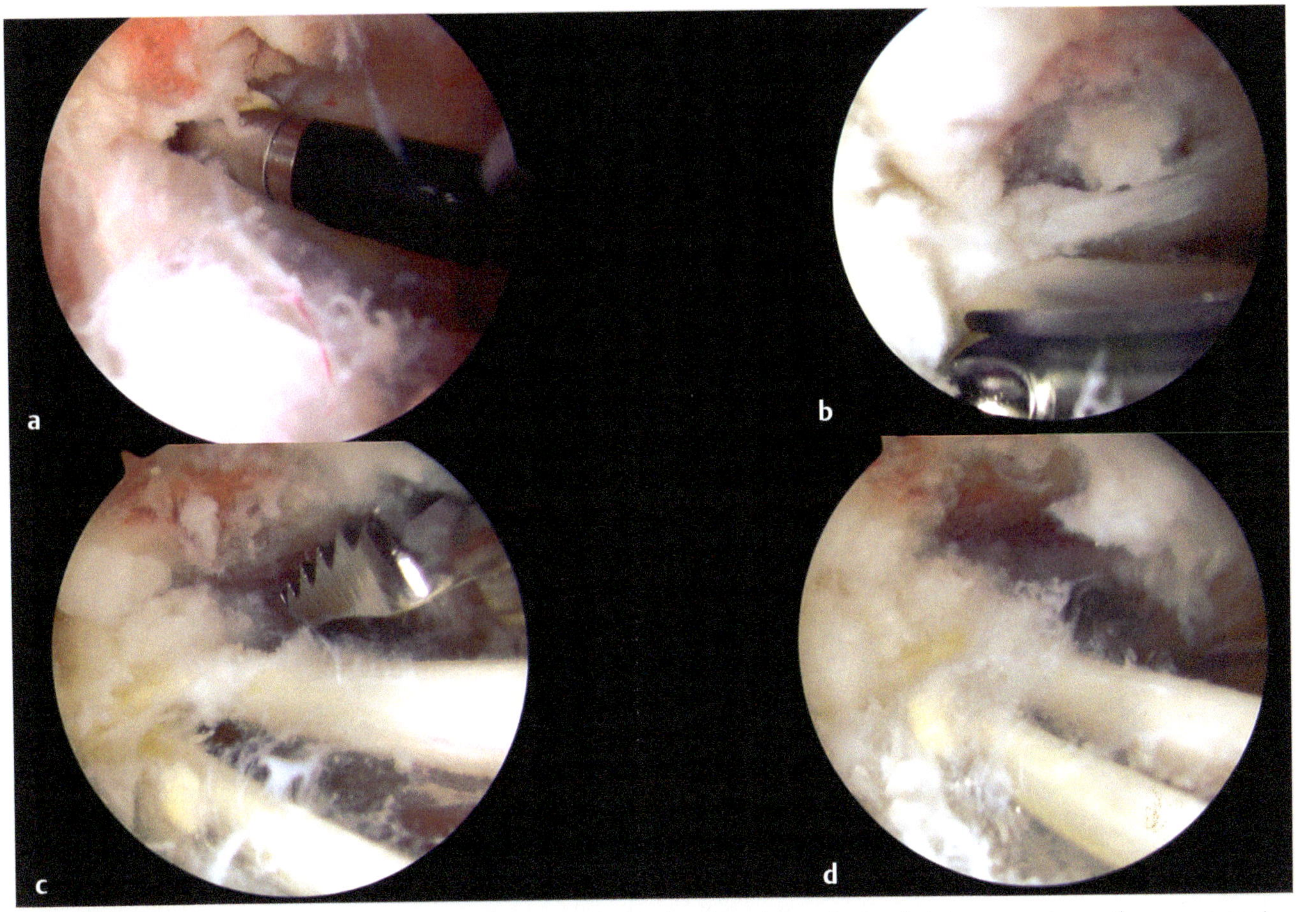

Fig. 38.3 (a) Inferior capsular release to access the axillary nerve. (b) The inferior humeral osteophyte is compressing on the nerve, a possible source of pain. (c) A rasp is used to smooth the resected surface. (d) Axillary nerve following completed neurolysis.

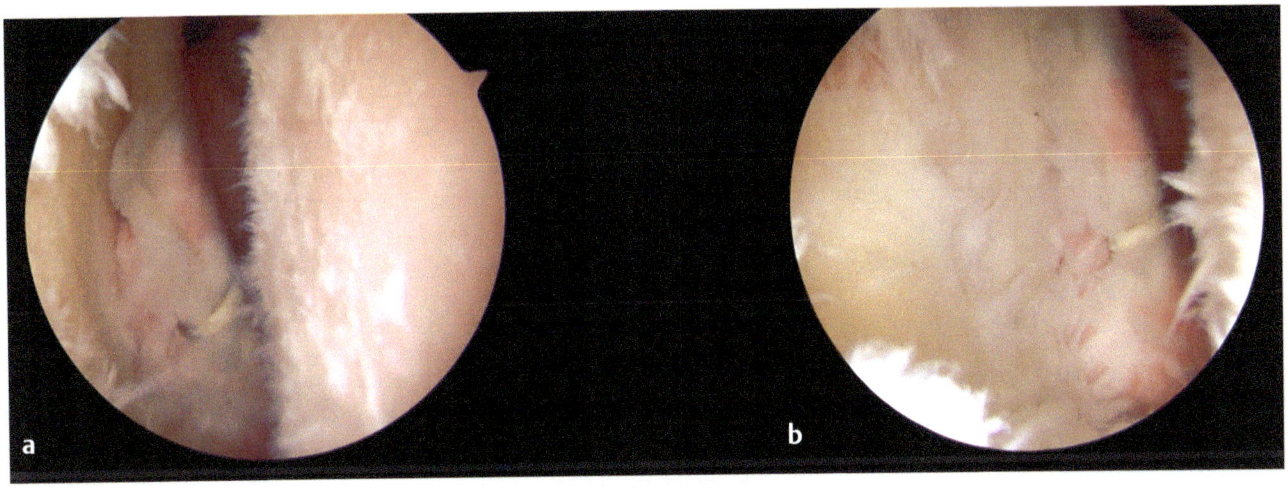

Fig. 38.4 (a) Osteoarthritis of the humeral head. (b) Osteoarthritis of the glenoid.

makes surgical intervention in the inferior capsular recess difficult and potentially dangerous.

38.6.1 Diagnostic Arthroscopy and Extensive Debridement

Upon entry into the glenohumeral joint, and after establishment of the standard viewing and working portals, a diagnostic arthroscopy is performed to evaluate the humeral and glenoid articular surfaces, the labrum, biceps tendon, rotator cuff, and capsuloligamentous structures. An extensive debridement is performed including loose body removal, chondroplasty, and synovectomy (**Fig. 38.4**, **Fig. 38.5**). Following debridement, preparation for microfracture of any small focal chondral lesions with stable chondral borders is undertaken. Microfracture is generally not performed until just prior to leaving the joint, and thus the nascent clot is not disrupted.[9]

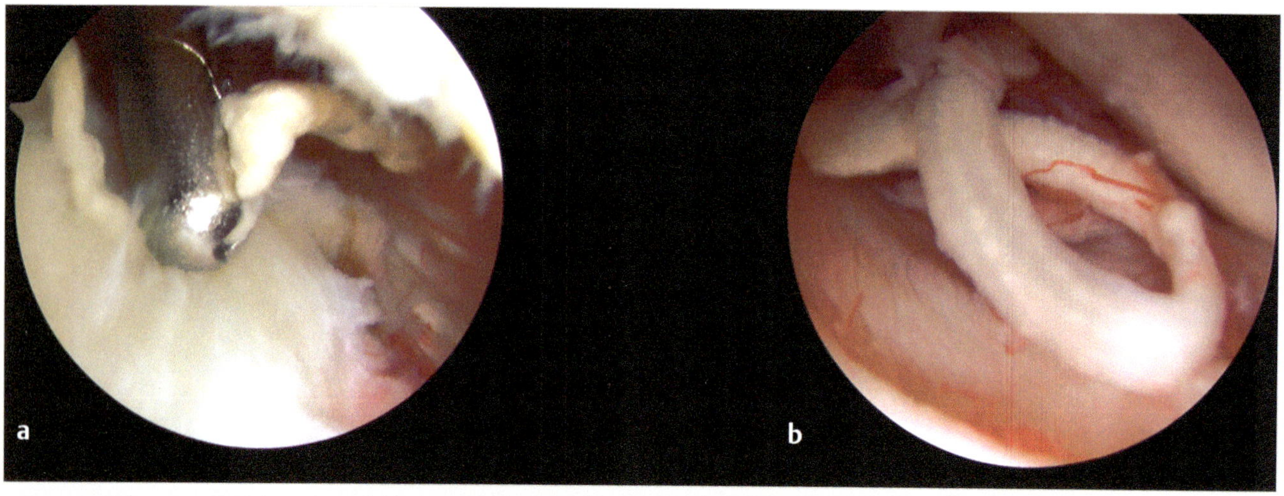

Fig. 38.5 (a) Removal of loose bodies with an arthroscopic grasper. (b) Foreign body from previous procedure in the capsular recess, a potential source of joint pain.

Chondral loose body removal is facilitated either by morcellation with an arthroscopic shaver and suction or by removal with an arthroscopic grasper (**Fig 38.5a**). Chondral surfaces that are unstable are stabilized via chondroplasty using a mechanical shaver. After addressing loose bodies (**Fig. 38.5**) and the chondral surfaces of the glenohumeral joint (**Fig. 38.4**), exuberant and hypertrophied synovitis can be addressed utilizing the radiofrequency (RF) electrocautery. The RF device is also utilized for release of rotator interval adhesions. The capsule is preserved at this point so as to avoid excessive fluid extravasation.

The long head of the biceps tendon is carefully assessed arthroscopically. In particular, the tendon is pulled into the joint with an arthroscopic probe and the length of the visualized tendon is examined for fraying, splits, tears, and tenosynovitis. When there is severe long head of the biceps tendon degeneration, biceps pulley incompetence, an hourglass deformity, or a superior labral anteroposterior (SLAP) injury, the long head of the biceps tendon is released and a tenodesis is subsequently performed after all the arthroscopic work is completed. Our preference is to perform a mini-open subpectoral biceps tenodesis with unicortical fixation with a polyetheretherketone (PEEK) tenodesis screw (Arthrex, Naples, FL) near the conclusion of the procedure.

38.6.2 Humeral Osteoplasty for Resection of the Inferior Humeral Osteophyte

Osteoarthritis of the shoulder is frequently associated with a large inferior humeral head osteophyte (known as the "goat's beard" deformity), which is readily identified radiographically[7] (**Fig. 38.2**). Preoperatively, if the patient has posterior or lateral shoulder pain corresponding to the axillary nerve distribution, displacement of the nerve on MRI of more than 5 mm, teres minor atrophy, a positive EMG for axillary neuropathy, or evidence of capsular encroachment at the time of arthroscopy, then an osteoplasty of the inferior humeral head, inferior capsulotomy, and axillary neurolysis are performed.[13]

To facilitate performing these procedures and to gain access to the inferior axillary capsular recess, an accessory posterior-inferolateral portal at the 7 o'clock position is created (**Fig. 38.1**). This accessory portal is located approximately 5 cm inferior to the posterolateral acromion. The portal is created under direct visualization with an 18-gauge spinal needle localized to the medial and central third of the inferior shoulder joint capsule, which is located anterior to the posterior band of the inferior glenohumeral ligament. Creation of this portal is done carefully to avoid iatrogenic injury to the axillary nerve. After marking the skin location of the portal based upon needle localization, only a superficial skin incision is made and the path into the joint is bluntly created through the soft tissues using a 2.6-mm switching stick. The path is bluntly dilated sequentially with cannula dilators. A self-retaining 8.25-mm cannula (Gemini Cannula, Arthrex) is used as this prevents back-out of the cannula with the potential to injure the axillary nerve. The self-retaining cannula also facilitates retraction of the joint capsule while allowing for large shavers, burrs, and curettes to be used to remove the hypertrophic bone from the inferior spur.

Removal of the inferior "goat's beard" osteophyte (**Fig. 38.2**) is performed to decompress the axillary nerve and facilitate motion by removing the mechanical block. An arthroscopic 5.5-mm bone-cutting shaver and burr with a hooded shield is used to resect the inferior osteophyte utilizing the established 7 o'clock position accessory portal. It is important to preserve the inferior capsular tissue during osteophyte resection, as the capsule provides a layer of protection for the axillary nerve, which runs close to this region. Furthermore, preservation of the inferior capsule prevents excessive fluid extravasation. Inferior humeral osteoplasty is aided by periodic fluoroscopic evaluation utilizing C-arm imaging while internally and externally rotating the arm (**Fig. 38.2**). Occasionally, it is helpful to utilize a curved curette to remove hypertrophic bone, especially in the anteroinferior region where motorized instrumentation is difficult to manipulate. The final resection surface is smoothed with a rasp (**Fig. 38.3c**).

38.6.3 Inferior Capsular Release and Axillary Nerve Neurolysis

The preoperative evaluation of the patient's shoulder motion is utilized to determine the extent of the shoulder joint capsular release. The release of the inferior joint capsule facilitates axillary neurolysis (**Fig. 38.3a**). Again, the inferior humeral head osteoplasty is completed prior to resection of the osteophyte to avoid iatrogenic injury to the axillary nerve and excessive fluid extravasation.

Capsulotomy is initiated in the inferior shoulder joint by the cannula insertion site and performed utilizing a hook-tip RF electrocautery device (CoolCut 90-degree hook tip; Arthrex). This transmits less energy and is less likely to injure the axillary nerve. Alternatively, arthroscopic scissors can be used to perform the capsulotomy. The capsulotomy should be performed under direct visualization using either the 30- or the 70-degree arthroscope.

The axillary nerve is typically found, on average, 2.5 mm from the inferior glenohumeral ligament, and an axillary neurolysis is performed bluntly under direct visualization with a probe and arthroscopic punches (**Fig. 38.3**). The neurolysis is initiated along the length of the nerve from proximal to distal. The proximal extent of the axillary nerve is first identified as it courses inferior to the subscapularis tendon. The distal extent of the nerve courses between the teres minor and major tendons. The nerve has numerous arborizations and care is taken to preserve these various innervations to the teres minor and deltoid musculature during blunt dissection and neurolysis. Once the axillary nerve is free from its overlying and surrounding soft tissue and bony impingement no longer occurs, the neurolysis is considered complete (**Fig. 38.3**).

38.6.4 Anterior and Posterior Capsular Releases

Anterior and posterior capsulotomies are then performed. Scar and synovitis are debrided from the rotator interval prior to the anterior capsule being divided from the rotator interval to the 5 o'clock position by visualizing from the standard posterior portal. All tissue is typically removed until the entire subcoracoid space is well visualized. Loose bodies are often found in the subscapularis recess. These should always be checked for on imaging and with direct arthroscopic visualization; when encountered, these loose bodies can be removed by enlarging the anterosuperior portal. An RF probe is then used to perform the capsulotomy lateral to the labrum at the capsulolabral junction. Care is taken during anterior capsulotomy to avoid damage to the subscapularis. The entire subcoracoid space is visualized and freed to restore the normal scapulohumeral motion interface.

The arthroscope is then repositioned to the anterior portal and a posterior capsular release is performed from the 7 o'clock to the 11 o'clock position. This is done at the capsulolabral junction to avoid injury to the tendinous insertion of the rotator cuff, which is more lateral. The arm should then be reexamined under anesthesia; adequate release of the capsule and resection of the inferior humeral head osteophyte should result in restored passive motion.

38.7 Microfracture (if Indicated)

After assessment and debridement of the glenohumeral joint and treatment of the inferior humeral osteophyte and release of the capsule, isolated or focal Outerbridge grade IV small chondral injuries (1–2 cm^2) with stable rims can be treated with microfracture. Our preferred technique for microfracture includes debriding the calcified cartilage layer with a curette, followed by perforation of the underlying subchondral bone with microfracture picks to a depth of 2 to 4 mm under arthroscopic visualization, using a power microfracture awl (Powerpick, Arthrex). The bone perforations should be 3 mm apart and evenly spaced throughout the cartilage defect. After completing the microfracture procedure, inflow of arthroscopic fluid is temporarily stopped and egress of fat droplets, blood, and marrow should be observed. The arthroscope is then removed from the joint to allow the clot to form. Microfracture, when needed, is performed last so that blood will not obscure visualization and so that the "superclot" can form in the defect.

38.7.1 Supplemental Procedures

Other pain generators about the shoulder joint that are often associated with glenohumeral arthritis are subcoracoid impingement, subacromial impingement, and biceps tendonitis, tearing, or subluxation. These entities are assessed preoperatively and intraoperatively and subcoracoid decompression, subacromial decompression, and subpectoral biceps tenodesis are performed based upon an individual patient's pathoanatomy.

Radiographic and intraoperative criteria for coracoplasty are a coracohumeral interval less than 8 mm in females and 10 mm in males. The interval is restored utilizing an arthroscopic burr to resect the coracoid. After successful coracoplasty, the coracoid is anteriorized, medialized, and superiorized.

The arthroscope is then inserted into the subacromial space through the posterior portal and subacromial bursectomy is performed. A modified cutting block technique using an arthroscopic burr can be utilized to address type III acromions or other impingement lesions identified. A thorough bursectomy is performed to restore the normal scapulohumeral motion interface.

Long head of the biceps pathology identified during glenohumeral arthroscopy is addressed via open subpectoral biceps tenodesis using a small incision in the axillary fold. The biceps tendon that was previously tenotomized is identified in the interval between the pectoralis major and the conjoint tendons; it is then affixed to the subpectoral humeral bone utilizing either a 7- or an 8-mm unicortical socket with PEEK tenodesis screw (Arthrex).

38.7.2 Manipulation under Anesthesia

Following all the releases and the subacromial arthroscopy with associated procedures, the shoulder is manipulated gently in all planes with internal and external rotation to restore full mobility.

38.8 Tips and Pearls

- Prior to sterile preparation, ensure that the humeral head osteophyte can be completely visualized utilizing fluoroscopy of the shoulder in internal and external rotation of the humerus.
- To gain access to the inferior axillary capsular recess, an accessory posterior-inferolateral portal at the 7 o'clock

position is created (**Fig. 38.1**). Only a superficial skin incision is made and the path into the joint is bluntly created using a 2.6-mm switching stick.
- A self-retaining cannula is used to prevent back-out of the cannula, thus avoiding injury to the axillary nerve.

38.9 What to Avoid

- Avoid entry into the subacromial or subcoracoid space and do not release the glenohumeral join capsule until after the inferior humeral head osteophyte is resected to avoid fluid extravasation.
- Axillary nerve neurolysis and capsular releases (**Fig. 38.3**) are performed prior to entry into the subacromial space to avoid excessive extravasation, as this makes surgical intervention in the inferior capsular recess difficult and potentially dangerous.
- Creation of the accessory posterior-inferolateral portal is done carefully under direct visualization with an 18-gauge spinal needle, followed by serial blunt dilation to avoid iatrogenic injury to the axillary nerve.

38.10 Complications

- Extreme care must be taken during the CAM procedure to avoid iatrogenic injury to the axillary nerve during establishment of the accessory portal, osteoplasty, and neurolysis.
- Patients for whom the CAM procedure does not provide sufficient pain relief will ultimately have to progress to TSA or hemiarthroplasty (provided their rotator cuff is intact and functional). Careful preoperative discussions need to occur so that the patients are adequately informed about the benefits and limitations of the procedure.

38.11 Postoperative Care

Rehabilitation is initiated immediately following surgery. The focus of rehabilitation is to improve or maintain the motion that was gained by the CAM procedure. Successful rehabilitation is aimed to prevent recurrent scarring and contraction, while improving upon glenohumeral and scapulothoracic mechanics. Our rehabilitation protocol for the CAM procedure follows three general phases, the first of which emphasizes passive and active shoulder motion during the first 6 weeks following surgery. The second phase of CAM rehabilitation focuses on strengthening the shoulder around 6 to 12 weeks postoperatively. The third and final CAM rehabilitation phase focuses most on functional return to activities, which is typically initiated 3 months postoperatively. We counsel our patients that maximal recovery and benefit is often seen 4 to 6 months postoperatively.

38.12 Conclusion

Arthroscopic management of shoulder arthritis is aimed at addressing various pain generators located about the degenerative shoulder joint. By systematically addressing the pain generators and pathophysiology, the patient who undergoes the CAM procedure should have restored shoulder motion and reduced pain. The CAM procedure does have some associated surgical risks; however, meticulous surgical technique helps prevent potential pitfalls and mitigates risk.[14] The CAM procedure does address axillary nerve compression, which differs from some previous arthroscopic approaches to GHOA.[11,12]

Previous research outcomes with minimum 2-year follow-up demonstrated 92% survivorship at 1 year and 85% at 2 years; American Shoulder and Elbow Surgeons scores improved from 58 to 83 points; pain significantly decreased with activities of daily living, work, recreation, and sleep; and median patient satisfaction was 9 out of 10.[15] At minimum 5-year follow-up, Mitchell et al demonstrated 76.9% survivorship for the CAM procedure.[16] When counseling patients preoperatively, it is important to indicate that the CAM procedure may delay progression to arthroplasty. However, approximately 23.1% of patients in our experience have GHOA progression despite undergoing the CAM procedure at 5-year follow-up.[16]

Based on previous literature, the CAM procedure is better suited for younger patients or those active older patients who desire a joint-preserving solution, whereas TSA may be of greater benefit to patients older than 65 years.[8] For patients between ages 47 and 65 years, the literature shows no difference between treatment strategies and clinical judgment should guide optimal management. Moreover, the treating surgeon should not have firm age cutoffs for the CAM procedure; instead, the surgeon should customize surgical intervention based upon the patient's pathology, function, comorbidities, and postsurgical demands.

References

1. Memel DS, Kirwan JR, Sharp DJ, Hehir M. General practitioners miss disability and anxiety as well as depression in their patients with osteoarthritis. Br J Gen Pract 2000;50(457):645–648
2. Kerr R, Resnick D, Pineda C, Haghighi P. Osteoarthritis of the glenohumeral joint: a radiologic-pathologic study. AJR Am J Roentgenol 1985;144(5):967–972
3. Deshmukh AV, Koris M, Zurakowski D, Thornhill TS. Total shoulder arthroplasty: long-term survivorship, functional outcome, and quality of life. J Shoulder Elbow Surg 2005;14(5):471–479
4. Kim SH, Wise BL, Zhang Y, Szabo RM. Increasing incidence of shoulder arthroplasty in the United States. J Bone Joint Surg Am 2011;93(24):2249–2254
5. Schairer WW, Nwachukwu BU, Lyman S, Craig EV, Gulotta LV. National utilization of reverse total shoulder arthroplasty in the United States. J Shoulder Elbow Surg 2015;24(1):91–97
6. George MS. Arthroscopic management of shoulder osteoarthritis. Open Orthop J 2008;2(1):23–26
7. Millett PJ, Gaskill TR. Arthroscopic management of glenohumeral arthrosis: humeral osteoplasty, capsular release, and arthroscopic axillary nerve release as a joint-preserving approach. Arthroscopy 2011;27(9):1296–1303
8. Spiegl UJ, Faucett SC, Horan MP, Warth RJ, Millett PJ. The role of arthroscopy in the management of glenohumeral osteoarthritis: a Markov decision model. Arthroscopy 2014;30(11):1392–1399
9. Millett PJ, Huffard BH, Horan MP, Hawkins RJ, Steadman JR. Outcomes of full-thickness articular cartilage injuries of the shoulder treated with microfracture. Arthroscopy 200.9;25(8):856–863

10. Warner BT, et al. Arthroscopic management of glenohumeral osteoarthritis: Prospective evaluation of factors associated with success. Paper presented at the Arthroscopy Association of North America Annual Meeting. Los Angeles, CA; 2015
11. Van Thiel GS, Sheehan S, Frank RM, et al. Retrospective analysis of arthroscopic management of glenohumeral degenerative disease. Arthroscopy 2010;26(11):1451–1455
12. Weinstein DM, Bucchieri JS, Pollock RG, Flatow EL, Bigliani LU. Arthroscopic debridement of the shoulder for osteoarthritis. Arthroscopy 2000;16(5):471–476
13. Millett PJ, Schoenahl JY, Allen MJ, Motta T, Gaskill TR. An association between the inferior humeral head osteophyte and teres minor fatty infiltration: evidence for axillary nerve entrapment in glenohumeral osteoarthritis. J Shoulder Elbow Surg 2013;22(2):215–221
14. Mook WR, Petri M, Greenspoon JA, Millett PJ. The comprehensive Arthroscopic Management procedure for treatment of glenohumeral osteoarthritis. Arthrosc Tech 2015;4(5):e435–e441
15. Millett PJ, Horan MP, Pennock AT, Rios D. Comprehensive Arthroscopic Management (CAM) procedure: clinical results of a joint-preserving arthroscopic treatment for young, active patients with advanced shoulder osteoarthritis. Arthroscopy 2013;29(3):440–448
16. Mitchell JJ, Horan MP, Greenspoon JA, Menge TJ, Tahal DS, Millett PJ. Survivorship and patient-reported outcomes after Comprehensive Arthroscopic Management of glenohumeral osteoarthritis: minimum 5-year follow-up. Am J Sports Med 2016;44(12):3206–3213

39 Deltopectoral Approach for Shoulder Arthroplasty

Wame N. Waggenspack, Jr. and T. Bradley Edwards

Abstract

The deltopectoral approach, utilizing the internervous plane between the deltoid (axillary nerve) and the pectoralis major (medial and lateral pectoral nerves), is the standard for shoulder arthroplasty, allows unhindered access to the anterior glenohumeral joint, and is fully extensile to the anterolateral approach to the humerus. Following a stepwise surgical technique allows reliable and reproducible humeral and glenoid exposure for optimal preparation and implantation of components. We present our preferred technique in this chapter.

Keywords: *surgical approach shoulder, deltopectoral approach, shoulder arthroplasty, reverse shoulder arthroplasty, total shoulder arthroplasty, open shoulder surgery*

39.1 Introduction

The deltopectoral approach is the workhorse approach in open shoulder surgery and is the standard approach for anatomic shoulder arthroplasty. Reverse shoulder arthroplasty may be performed through either the deltopectoral approach or the anterosuperior approach, each with advantages and disadvantages. The anterosuperior approach uses a deltoid split, which violates the primary arm elevator, and is not extensile.

We prefer to use the deltopectoral approach for all shoulder arthroplasty for several reasons. It provides reliable and uncompromised access to the anterior shoulder and excellent glenoid exposure with proper capsular release and humeral head retraction without potential compromise of deltoid function. In addition, this approach is fully extensile into the anterolateral humerus approach. We describe our preferred stepwise surgical technique to reliably achieve adequate exposure for humeral and glenoid preparation and component implantation.

39.2 Operating Room Setup and Patient Positioning

Shoulder arthroplasty is performed under general anesthesia. It is important for the patient to be kept fully relaxed by anesthesia until implantation of components is complete to allow uniform assessment of soft-tissue tension during trialing. We prefer to have the operating room setup so that the operative extremity is opposite the sterile field. This allows the surgical technician to act as a second assistant. The patient is positioned in the modified beach-chair position. A small folded sheet should be placed under the patient at the medial scapular border to stabilize the scapula for the glenoid portion of the procedure. The patient must be positioned sufficiently near the edge of the table to allow for full extension and adduction of the surgical arm, which is essential for humeral preparation. The arm is then prepped and draped, and the axilla sealed off from the surgical field with a barrier drape (**Fig. 39.1**).

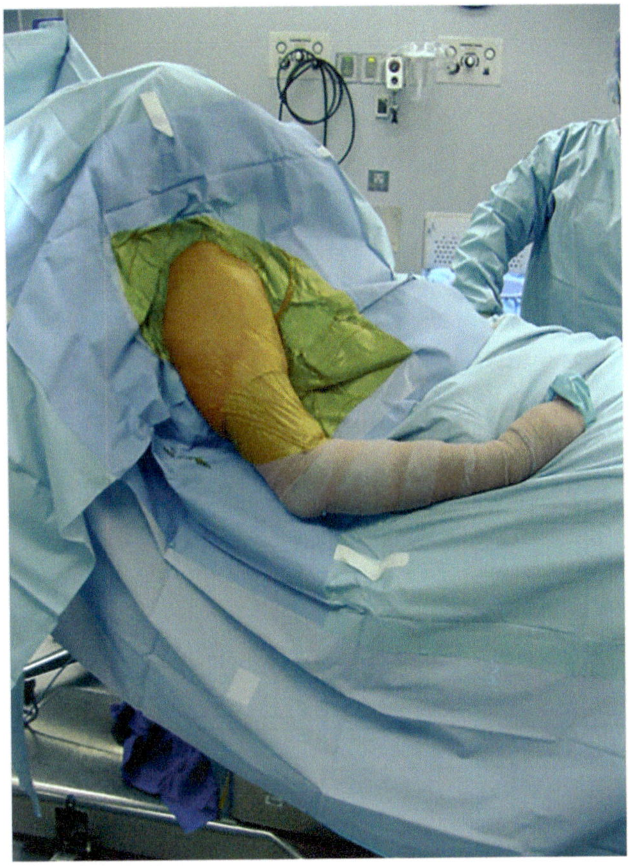

Fig. 39.1 Patient is positioned in the modified beach-chair position with the operative side opposite the sterile field. A barrier drape should be used to seal the axilla.

39.3 Operative Technique

39.3.1 Anatomy

The deltopectoral approach uses the internervous plane between the deltoid muscle, innervated by the axillary nerve, and the pectoralis major muscle, innervated by the medial and lateral pectoral nerves. The surgical approach begins with identification of the topographic anatomy of the shoulder. The coracoid process is typically readily palpable except in very obese patients or patients who have previously undergone a procedure involving the coracoid process. In thinner and muscular patients, the deltopectoral interval may be directly palpated to help guide the orientation of the skin incision, which extends approximately 10 to 15 cm distal and lateral from the coracoid (**Fig. 39.2**). The approach is also fully extensile to the anterolateral approach to the humerus if needed.

39.3.2 Superficial Dissection

With the arm in neutral rotation and adducted position, a no. 10 scalpel is used to sharply incise only the skin. Needle elec-

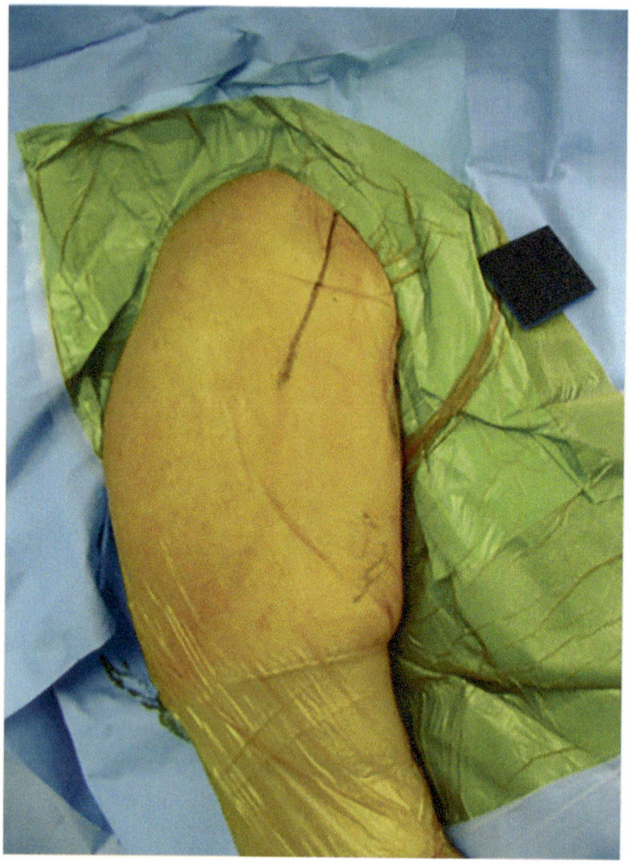

Fig. 39.2 The deltopectoral interval is marked beginning at the coracoid and extending 10 to 15 cm distal and lateral using the anterior border of the deltoid muscle as a guide if palpable.

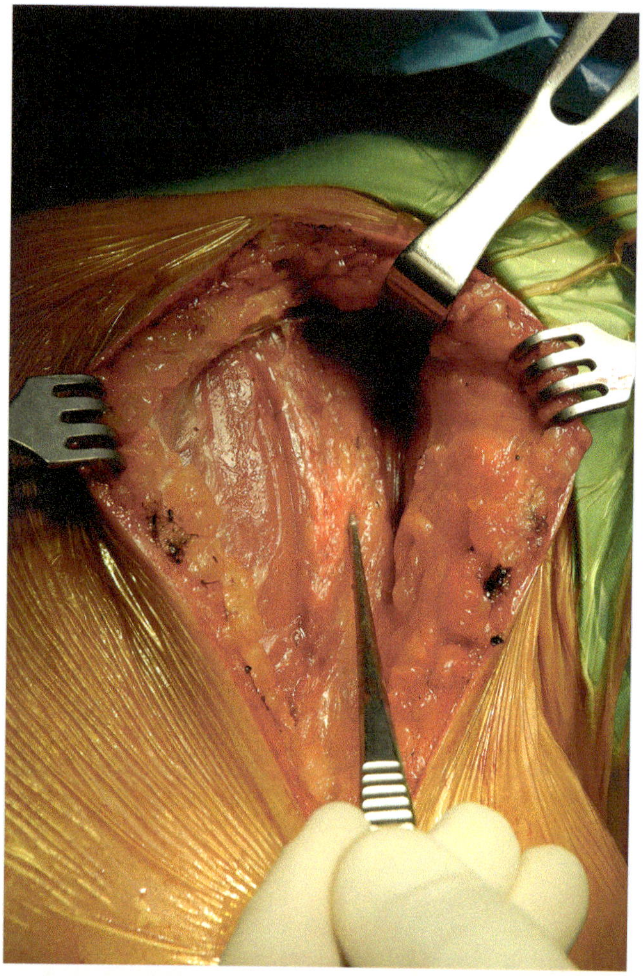

Fig. 39.3 The cephalic vein marks the deltopectoral interval and typically is located in a layer of fat between the deltoid and pectoralis major muscles.

trocautery is then used for subcutaneous dissection and most of the deep dissection throughout the procedure. Maintaining meticulous hemostasis with the initial dissection is important to prevent bleeding from the superficial vessels. Medium skin rakes are used to retract and tension the subcutaneous tissue. The dissection continues through the deltopectoral fascia to expose the cephalic vein, which identifies the interval between the deltoid and the pectoralis major muscles. The vein is surrounded by a layer of fat and typically easily identified. If difficulty is encountered due to a congenitally small or absent vein, a small triangular area devoid of muscle proximally at the coracoid allows identification of the interval (**Fig. 39.3**).

The cephalic vein is then dissected free of the pectoralis major muscle with Metzenbaum scissors, and may be taken either medially or laterally depending on surgeon preference. We prefer to retract the vein laterally, as most branches from the cephalic vein are deltoid based and retracting the vein medially may disrupt these branches and introduce unwanted hemorrhage. The deltoid and pectoralis major muscles are then retracted with the Army Navy retractors and a self-retaining retractor placed to develop the interval. The superior centimeter of the pectoralis major may be released sharply to enhance exposure of the inferior subscapularis, anterior circumflex vessels, and axillary nerve. Curved Mayo scissors are used to bluntly dissect superior to the coracoid and a Hohmann-type retractor is placed in the space to complete the initial exposure (**Fig. 39.4**).

39.3.3 Deep Dissection

The arm is then abducted and externally rotated. The clavipectoral fascia is divided sharply with electrocautery at the apex of the coracoacromial and conjoined tendon insertions on the coracoid, and dissection is continued distally along the lateral border of the conjoined tendon. The arm is then brought back into the neutral position. A narrow Richardson retractor is placed to retract the conjoined tendon medially and expose the subscapularis and anterior humeral circumflex vessels. Overzealous retraction of the conjoined tendon should be avoided to prevent injury to the musculocutaneous nerve that passes deep to the conjoined tendon and enters the biceps muscle approximately 5 to 8 cm distal to the coracoid. We do not use a self-retaining retractor deep to the conjoined tendon for this reason.

The anterior circumflex artery and its two partner veins ("three sisters") are then identified at the inferior border of the subscapularis and suture ligated. We use a dyed no. 0 braided, absorbable suture and place the sutures on either side of the anatomic neck of the humerus, leaving a 1-cm space between them. Care should be taken when ligating the vessels to avoid

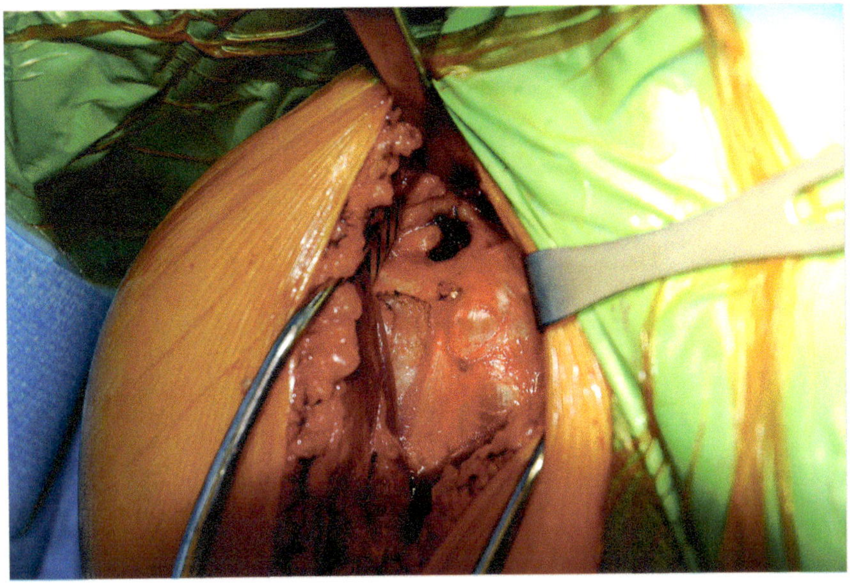

Fig. 39.4 Completed superficial exposure with the deltopectoral retractor in place. A Hohmann-type retractor placed superior to the coracoid process considerably increases exposure.

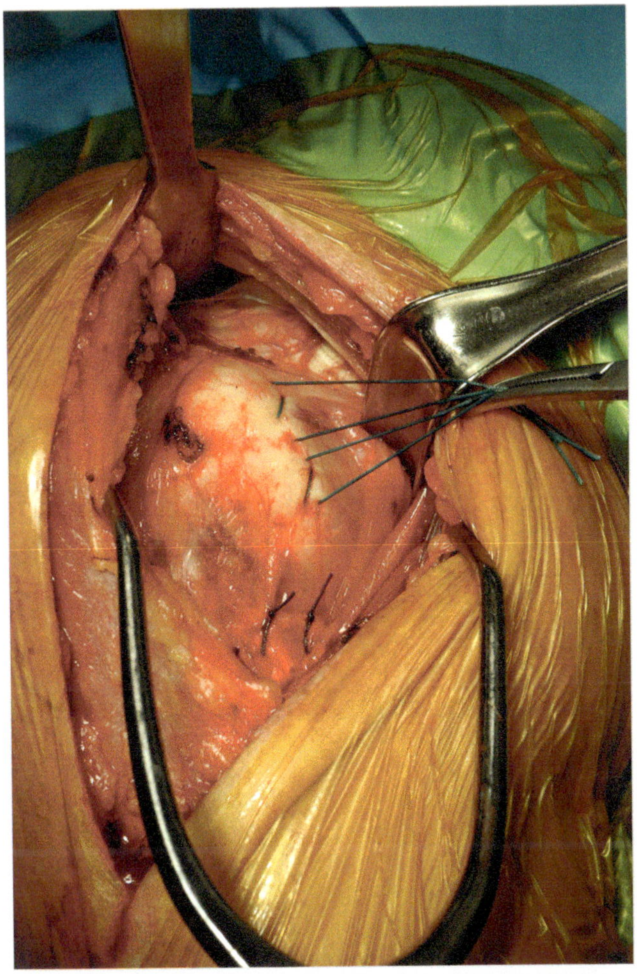

Fig. 39.5 The subscapularis is tagged with no. 1 heavy braided suture prior to tenotomy.

taking a large bite of tissue, which would place the axillary nerve located immediately inferior and deep to the vessels at risk.

Two stay sutures are placed in the superior and inferior subscapularis using heavy a no. 1 braided, nonabsorbable suture double-passed through the tendon (**Fig. 39.5**). Curved Mayo scissors are then passed tangentially and just superior to the subscapularis tendon to open the glenohumeral joint through the rotator interval. Arthrotomy of the glenohumeral joint is typically marked by an egress of synovial fluid. The superior border of the subscapularis is identified in preparation for release, and the arm is brought into an adducted and neutral or slightly externally rotated position.

39.3.4 Subscapularis Management

Various techniques for accessing the anterior shoulder during arthroplasty have been described, including complete and partial subscapularis tenotomy, subscapularis peel, lesser tuberosity osteotomy, and access solely through the rotator interval. We perform a complete subscapularis tenotomy. This allows unhindered access to the shoulder joint and release of subscapularis and capsular contractures frequently present in patients undergoing shoulder arthroplasty. In addition, tenotomy does not disrupt the osseous anatomy of the proximal humerus as with a lesser tuberosity osteotomy.

The tenotomy is performed by placing Ferris-Smith forceps into the opening in the rotator interval to identify the superior border of the subscapularis and place it under slight tension. A fresh no. 10 scalpel is used to perform a subscapularis tenotomy of the superior two-thirds along the anatomic neck of the humerus. It is critical to perform the tenotomy lateral enough to avoid the musculotendinous junction but medial enough to leave a cuff of tissue for adequate repair after implantation of the prosthesis. The inferior one-third of the subscapularis is more muscular, and is released using the electrocautery dissecting between the previously placed dyed absorbable sutures in the anterior humeral circumflex vessels. The inferior capsule is then released from the humerus using the electrocautery as the assistant gradually externally rotates the arm (**Fig. 39.6**).

39.3.5 Capsular Release

A Trillat-type or other humeral head retractor is placed by externally rotating the humerus and placing the retractor as the humerus is internally rotated back to neutral and the humeral

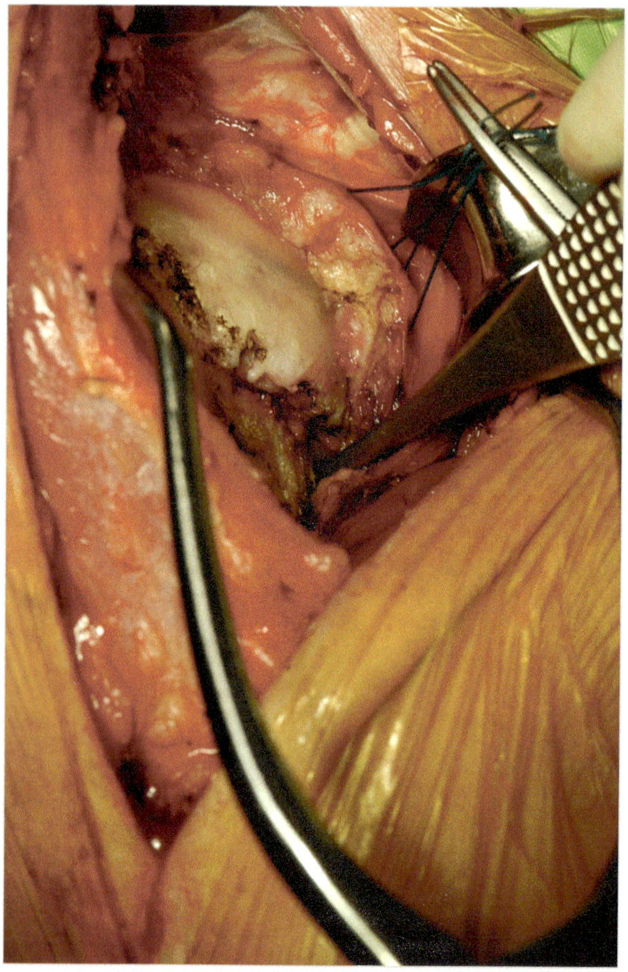

Fig. 39.6 Initial subscapularis tenotomy is performed with a long-handled scalpel, and completed using the electrocautery. The inferior capsule is released from the humeral neck as the assistant gradually externally rotates the arm. The release is adequate once the humeral head is easily dislocated.

head retracted posteriorly. We then perform a sequential release of the glenohumeral ligaments. The superior glenohumeral ligament is identified in the rotator interval at the superior border of the subscapularis and sharply divided using the curved Mayo scissors aimed toward the glenoid with the tips pointing slightly downward. Turning the tines inferiorly between the subscapularis and capsule to palpate a thickening of the capsule allows identification of the middle glenohumeral ligament, which is released parallel to the anterior border of the glenoid. The curved Mayo scissors are then used to bluntly dissect the plane between the inferior subscapularis muscle and the inferior capsule, and the inferior glenohumeral ligament is divided sharply with the tines pointed slightly superior and anterior to the glenoid. This technique allows complete release of the glenohumeral ligaments without putting the axillary nerve at risk (**Fig. 39.7**).

The intra-articular subscapularis recess is readily accessible after glenohumeral ligament release, and should be inspected for loose bodies. These are typically osseous and visible on preoperative radiographs. We routinely remove all loose bodies. A Cobb elevator may be used to bluntly release any remaining adhesions.

The subscapularis should have significantly increased excursion after release, and is tucked into the subscapularis fossa

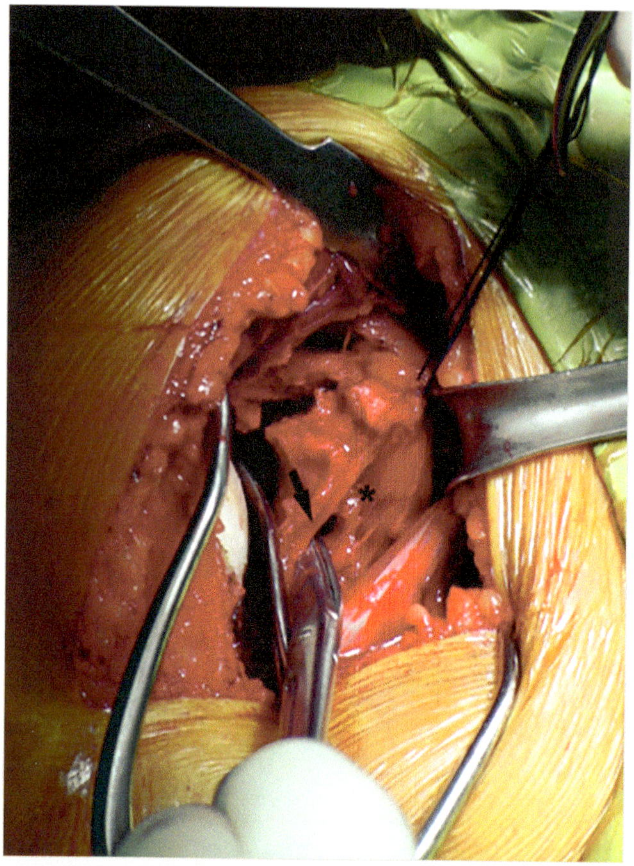

Fig. 39.7 The inferior glenohumeral ligament is released sharply with the Mayo scissors. Developing a plane between the capsule and muscular inferior subscapularis prior to release protects the axillary nerve.

with a sponge. An anterior glenoid retractor is placed to hold the subscapularis in the fossa and expose the anterior glenoid. This retractor remains in place until the end of the surgery, and it is critical for the surgical team to confirm sponge removal prior to the end of the case.

39.3.6 Glenoid Exposure

Obtaining adequate visualization of the osseous glenoid can be challenging for even the most experienced shoulder surgeon. However, glenoid exposure can be simplified and reliably achieved in our experience by performing a stepwise capsular release. With the humeral head retracted posteriorly, the remaining anterior labrum is excised with the needle electrocautery from the base of the coracoid process to the 5 o'clock position in a right shoulder (the 7 o'clock position in a left shoulder) to expose the osseous anterior glenoid margin.

Release of the inferior capsule off the glenoid rim is critical to obtaining exposure for glenoid component implantation, and is performed using the needle electrocautery with the tip in contact with bone at all times to protect the axillary nerve. The release is extended medially enough to the completely transect the capsule. Visualization of triceps muscle fibers or the axillary scapular border indicates sufficient capsular dissection.

The extent of the posterior release performed last is dependent on preoperative posterior subluxation. In patients without posterior subluxation, the clockwise capsular release should

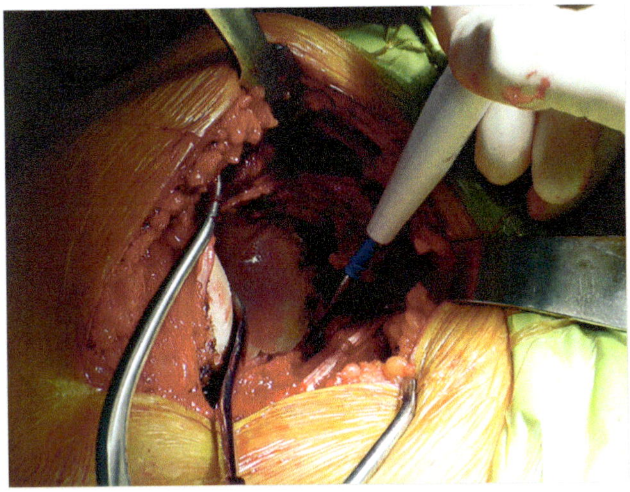

Fig. 39.8 The deep exposure is completed with excision of the anterior labrum and release of the inferior capsule from the glenoid.

be continued at the 8 o'clock position in a right shoulder (the 4 o'clock position in a left shoulder). However, patients with preoperative posterior subluxation often have distended posterior capsule and the release should only be performed at the 6 o'clock position initially to avoid further compromise of the soft-tissue structures, though it may be extended as necessary if exposure is still inadequate during glenoid preparation and implantation. We use a Cobb elevator to evaluate the adequacy of the capsular release. This completes the exposure prior to implantation of components (**Fig. 39.8**).

39.4 Tips and Pearls

39.4.1 Operating Room Setup and Patient Positioning

- Keep the patient completely relaxed until implantation of components is complete for uniform assessment of soft-tissue tension.
- The patient should be positioned far enough toward the edge of the bed that the arm can be fully adducted and extended to allow optimal humeral preparation and component implantation.

39.4.2 Superficial Dissection

- Maintaining meticulous hemostasis with the initial dissection will minimize bleeding of the superficial vessels throughout the case.
- Retracting the cephalic vein laterally with the deltoid avoids injury to the multiple deltoid-based branches off the vein.

39.4.3 Deep Dissection

- Avoid overzealous retraction of the conjoined tendon, which can put the musculocutaneous nerve at risk.
- Identification and ligation of the anterior circumflex artery and veins ("three sisters") is important for hemostasis and to mark the inferior extent of the subscapularis.

39.4.4 Subscapularis Management

- We prefer to perform a complete subscapularis tenotomy. It is critical to maintain a sufficient cuff of tendon laterally for transosseous repair after component implantation.

39.4.5 Capsular Release

- Use curved Mayo scissors to develop the plane between capsule and subscapularis to allow complete release of the glenohumeral ligaments while avoiding injury to the axillary nerve.
- Inspect the subscapularis fossa for loose bodies and remove them if present.

39.4.6 Glenoid Exposure

- Maintain the tip of the electrocautery in contact with the osseous glenoid at all times to avoid injury to the axillary nerve while releasing the capsule from the glenoid.

Suggested Reading

Gartsman GM, Edwards TB, eds. Shoulder Arthroplasty. Philadelphia, PA: Saunders Elsevier; 2008

40 Humeral Resurfacing Arthroplasty

Daniel E. Davis and Matthew L. Ramsey

Abstract
Humeral head arthrosis may occur due to a variety of pathologies. If this presents itself in young patients without glenoid articular changes, a resurfacing arthroplasty of the humeral head may be indicated. The large benefit of this operation is to preserve metaphyseal bone as these patients are at higher risk of requiring further arthroplasty procedures. This chapter will review the indications and techniques of performing this operation.

Keywords: *shoulder arthritis, humeral AVN, post-traumatic arthritis, humeral resurfacing, unipolar lesions*

40.1 Goals of Procedure

Arthritic changes of the humeral head articular cartilage may occur through degenerative, inflammatory, traumatic, or iatrogenic mechanisms.[1] When this occurs in younger patients and broadly affects the articular surface, surgical management is challenging. If possible, in a young patient population, maintenance of the native glenoid is preferred in order to avoid early replacement of the glenoid.[2]

The goal of any arthroplasty procedure is to relieve pain and improve function. Humeral head resurfacing achieves these goals by replacing the arthritic or damaged cartilaginous surface. The glenoid is not typically addressed with humeral head resurfacing. However, management of glenoid sided bone and cartilage involvement are not precluded with humeral head resurfacing.

New stemless implants have recently been introduced, which can accomplish the same goal of humeral arthroplasty without the need for stem introduction into the metaphysis or diaphysis. These do, however, require resection of the head and therefore sacrifice more metaphyseal bone than a humeral resurfacing implant. This chapter will focus on humeral resurfacing.

40.2 Advantages

The main advantage of resurfacing the humeral head is the ability to re-create the native anatomy of the proximal humerus independent of the humeral canal. Since the resurfacing component is a shell configuration, it allows for minimal bone resection. The lack of an intramedullary stem allows the surgeon to place the implant in the precise position without being limited by the relationship of the intramedullary canal to the articular surface. The ability to minimize bone resection of the proximal humerus and avoid instrumentation of the humeral canal may facilitate future reconstructive procedures such as arthrodesis or further arthroplasty.[3]

40.3 Indications

Humeral head resurfacing is indicated for young patients (<60 years old), who have significant pain and dysfunction from cartilage compromise of the humeral head. It is preferred that the glenoid articular cartilage is maintained and that the humeral head remains concentric on the glenoid on both anteroposterior (AP) and axillary views. Patients with posttraumatic arthritis and disruption of the relationship of the humeral head to the diaphysis also benefit from a resurfacing procedure. When the relationship of the humeral canal and head precludes stemmed arthroplasty, humeral head resurfacing is preferred to tuberosity osteotomy. Avascular necrosis (AVN) with articular collapse involving greater than 40% of the humeral articular surface is another indication for humeral resurfacing. However, in these cases it is important that at least 60% of the subchondral bone be of good quality in order to support the resurfacing prosthesis.[4] Finally, a rare indication for resurfacing is a large, engaging Hill–Sachs defect secondary to instability, which takes up more than 40% of the humeral head surface. Generally, these defects may be treated with partial head replacement or allograft reconstruction; however, occasionally a complete resurfacing may be needed.

40.4 Contraindications

Resurfacing of the humeral head should be avoided in patients with deficiency of more than 60% of the humeral head or poor subchondral bone. Resurfacing of the humerus should also be avoided in the setting of acute three- and four-part fractures of the proximal humerus, as the implant will not have appropriate bony support in the face of tuberosity involvement. While glenoid arthrosis is not an absolute contraindication to resurfacing, it should be avoided in this situation as the patient may continue to experience glenoid-based pain. Glenoid resurfacing can be performed in the setting of humeral head resurfacing (**Fig. 40.1**). However, the retained portion of the humeral head limits glenoid exposure.

40.5 Preoperative Preparation/ Positioning

A thorough history and orthopaedic evaluation should be undertaken initially to establish the correct diagnosis. A complete radiographic examination should also be performed including AP views of the glenohumeral joint in the plane of the scapula with the humerus in internal and external rotation as well as an axillary view and a scapular Y view. The AP views help assess the quality of the joint space as well as presence of osteophytes and location of the humerus with respect to the glenoid. The lateral and axillary views are key to evaluate posterior subluxation of the humerus, version of the glenoid, and posterior glenoid wear. A CT scan may also be useful for a more detailed evaluation of the glenoid if there is any concern for extensive disease on the plain radiographs. Finally, if there is any concern for rotator cuff disease, an MRI should be obtained to confirm the integrity of the rotator cuff tendons.

As with other arthroplasty procedures, we prefer to perform the procedure in the beach-chair position in 30 degrees of elevation. Sterile preparation and draping is done in the standard fashion with the arm held in a positioning device (**Fig. 40.2**).

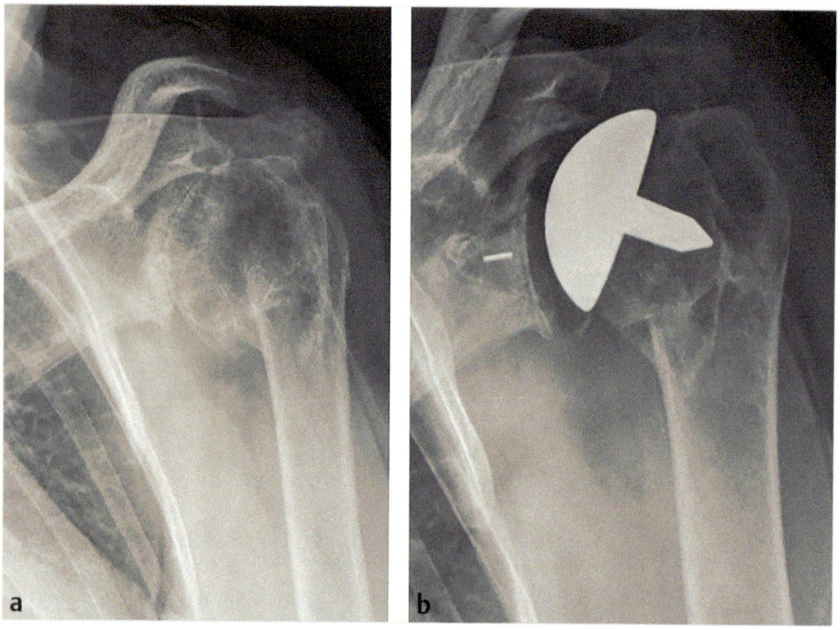

Fig. 40.1 (a) Preoperative radiograph of a patient with a mal-united proximal humerus fracture with associated posttraumatic arthritis. (b) Postoperative radiographs following resurfacing total shoulder replacement.

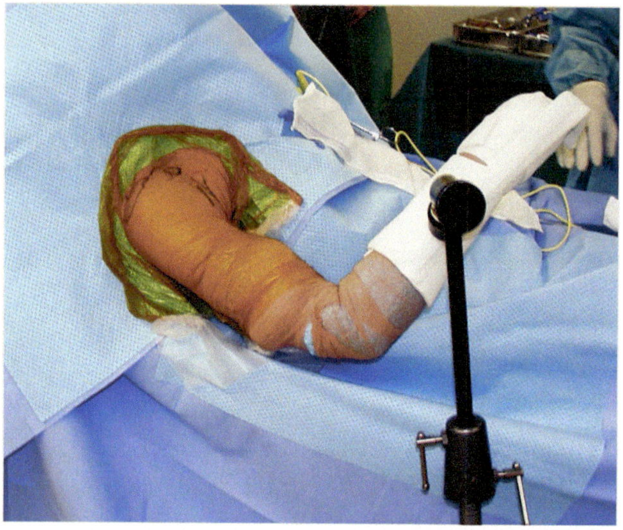

Fig. 40.2 The beach-chair position utilized for resurfacing shoulder replacement.

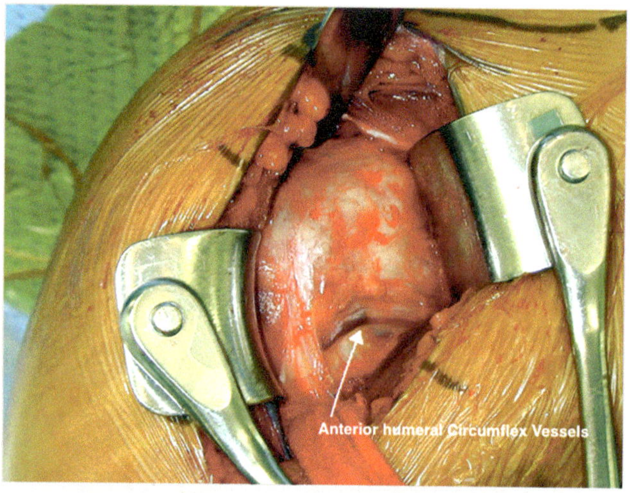

Fig. 40.3 Intraoperative photograph demonstrating the subscapularis and overlying anterior humeral circumflex vessels.

40.6 Operative Technique

While a subscapularis sparing approach through the rotator interval has been proposed for this procedure, we prefer to use the standard deltopectoral approach with a lesser tuberosity osteotomy. After the shoulder has been prepped and draped, an incision is made beginning at the coracoid directed toward the insertion of the deltoid. The incision is generally approximately 10 cm; however, the length is primarily dictated by the size of the patient and the amount of exposure required. With a no. 15 blade, the skin is incised just through the dermis. Electrocautery is then used to control the skin bleeders and complete the incision through the dermis to the subcutaneous fat. The cephalic vein is identified and dissected and can be retracted either medially or laterally. Medial retraction limits trauma to the vein throughout surgery but requires ligation of the feeder vessels from the anterior deltoid. The deltopectoral interval is an internervous plane between the deltoid (axillary nerve) and the pectoralis major (lateral and medial pectoral nerves). This interval is developed allowing identification and dissection of the subdeltoid and subacromial spaces. The subdeltoid space is then bluntly defined laterally just above the deltoid insertion. The coracoacromial ligament is identified at the lateral tip of the coracoid. Dissection under the coracoacromial ligament allows the subacromial space to be developed. It is critical to develop the entire subacromial and subdeltoid spaces to the posterior aspect of the shoulder. A deltoid retractor is placed superolateral to the humeral head and a Kolbel retractor is placed below the deltoid and the pectoralis major.

The clavipectoral fascia is incised lateral to the conjoint tendon and the axillary and musculocutaneous nerves are palpated deep to this structure. The Kolbel retractor is repositioned to retract the conjoint tendon avoiding excessive retraction on the conjoint tendon (**Fig. 40.3**). The anterior humeral circumflex vessels are ligated or cauterized. The biceps tendon sheath is incised and a soft-tissue tenodesis is performed to the superior margin of the tendon of the pectoralis major. The proximal portion of the tendon is excised through the rotator interval. The intertubercular groove is then cleared of the overlying soft tissue and bleeding is controlled.

The superior insertion of the subscapularis is identified to direct the depth and direction of the osteotomy. For total joint arthroplasty, we generally take an approximately 10-mm osteotomy; however, when planning a resurfacing procedure we take a thinner osteotomy, approximately 5 mm, to preserve as much subchondral metaphyseal bone as possible. The lesser tuberosity osteotomy is performed and the capsule is released from the rotator interval to the posteroinferior aspect of the humerus.

The humeral head is dislocated with external rotation and extension and soft-tissue retractors are placed (**Fig. 40.4**). Proper preparation of the humeral head for resurfacing depends on identifying normal anatomic landmarks at the anatomic neck. The insertion of the posterosuperior rotator cuff is defined and inspected to ensure an intact cuff.

A rongeur is used to circumferentially remove osteophytes at the margin of the articular surface. Inferiorly, the osteophyte is removed until the native capsular insertion is identified (**Fig. 40.5**). Following removal of the osteophytes, the premorbid structure of the humeral articular surface is reestablished. This is critical to appropriate sizing of a humeral resurfacing implant.

The bone of the humeral head is evaluated to be sure that there is adequate support for the resurfacing implant. After all osteophytes are removed, a humeral head sizer is used to measure the humeral head. The inferior portion of the sizer should seat to the articular margin established after osteophyte removal (**Fig. 40.6**). If the sizer does not fully seat to the articular margin, a deeper humeral head reamer may be necessary. If the sizer is placed appropriately on the articular surface, there will be no asymmetry between the superior and inferior articular margins or the anterior and posterior margins.

A guide pin is placed through the humeral sizer making sure that the lateral humeral cortex is penetrated (**Fig. 40.7**). This provides greater stability of the pin during humeral reaming. A finger should be placed in the subdeltoid space against the lateral humeral cortex to avoid overpenetration of the cortex. The appropriate-sized humeral head shaper is placed over the guide wire and the proximal humerus is prepared. The serrated teeth at the margins of the reamer may undercut the bone in the proximal humerus. Care must be taken not to ream the proximal humeral bone below the rotator cuff attachments. Any undercut bone at the periphery can be removed with a rongeur maintaining the bone at the cuff attachments.

The appropriate trial component corresponding to the shaper used is inserted to assess the adequacy of the proximal humerus bone preparation. The trial must seat fully without any gap between the trial and the proximal humerus (**Fig. 40.8**).

At this point, the glenoid should be inspected for cartilage integrity. The prepared proximal humerus is protected with the humeral trial. All retractors are removed and the humerus is internally rotated and reduced. The trial is left to protect the humeral cancellous bone, but it is also important to protect the glenoid from the trial implant. A Fukuda ring retractor is inserted posterior to the glenoid to retract the humeral head

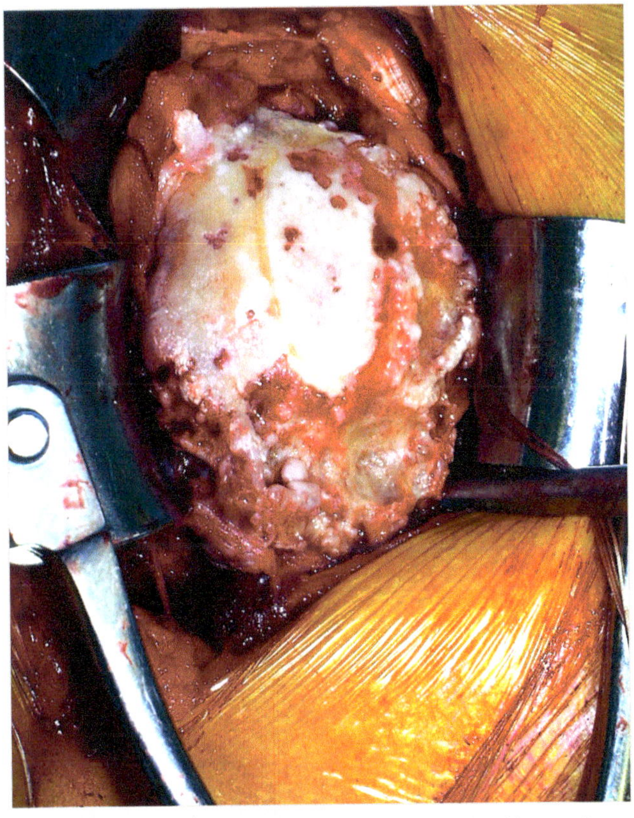

Fig. 40.4 Intraoperative photograph of the dislocated humeral head. Note the abundant peripheral osteophytes.

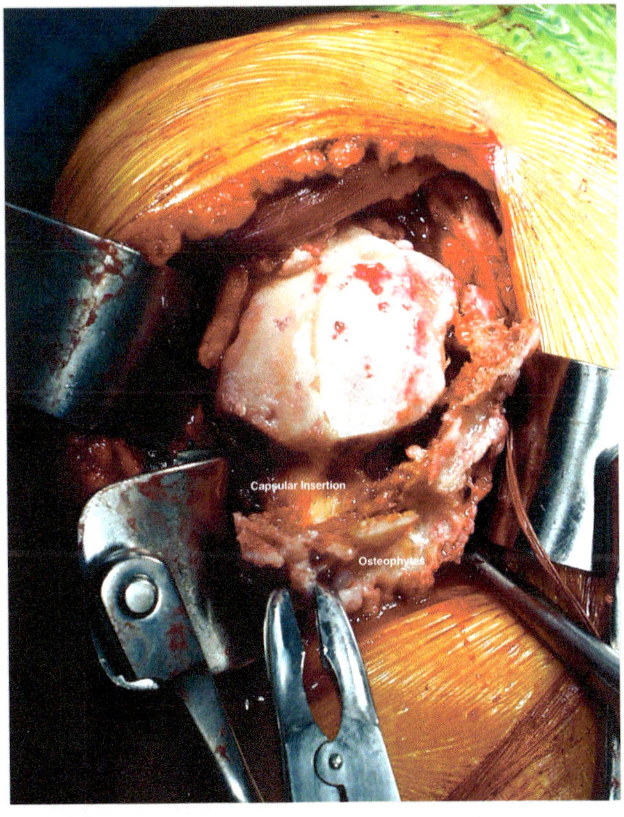

Fig. 40.5 Intraoperative photograph during osteophyte excision. Note the osteophytes have been excised to the native capsular insertion.

being cautious not to damage the glenoid cartilage. At this point, the remaining stump of the biceps tendon should be removed so it does not impinge within the joint. The labrum is maintained if it is structurally intact but is resected if compromised.

The shoulder is reduced and assessed for stability. We prefer to test with the humerus elevated to 30 degrees in the plane of the scapula. A posteriorly directed force is applied to the head; an appropriately sized implant should subluxate posteriorly no more than 50% and return to the glenoid once the displacement force is withdrawn.

The humerus is again dislocated and retractors are placed. The wound is irrigated. Three drill holes are made in the bicipital groove about the bed of the lesser tuberosity osteotomy. Sutures are placed for subscapularis repair before the final implant is impacted.

The final component is prepared for implantation. If there is any irregularity of the prepared proximal humeral surface, bone graft from the proximal humerus reaming is packed into the backside of the component (**Fig. 40.9**). The final component is impacted onto the prepared surface of the proximal humerus and the shoulder is reduced (**Fig. 40.10**).

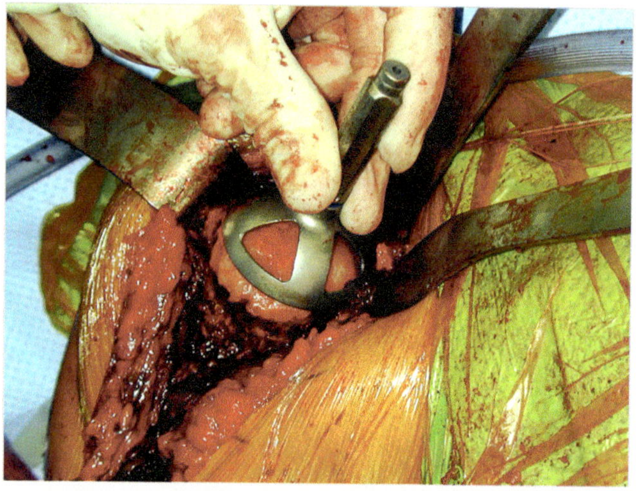

Fig. 40.6 Intraoperative photograph showing the position of the humeral sizer to reestablish appropriate inclination and version.

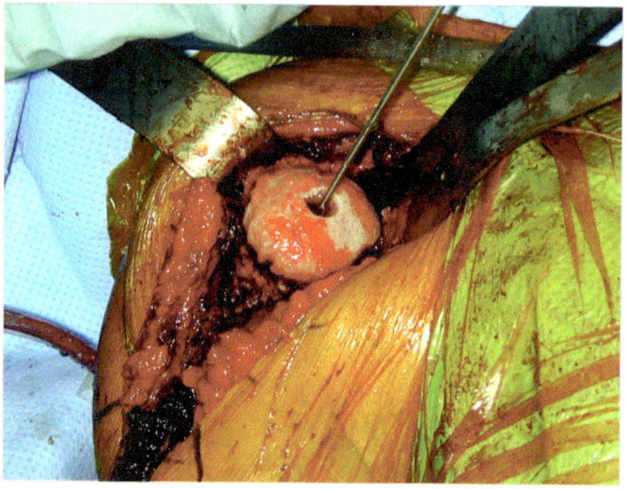

Fig. 40.7 Intraoperative photograph following placement of the humeral guide pin.

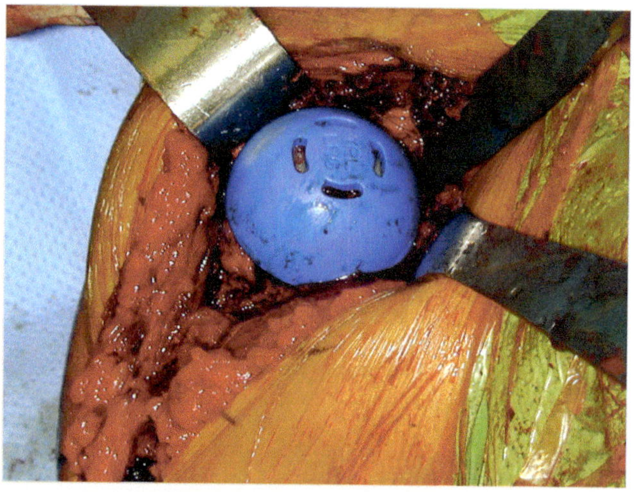

Fig. 40.8 Intraoperative photograph with the resurfacing trial component in place. The trial re-creates the premorbid head height, version, and inclination.

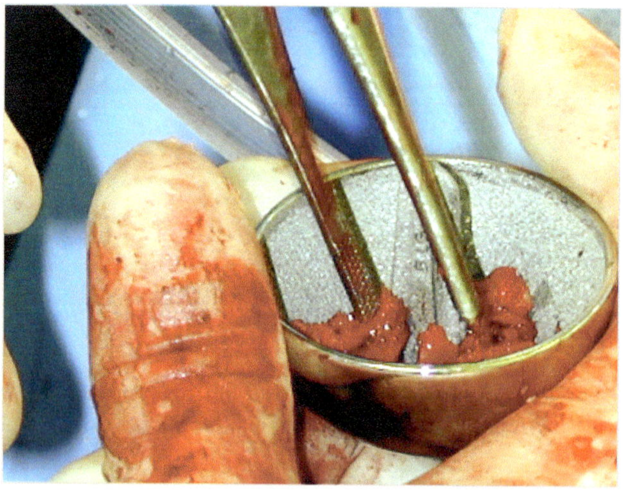

Fig. 40.9 Intraoperative photograph showing morselized bone graft being placed behind the component.

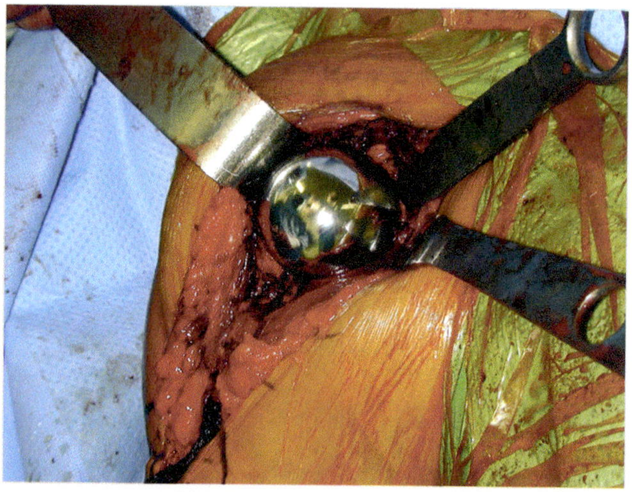

Fig. 40.10 Intraoperative photograph following placement of the final component.

The sutures are passed medial to the lesser tuberosity in the subscapularis tendon and tied to reduce the tuberosity. The rotator interval is closed laterally with the arm in 30 degrees of external rotation to avoid loss of motion. The deltopectoral interval is closed with interrupted 0 Vicryl suture and the subcutaneous and cutaneous layers are closed. A drain may or may not be used depending on surgeon preference and on a case-by-case basis.

40.7 Tips and Pearls/Expert Suggestions

- Remove all osteophytes down to the capsular reflection at the anatomic neck.
- Minimize the size of the lesser tuberosity osteotomy.
- Be sure the guide pin is seated in the lateral cortex without pass pointing near the axillary nerve.
- When reaming the humeral head, be sure to ream all the way to the anatomic neck without undermining the rotator cuff insertion.
- Ensure head size is flush with the cortex without being undersized or overhanging.

40.8 What to Avoid

- Protection of the glenoid cartilage is necessary to avoid iatrogenic chondral damage.
- A large osteotomy risks losing more metaphyseal bone stock than desirable for supporting a resurfacing prosthesis.
- Undermining of the rotator cuff with the reamer puts the cuff tissue at risk of failure.
- Overstuffing the joint risks damage to the rotator cuff as well as increased pressure on the intact glenoid cartilage.

40.9 Complications/Bailout/ Salvage

The benefit of a resurfacing procedure is the large number of bailout options in the face of failure. Major complications that may occur after this operation include implant loosening, advanced glenoid wear, rotator cuff failure, and infection. If there is still a viable, intact rotator cuff, revision of the prosthesis may be done if the glenoid is still in good condition. Otherwise, the implant may also be converted to an anatomic total shoulder. If the implant is loose, it is advisable to convert to a stemmed or metaphyseal fit implant to gain greater stem stability. In the setting of infection, debridement and removal of all implants is generally advisable, followed by a course of IV antibiotics for 6 weeks. In the case of cuff failure or revision after infection, a reverse total shoulder may be the only reconstruction option for a functional shoulder. If the patient's age precludes a reverse total shoulder arthroplasty, glenohumeral arthrodesis may be an option, which is a benefit of the bone preservation provided by the resurfacing procedure.

40.10 Postoperative Care

Depending on the patient and the surgeon preference, this procedure may be done on an outpatient or overnight inpatient stay. At this point, we prefer one night stay for pain control and patient comfort. Patients are discharged in a sling and prior to discharge are taught passive exercises with external rotation limited to 30 degrees and supine forward elevation limited to 130 degrees. The first post-op visit is at 2 weeks for a wound check and radiographs. At that point, the passive exercises are advanced to 40 degrees external rotation and 140 degrees elevation, and some freedom from the sling for waist-level activities is given. At 6 weeks post-op, the sling is permanently removed and patient is advanced to further increases in active-assisted range of motion and incremental strengthening. By 3 months, formal therapy is generally completed with subsequent follow-up visits at 6 months and 1 year.

References

1. Burgess DL, McGrath MS, Bonutti PM, Marker DR, Delanois RE, Mont MA. Shoulder resurfacing. J Bone Joint Surg Am 2009;91(5):1228–1238
2. Jensen KL. Humeral resurfacing arthroplasty: rationale, indications, technique, and results. Am J Orthop 2007;36(12, Suppl 1):4–8
3. Pearl ML. Proximal humeral anatomy in shoulder arthroplasty: Implications for prosthetic design and surgical technique. J Shoulder Elbow Surg 2005;14(1, Suppl S): 99S–104S
4. Levy O, Copeland SA. Cementless surface replacement arthroplasty of the shoulder. 5- to 10-year results with the Copeland mark-2 prosthesis. J Bone Joint Surg Br 2001;83(2):213–221

41 Subscapularis Management in Shoulder Arthroplasty: Tenotomy, Peel, and Osteotomy

Samuel R.H. Steiner, Heather M. Menzer, Stephen F. Brockmeier, and Brian C. Werner

Abstract

Subscapularis takedown and management, whether by tenotomy, peel, or osteotomy, is a critical step in total shoulder replacement (TSR). Only by doing so can adequate exposure to the glenohumeral joint be achieved through the standard deltopectoral approach. Although not as important in reverse shoulder arthroplasty, restoration of a functioning subscapularis is vital in anatomic TSR in order to provide stability and maintain motion, thereby improving postoperative outcome scores. With pros and cons to each method of managing the subscapularis, it is imperative that the surgeon understand the principles for each technique and has them in his or her repertoire.

Keywords: *total shoulder arthroplasty, reverse total shoulder arthroplasty, subscapularis tendon, subscapularis peel, subscapularis tenotomy, lesser tuberosity osteotomy*

41.1 Goals of Procedure

41.1.1 Restoration of Subscapularis

Surgical exposure to the glenohumeral (GH) joint in total shoulder replacement (TSR) requires takedown of the subscapularis tendon at its insertion, which can be performed using various techniques, which include tenotomy, tendon peel, and lesser tuberosity osteotomy (LTO). Preoperative planning of the exposure is important so that the subscapularis tendon can be addressed appropriately at the end of the case. Adequate mobilization of the tendon is also important, as preoperative internal rotation contractures are common in GH osteoarthritis. The purpose of repair is to restore subscapularis function, thereby providing stability and motion to the shoulder postoperatively.

41.2 Advantages

41.2.1 Stability

The subscapularis tendon resists anterior translation of the humeral head relative to the glenoid. An intact tendon reduces the risk of postoperative anterior instability. It also creates a concentric joint and distributes polyethylene contact surface area. Several studies have demonstrated increased risk of anterior instability after both conventional and reverse TSR in patients without an intact subscapularis tendon.[1-5] Some recent data suggest that an intact subscapularis may not be necessary after reverse TSR and does not result in increased instability rates.[6]

41.2.2 Motion

Repair of the subscapularis tendon theoretically restores the subscapularis's main function of internal rotation. This is particularly important to patients as it allows for reaching into the back pocket and tucking in a shirt. The subscapularis also draws the humeral head forward and downward when the arm is raised. By providing a stable and balanced joint, a restored subscapularis improves the function of the deltoid and other rotator cuff muscles.

41.2.3 Improved Outcomes

Patients with an intact subscapularis after TSR, compared to those without an intact or functioning muscle, report improved Disabilities of the Arm, Shoulder, and Hand (DASH) scores[7] and patient-reported outcomes.[2,8,9] Subscapularis tendon management in TSR yields similar overall patient outcome scores, and no specific technique is considered superior.[10] Several studies report excellent or satisfactory outcome after subscapularis tenotomy and repair.[11-14] Caplan et al reported normal belly press at final follow-up after tendon-to-tendon repair,[15] though Miller et al report 65% altered subscapularis function with this technique.[9]

LTO provides anatomic repair of the lesser tuberosity footprint and reliable bone-to-bone healing.[5] Initial fixation of LTO is stronger[16-18]; however, biomechanical studies demonstrate similar long-term outcomes between each repair technique.[10,16-20]

41.3 Disadvantages

41.3.1 Challenges with Mobilization

Complete mobilization of the subscapularis is important in the exposure of the glenoid as well as the ability to repair the tendon upon completion of the TSR. Preoperative contractures as well as implant lateralization can make it difficult to obtain an anatomic subscapularis repair. This can be problematic in LTO repairs. Tenotomies and peel techniques can be medialized to the anterior humeral neck osteotomy if needed.

41.3.2 Subscapularis and Reverse Total Shoulder Replacement

Subscapularis repair may not always be advantageous after reverse TSR. A recent biomechanical study reported that concomitant subscapularis repair with reverse shoulder arthroplasty (RSA) created a biomechanically unfavorable condition during arm elevation, due to an increase in the force required by the deltoid and posterior rotator cuff.[21] They also found significantly increased joint reaction forces when the subscapularis was repaired.[21] Giles et al confirmed these findings in another cadaveric study and concluded that rotator cuff repair, especially in conjunction with glenosphere lateralization, produced an antagonistic effect that increased deltoid and joint loading.[22]

41.4 Indications

Subscapularis repair should be performed in all cases of anatomic TSR. The tendon should be thoroughly evaluated, both preoperatively and intraoperatively, for integrity and quality. If it is determined that the tendon can be reapproximated, subscapularis repair is performed following TSR implantation. If the tendon cannot be appropriately mobilized, or is torn and not reparable, reverse TSR should be considered. For reverse TSR, recent evidence suggests that routine repair is not necessary for stability or postoperative function, and may at times be deleterious. In the setting of reverse TSR, if the tendon can be adequately repaired without undue tension, is of good quality, and the glenosphere is not significantly lateralized, repair can be considered at the conclusion of implantation.

41.5 Contraindications

In anatomic total shoulder arthroplasty (TSA), as inadequate or failed healing of the subscapularis tendon has been associated with worse patient outcomes,[23] repair is appropriate for all cases. If there is tendon attrition, poor tendon quality, the tendon is irreparable intraoperatively, or the tendon does not reapproximate despite adequate release, the patient should be converted to a reverse TSR implant. For reverse TSR, recent evidence suggests that repairing the subscapularis has no appreciable effect on complication rate, dislocation events, or range-of-motion gains and pain relief.[6]

41.6 Preoperative Preparation/ Positioning

41.6.1 Imaging

Standard X-rays of the shoulder obtained preoperatively need to include an axillary view. This is assessed for anterior humeral head subluxation, which would indicate incompetence of the subscapularis. It is not routine at our institution to obtain an MRI or CT scan prior to every TSR. When advanced imaging is obtained, however, the subscapularis tendon is inspected for partial or complete tearing. The muscle is evaluated for fatty degeneration and staged according to the Goutallier classification.[24]

41.6.2 Positioning

A regional block is performed preoperatively. General anesthesia is administered and the patient is positioned in the modified beach-chair position. We prefer to use a pneumatic articulating device (spider limb positioning system, Smith & Nephew) to securely hold and adjust arm position during the procedure.

41.7 Operative Technique

41.7.1 Approach

A standard deltopectoral incision is made starting from the tip of the coracoid distally to the deltoid insertion. The cephalic vein is identified between the deltoid and pectoralis major, and mobilized laterally with the deltoid. The interval can be developed by blunt digital release of adhesions and retractors can be placed under the deltoid and conjoined tendon (**Fig. 41.1**). This exposes the underlying subscapularis tendon and its insertion on the lesser tuberosity. The long head of the biceps tendon can be identified in the bicipital groove, lateral to the lesser tuberosity. The biceps is released from its sheath and tenodesed to the superior border of the pectoralis major (**Fig 41.2**). Proximally Mayo scissors are advanced along the biceps tendon as they course through the rotator interval with the tips aiming toward the base of the coracoid process. This releases the coracohumeral ligament, which defines the superior border of the subscapularis. Caution is taken to preserve the coracoacromial ligament. The anterior humeral circumflex artery and veins, so-called the three sisters, mark the inferior border of the subscapularis tendon and can be either ligated or cauterized. A heavy suture is used to tag the subscapularis tendon several centimeters medial to its insertion.

41.7.2 Subscapularis Takedown

Tenotomy

Once traction sutures are placed into the tendon, a scalpel or electrocautery device can be used to perform a tenotomy approximately 1 cm medial to the lesser tuberosity insertion

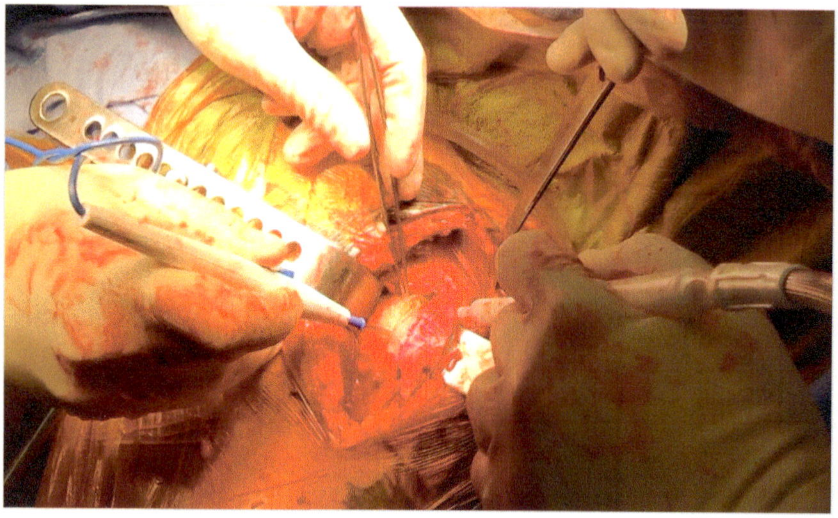

Fig. 41.1 Total shoulder arthroplasty (TSA) of the left shoulder through a deltopectoral approach. Retractors are placed around the deltoid laterally and the conjoined tendon medially. The medial insertion of the subscapularis is marked (*solid line*) and approximately 1 cm medial to this the tendon is incised longitudinally, either sharply or with electrocautery.

leaving enough tendon at the insertion to perform a tendon-to-tendon suture repair upon completion of the TSR. This is performed with the arm in neutral or slight external rotation using heavy, nonabsorbable sutures. Transosseous repair may be performed to augment the tendon-to-tendon repair if necessary. A partial tenotomy, leaving the superior 30 to 50% of the tendon fibers intact, has been described to help preserve postoperative function; however, this limits surgical exposure of the TSR.[25,26]

Peel

In the peel technique, the entire insertion of the subscapularis tendon is removed from the bone using a scalpel or electrocautery device after being tagged with a traction suture. The tendon is mobilized and retracted during the case. Heavy, nonabsorbable sutures are then used to repair the tendon through a series of bone tunnels at the insertion on the medial aspect of the bicipital groove (**Fig 41.3**). The repair can also be medialized to the anterior humeral neck osteotomy in the cases with the presence of preoperative internal rotation contracture or if lateralization of implants was performed.

Lesser Tuberosity Osteotomy

The arm is positioned in slight internal rotation and the lesser tuberosity is osteotomized with the use of a sagittal saw starting in the bicipital groove and aiming medially. The goal is to remove a 3- to 5-mm-thick wafer of lesser tuberosity. The osteotomy is completed with a 1-inch curved osteotome (**Fig 41.4**). With the osteotomy complete, if the subscapularis does not mobilize, position the arm in external rotation

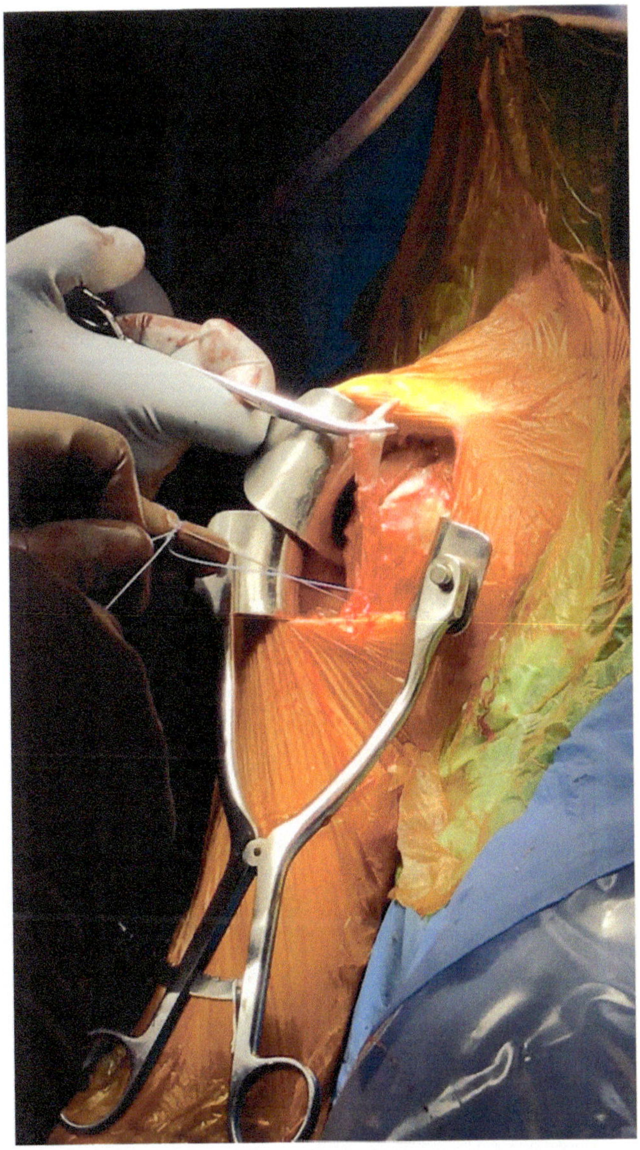

Fig. 41.2 The long head of the biceps tendon (grasped with a tonsil), after already being released from its insertion, is tenodesed to the superior margin of the pectoralis major tendon. This can also be performed prior to release of the biceps tendon from its insertion in order to aid in tensioning

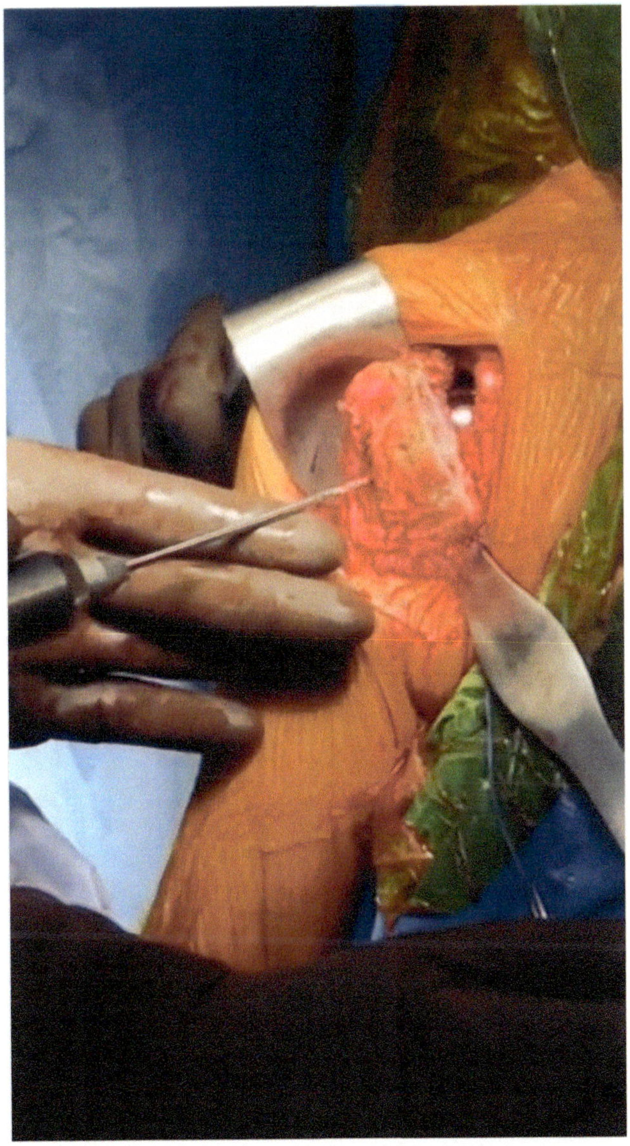

Fig. 41.3 Bone tunnels, just large enough to accommodate heavy, nonabsorbable suture needles, are drilled into the humeral canal starting at the medial border of the bicipital groove. If the subscapularis cannot be reapproximated to its anatomic location, the tunnels can be positioned more medially.

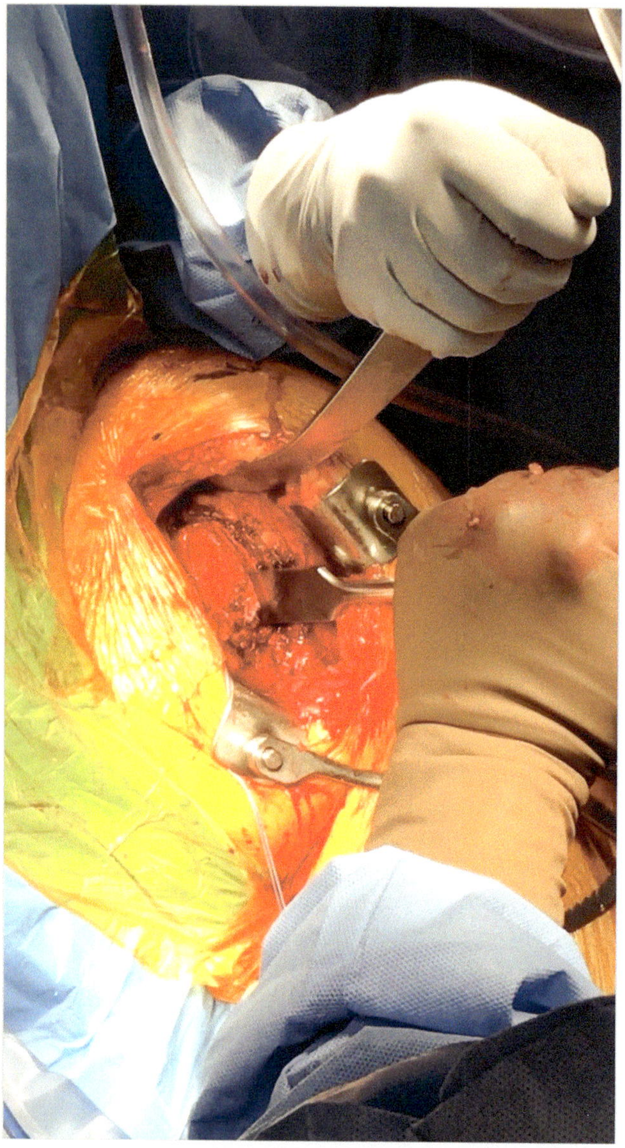

41.4 After using a sagittal saw to begin the lesser tuberosity osteotomy, it is completed with a 1-inch curved osteotome.

to place tension on any soft-tissue attachments. Identify the axillary nerve and protect it. Use electrocautery to release any soft-tissue attachments hindering mobilization without violating the subscapularis tendon.

With the subscapularis tendon mobilized, the humerus and glenoid are prepared in the standard fashion. Just prior to final humeral component placement, a 2-mm drill is used to create three drill holes starting in the bicipital groove and exiting within the canal. Three no. 5 FiberWire sutures (Arthrex, Naples, FL) are passed lateral to medial through the tunnels with corresponding sutures clamped to each other for later identification. The needles are left in place for later use. Any slack is removed from the sutures and the humeral stem implanted anterior in relation so that the sutures are wrapped around the stem. This mitigates the risk of suture cutout. The three sutures are then passed through the tendon just medial to the bony wafer. The most superior and inferior sutures are passed in a modified Mason–Allen technique. The middle suture is passed in simple fashion and is the first to be tied down, reapproximating the lesser tuberosity wafer back to its anatomic position. After the first throw, a Webster needle holder is used to hold the knot in place prior to the second throw, thereby ensuring an air knot does not occur. The remaining sutures are then tied in similar fashion. With the subscapularis tendon reapproximated, no. 2 Ti-Cron sutures (Covidien, New Haven, CT) are placed in the far lateral aspect of the rotator interval, reapproximating the supraspinatus to the subscapularis.

41.8 Tips and Pearls

- When performing a peel tenotomy, start directly adjacent to the medial border of the bicipital groove in an attempt not to leave any tendon behind.
- If there is a concern about overtensioning the subscapularis tendon, performing a peel tenotomy will allow for medialization and proper tensioning of the tendon during repair.
- Ideal fragment size for LTO is 3 to 5 mm.
- A strong, anatomic repair is required to achieve optimal outcomes.

41.9 What to Avoid

- Excising tendon during takedown of the subscapularis.
- Performing an excessively large LTO as this may increase risk of calcar fracture.
- Overtensioning the subscapularis tendon.

41.10 Rehabilitation

Although rehabilitation regimens may vary by surgeon, postoperative rehabilitation after subscapularis takedown should initially not exceed passive external rotation beyond what was obtained in the operating room. At our institution, we typically initially limit external rotation to a maximum of 20 degrees. A cadaveric study demonstrated that forward flexion and scapular plane elevation (scaption) do not increase tension on the subscapularis tendon and thus do not need to be limited after TSR, while external rotation and abduction should be restricted.[27]

References

1. Chalmers PN, Rahman Z, Romeo AA, Nicholson GP. Early dislocation after reverse total shoulder arthroplasty. J Shoulder Elbow Surg 2014;23(5):737–744
2. Edwards TB, Williams MD, Labriola JE, Elkousy HA, Gartsman GM, O'Connor DP. Subscapularis insufficiency and the risk of shoulder dislocation after reverse shoulder arthroplasty. J Shoulder Elbow Surg 2009;18(6):892–896
3. Oh JH, Shin SJ, McGarry MH, Scott JH, Heckmann N, Lee TQ. Biomechanical effects of humeral neck-shaft angle and subscapularis integrity in reverse total shoulder arthroplasty. J Shoulder Elbow Surg 2014;23(8):1091–1098
4. Trappey GJ IV, O'Connor DP, Edwards TB. What are the instability and infection rates after reverse shoulder arthroplasty? Clin Orthop Relat Res 2011;469(9):2505–2511
5. Defranco MJ, Higgins LD, Warner JJ. Subscapularis management in open shoulder surgery. J Am Acad Orthop Surg 2010;18(12):707–717

6. Clark JC, Ritchie J, Song FS, et al. Complication rates, dislocation, pain, and postoperative range of motion after reverse shoulder arthroplasty in patients with and without repair of the subscapularis. J Shoulder Elbow Surg 2012;21(1):36–41
7. Jackson JD, Cil A, Smith J, Steinmann SP. Integrity and function of the subscapularis after total shoulder arthroplasty. J Shoulder Elbow Surg 2010;19(7):1085–1090
8. Miller BS, Joseph TA, Noonan TJ, Horan MP, Hawkins RJ. Rupture of the subscapularis tendon after shoulder arthroplasty: diagnosis, treatment, and outcome. J Shoulder Elbow Surg 2005;14(5):492–496
9. Miller SL, Hazrati Y, Klepps S, Chiang A, Flatow EL. Loss of subscapularis function after total shoulder replacement: a seldom recognized problem. J Shoulder Elbow Surg 2003;12(1):29–34
10. Shields E, Ho A, Wiater JM. Management of the subscapularis tendon during total shoulder arthroplasty. J Shoulder Elbow Surg 2017;26(4):723–731
11. Adams JE, Sperling JW, Schleck CD, Harmsen WS, Cofield RH. Outcomes of shoulder arthroplasty in Olmsted County, Minnesota: a population-based study. Clin Orthop Relat Res 2007;455(455):176–182
12. Cofield RH. Total shoulder arthroplasty with the Neer prosthesis. J Bone Joint Surg Am 1984;66(6):899–906
13. Foruria AM, Sperling JW, Ankem HK, Oh LS, Cofield RH. Total shoulder replacement for osteoarthritis in patients 80 years of age and older. J Bone Joint Surg Br 2010;92(7):970–974
14. Neer CS II, Watson KC, Stanton FJ. Recent experience in total shoulder replacement. J Bone Joint Surg Am 1982;64(3):319–337
15. Caplan JL, Whitfield B, Neviaser RJ. Subscapularis function after primary tendon to tendon repair in patients after replacement arthroplasty of the shoulder. J Shoulder Elbow Surg 2009;18(2):193–196, discussion 197–198
16. Fishman MP, Budge MD, Moravek JE Jr, et al. Biomechanical testing of small versus large lesser tuberosity osteotomies: effect on gap formation and ultimate failure load. J Shoulder Elbow Surg 2014;23(4):470–476
17. Krishnan SG, Stewart DG, Reineck JR, Lin KC, Buzzell JE, Burkhead WZ. Subscapularis repair after shoulder arthroplasty: biomechanical and clinical validation of a novel technique. J Shoulder Elbow Surg 2009;18(2):184–192, discussion 197–198
18. Van den Berghe GR, Nguyen B, Patil S, et al. A biomechanical evaluation of three surgical techniques for subscapularis repair. J Shoulder Elbow Surg 2008;17(1):156–161
19. Giuseffi SA, Wongtriratanachai P, Omae H, et al. Biomechanical comparison of lesser tuberosity osteotomy versus subscapularis tenotomy in total shoulder arthroplasty. J Shoulder Elbow Surg 2012;21(8):1087–1095
20. Van Thiel GS, Wang VM, Wang FC, et al. Biomechanical similarities among subscapularis repairs after shoulder arthroplasty. J Shoulder Elbow Surg 2010;19(5):657–663
21. Hansen ML, Nayak A, Narayanan MS, et al. Role of subscapularis repair on muscle force requirements with reverse shoulder arthroplasty. Bull Hosp Jt Dis (2013) 2015;73(1, Suppl 1):S21–S27
22. Giles JW, Langohr GD, Johnson JA, Athwal GS. The rotator cuff muscles are antagonists after reverse total shoulder arthroplasty. J Shoulder Elbow Surg 2016;25(10):1592–1600
23. Buckley T, Miller R, Nicandri G, Lewis R, Voloshin I. Analysis of subscapularis integrity and function after lesser tuberosity osteotomy versus subscapularis tenotomy in total shoulder arthroplasty using ultrasound and validated clinical outcome measures. J Shoulder Elbow Surg 2014;23(9):1309–1317
24. Goutallier D, Postel JM, Bernageau J, Lavau L, Voisin MC. Fatty muscle degeneration in cuff ruptures. Pre- and postoperative evaluation by CT scan. Clin Orthop Relat Res 1994(304):78–83
25. Savoie FH III, Charles R, Casselton J, O'Brien MJ, Hurt JA III. The subscapularis-sparing approach in humeral head replacement. J Shoulder Elbow Surg 2015;24(4):606–612
26. Kummer FJ, Mahoney AP, Onyekwelu I, Kwon YW. Partial subscapularis release for total shoulder arthroplasty: a biomechanical comparison of two techniques. Bull Hosp Jt Dis (2013) 2014;72(4):259–262
27. Wright T, Easley T, Bennett J, Struk A, Conrad B. Shoulder arthroplasty and its effect on strain in the subscapularis muscle. Clin Biomech (Bristol, Avon) 2015;30(4):373–376

42 Total Shoulder Arthroplasty

Lawrence V. Gulotta

Abstract
Total shoulder arthroplasty is a safe and effective means to improve pain and dysfunction for patients with glenohumeral joint arthritis. Meticulous attention to soft tissue dissection is necessary to ensure adequate visualization for proper implantation, and for adequate balance postoperatively. Exposure of the glenoid starts with steps taken on the humerus, and include: 1) generous inferior capsule release off of the humerus; 2) adequate humeral head cut; 3) removal of all humeral head osteophytes; and 4) release of all subacromial and subdeltoid adhesions.

Keywords: *total shoulder arthroplasty, total shoulder replacement, shoulder osteoarthritis, glenohumeral joint osteoarthritis*

42.1 Goals of Procedure

- **Function**: Neer et al demonstrated total shoulder arthroplasty (TSA) to be a successful and reproducible procedure to restore function, even in its most seminal form.[1] More modern, short-term studies have improved functional outcomes, now with good to excellent results in up to 92 to 93% of patients postoperatively.[2,3] Metrics such as activity, return to sport, mobility, and strength are all significantly impro ved.[2,4,5] TSA has also been shown to improve quality-of-life metrics, as well as overall physical well-being.[6,7] Long-term studies have shown the durability of patients' functionality, remaining significantly improved for more than a decade.[8] Patient satisfaction reported in the literature is excellent, ranging from 86 to 100%.[1,5,8,9] Finally, long-term studies have reported excellent survivorship, as high as 87 to 88% at 15 years postoperatively.[10,11]
- **Pain relief**: Improvement in shoulder pain has been consistently demonstrated in the TSA literature.[1,2,8,12,13] Significant pain reduction is evident as early as 6 months postoperatively, improving until 1 year.[8,14] While shoulder pain relief does diminish trivially with long-term follow-up, significant pain reduction has been shown to have excellent durability, with data supporting improvement for at least 15 years.[4,8]
- **Shoulder range of motion (ROM)**: Patients gain and maintain significant shoulder ROM postoperatively after TSA.[4,9,10,15] A 15-study meta-analysis of ROM after TSA found flexion and external rotation improved 53 and 34 degrees, respectively.[9] When 1,800 patients were pooled, average flexion and external rotation after TSA was 141 and 34 degrees, respectively.[9] The maintenance of the ROM over time is also exceptional, with ROM in shoulder flexion, abduction, and external rotation significantly improved over a decade from the index surgery.[4,8]

42.2 Indications

- Advanced glenohumeral joint degeneration from osteoarthritis (OA), inflammatory arthropathies, trauma, and osteonecrosis.
- Intact and functional rotator cuff.

42.3 Contraindications

- Active or recent infection.
- Irreparable rotator cuff injury.
- Paralysis of the rotator cuff and deltoid musculature.
- Severe medical comorbidity burden precluding surgical intervention.

42.4 Preoperative Preparation/ Positioning

42.4.1 Clinical Evaluation

- A thorough history and physical examination should be conducted. This should include the intensity of pain, duration of symptoms, and secondary loss of function. Typical conservative treatments for glenohumeral degeneration include physical therapy, activity modification, and intra-articular injections.
- Physical examination should rule out cervical radiculopathy. Focused examination on active and passive ROM should be noted, with global ROM loss characteristic. Rotator cuff strength should be noted.

42.4.2 Imaging

- Radiographs: anteroposterior (AP), scapular outlet, and axillary views should be obtained. AP views should be assessed for superior humeral head migration, which can be seen in the setting of rotator cuff tears. The AP view may also be used to template the humeral stem. The axillary view allows for evaluation of posterior glenoid wear. The position and severity of osteophytes and loose bodies are also noted.
- CT: Evaluate for glenoid eccentric wear, retroversion, and other bony abnormalities. 3D reconstructions may provide further understanding.
- MRI: MRI may be helpful to evaluate patients in whom a rotator cuff injury is suspected, that is, evidence of superior escape on radiographs, or history of prior surgery.

42.4.3 Regional Anesthesia

- If not contraindicated, the authors prefer regional anesthesia for muscle paralysis and immediate postoperative pain control.

42.4.4 Positioning

- Beach chair: Instead of the upright position typically used in arthroscopy, the patient is placed in 45 degrees of reverse Trendelenburg and 15-degree airplane away from the affected side for a more ergonomic position for the surgeon and assistants (**Fig. 42.1**).

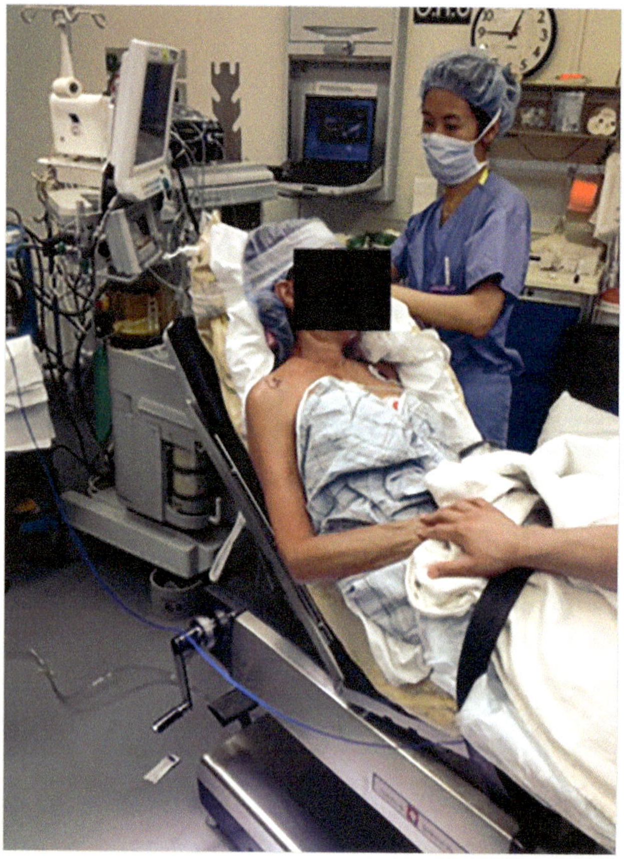

Fig. 42.1 Positioning.

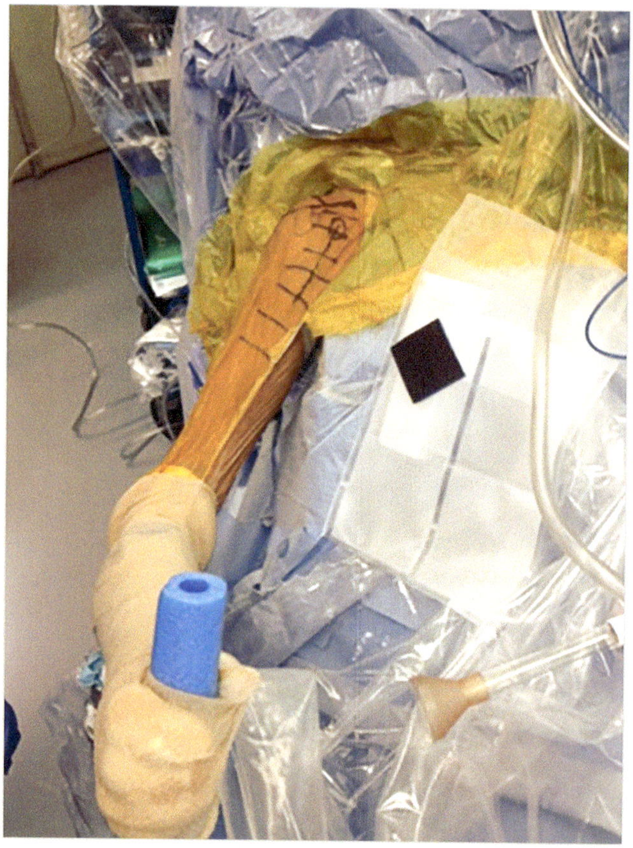

Fig. 42.2 Draping and incision.

- Beanbag: We prefer to use a beanbag to position the patient. A large beanbag spans from the head to the hip. The beans are molded around the head to hold the neck in neutral flexion–extension, tilt, and rotation. The beans are molded around the affected shoulder; contouring the beans to be 2 cm lateral to the medial scapular border allows the arm to be free, and stabilizes the scapula to reduce scapular motion while the glenoid is addressed intraoperatively. The beans are then driven back along the lumbar region so the arm can be adducted, extended, and externally rotated freely. This step is confirmed prior to the case initiation as it is critical to dislocate the humerus.
- Hydraulic arm positioner: This maintains arm position throughout the procedure.
- Draping: The arm and shoulder girdle are draped extending to the medial clavicle. The acromion, clavicle, and coracoid should be visible. We use a mesentery-style draping, sealing the axilla and all drapes (**Fig. 42.2**).
- All bony prominences are well padded as needed.

42.5 Operative Technique

42.5.1 Deltopectoral Approach

- Anatomic landmarks: The acromion, distal clavicle, acromioclavicular joint, and coracoid process are marked on the shoulder with a surgical pen.
- Incision: We make a more oblique incision for the deltopectoral approach than standard, extending from the tip of the coracoid to the deltoid insertion centered on the humerus (**Fig. 42.2**).
- Skin and subcutaneous dissection:
  - Position the arm in 20 degrees of forward flexion and neutral rotation to relax the interval. Avoid arm extension.
  - Skin incision is made with a no. 10 blade, through the epidermis to the level of subcutaneous fat. We then switch to electrocautery given the vascularity of the area. Dissection is carried down to the level of the deltoid fascia.
  - Gelpi retractors are placed superiorly and inferiorly in the incision to aid in dissection. Lifting superficially will allow an easy plane of dissection.
  - Developing the deltopectoral interval:
    - Identification of the interval almost always requires medial dissection. Dissect medial across the deltoid fascia until the fat stripe is revealed. Continue the dissection 2 cm medial to the fat stripe.
    - Unroof the fat stripe; curved Mayo scissors are used to carefully open the deltopectoral fascia superficial in the fat stripe. If not immediately visible, the cephalic vein will be deep in the fat stripe.
    - Use the curved Mayo scissors to develop a plane medial to the cephalic vein, taking the vein lateral with the deltoid. Be aware there may be many tributaries to the cephalic that can be ligated with electrocautery. These are typically seen at the tip of the coracoid. Replace the Gelpi retractors deep to the cephalic vein in the aperture

being developed. This will facilitate the identification of crossing vessels and separation of the interval.

- Subdeltoid preparation:
  - Reposition the arm in 60 degrees of abduction to relax the deltoid.
  - Place a large Richardson retractor under the deltoid.
  - Release the subdeltoid adhesions. This can be done bluntly with a finger, a Darrach retractor, or carefully with electrocautery. First, clear anteriorly under the deltoid, and continue lateral and posteriorly. Continue with the lysis until a Brown retractor can be easily placed behind the head, subluxing it anteriorly.
  - Pitfalls:
    i. Avoid damage to the axillary nerve as it wraps under the deltoid posteriorly. A tug test can be used to confirm the location of the axillary nerve.[16]
    ii. Preserve the coracoacromial ligament for anatomic TSA.
- Biceps and rotator interval identification:
  - Position the arm back in adduction at the patient's side. Palpate the lesser tuberosity, greater tuberosity, and biceps groove. The rotation of the arm should be adjusted so the biceps groove lies directly in front of the surgeon.
  - Identify the biceps tendon as it enters the groove inferiorly. Unroof the biceps tendon with electrocautery.
  - Once the biceps tendon is exposed, remove the tendon out of the groove with Mixter right angle forceps. The long head of the biceps is then tenodesed to the pectoralis major tendon with nonabsorbable sutures in a figure-of-8 configuration.
  - Transect the biceps tendon just cephalad to the tenodesis sutures.
  - Follow the biceps groove into the rotator interval from distal to proximal. We use curved Mayo scissors to incise the rotator interval. Stay on the medial aspect of the biceps groove to avoid errant supraspinatus injury. The Mayo scissors should easily transect the rotator interval; if the tissue is difficult to cut, this may indicate errant dissection into the rotator cuff.
- Anterior humeral circumflex vessels (the three sisters):
  - Identify the vessels at the inferior aspect of the subscapularis insertion and ligate these with electrocautery. External rotation of the shoulder can facilitate exposure of the vessels.
- Lesser tuberosity osteotomy (LTO):
  - Using electrocautery, clear the floor of the biceps groove near the subscapularis insertion.
  - Using an osteotome, cut a 5-mm wafer of bone starting in the floor and medial wall of the biceps groove, aimed directly medial.
  - Continue dissection medially on the superior and inferior border of the lesser tuberosity, mobilizing the subscapularis tendon and capsule.
  - Tag the upper and lower borders of the subscapularis tendon with nonreabsorbable suture.
- Capsular release:
  - Externally rotate the arm.
  - Perform a generous capsular release off the humeral neck. Start anteriorly and extend inferiorly. Take care to avoid the insertion of the latissimus dorsi as it inserts on the anterior humerus just inferior to the capsule.
  - Release the capsule to the 6 o'clock position on the humerus.

• **Humeral preparation:**
- Dislocation: In concert, bring the arm into adduction and external rotation.
- Retractor placement:
  - Place a Brown retractor laterally behind the head, a Bennett retractor medially around the head, and a Darrach retractor posterior to the head. Take care not to lever on the acromion excessively, as this may cause an iatrogenic fracture (**Fig. 42.3**).
- Neck cut:
  - Use the cutting guide to template the cut confirming version. Score the neck with electrocautery. Using the insertion of the supraspinatus and infraspinatus will approximate the angle of the cut.
  - Complete the cut with a saw.
  - Remove osteophytes with a rongeur, especially of the inferior neck.
- Humeral preparation:
  - The initial entry reamer may be sunk on power and continued until two sizes under the preoperative template size.
  - Hand ream the final sizes until a good cortical fit is felt, and harder cortical bone can be seen in the reaming flutes.

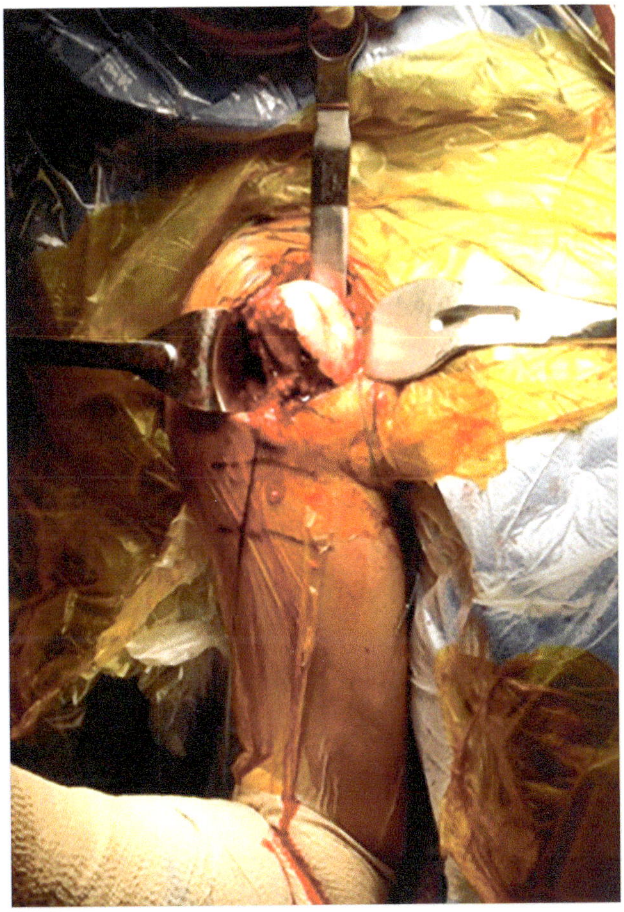

Fig. 42.3 Humeral exposure.

  - Complete broaching: We start three sizes down from the reaming size (8-9-10, for a reamed 10). Mallet the broach to the appropriate height, matching version of the neck cut.
  - Avoid overstuffing the humeral canal. In most press-fit humeral systems, the final implant has a larger diameter than the corresponding broach. If between broaches, it is advisable to go with the smaller broach to avoid iatrogenic humeral fracture.
  - When complete, place a humeral cap to protect the soft bony surface.

- **Glenoid Preparation:**
  - Internally rotate the arm, and translate the humerus posteriorly to expose the glenoid.
  - Retractors:
    - An anterior hip retractor is placed behind the posterior glenoid. Alternatively, a Bankart or a Fukuda retractor can be placed posteriorly.
    - A pointed Hohmann retractor is placed on top of the glenoid, just behind the origin of the long head of the biceps; take care not to injure the suprascapular nerve by avoiding placing the retractor too deep. The pointed Hohmann retractor will serve as the 12 o'clock position reference. Once placed, resect the biceps.
    - A two-pronged capsule retractor such as a large Bankart retractor is placed anteriorly (**Fig. 42.4**).
  - Anterior capsulectomy and subscapularis release:
    - Follow the upper border of the subscapularis back to the glenoid. Pull tension on the subscapularis tagging sutures to dissect between the middle glenohumeral ligament (MGHL) and the subscapularis with electrocautery. This will facilitate placement of the two-pronged capsule retractor.
    - Resect the anterior capsule and MGHL.
    - Beware of the axillary nerve as it dives inferior to the muscle belly of the subscapularis.

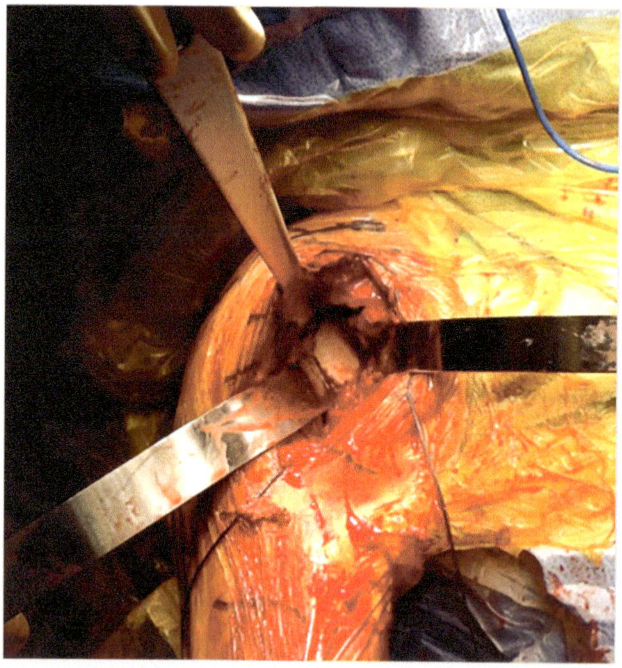

Fig. 42.4 Glenoid exposure.

    - Free the subscapularis from the capsule posteriorly, and from the coracoid superiorly.
    - Remove loose bodies from the subcoracoid recess if present. Forward flexing the arm can relax the conjoined tendon to facilitate removal of these loose bodies.
  - Labral resection:
    - Using electrocautery, score the outer rim of the glenoid circumferentially.
    - Take care when dissecting the inferior labrum so as to not injure the axillary nerve. Place your finger or forceps on the inferior capsule to tension the capsule, pulling this away from the glenoid, and release the labrum.
    - Starting the labral resection at the 12 o'clock position where the dissection is easier and placing an Alice clamp to provide tension on the labrum may facilitate this step.
    - In patients with posterior glenoid erosion or posterior humeral subluxation, take care not to release the posterior capsule when removing the posterior labrum as this may lead to postoperative instability.
  - Remove osteophytes: Use a rongeur or osteotome to resect osteophytes.
  - Orient: Mark a 12 o'clock to 6 o'clock position line in the glenoid with electrocautery. Mark the 9 o'clock to 3 o'clock position line. The intersection of the lines approximates the central glenoid where the peg or keel will seat.
  - Place the alignment guide for the respective system.
  - Ream away the remaining glenoid cartilage to bleeding bone. Eccentric reaming of the anterior glenoid bone stock may be necessary to avoid placing the component in retroversion.
  - Trial the component: The trial should sit flush on the reamed glenoid surface; resurface as needed.
    - Pearls:
      i. Perform minimal reaming so that implant is seated on hard subchondral bone, and not on soft cancellous bone.
      ii. For cementing, copiously irrigate with a pulse lavage to remove all debris. Apply cement, impact the glenoid component, and clear excess cement with curettes and forceps. Maintain pressure on the component through a finger or an instrument as the cement hardens.

- **Humeral component:**
  - Insert the humeral trial component, taking care to dial in the correct version.
  - Reduce the humeral component and check soft-tissue tensioning and component stability.
    - Tips:
      i. There should be approximately 50% translation when shucking the components in the AP plane. There should be a solid endpoint to posterior translation.
      ii. Forward flex the arm to 90 degrees and confirm the component does not dislocate posteriorly or inferiorly; advanced primary OA may predispose to posterior instability.
      iii. If too much laxity, upsize the head component.
      iv. If cementing, place a cement restrictor, pulse irrigate, dry with vaginal packing, or endosteal suction, with care to reproduce the correct version and height.
  - Drill three bone tunnels in the biceps groove (proximal, middle, and distal) for suture passage and approximation of the LTO.

- Impact the final stem prosthesis with care to dial in correct version, which is somewhere between 20 and 40 degrees of retroversion depending on the patient's anatomy and native version.
- Complete the suture repair of the LTO.
- Check the ROM of the prosthesis with care to observe your lesser tuberosity repair; the repair and prosthesis should move as a single unit.

- **Closure:**
  - Copious pulse irrigation.
  - Close the deltopectoral with a running nonreabsorbable suture—tagging the interval for later revision surgery if necessary.
  - Layered closure: running 0 Vicryl suture for fascia of Scarpa, 2–0 Vicryl for the subdermal layer, and 2–0 Prolene with escape stitch.
  - Sterile dressing.
  - Sling with abduction wedge applied in the OR.

42.6 Tips and Pearls/Expert Suggestions

Four tips for glenoid exposure:

- Adequately release the subdeltoid and subacromial adhesions.
- Release the capsule from the humerus to the 6 o'clock position.
- Cut the humeral head at the level of the supraspinatus insertion. Do not undercut the humeral head. Use the calcar planar to ensure adequate head resection.
- Remove all of the osteophytes of the humerus.

42.7 Complications/Bailout/Salvage

- Glenoid component failure and aseptic loosening:
  - Aseptic loosening may result from component malpositioning or insufficient bone stock for fixation. Thoughtful preoperative templating on axial imaging can help guide component version intraoperatively, as well as the need and location for autograft. Significant time should be spent on exposure of the glenoid to guide eccentric reaming if needed.
- Axillary nerve injury:
  - Caution must be taken during the anteroinferior capsule release.
- Intraoperative fracture:
  - Careful reaming and broaching should be performed when preparing the humerus.
  - Spiral humeral fractures can be caused from torque while positioning the arm.
  - Thorough capsular release and the use of a bone hook may facilitate positioning.
- Rotator cuff injury:
  - Care should be taken during the humeral head osteotomy to cut just proximal to the insertion of the rotator cuff tendons.
  - If rotator cuff tear is encountered at the time of surgery, either repair with sutures through drill holes in the greater tuberosity in younger, more active patients or convert to reverse shoulder replacement in older, more sedentary individuals.
- Instability:
  - Anterior instability:
    - Abnormal version may predispose the prosthesis for anterior instability. Stem revision is indicated if found to be the etiology.
    - Subscapularis insufficiency: Conservative therapy, tendon repair, or reconstruction with allograft can be attempted. Use of an LTO may abrogate this complication.
  - Superior instability:
    - Failure of the rotator cuff or loss of the force couple between the deltoid and rotator cuff can cause superior migration.
    - Physical therapy may be trialed, as well as rotator cuff repair, with salvage being conversion to a reverse shoulder arthroplasty.
  - Posterior instability:
    - It is often associated with excessive glenoid retroversion, with revision indicated. Capsular imbrication may be necessary if attenuation has occurred.
- Stiffness:
  - Stiffness may result from oversized components, soft-tissue imbalance, or poor therapy. Revision of component size, and procedures to rebalance the soft tissues, including anterior capsular and rotator interval release, may be indicated.
- Infection:
  - Arthroscopic culture is more sensitive than aspiration. Anaerobic culture bottles in addition to standard cultures should be held for 14 days for *Propionibacterium acnes*.

42.8 Postoperative Care

- The operative shoulder is placed in a shoulder immobilizer with an abduction wedge.
- Standard AP radiograph of the operative shoulder is performed in the postanesthesia care unit (PACU).
- Physical therapy is initiated immediately following surgery with Codman's pendulum exercises, forward elevation to 90 degrees, and external rotation to neutral.
- Patients are typically discharged on postoperative day 1 (POD1) or POD2, depending on their progression and perioperative pain control.
- Postoperative evaluation should include radiographs of the operative shoulder and clinical evaluation for ROM postoperatively.

References

1. Neer CS II, Watson KC, Stanton FJ. Recent experience in total shoulder replacement. J Bone Joint Surg Am 1982;64(3):319–337
2. Edwards TB, Kadakia NR, Boulahia A, et al. A comparison of hemiarthroplasty and total shoulder arthroplasty in the treatment of primary glenohumeral osteoarthritis: results of a multicenter study. J Shoulder Elbow Surg 2003;12(3):207–213

3. Adams JE, Sperling JW, Schleck CD, Harmsen WS, Cofield RH. Outcomes of shoulder arthroplasty in Olmsted County, Minnesota: a population-based study. Clin Orthop Relat Res 2007;455(455):176–182
4. Sowa B, Bochenek M, Bülhoff M, et al. The medium- and long-term outcome of total shoulder arthroplasty for primary glenohumeral osteoarthritis in middle-aged patients. Bone Joint J 2017;99-B(7):939–943
5. Garcia GH, Liu JN, Mahony GT, et al. Hemiarthroplasty versus total shoulder arthroplasty for shoulder osteoarthritis: a matched comparison of return to sports. Am J Sports Med 2016;44(6):1417–1422
6. Lo IKY, Litchfield RB, Griffin S, Faber K, Patterson SD, Kirkley A. Quality-of-life outcome following hemiarthroplasty or total shoulder arthroplasty in patients with osteoarthritis. A prospective, randomized trial. J Bone Joint Surg Am 2005;87(10):2178–2185
7. Carter MJ, Mikuls TR, Nayak S, Fehringer EV, Michaud K. Impact of total shoulder arthroplasty on generic and shoulder-specific health-related quality-of-life measures: a systematic literature review and meta-analysis. J Bone Joint Surg Am 2012;94(17):e127
8. Raiss P, Bruckner T, Rickert M, Walch G. Longitudinal observational study of total shoulder replacements with cement: fifteen to twenty-year follow-up. J Bone Joint Surg Am 2014;96(3):198–205
9. Radnay CS, Setter KJ, Chambers L, Levine WN, Bigliani LU, Ahmad CS. Total shoulder replacement compared with humeral head replacement for the treatment of primary glenohumeral osteoarthritis: a systematic review. J Shoulder Elbow Surg 2007;16(4):396–402
10. Deshmukh AV, Koris M, Zurakowski D, Thornhill TS. Total shoulder arthroplasty: long-term survivorship, functional outcome, and quality of life. J Shoulder Elbow Surg 2005;14(5):471–479
11. Torchia ME, Cofield RH, Settergren CR. Total shoulder arthroplasty with the Neer prosthesis: long-term results. J Shoulder Elbow Surg 1997;6(6):495–505
12. Stewart MP, Kelly IG. Total shoulder replacement in rheumatoid disease: 7- to 13-year follow-up of 37 joints. J Bone Joint Surg Br 1997;79(1):68–72
13. Gartsman GM, Roddey TS, Hammerman SM. Shoulder arthroplasty with or without resurfacing of the glenoid in patients who have osteoarthritis. J Bone Joint Surg Am 2000;82(1):26–34
14. Sandow MJ, David H, Bentall SJ. Hemiarthroplasty vs total shoulder replacement for rotator cuff intact osteoarthritis: how do they fare after a decade? J Shoulder Elbow Surg 2013;22(7):877–885
15. van den Bekerom MPJ, Geervliet PC, Somford MP, van den Borne MPJ, Boer R. Total shoulder arthroplasty versus hemiarthroplasty for glenohumeral arthritis: a systematic review of the literature at long-term follow-up. Int J Shoulder Surg 2013;7(3):110–115
16. Flatow EL, Bigliani LU. Tips of the trade. Locating and protecting the axillary nerve in shoulder surgery: the tug test. Orthop Rev 1992;21(4):503–505

43 Stemless Anatomic Shoulder Replacement

André Thès and Philippe Hardy

Abstract

Stemless reverse shoulder arthroplasty is a relatively new system designed to reduce stem-related complications such as periprosthetic fractures or difficult revisions. It is also associated with decreased operating time and a more anatomical positioning of the prosthesis. They can be useful in posttraumatic arthritis especially when there is tuberosity malunion. They are contraindicated in case of a poor bone stock in the humeral head that must be evaluated pre- and perioperatively and like others anatomic total shoulder arthroplasty in case of a rotator cuff tear especially because the humeral head resection is driven by the supraspinatus tendon.

Keywords: *total shoulder arthroplasty, stemless, surgical technique, malunion, posttraumatic arthritis*

43.1 Goals of Procedure

The anatomic shoulder arthroplasty aims to reduce the pain and preserve or enhance the mobility of the shoulder in patients suffering from end-stage shoulder arthritis without rotator cuff tear (RCT). Conservative management (such as physical therapy, medication, or cortisone injections) should precede any shoulder replacement. Stemless anatomic shoulder arthroplasty (**Fig. 43.1**) is a relatively new system designed to reduce stem-related complications, such as periprosthetic fractures or difficult revisions.

43.2 Advantages

The main improvement of the stemless shoulder arthroplasty is preserving bone stock in the humeral medullary canal. The position of the humeral anchor is independent of the location of the humeral canal, allowing for an anatomically driven reconstruction. The principle is to use an easily revisable prosthesis instead of a convertible one. The landmarks are the rotator cuff tendons. It is a soft tissue–driven implantation. These prostheses provide similar clinical outcomes compared to stemmed prosthesis with numerous advantages, such as decreased operating time, more anatomical placement, decreased intraoperative complications, less intraoperative blood loss, decreased risk of periprosthetic fracture, and, if necessary, easier revisions.[1-3] Minimal blood loss and a nonviolated humeral canal have led us to perform this surgery in an outpatient protocol.

43.3 Indications

Stemless anatomic shoulder replacement has the same indications as stemmed arthroplasty. The main indication for its use is glenohumeral osteoarthritis in the presence of a normal rotator cuff. Clearly, the proximal metaphysis has to be intact with sufficient bone stock. Evaluation of bone quality is crucial as it is highly correlated to the initial stability of the implant. This type of prosthesis is very helpful in posttraumatic arthritis with or without necrosis. In these cases, the anatomy is severely disturbed by tuberosity malunions. When the anatomy is severely disturbed by tuberosity malunions the results of anatomical implants associated with tuberosity osteotomies are poor.4 In these cases a reverse shoulder arthroplasty would be the good option and the stemless humeral implant allows to compose with the malunion.[5] (**Fig. 43.2**).

43.4 Contraindications

An RCT and active infection are classic contraindications to anatomical shoulder replacement. Many authors recommend

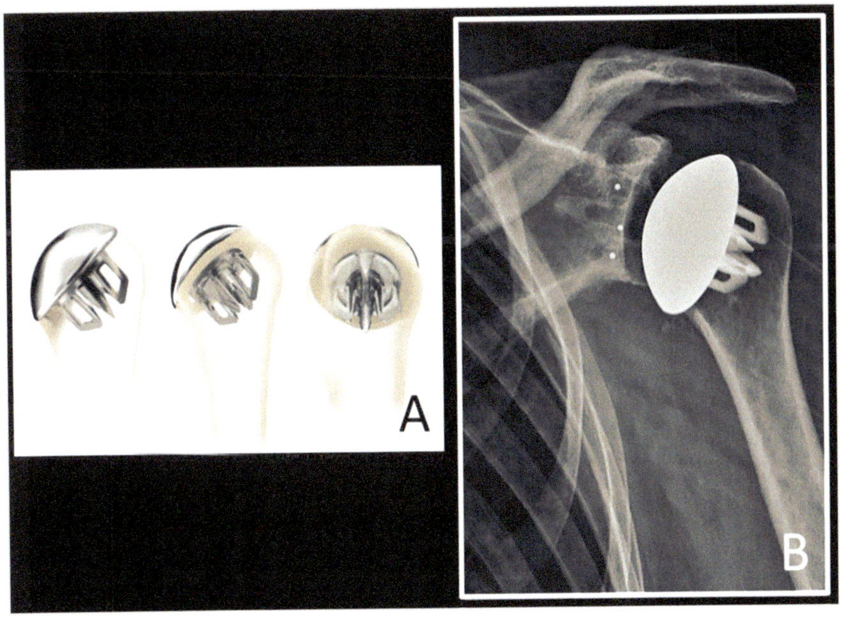

Fig. 43.1 (a, b) The Sidus Stem-free anatomical prosthesis (Zimmer Biomet).

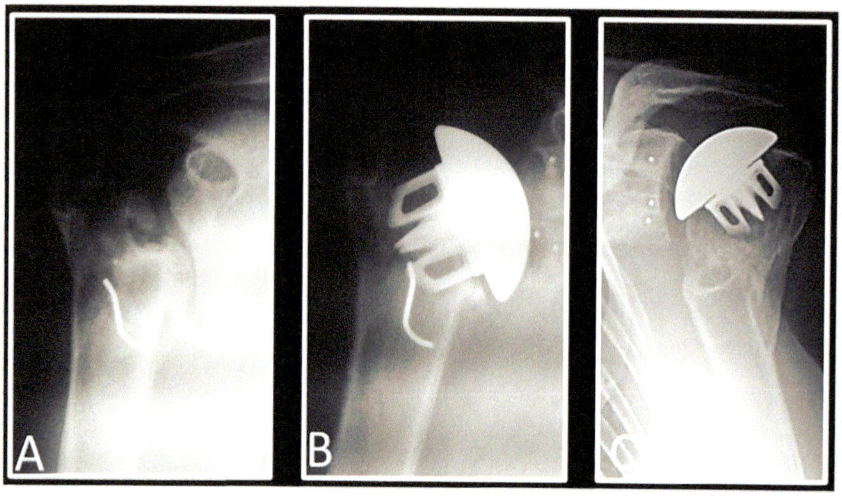

Fig. 43.2 (a) X-ray of a posttraumatic humeral head necrosis with tuberosities malunion. (b) After implantation of a stemless anatomic total arthroplasty. (c) Stemless anatomic total arthroplasty implanted on a proximal humeral metaphysis malunion.

reverse shoulder arthroplasty in B2- or C-type glenoid. Stemless arthroplasty has a specific contraindication related to the fixation of the humeral component. Primary stability is achieved with fins and press-fit impaction inside the spongy bone. A hydroxyapatite coating with titanium porous or trabecular metal permits secondary osteointegration. To avoid secondary displacement, the bone quality needs to be sufficient. Osteoporosis, a severe osteopenia or large cysts or tuberosity nonunions are contraindications to stemless implants (**Fig. 43.5a**). Pre- and perioperative evaluation of the bone quality is therefore of great importance.

43.5 Preoperative Preparation/ Positioning

The preoperative planning includes standard X-rays and either an MRI or a CT arthrogram of the shoulder. Contraindications to the stemless implants must be eliminated with these examinations. One should evaluate the bone stock in the humeral metaphysis and the glenoid wear. The presence of large osteophytes should also be noted. The rotator cuff is also evaluated. An RCT is an absolute contraindication to the total anatomic shoulder replacement.

The patient is positioned in the beach-chair position and the use of a pneumatic arm holder is helpful. A stemmed prosthesis should always be available as a backup if a poor bone quality is discovered during surgery.

43.6 Operative Technique

43.6.1 Approach

A standard deltopectoral approach is used leaving the cephalic vein attached to the deltoid. The conjoined tendon, the subscapularis muscle, and the insertion of the pectoralis major are exposed. A modified Brown retractor is placed laterally protecting the deltoid muscle.

A vertical tenotomy of the subscapularis muscle tendon is made 1 cm medial to the bicipital groove. The humeral head is exposed with progressive external rotation and capsular release from the anatomic neck. A lesser tuberosity osteotomy could be performed with the risk of compromising the initial

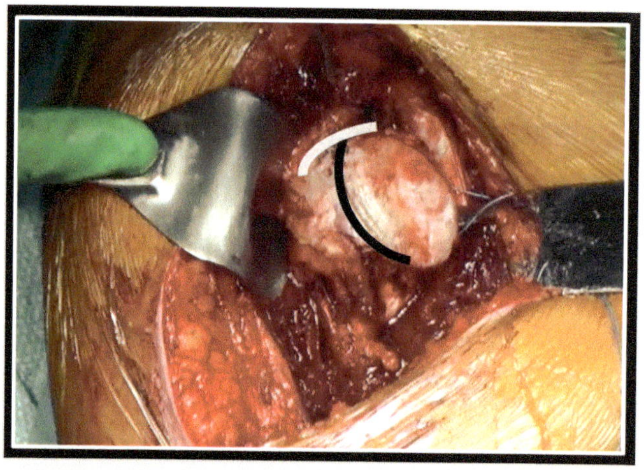

Fig. 43.3 Exposition of the humeral head. The white line represents the insertion of the supraspinatus tendon and the black line is the estimated cut, flush to the supraspinatus tendon.

stability of the stemless implant. If this option is chosen, the size of the osteotomized fragment should be minimal. Another option is to detach the tendon from the lesser osteotomy with bone chips. Our preferred technique remains vertical tenotomy. The long head of the biceps is cut at its glenoid insertion. We prefer tenotomy rather than tenodesis in most of the patients.

43.6.2 Humeral Head Resection

The humeral osteophytes are removed with chisels and rongeurs, but care must be taken to preserve the cortical bone of the humeral metaphysis. A Fukuda retractor is then placed in the medial position between the head and the glenoid to bring out the humeral head (**Fig. 43.3**). Then a small Hohmann retractor is placed just under the supraspinatus tendon, which is the most important landmark for the head cut. It is very important to expose clearly the insertion of the supraspinatus tendon. This will be our landmark for the cutting guide.

The ancillary system helps position the insertion of a first K-wire, thus bringing the anatomical retroversion to the cut (**Fig. 43.4**). This first K-wire follows the insertion of the supraspinatus tendon. The cutting guide is then positioned on the K-wire. This resection guide has a tip with a 135-degree angle that should be aligned to the humeral axis. Two or more

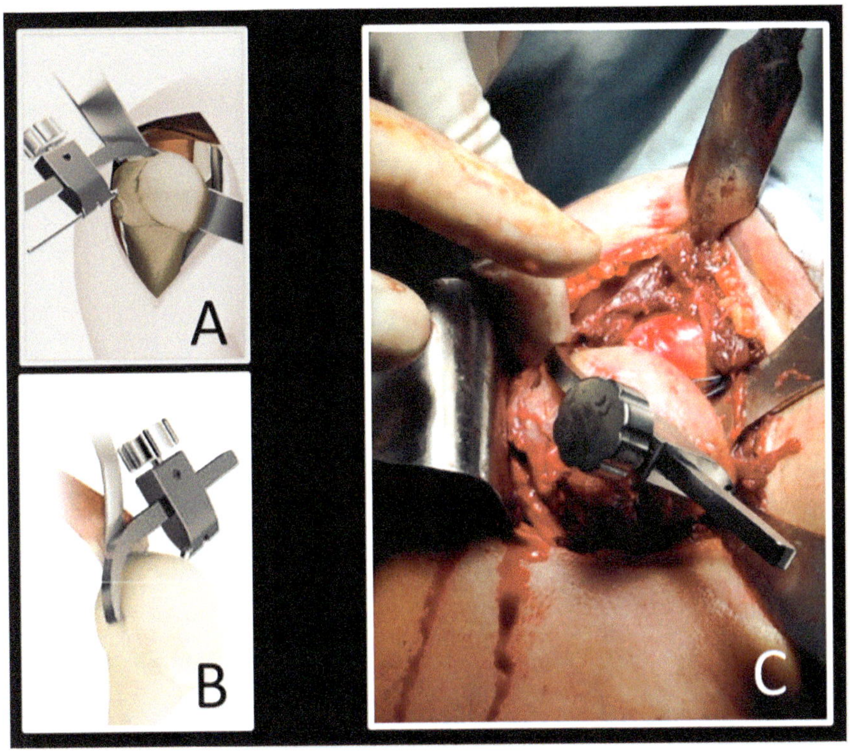

Fig. 43.4 (a) Positioning of the first K-wire gives the retroversion of the cut. (b) Posterior view of the ancillary system. (c) Operative view.

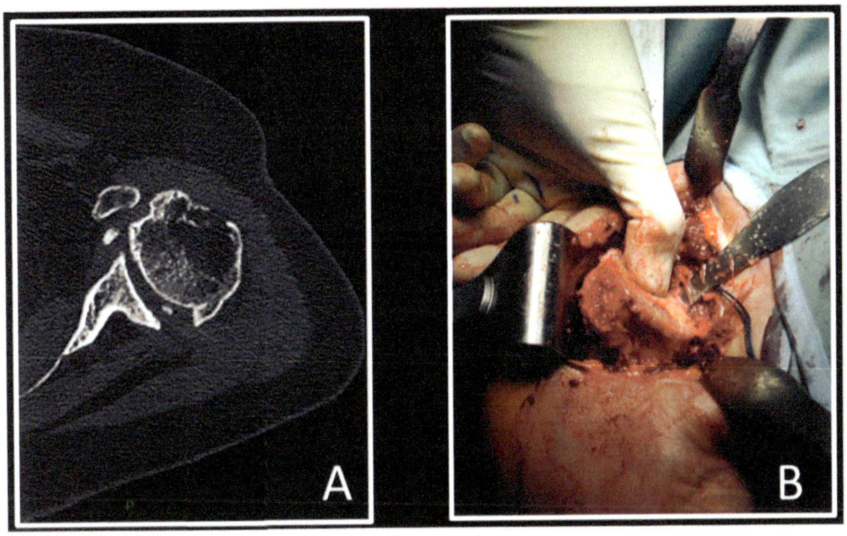

Fig. 43.5 (a) A large bone cyst in the humeral head contraindicates the implantation of a stemless prosthesis. (b) The "thumb test" permits perioperative evaluation of the bone quality.

K-wires are then added. The humeral head is then resected. The cut of the head must finish just at the insertion of the supraspinatus tendon and should be in contact with the K-wires.

After removing the cutting guide and the K-wires, the bone quality is assessed with the "thumb test" (**Fig. 43.5b**). The compaction of the metaphyseal bone under a light pressure of the thumb is a simple test to detect poor bone quality. If the head cancellous bone is easily depressed, a stemmed implant should be used. If no compaction occurs, the bone quality is good enough to use a stemless implant. Then, the anterior and superior cortex of the humeral head is protected with a humeral cut protector.

43.6.3 Glenoid Preparation

The arm is put in small internal rotation and small abduction. The Fukuda retractor is put behind the glenoid, a Hohmann retractor at the superior part, and another at the anterior part. Capsulectomy is performed by staying inside the joint, in contact with the bone, preserving the axillary nerve (limit the abduction, arm in extension, and stay close to the glenoid bone).

The glenoid is then prepared according to the implant used. A self-retaining glenoid retractor is used to expose the glenoid fossa (**Fig. 43.6**). Reaming of the glenoid cartilage shall not exceed the subchondral bone and it should be in most of the glenoid more anterior than posterior and more inferior than superior. Our preference goes to an all-polyethylene cemented pegged glenoid. The holes are coned and then the glenoid is washed with pulsatile lavage and dried. Cement is put inside the holes and compacted with a dedicated instrument. More cement is added inside the holes but not on the glenoid surface. Cement is applied to the backside of the glenoid implant, but the less possible and is then impacted. Excess cement is removed by pushing it to the anterior part of the glenoid so that it prevents pullout of the glenoid implant. Likewise, the removal of the posterior retractor should be done by pulling on the humeral head.

43.6.4 Humeral Implant Positioning and Anchor Size Determination

The arm is held in external rotation and adduction. A Fukuda retractor is put between the head and the glenoid and the Brown retractor under the deltoid. Head size was determined using trial heads. The rest of the procedure will be driven by trial implants. The size of the head is chosen so that it is flush with the superior (insertion of the supraspinatus tendon) and the anterior cortical rims (**Fig. 43.7a**).

A large central pin is then inserted through the selected trial head and clamped into the lateral cortex of the humerus but not further. The bone quality is checked again by gently moving the central pin. If there is a large movement, the bone quality might not be good enough for a stemless implant.

The size of the anchor is then determined using the reamers. No cortical bone should be seen inside the reamer windows (**Fig. 43.7b**). The largest size must be used to permit the best fixation, but the anchor shall not involve the cortical bone. A 2-mm-thick reaming is performed. This stemless implant allows minimal bone removal from the proximal humeral bone stock. Countersink the metaphysis with the corresponding reamer and then prepare the fin insertions with the impactor over the central pin.

Then the anchor is impacted in the prepared cuts flush with the humeral cut (**Fig. 43.7c**). The central pin is removed and the definitive head is impacted. If needed, a trial could be made with the trial head on the definitive anchor.

Remove any residual osteophytes or any bone extending beyond the periphery of the humeral head with a rongeur, especially in the medial aspect of the humeral head to prevent impingement with the glenoid. A trial glenoidal implant could be of help in order to avoid any bony impingement (**Fig. 43.8a**).

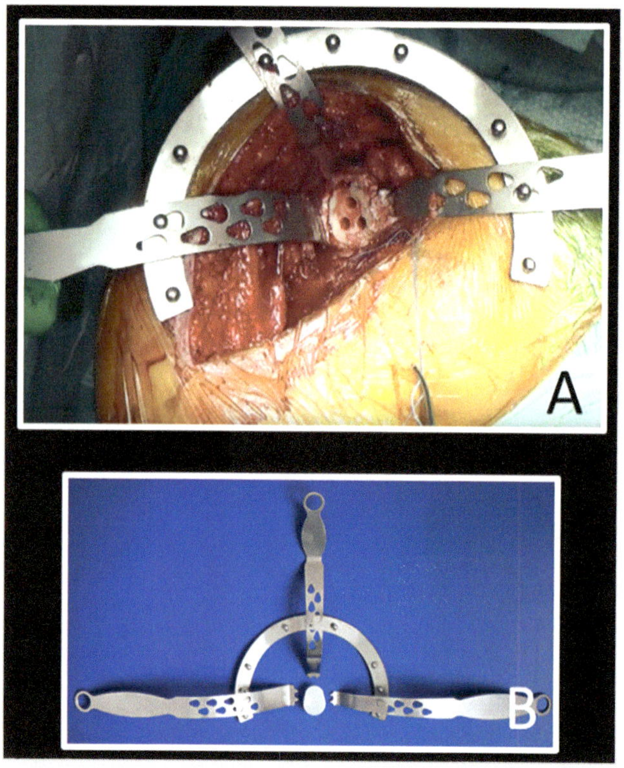

Fig. 43.6 Exposition of the glenoid **(a)** after capsulectomy and glenoid preparation is facilitated with a self-retaining retractor **(b)** (Arceau B2M Ready, Surginov).

43.6.5 Prosthesis Reduction and Closure

Reduction is achieved in internal rotation after removing the retractors. Before closing the joint, the subscapular muscle might be released anteriorly and posteriorly. When free enough, the subscapularis tendon is repaired using a double running suture with a no. 2 FiberWire (Arthrex) or equivalent. The interval rotator is not closed. After skin closure and dressing, the arm is held in a sling.

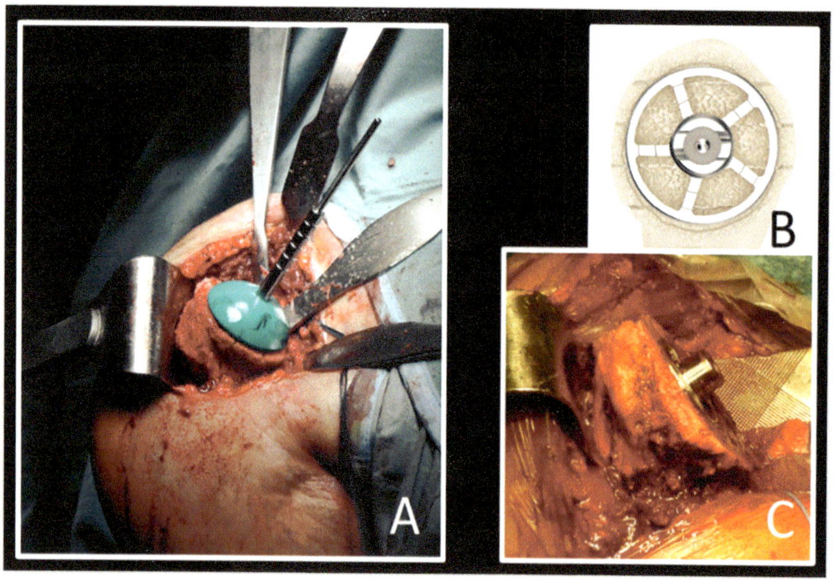

Fig. 43.7 **(a)** Operative view of the positioning of the trial head. **(b)** No cortical bone is seen through the reamer window. **(c)** The anchor is impacted flush to the cortical bone.

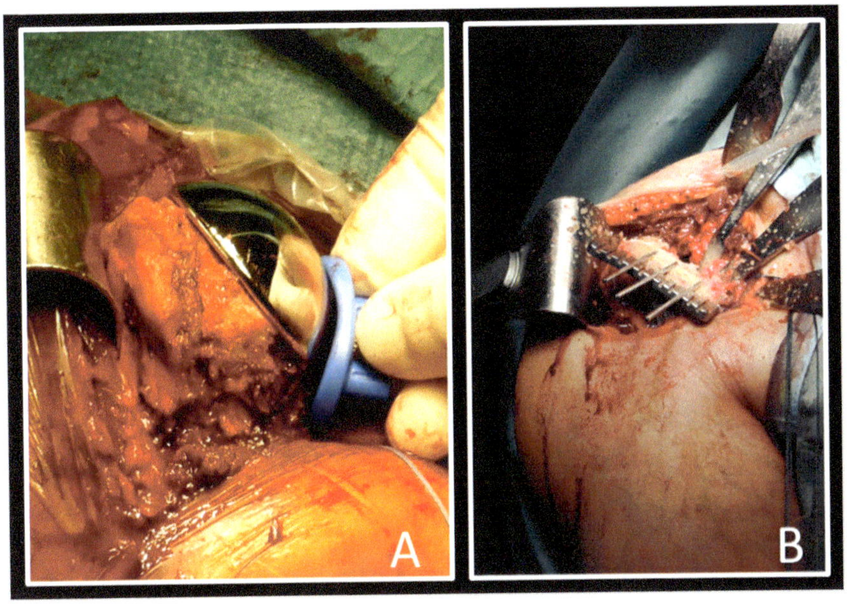

Fig. 43.8 **(a)** A glenoid trial is used to look for impingement with osteophytes or cortical bone on the medial aspect of the humeral head. **(b)** Overhanging of the humeral head is prevented by making a cut flush to the K-wires.

43.7 Tips and Pearls/Expert Suggestions

Positioning of the humeral cut is guided by soft tissues. The supraspinatus tendon insertion is the main landmark and must be well exposed.

The cut must be flush to the K-wires. Care must be taken to cut the anterior part as much as the posterior, preventing a bad positioning of the anchor (**Fig. 43.8b**).

43.8 What to Avoid

Overhanging of the humeral head should be avoided by using the thinnest humeral head for the chosen size.

43.9 Complications/Bailout/Salvage

Always have a stemmed implant in the OR if the bone quality appears to be insufficient.

43.10 Postoperative Care

- Sling immobilization for 1 month.
- Passive rehabilitation in flexion, avoiding external rotation for 1 month to protect the subscapularis tendon repair.

References

1. Habermeyer P, Lichtenberg S, Tauber M, Magosch P. Midterm results of stemless shoulder arthroplasty: a prospective study. J Shoulder Elbow Surg 2015;24(9):1463–1472
2. Maier MW, Lauer S, Klotz MC, Bülhoff M, Spranz D, Zeifang F. Are there differences between stemless and conventional stemmed shoulder prostheses in the treatment of glenohumeral osteoarthritis? BMC Musculoskelet Disord 2015;16:275
3. Berth A, Pap G. Stemless shoulder prosthesis versus conventional anatomic shoulder prosthesis in patients with osteoarthritis: a comparison of the functional outcome after a minimum of two years follow-up. J Orthop Traumatol 2013;14(1):31–37
4. Moineau G, McClelland WB Jr, Trojani C, Rumian A, Walch G, Boileau P. Prognostic factors and limitations of anatomic shoulder arthroplasty for the treatment of posttraumatic cephalic collapse or necrosis (type-1 proximal humeral fracture sequelae). J Bone Joint Surg Am 2012;94(23):2186–2194
5. Ballas R, Teissier P, Teissier J. Stemless shoulder prosthesis for treatment of proximal humeral malunion does not require tuberosity osteotomy. Int Orthop 2016;40(7):1473–1479

44 Patient-Specific Instrumentation Facilitates Glenoid Replacement in Shoulder Arthroplasty

Bradley Jaquith and Thomas (Quin) Throckmorton

Abstract
Patient-specific instrumentation improves accuracy of glenoid replacement in anatomic and reverse total shoulder arthroplasty and is especially useful in cases of glenoid deformity where traditional methods may be inadequate. Patient-specific targeting guides are developed based on preoperative 3D CT scans using modeling software. These guides allow more accurate placement of the glenoid guide pin, which aids in reaming the glenoid in correct version and inclination. Improved glenoid component positioning may improve implant stability, longevity, and function.

Keywords: *patient-specific instrumentation, shoulder arthroplasty, glenoid deformity*

44.1 Introduction

Accurate glenoid component placement is an important technical goal in shoulder arthroplasty. Multiple biomechanical studies have shown that glenoid component malposition in either version or inclination leads to compromised fixation and stability.[1–6] Glenoid component malposition also has clinically significant implications for implant longevity and function.[7–9] Standard methods to address glenoid wear patterns include eccentric reaming, bone grafting, and augmented components. In shoulders with glenoid deformity, these methods often are technically difficult and can lead to glenoid component malposition and early aseptic loosening. To prevent glenoid component malposition, CT scans have been used to develop patient-specific guides to improve the accuracy of glenoid component placement. Compared with traditional instrumentation, patient-specific guides have been shown to improve the accuracy of version and inclination and to reduce significant outliers in a cadaver study of 70 arthritic shoulders.[10] We describe our surgical technique with patient-specific instrumentation (PSI) in shoulder arthroplasty with specific tips and pearls.

44.2 Preoperative Planning

Standard preoperative planning begins with a radiographic examination of the shoulder. Our standard shoulder series includes anteroposterior (AP), true AP (Grashey), and axillary lateral views. The axillary lateral view provides information about the glenoid wear pattern and version of the glenoid. The true AP view provides an idea of the glenoid inclination. If rotator cuff function is in question, MRI, CT arthrography, or ultrasound can provide information to aid in deciding between an anatomic and a reverse shoulder arthroplasty.

Plain radiographs frequently are inadequate for characterization of glenoid wear patterns because of interference from the axillary soft tissues. Therefore, CT scans are often obtained for further evaluation of glenoid anatomy and for consideration of PSI. Multiple implant companies have 3D glenoid component planning guides with PSI (**Table 44.1**). The CT protocol used at our institution is in accordance with the patient-specific guide protocol and uses soft-tissue algorithms and 0.625 × 0.625 mm slices at 120 kVp. Patients are placed supine in the CT scanner with the arm externally rotated (palm up). 2D DICOM (digital imaging and communications in medicine) images are segmented to create a 3D representation of the patient's scapula. The Signature planning technique uses the 3D CT imaging to plan implantation in neutral version based on the method of Friedman et al.[11] This method aligns the implant version by aiming toward the medial border of the scapula and is defined as an anatomic version. Glenoid inclination is planned preoperatively in neutral inclination based on the methods of Churchill et al[12] and De Wilde et al[13]; an average of the results from both groups (8 degrees inclined from the anatomic axis projecting

Table 44.1 Available patient-specific instrumentation (PSI) for glenoid component placement

Company	System	Features
Zimmer Biomet	Signature Personalized Patient Care Glenoid System	Web-based portal where surgeon can develop preoperative plan after uploading CT scan. PSI guide developed based on plan for glenoid guide pin placement. Guide includes pin placement for anatomic and reverse total shoulder arthroplasty.
Zimmer	Zimmer PSI Shoulder System	Software-based 3D modeling system where surgeon uploads CT scan and develops preoperative plan. Guide developed based on plan for glenoid guide pin placement. Used only for reverse total shoulder arthroplasty.
DJO Global	Match Point System	Software-based 3D modeling system in which surgeon uploads CT scan and develops preoperative plan. Guide developed based on plan for glenoid guide pin placement. Separate guides for anatomic and reverse total shoulder arthroplasty.
Tornier	Blueprint 3D planning + PSI	Software-based 3D modeling system in which surgeon uploads CT scan and develops a preoperative plan. Guide developed based on plan for glenoid guide pin placement.
Arthrex	Glenoid Intelligent Reusable Instrument System	CT scan submitted to company and Ortho Vis 3D modeling software used to develop preoperative plan by engineers to be reviewed by surgeon. Custom model and instrumentation then developed for use in placing glenoid guide pin. Available for anatomic and reverse total shoulder arthroplasty.

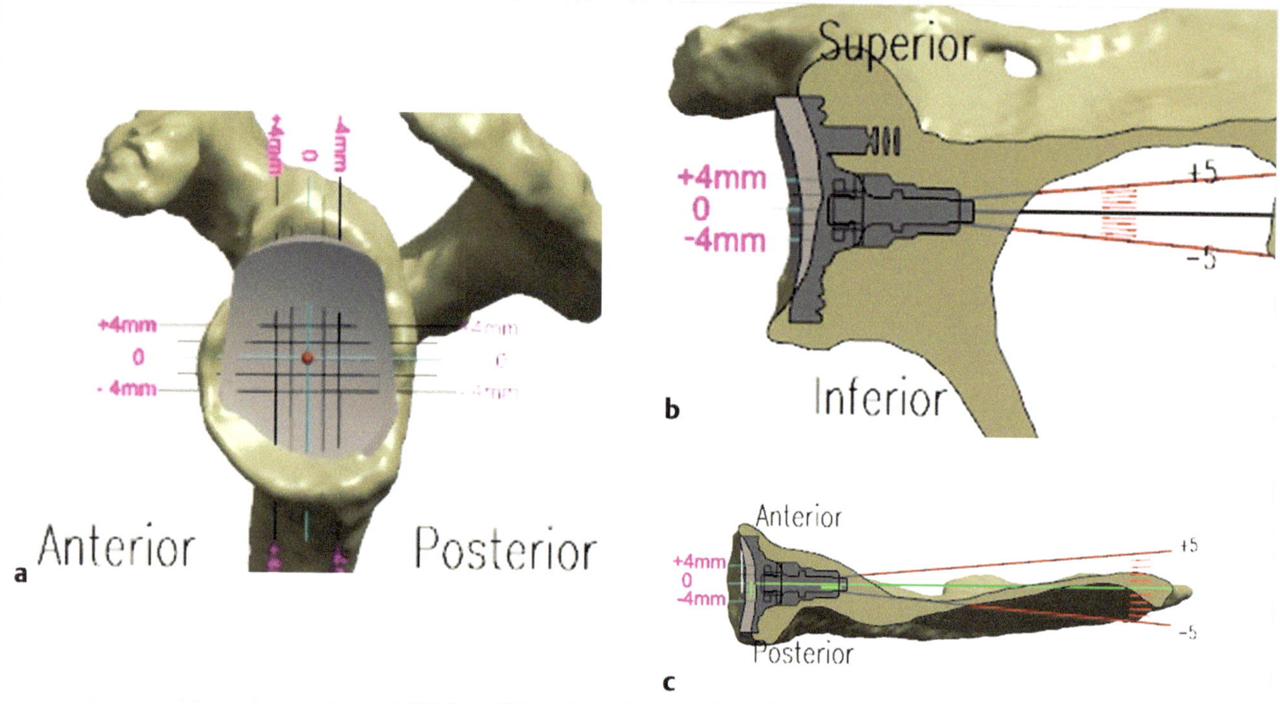

Fig. 44.1 Preoperative plan for anatomic total shoulder arthroplasty.

perpendicular to the medial border of the scapula) was used. A web-based portal is used by the surgeon to review and plan the starting point for guide pin placement (**Fig. 44.1**). Anatomic total shoulder implants are placed in the center of the glenoid based off the anteroposterior and superoinferior measurements of the glenoid. Placement of the baseplate components in reverse total shoulder arthroplasty is planned for the anteroposterior center of the glenoid, but positioned slightly inferior such that the inferior aspect of the baseplate is flush with the inferior glenoid rim. The position and orientation of the implants can be changed by the surgeon on the web-based portal and submitted to the implant company for review and creation of the guide. The patient-specific guide and a bone model of the scapula for reference are then produced (**Fig. 44.2**).

The importance of careful preparation and planning by the surgeon cannot be overstated. Only by studying the CT scan and truly understanding the glenoid deformity can an effective plan be generated. Surgeons are specifically discouraged from simply applying default values without further evaluation.

44.3 Surgical Technique

A standard deltopectoral approach is used and the humeral head is cut based on preoperative templating. After the humerus is prepared, the glenoid face is exposed. The soft tissues on the anterior aspect of the glenoid (capsule and labrum) are resected from the coracoid base to the 6 o'clock position. Using electrocautery to remove the soft tissue from the glenoid rim helps preserve the bony landmarks and create a clean surface for guide registration. Care must be taken to preserve the axillary nerve as it courses near the anteroinferior aspect of the glenoid. After dissection of the capsulolabral complex to the bone, the patient-specific targeting guide is applied and registers off the anterior aspect of

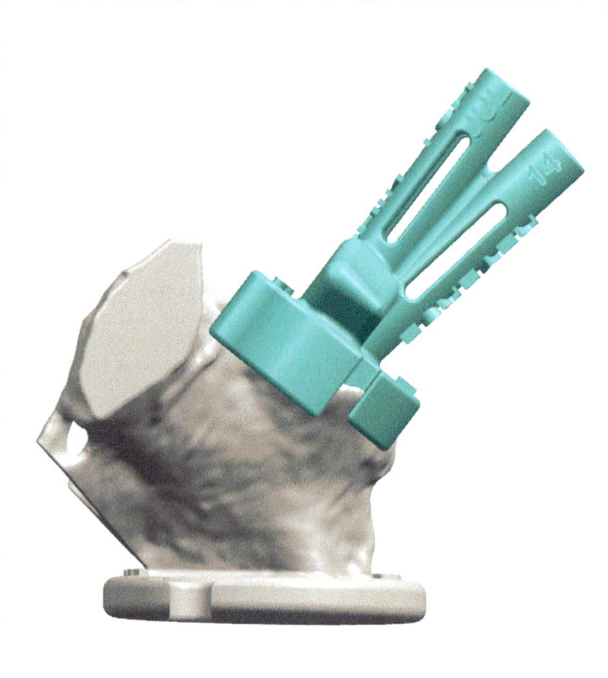

Fig. 44.2 A computer model of the glenoid with patient-specific targeting guide fitted on the anterior glenoid.

the glenoid (**Fig. 44.3**). When the guide registers correctly, a firm grip is felt on the anterior glenoid rim and contour of the glenoid face. There should be no toggle or shifting of the guide if it is correctly placed. Osteophytes should be left in place as the guide is designed to register off of them. The guide pin is then placed with a trajectory in neutral version and inclination for an ana-

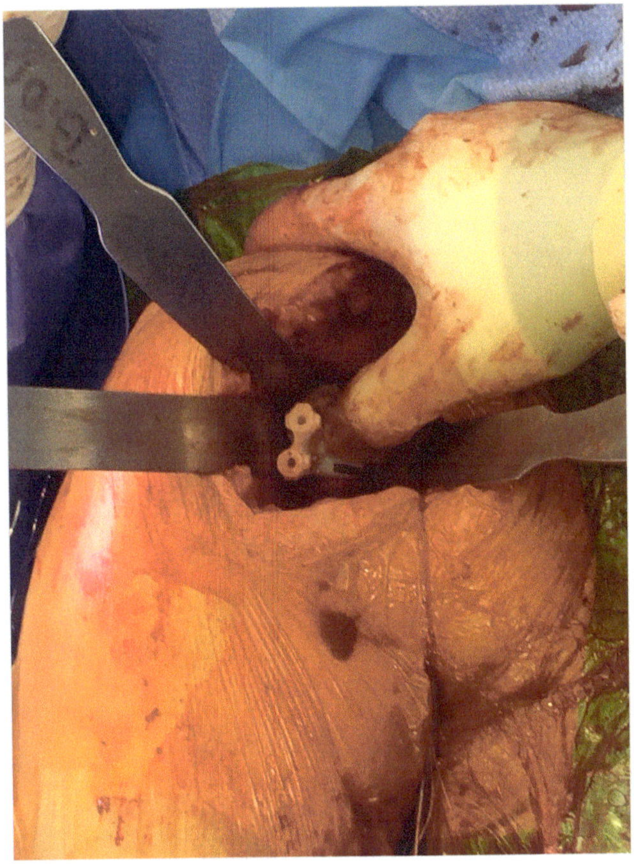

Fig. 44.3 Placement of the guide on the glenoid face.

tomic total shoulder arthroplasty (TSA) and with 10 degrees of inferior tilt and neutral version for reverse total shoulder arthroplasty (RTSA; **Fig. 44.4**). The glenoid is then reamed and components are implanted in standard fashion.

44.4 Indications for Patient-Specific Instrumentation

Patient-specific targeting guides have created a reproducible technique to improve glenoid component positioning in shoulder arthroplasty.[14] However, in an era of value-based medical care, it is important to understand that not all patients are optimal candidates for this technology. Specifically, the cost of custom, patient-specific guides is often cited as excessive for most standard shoulder arthroplasty cases. Alternatively, generic, reusable targeting guides have been found to have accuracy in glenoid version approaching that of PSI.[15] We, therefore, reserve patient-specific guides for shoulder with advanced glenoid deformity, usually more than 15 degrees (**Fig. 44.5**) where PSI can reduce outliers and significant component malposition.[10]

44.5 Conclusion

PSI is an effective tool to ensure proper glenoid component position in shoulder arthroplasty. While not a panacea or substitute for careful preoperative planning, it is effective to reduce component malposition, primarily in shoulders with significant glenoid wear. Meticulous dissection of the glenoid vault to ensure proper guide registration is crucial to technical success.

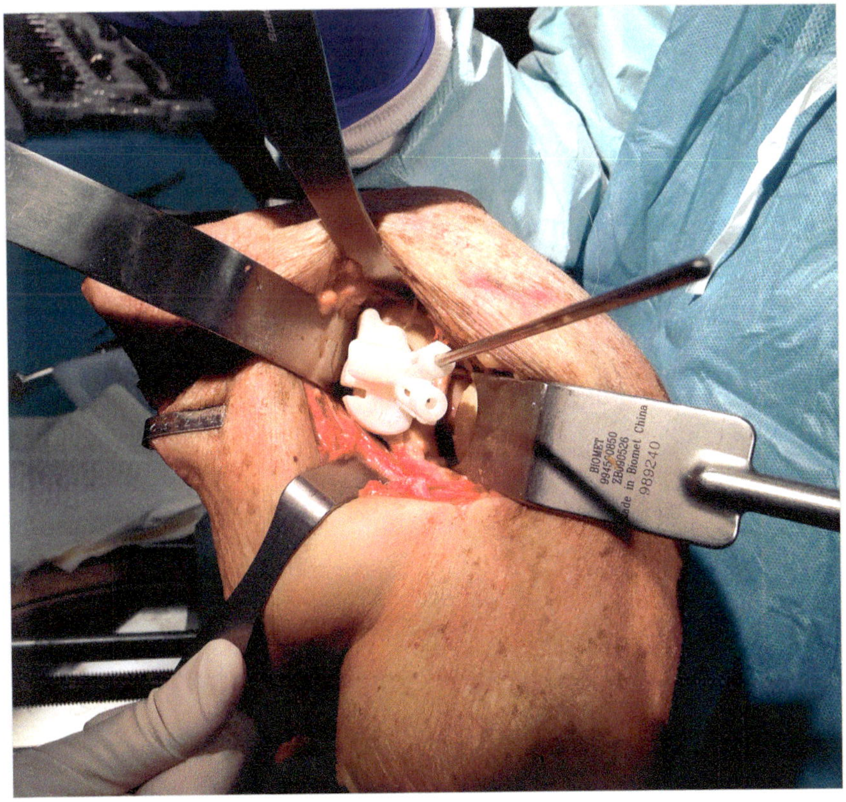

Fig. 44.4 Placement of the guide pin in the superior hole for an anatomic shoulder arthroplasty in a cadaver specimen. The inferior pin can be used for a reverse total shoulder arthroplasty.

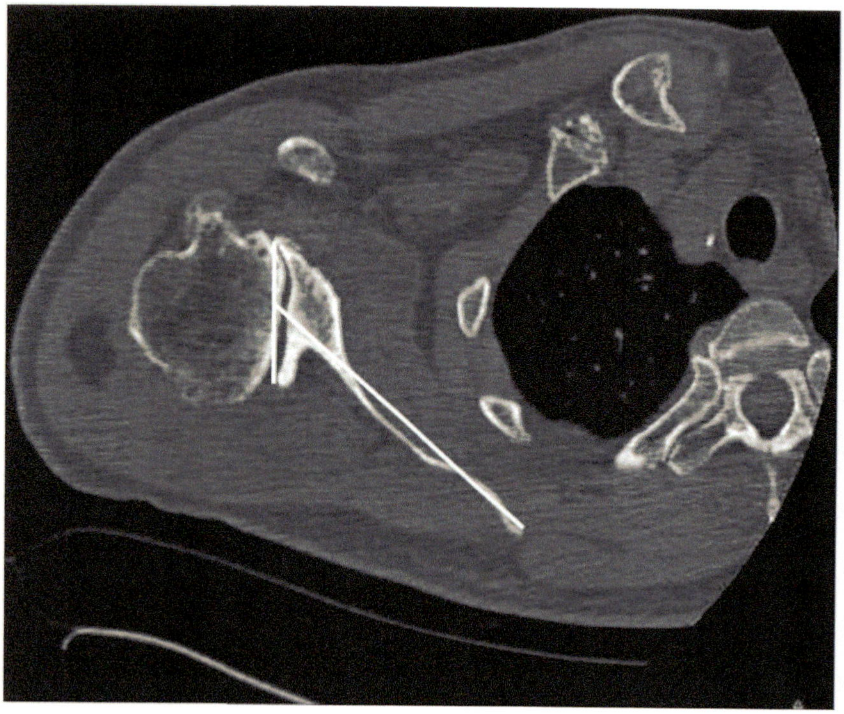

Fig. 44.5 Example of advanced glenoid deformity where patient-specific instrumentation is useful.

References

1. Hopkins AR, Hansen UN, Amis AA, Emery R. The effects of glenoid component alignment variations on cement mantle stresses in total shoulder arthroplasty. J Shoulder Elbow Surg 2004;13(6):668–675
2. Mansat P, Briot J, Mansat M, Swider P. Evaluation of the glenoid implant survival using a biomechanical finite element analysis: influence of the implant design, bone properties, and loading location. J Shoulder Elbow Surg 2007;16(3, Suppl):S79–S83
3. Nyffeler RW, Sheikh R, Atkinson TS, Jacob HAC, Favre P, Gerber C. Effects of glenoid component version on humeral head displacement and joint reaction forces: an experimental study. J Shoulder Elbow Surg 2006;15(5):625–629
4. Oosterom R, Rozing PM, Bersee HEN. Effect of glenoid component inclination on its fixation and humeral head subluxation in total shoulder arthroplasty. Clin Biomech (Bristol, Avon) 2004;19(10):1000–1008
5. Shapiro TA, McGarry MH, Gupta R, Lee YS, Lee TQ. Biomechanical effects of glenoid retroversion in total shoulder arthroplasty. J Shoulder Elbow Surg 2007;16(3, Suppl):S90–S95
6. Suárez DR, van der Linden JC, Valstar ER, et al. Influence of the positioning of a cementless glenoid prosthesis on its interface micromotions. Proc Inst Mech Eng H 2009;223(7):795–804
7. Favre P, Sussmann PS, Gerber C. The effect of component positioning on intrinsic stability of the reverse shoulder arthroplasty. J Shoulder Elbow Surg 2010;19(4):550–556
8. Gutiérrez S, Greiwe RM, Frankle MA, Siegal S, Lee WE III. Biomechanical comparison of component position and hardware failure in the reverse shoulder prosthesis. J Shoulder Elbow Surg 2007;16(3, Suppl):S9–S12
9. Ho JC, Sabesan VJ, Iannotti JP. Glenoid component retroversion is associated with osteolysis. J Bone Joint Surg Am 2013;95(12):e82
10. Throckmorton TW, Gulotta LV, Bonnarens FO, et al. Patient-specific targeting guides compared with traditional instrumentation for glenoid component placement in shoulder arthroplasty: a multi-surgeon study in 70 arthritic cadaver specimens. J Shoulder Elbow Surg 2015;24(6):965–971
11. Friedman RJ, Hawthorne KB, Genez BM. The use of computerized tomography in the measurement of glenoid version. J Bone Joint Surg Am 1992;74(7):1032–1037
12. Churchill RS, Brems JJ, Kotschi H. Glenoid size, inclination, and version: an anatomic study. J Shoulder Elbow Surg 2001;10(4):327–332
13. De Wilde LF, Verstraeten T, Speeckaert W, Karelse A. Reliability of the glenoid plane. J Shoulder Elbow Surg 2010;19(3):414–422
14. Throckmorton TW, Vogt W, Wasmaier J, Hurst JM, Frostick S, Sperling JW. Patient-specific targeting guides for glenoid component placement in shoulder arthroplasty: technique and initial clinical experiences. Tech Shoulder Elbow Surg 2014;15(4):103–108
15. Mulligan RP, Azar FM, Throckmorton TW. Is a generic targeting guide useful for glenoid component placement in shoulder arthroplasty? J Shoulder Elbow Surg 2016;25(4):e90–e95

45 Posterior Glenoid Wear in Total Shoulder Replacement: Eccentric Reaming

Lauren Casnovsky, Edward Craig, and Alicia K. Harrison

Abstract

Eccentric reaming is a common technique in addressing posterior glenoid wear during total shoulder replacement. Posterior glenoid wear is a well-described pattern of glenohumeral arthritis and is one of the hallmarks of primary osteoarthritis of the shoulder. Early on in the process, with less severe glenoid wear, the arthritic humeral head remains well centered on the glenoid. As a greater degree of wear occurs, increasing amounts of humeral head posterior subluxation complements this pathology. This is frequently accompanied by posterior capsular incompetence and can be a challenge to a successful anatomic total shoulder arthroplasty. It has been widely demonstrated that the degree of glenoid retroversion and posterior humeral subluxation have great impacts on the success rates of shoulder replacements.[2] By eccentrically reaming the anterior cortex in patients with 5 to 10 degrees of retroversion, the glenoid version is corrected to an anatomic neutral version position. Where appropriate, eccentric reaming avoids the need for more technically complex procedures such as glenoid bone grafts or augmented glenoid components for use in anatomic arthroplasty. Although eccentric reaming of the glenoid is a common technique in total shoulder arthroplasty, there are also risks associated with the practice. Because of the "funnel" shape of the glenoid vault, one must be careful to avoid aggressive over-reaming of the anterior cortex, due to the risk of cortical perforation, loosening of the future implant, and even implant failure. The authors have identified various tricks for successful asymmetric reaming and avoidance of potential complications.

Keywords: *eccentric reaming, posterior subluxation, glenohumeral arthritis, total shoulder arthroplasty*

45.1 Goals of Procedure

Eccentric reaming is a common technique in addressing posterior glenoid wear during total shoulder replacement. Walch et al classified the patterns of acquired glenoid retroversion, as seen in **Fig. 45.1**.[1] The goals of eccentric reaming are to establish relatively normal version of the glenoid without sacrificing subchondral bone for implant placement, permitting an anatomic arthroplasty to more predictably remain centered. This is a frequent challenge as the degree of retroversion has a large impact on the success of total shoulder replacements.[2]

45.2 Advantages

There are several advantages to eccentrically reaming the glenoid during total shoulder arthroplasty. Glenoid version may be corrected to a more anatomical position, permitting the utilization of a standard glenoid implant, without

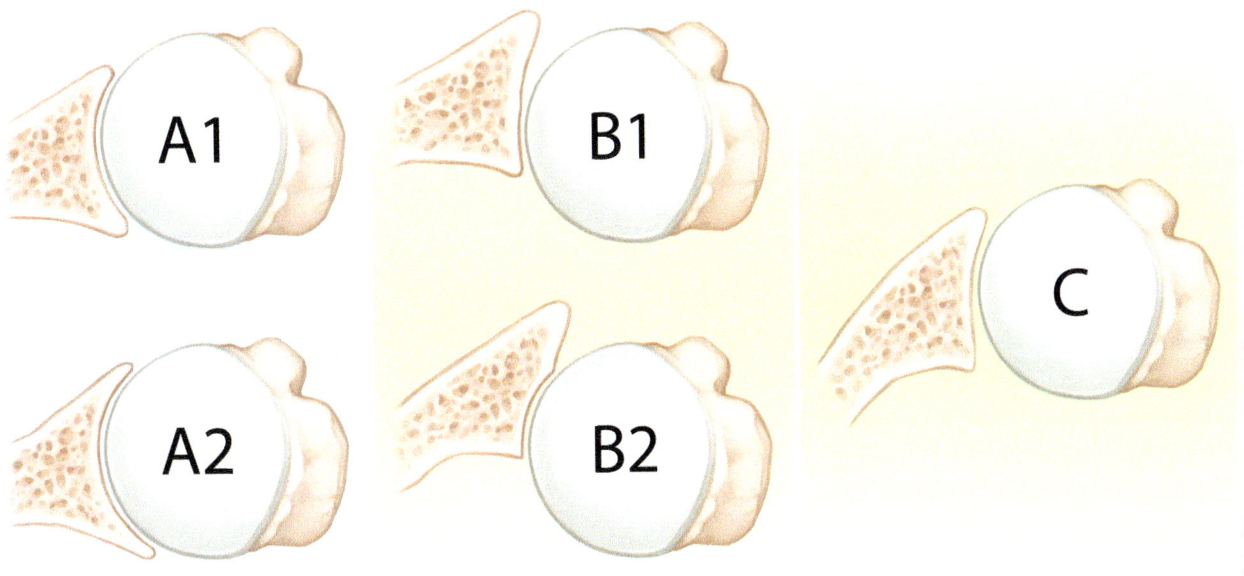

Fig. 45.1 Walch's classification.

having to utilize graft, augmented implant, or a more constrained (reverse) implant. However, it has been shown that as the glenoid retroversion increases, asymmetric reaming becomes less feasible without compromising glenoid integrity. In a study of eight cadaveric scapulae, Gillespie et al simulated posterior glenoid wear in 5-degree increments. By eccentrically reaming glenoid specimens with greater than 15 degree of retroversion, placement of a pegged glenoid was not possible in 50% of the specimens due to inadequate bone stock, peg penetration, or both.[3]

Eccentric reaming is also used to correct posterior humeral subluxation when associated with glenoid retroversion, though, on occasion, posterior capsular plication is an additional technical option. Habermeyer et al evaluated 77 patients undergoing primary total shoulder arthroplasty to determine whether eccentric reaming could correct posterior subluxation. Postoperatively, no posterior subluxation was observed and 86% of the humeral heads were centered.[4] Gerber et al followed 33 patients undergoing total shoulder replacement whose preoperative subluxation index averaged 71% and preoperative glenoid retroversion was 18 degrees. Eccentric reaming of the glenoid was able to restore version within 0 to 10 degrees and subluxation was corrected in 21 patients. In addition, patient constant scores, age-adjusted constant scores, and subjective shoulder values improved postoperatively.[5]

Bone graft augmentation has been described as one approach for correcting excessive glenoid retroversion.[6] Eccentric reaming may be less technically demanding than bone grafting and is not associated with the same significant postoperative complications. Clinical results for glenoid bone grafting have been mixed and are associated with glenoid component failure, graft complications, and instability.[7]

In the presence of significant posterior bone loss, failure to make corrections in an attempt to normalize version may result in a variable amount of the glenoid component remaining unsupported by bone. One additional technical tip may be the use of a glenoid component sized slightly smaller than one fitting the native glenoid exactly. A smaller sized glenoid may well result in more uniform support on subchondral bone.

45.3 Indications

Eccentric reaming of the glenoid can be used in patients who have symptomatic glenohumeral arthritis with up to 10 to 15 degrees of glenoid retroversion.

Implant selection is an important consideration when selecting a version correcting technique. Implant designs have differing fixation designs: keeled, inline peg, out-of-line peg, or even hybrid implants, combining poly peg and ingrowth central fixation devices. Keeled and inline pegs may be more amenable to use with asymmetric reaming techniques when compared with out-of-line components. Out-of-line pegs sometimes are associated with perforation of the cortex, as the anterior and posterior peg preparation is in bone where there is less depth. Using a slightly smaller size glenoid may make this less of a problem. In addition, depending on how many points of fixation the particular implant design has, perforation of an anterior or a posterior peg hole is rarely a significant problem, and implant choice should take into consideration that argument that peg fixation, either inline or out of line, may more effectively resist pullout forces.

45.4 Contraindications

Although asymmetric reaming can be used in the majority of glenoid preparations, it has been widely demonstrated that this technique should not be employed in the cases with greater than 15 degrees of glenoid retroversion if one's goal is to normalize the glenoid version. Asymmetric reaming with greater degrees of glenoid retroversion may make normalization of the version impossible without compromising bone support.

45.5 Preoperative Preparation/ Positioning

Thoughtful imaging prior to total shoulder arthroplasty allows for accurate preoperative planning and evaluation of the glenoid bone stock. Radiographs of the glenohumeral joint should include the following views: anteroposterior in the plane of the scapula, standard anteroposterior, scapular Y, and axillary. Furthermore, CT, with or without 3D reconstruction and humeral head subtraction, or MRI scans prove helpful in determining the degree of glenoid retroversion and precise imaging of the patient anatomy, an essential element in surgical planning (**Fig. 45.2**). By evaluating these preoperative images, and precisely measuring glenoid axis and retroversion, one is able to determine whether or not eccentric reaming alone can be used to correct the glenoid deficiency. In some arthroplasty systems, patient-matched instrumentation may be helpful for glenoid preparation.

The patient should be positioned in a standard beach-chair position with all bony prominences padded. The patient's head is placed in a headrest taking care to keep the neck in a neutral position. The shoulder and extremity are draped widely such that the entire field is exposed.

45.6 Operative Technique

A standard deltopectoral approach is undertaken. The long head of the biceps is tenotomized with or without a plan for later tenodesis, as this more easily permits humeral extension for access to humeral shaft. The anterior circumflex vessels are then ligated or cauterized. The joint is then entered via a subscapularis tenotomy, subscapularis subperiosteal peel, or lesser tuberosity osteotomy. Knowledge of axillary nerve anatomy is essential for protection of this important structure. Direct visualization, surgical palpation, and the axillary nerve tug test are methods that may be utilized throughout the exposure and during the procedure to ensure nerve integrity and minimize the chance of direct or indirect injury, particularly during capsular releases.

After humeral preparation, the glenoid is exposed. Sufficient glenoid exposure encompasses many steps, including adequate anesthesia, blunt release of subdeltoid and subacromial adhesions and scar, complete subscapularis division, complete humeral head osteophyte removal, capsular releases anteriorly

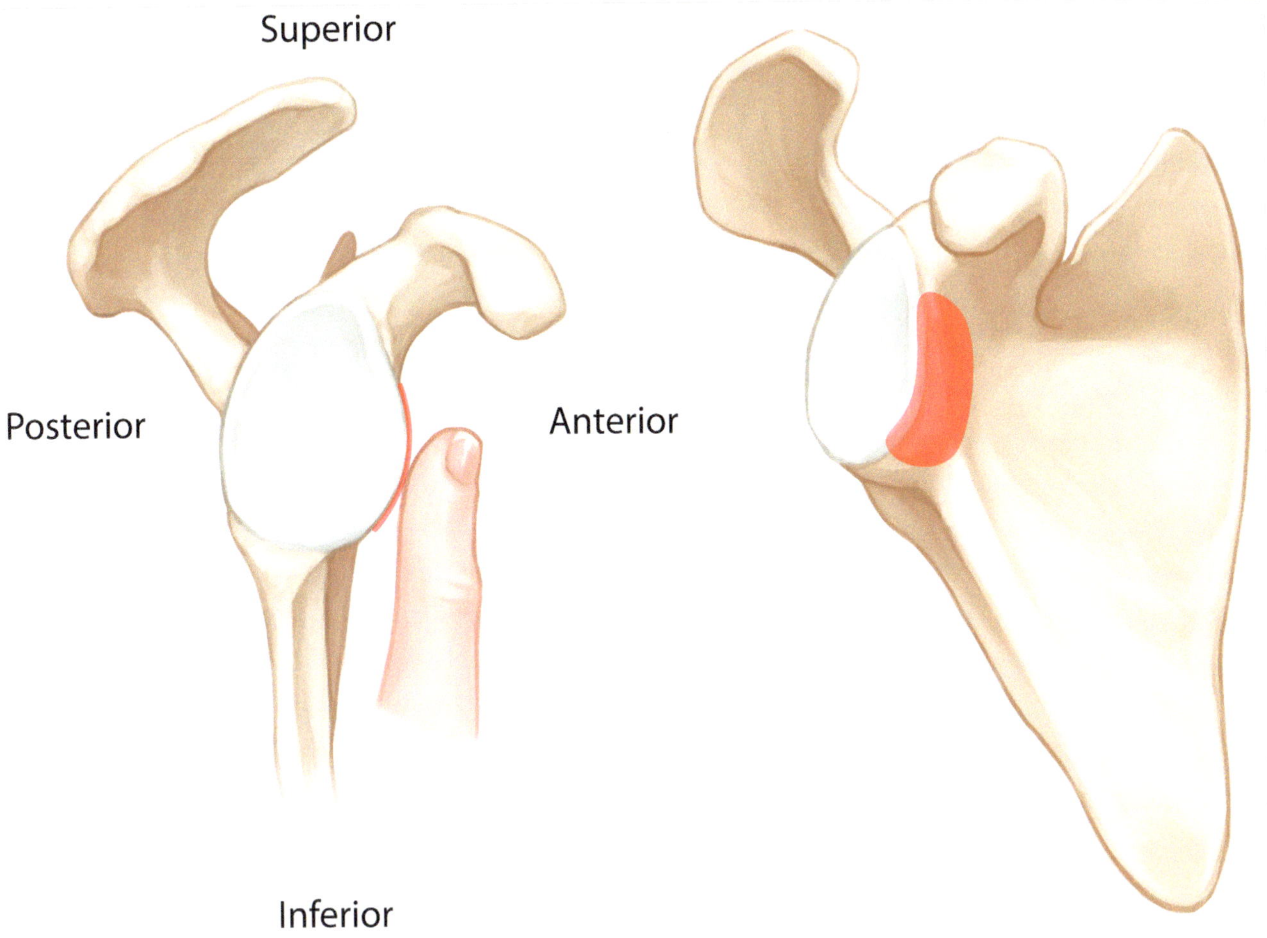

Fig. 45.2 MRI axillary sequence demonstrating selective posterior glenoid wear. This wear pattern increases the glenoid retroversion and can be corrected with reaming.

and inferiorly, and sufficient humeral head removal. Good retraction is essential to adequately visualize the glenoid vault, and optimal retractor position usually entails one anteriorly between the subscapularis and the anterior glenoid, one posteriorly behind the glenoid rim, and one superiorly at the base of the coracoid process. Thorough capsular releases both improve glenoid exposure and favor optimal postoperative motion. Next, the labrum is removed circumferentially and all remaining glenoid articular cartilage is removed. Thorough labrum and cartilage removal permits the surgeon to obtain a clear picture of the existing bony anatomy. After the glenoid is adequately debrided, the surgeon must obtain an understanding of the existing version and understand the degree of correction required. At this point in the procedure, it may be helpful to once again look at the preoperative images, confirming preoperatively anticipated deformity with observed surgical anatomy. The authors favor a technique whereby the surgeon places a finger along the anterior glenoid neck to assess the existing glenoid version (**Fig. 45.3**). By drilling the initial central pin toward the surgeon's fingertip on the glenoid neck, the arthroplasty version can be set to neutral. The surgeon then places the glenoid reamer in this same orientation and the anterior lip of the glenoid is planed down. One must take care not to ream too aggressively as the glenoid bone stock can be compromised. Once reaming is completed (**Fig. 45.4**), the surgeon completes drilling and instrumentation for the selected component. A trial component may be placed in order to confirm stability. Once trialing is successful and the components are selected, the final implants are inserted. The type of fixation and the number and orientation of pegs will be system dependent. A variable amount of cement is utilized, depending on design. Some designs require little cement in each of the peg holes, while some designs are expected to be accompanied by a cement mantle for optimal fixation. Even if utilizing a cement mantle, a thin layer of cement is usually all that is required. Care is taken to ensure there is no cement buildup beneath the face of the final glenoid component. This may reduce the implant stability, produce cracking of the cement mantle, loss of implant support, and lead to failure.

45.7 Tips and Pearls/Expert Suggestions

Using an index finger along the anterior glenoid neck may assist in achieving the correct version.

Implant selection is important, and specific knowledge of the method and points of optimal fixation are important. Some

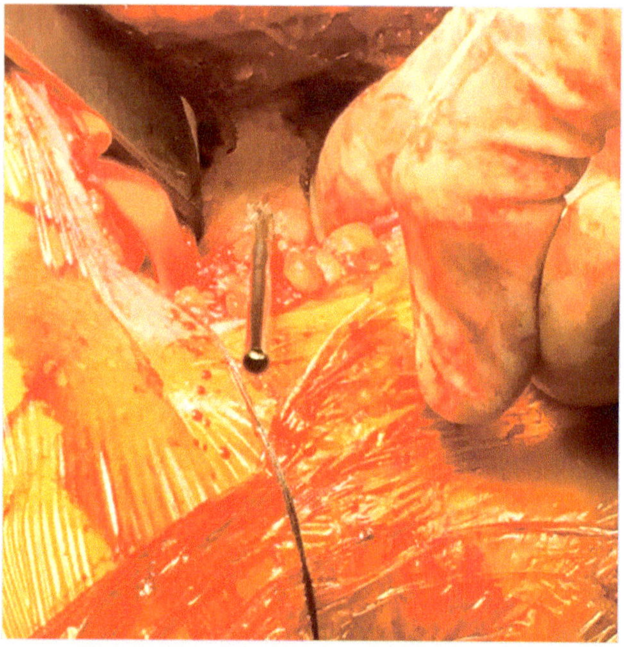

Fig. 45.3 Finger along glenoid neck guiding central pin placement.

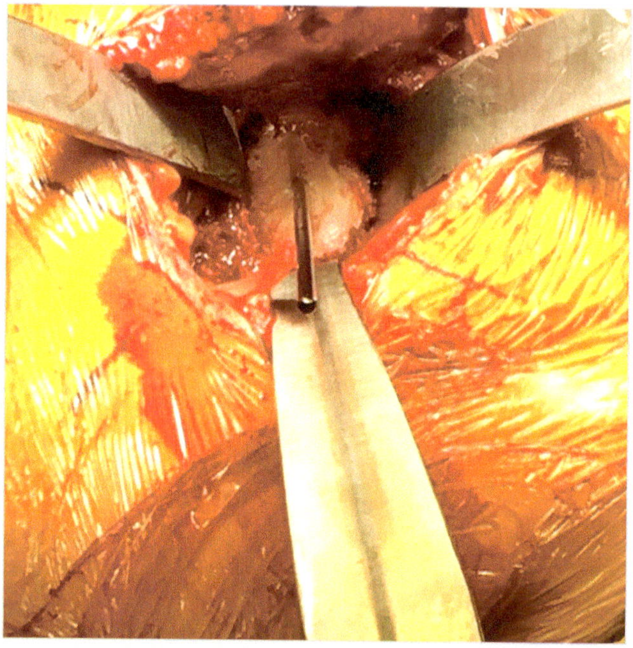

Fig. 45.4 After reaming of the glenoid is completed.

surgeons favor a glenoid component with inline pegs or a keel when the surgeon anticipates maximizing the eccentric reaming technique, though to a great extent, precise glenoid instrumentation optimizes fixation whatever the design.

45.8 What to Avoid

Overly aggressive reaming should be avoided due to the risk of reducing the subchondral bone needed for implant support. Additionally, medializing the joint line may compromise the rotator cuff function. Using excessive cement beneath the glenoid implant should also be avoided, as this can cause cement cracking, loss of support, implant loosening, and failure. Furthermore, overly aggressive soft-tissue release can cause implant instability. While it is typical to release anterior and inferior capsule, it is usually wise to avoid posterior capsular release, as posterior bone loss, posterior capsular stretching, preoperative humeral posterior subluxation, and intraoperative posterior capsular release are a recipe for posterior implant instability.

45.9 Complications/Bailout/ Salvage

There are several complications associated with aggressive eccentric reaming: cortical perforation, excessive medialization of the joint line, and joint instability. In the case of cortical perforation, one may impact a salvage bone graft (autograft from the humeral head cut) to prevent cement extrusion. Where the surgeon is concerned about joint line medialization, convert to the use of an augmented glenoid component. The surgeon should always carefully assess joint stability prior to finalizing all components. If the anterior glenoid has been excessively reamed and the version overcorrected, anterior instability may occur. In such a setting, the glenoid version must be corrected to neutral.

Many implant systems are now platform systems, with the ability to decide on an anatomic or reverse prosthesis intraoperatively after humeral osteotomy and glenoid preparation. Although it is usually more difficult to convert a fully implanted anatomic glenoid to a reverse prosthesis, system flexibility, precise instrumentation, and universal system compatibility usually permit this conversion if necessary for ultimate implant stability.

45.10 Postoperative Care

During the first week postoperatively, patients can remove their sling to shower and do pendulum exercises. They may also work on passive supine forward elevation in the scapular plane to approximately 140 degrees and supine passive external rotation at the side to 40 degrees. No internal rotation up the back for approximately 6 to 12 weeks.

At 6 weeks postoperatively, patients may discontinue their sling and use the arm for light activities of daily living. Rehab also includes isometric rotator cuff and deltoid exercises.

At 12 weeks, patients increase theraband resistance for rotator cuff and deltoid exercises.

Activities are typically limited for approximately 4 to 6 months.

At 6 months postoperatively, restrictions are lifted other than the lifetime restrictions that include no repetitive lifting more than 50 lbs and no repetitive vibratory activity such as chopping wood, jackhammer, etc.

References

1. Walch G, Badet R, Boulahia A, Khoury A. Morphologic study of the glenoid in primary glenohumeral osteoarthritis. J Arthroplasty 1999;14(6):756–760

2. Iannotti JP, Norris TR. Influence of preoperative factors on outcome of shoulder arthroplasty for glenohumeral osteoarthritis. J Bone Joint Surg Am 2003;85-A(2):251–258
3. Gillespie R, Lyons R, Lazarus M. Eccentric reaming in total shoulder arthroplasty: a cadaveric study. Orthopedics 2009;32(1):21
4. Habermeyer P, Magosch P, Lichtenberg S. Recentering the humeral head for glenoid deficiency in total shoulder arthroplasty. Clin Orthop Relat Res 2007;457(457):124–132
5. Gerber C, Costouros JG, Sukthankar A, Fucentese SF. Static posterior humeral head subluxation and total shoulder arthroplasty. J Shoulder Elbow Surg 2009;18(4):505–510
6. Neer CS II, Morrison DS. Glenoid bone-grafting in total shoulder arthroplasty. J Bone Joint Surg Am 1988;70(8):1154–1162
7. Stephens SP, Paisley KC, Jeng J, Dutta AK, Wirth MA. Shoulder arthroplasty in the presence of posterior glenoid bone loss. J Bone Joint Surg Am 2015;97(3):251–259

46 Posterior Glenoid Wear in Anatomic Total Shoulder Replacement: Augmented Polyethylene Glenoid Component

Jason C. Ho, Richard Puzzitiello, Joseph P. Iannotti, and Eric T. Ricchetti

Abstract
Posterior glenoid bone loss in glenohumeral osteoarthritis is a difficult problem to treat with anatomic total shoulder arthroplasty, and techniques using standard all-polyethylene glenoid components may not be biomechanically and clinically optimal. Posterior augmented all-polyethylene glenoid components have recently been introduced as an alternative treatment option and have shown promising results both biomechanically and clinically. However, when using augmented glenoid components, appropriate preoperative planning using 3D imaging and templating, adequate glenoid exposure and preparation, and knowledge of potential pitfalls and complications are paramount for good clinical outcomes.

Keywords: *augmented glenoid, posterior glenoid bone loss, preoperative planning, preoperative templating*

46.1 Goals of Procedure

The presence of posterior bone loss in advanced glenohumeral osteoarthritis (OA) results in increased retroversion and often a biconcave (B2) glenoid. This presents a particularly difficult problem when treating glenohumeral OA with anatomic total shoulder arthroplasty (TSA). Treatment goals of advanced glenohumeral OA with asymmetric bone loss using anatomic TSA include (1) correction of glenoid bony deformity to restore the patient's native version and inclination, (2) restoration of the location of the native joint line, (3) balancing of the soft tissues, and (4) centering of the humeral head. This chapter will focus on use of the augmented glenoid component and its ability to restore native glenohumeral anatomy (version, inclination, and location of the joint line) in anatomic TSA when posterior bone loss is present.

46.2 Advantages

The correction of pathologic version and posterior glenoid bone loss in shoulder arthroplasty has been shown to improve outcomes by balancing forces across the shoulder joint and re-creating an anatomic alignment of the humeral head and glenoid. Correction of increased glenoid retroversion has been proposed by reaming the high side, bone grafting, or using an augmented glenoid component.

Reaming the high side in cases with moderate to severe posterior glenoid bone loss to match native version can cause significant joint line medialization with increased risk of peg perforation, loss of the stronger cortical bone, and decreased tensioning of the soft tissues. Alternatively, reaming the glenoid in its pathologic plane will result in excessive retroversion of the glenoid component, which can lead to increased rates of osteolysis, and potential component loosening when placed in greater than 15 degrees of retroversion.[1–6] In contrast, use of bone graft with a standard glenoid component allows correction of version and maintenance of joint line when addressing advanced posterior glenoid bone loss. However, this procedure is technically more difficult to obtain stability of the bone graft and the implant, as stability of the polyethylene component requires bone incorporation. A few level IV clinical studies have demonstrated good clinical success, but a high incidence of radiolucency and complications associated with graft preparation, fixation, and incorporation have been reported.[7–11]

A recent alternative to correcting severe pathologic glenoid deformity during anatomic TSA has been the use of an augmented polyethylene glenoid component. A variety of augmented polyethylene glenoid designs have been evaluated biomechanically in the recent literature and three are currently commercially available (**Fig. 46.1**). Biomechanical, computa-

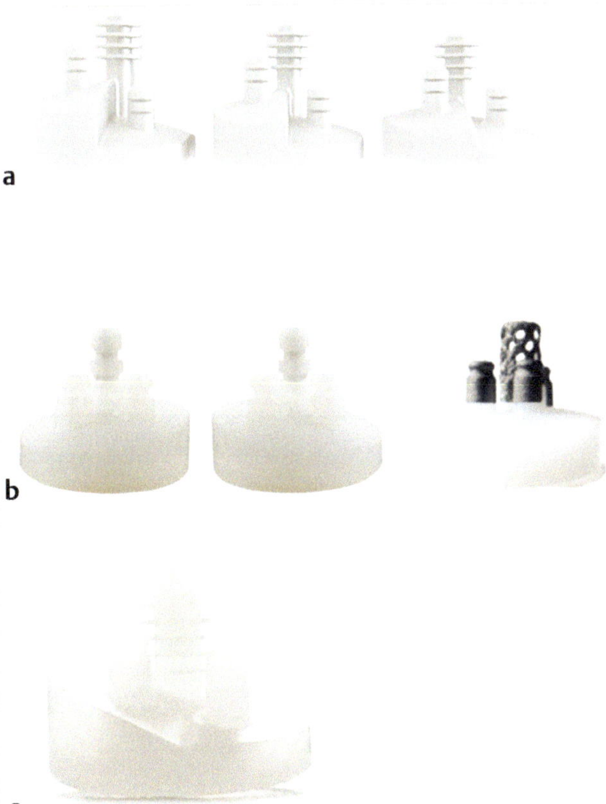

Fig. 46.1 **(a)** Global StepTech +7, +5, and +3 mm augmented stepped glenoids from Depuy Synthes. **(b)** Equinoxe Posterior Augment wedge glenoid for right and left, and with metal-coated pegs from Exactech (Gainesville, FL). **(c)** Aequalis Perform + posterior half-wedge augmented glenoid from Wright Medical Group N.V. (Memphis, TN).

tional, and now clinical data have demonstrated the benefits of the use of augmented polyethylene glenoids when addressing significant posterior glenoid wear and deformity. These studies have shown improved clinical function and outcome scores, and the ability to restore native glenoid anatomy (version, joint line, and humeral head centering).[1-14]

46.3 Indications

The primary indication for an augmented glenoid component is glenohumeral OA with an intact rotator cuff and posterior glenoid bone loss not correctable with a standard component. This is primarily determined through preoperative 3D planning using a thin-cut CT scan and associated Food and Drug Administration (FDA) approved planning software. Prior literature has shown a high (16%) revision rate in B2 glenoids treated with standard glenoid components at an average of 77 months (14–180 months) of follow-up.[15] We believe an augmented glenoid component is a reliable option for joint line restoration, version correction, and centering of the humeral head for B2 glenoids, and there is early literature supporting this claim.[13,14] Currently, the B2 glenoid is the most common pattern of moderate to severe bone loss in which we utilize an augmented glenoid component.

46.4 Contraindications

Contraindications to use of an augmented glenoid component include rotator cuff deficiency and very severe bone loss. With the advances in preoperative planning and implant designs, we have identified potential limitations to the use of augmented glenoids when bone loss or retroversion is very severe (e.g., B3- or C-type glenoids). In these cases of advanced bone loss or pathology, reverse TSA with or without bone grafting may be a more reliable option for implant stability and longevity.

46.5 Preoperative Preparation/ Positioning

46.5.1 Preoperative Planning

Currently, we use 3D CT imaging for preoperative planning in cases of moderate or severe posterior glenoid bone loss, as this allows more precise determination of the optimal implant choice based on the degree of pathologic correction and joint line restoration that is possible with augmented or standard glenoid components (**Figs. 46.2, 46.3**). Prior studies have shown that using 3D CT preoperative planning can help predict the amount of correction achievable using standard and augmented glenoids and improves glenoid implant positioning postoperatively.[16-18]

46.5.2 Perioperative Preparation

A combination of general and regional anesthesia is used and prophylactic antibiotics are given prior to all TSAs. The patient is placed in the beach-chair position at 45 degrees. We assess the shoulder for range of motion to allow maximal adduction and hyperextension to obtain optimal exposure for the humerus and glenoid, and then the patient is prepped and draped, and the arm is placed in an arm holder.

46.6 Operative Technique

The standard deltopectoral approach that is described elsewhere in this volume is utilized to perform the procedure. We mobilize the subscapularis with a lesser tuberosity osteotomy. This allows freeing of the subscapularis from the underlying capsule and bone-to-bone healing of the subscapularis repair. The capsule is released along the anatomic neck of the humeral head (**Fig. 46.4a**) and release of the inferior capsule as posterior as possible is important for increased glenoid exposure, as this allows for increased posterior retraction of the humerus. The humeral head is then dislocated, the anatomic neck cleaned of any osteophytes and marked, and the humeral head is cut in approximately 20 to 30 degrees of retroversion, exiting approximately 2 to 3 mm above the superior and posterior rotator cuff reflection (**Fig. 46.4b–d**).

Appropriate glenoid exposure is crucial to achieving optimal preparation of the glenoid for placement of an augmented glenoid component. A glenoid retractor is placed along the posterior inferior border of the glenoid to displace the humerus posteriorly out of the visual field. Another glenoid retractor is placed anteriorly for exposure of the anterior glenoid rim and to protect the axillary nerve. We routinely perform a resection of the anterior and inferior joint capsule to maximize glenoid exposure. The subscapularis and anterior capsular plane is developed, and the entire anterior and inferior capsule and labrum is excised (**Fig. 46.5**). This can be performed without concern for injury to the axillary nerve with appropriate identification of the nerve and protection with retractors. The posterior capsule is released if needed, and the posterior labrum is excised from the posterior glenoid rim. A superior glenoid retractor is then placed to achieve complete visualization of the glenoid face, and the posterior glenoid bone loss can be inspected (**Fig. 46.6a, b**).

The centering guide pin is placed (**Fig. 46.6c**) using standard or patient-specific instrumentation in a manner defined by the 3D preoperative planning software. When using the posterior step augmented glenoid (StepTech, DePuy Synthes, Warsaw, IN), the glenoid reamer is set over the guide pin, and the anterior glenoid is reamed to a level defined by the planning software and the shape of the augmented glenoid component (**Figs. 46.2, 46.3, 46.6d**). The centering hole for the anchor peg glenoid is then drilled over the guide pin, after which the guide pin is removed and the reaming guide for the posterior glenoid is placed over the prepared surface of the anterior glenoid (**Fig. 46.6e**). For a posterior step augmented glenoid, a guided reamer supplied by the manufacturer and a high-speed burr (**Fig. 46.6e**) are used to prepare the posterior half of the glenoid. The high-speed burr can be very useful to ream centrally, where the majority of bone is removed to create the posterior step cut (**Fig. 46.2e**), with the guided reamer used to finish the step cut and create a smooth transition moving from centrally to the peripheral posterior glenoid edge. The peripheral holes for the anchor peg glenoid are next drilled with a guide, and the glenoid trial is placed to ensure appropriate seating of the component both anteriorly and posteriorly (**Fig. 46.6f**). The peg holes are irrigated and dried, with the peripheral holes filled with pressurized cement and the grooves of the center peg filled with cancellous bone graft before final impaction of the glenoid (**Fig. 46.6g–i**).

After the glenoid component is placed, we proceed with the humeral canal preparation and component placement. Completion of humeral component implantation is performed according to the appropriate technique of the selected implant and is described in detail in preceding chapters. The trial humeral implant should be reduced to assess for proper soft-tissue tensioning prior to placement of the final implant. Subscapularis repair is described in detail in preceding chapters.

46.7 Tips and Pearls/Expert Suggestions

Exposure of the glenoid is crucial in glenoid preparation for augmented glenoids. This includes proper retractor placement and appropriate capsular releases off the humerus and glenoid.

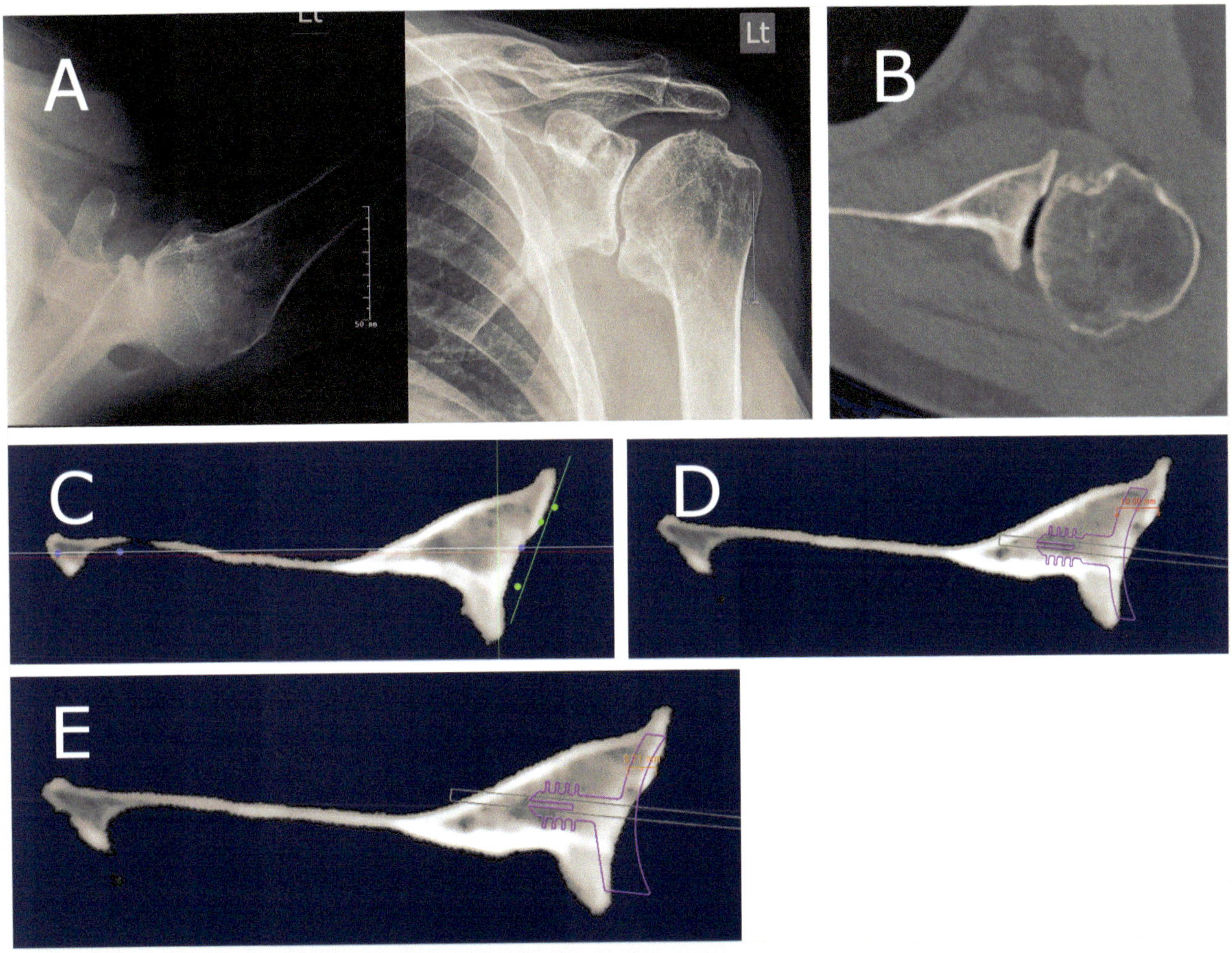

Fig. 46.2 **(a)** Preoperative axillary and true anteroposterior (AP) radiographs of a B2 glenoid. **(b)** Preoperative CT axial cut of the same B2 glenoid showing biconcavity and posterior subluxation of the humeral head. **(c)** Once the CT is placed in the 3D planning software, the scapular (*white line*) and glenoid (*green line*) planes are defined to determine glenoid measurements, with this B2 glenoid showing 20.5 degrees of retroversion and 4.6 degrees of inclination. Implant trialing can then be performed in the planning software to determine the component that best corrects pathologic version, while restoring or maintaining the joint line. The axial CT cuts show **(d)** a standard glenoid component compared to **(e)** a +5-mm augmented glenoid component with center guide pin (*gray bar*). Both components are placed to correct retroversion to 6 degrees, but 5 mm more reaming is required for complete backside seating of the standard component, leading to significant joint line medialization. The standard component also has to be placed more posteriorly to avoid anterior component overhang. Once the augmented component is selected, the depth of reaming can be defined both anteriorly and posteriorly.

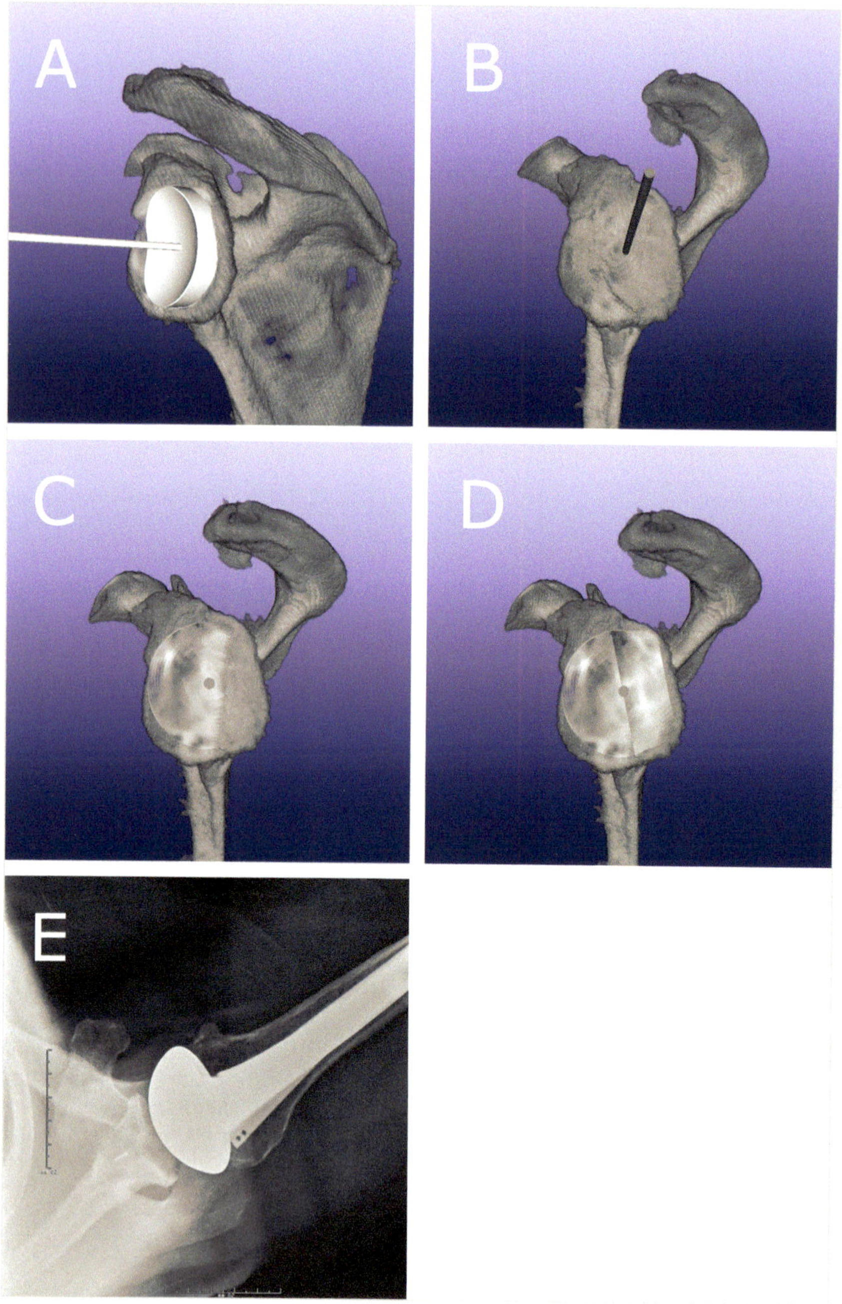

Fig. 46.3 Once an augmented component is selected, the 3D reconstructed scapula can be viewed to show **(a)** the implant and **(b)** the location and trajectory of the center guide pin. Noting the location of the guide pain in relation to the biconcavity is helpful in confirming the correct guide pin position at the time of surgery. Views of the location of **(c)** anterior and **(d)** posterior reaming are also helpful to confirm reaming is performed correctly at the time of surgery. **(e)** Postoperative axillary radiograph showing restoration of joint line and centering of the humeral head.

Depending on the amount of posterior humeral head subluxation and patient size, posterior glenoid exposure may be more difficult. Large male patients may have a large deltoid that makes this exposure difficult or a tight posterior capsule may be present. Typically the posterior subluxation of the humeral head in B2 glenoids creates a loose posterior capsule, but that is not always the case. Whether a posterior capsular release needs to be done is dependent on the amount of humeral head subluxation, soft-tissue laxity, and the other capsular releases or excisions performed. A full anterior and inferior capsulectomy and circumferential removal of the labrum are important for maximal glenoid exposure that allows for unhindered glenoid preparation (**Figs. 46.5, 46.6**). Inadequate exposure may lead to poor glenoid preparation and poor seating of the augmented glenoid component.

When preparing the sclerotic posterior glenoid for the augmented glenoid component, under-reaming will cause the implant to not fully seat. The use of a high-speed burr is helpful in the initial shaping of the posterior glenoid and removal of bone, followed by use of the manufacturer's reamer to finish the step cut, and ensures adequate seating of the implant. If the manufacturer-provided tools alone cannot completely ream to allow full backside implant seating, the burr is also a useful adjunct to correct any imperfections or remove residual osteophytes. Preoperative 3D planning and templating is also helpful in defining which osteophyte to remove.

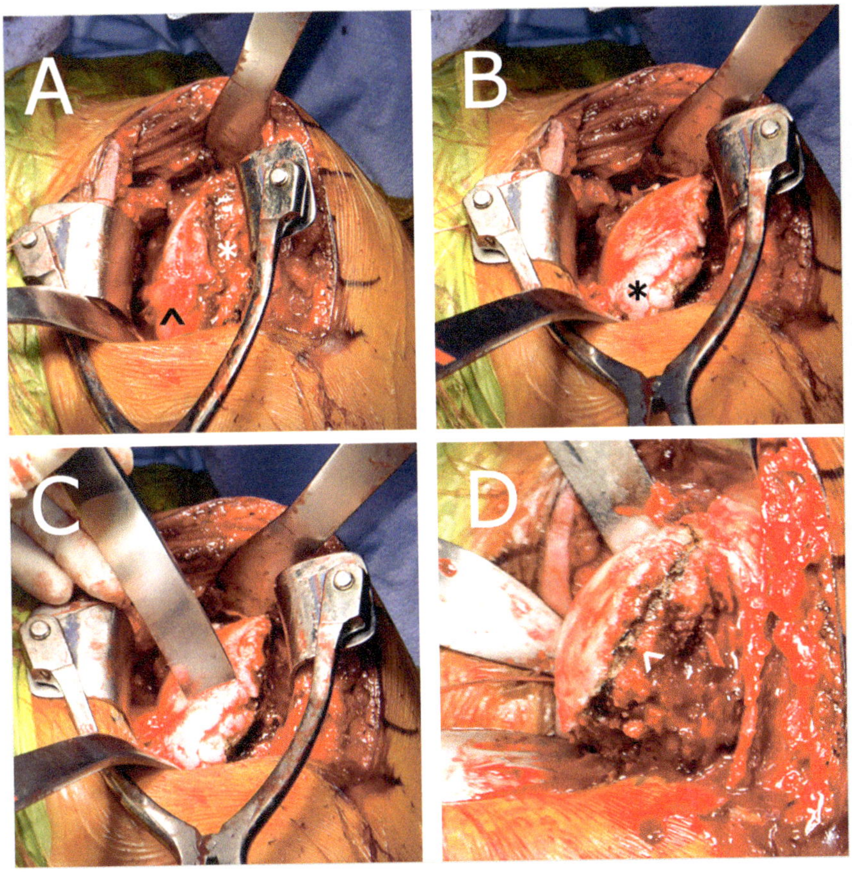

Fig. 46.4 **(a)** Exposed humeral head prior to dislocation showing lesser tuberosity osteotomy footprint (*white* *) and inferior capsule (*black* ^) prior to release. **(b)** The humeral head has been dislocated, showing the inferomedial osteophyte (*black* *) that is obscuring the anatomic neck and medial calcar of the humerus. **(c)** Osteophyte being removed with an osteotome in line with the inferior neck of the humeral head. **(d)** Once all osteophytes are removed from the periphery of the humeral head, the anatomic neck can be appropriately visualized and marked (*white* ^ showing Bovie line) prior to making the humeral head cut.

46.8 What to Avoid

Release of the posterior capsule is only performed in a B2 glenoid when an augmented glenoid component is used to restore anatomic version without medialization of the native joint line. If the posterior capsule is released and there is residual glenoid retroversion or medialization of the joint line, then posterior instability of the humeral head is much more likely. Excessive reaming of the posterior glenoid should also be avoided to prevent inadequate bone support for the augmented component. For a stepped augment, very little or no bone is removed from the posterior glenoid rim, with the majority of the bone removed more centrally in creating the posterior step (**Fig. 46.2e**). Preoperative 3D planning and templating is helpful to define the correct depth of reaming by choosing the appropriate size of the posterior augment. Choosing an augment that is too small may lead to incomplete pathologic correction, while choosing an augment that is too large may lead to excessive reaming that results in peg perforation and inadequate bone support for the implant. Finally, when removing the posterior retractor from the posterior inferior glenoid after glenoid implantation, one must be careful not to catch the implant in the retractor, as it can be pulled out or loosened.

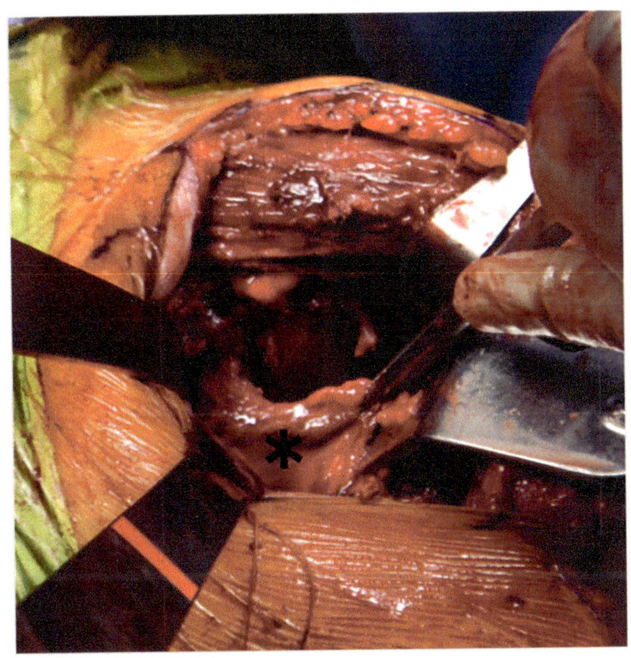

Fig. 46.5 Isolation of the anterior inferior capsule (*asterisk*) prior to resection to aid in glenoid exposure.

46.9 Complications/Bailouts/Salvage

A devastating complication during this procedure is a glenoid rim fracture during glenoid preparation. This may occur due to excessive posterior glenoid reaming or excessive pathologic bone loss. Preoperative 3D planning is key to avoiding this scenario, as it shows how much glenoid is available for reaming, if an augmented component is feasible, and the appropriate

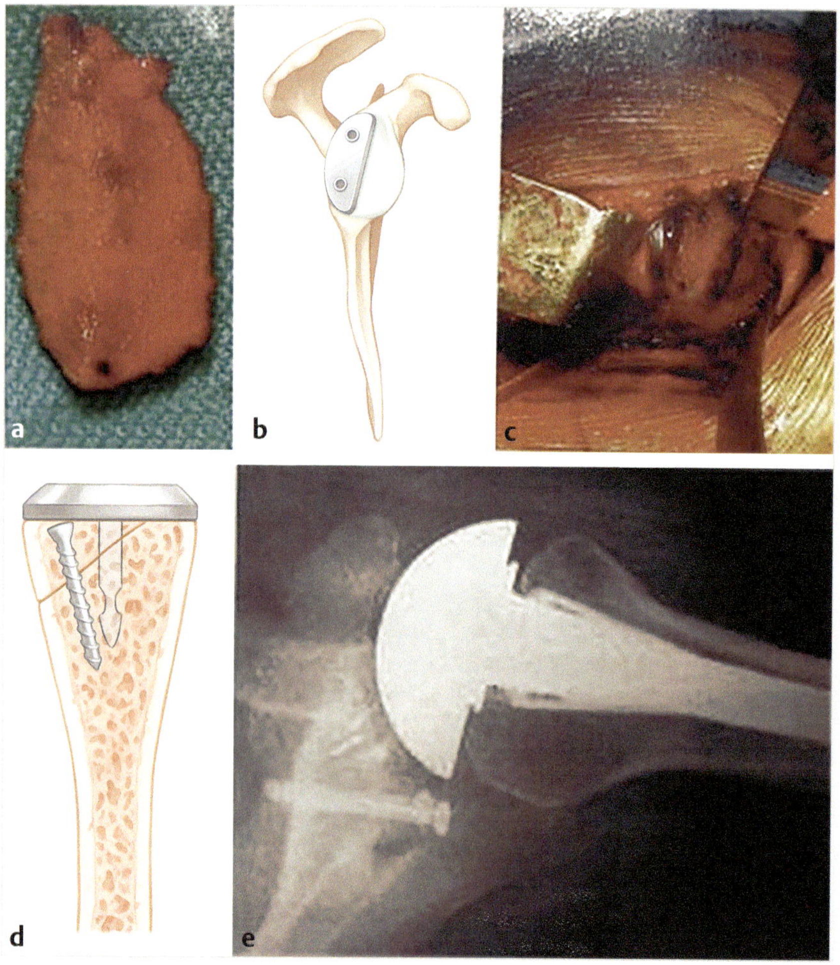

Fig. 47.5 Onlay technique. **(a)** Humeral head graft prepared for implantation. **(b)** Schematic depicting sagittal view of completed onlay technique. **(c)** Intraoperative view of graft fixation. **(d)** Schematic depicting lateral view of completed onlay technique. **(e)** X-ray post fixation of graft using onlay technique.

perpendicular to the glenoid axis in the neutral position. The high side is then slightly reamed to create a flat surface for lateral attachment of the bone graft (**Fig. 47.5**).

Next, the defect surface is prepared with light burring to create a bleeding surface. The humeral head is prepared and contoured to fit the defect. The graft is placed to re-create a flush surface with the anterior glenoid. The graft is fixed with 3.5-mm screws over the previously placed guide wires. We prefer to use an arthroscopic cannula posteriorly to allow easier access for instrumentation and to improve pin access for pin and screw placement. With the graft well fixed, the glenoid component is cemented into place in a standard fashion.

47.3 Tips and Pearls

- If instability persists during trial reduction prior to final humeral component placement, humeral head component offset or sizing and, in rare patients, possible posterior capsular plication may be considered

47.4 What to Avoid/Pitfalls

- Inadequate graft preparation and/or graft fixation will likely result in failure of graft and loss of fixation of the glenoid component.
- Ensure that there is sufficient bone stock left after making the step cut in the glenoid for central peg placement within the native glenoid vault.
- Preoperative planning helps prevent this from occurring.
- When reaming the glenoid after graft placement, take caution to not over-ream beyond the posterior screws.
- Be cognizant of poor bone quality.
- Be cognizant of severe cavitary glenoid defects that may require a shape allograft (**Fig. 47.6**).
- Be cognizant of patients with extensive bone loss that may require reverse shoulder arthroplasty or hemiarthroplasty for optimal results (**Fig. 47.7**).

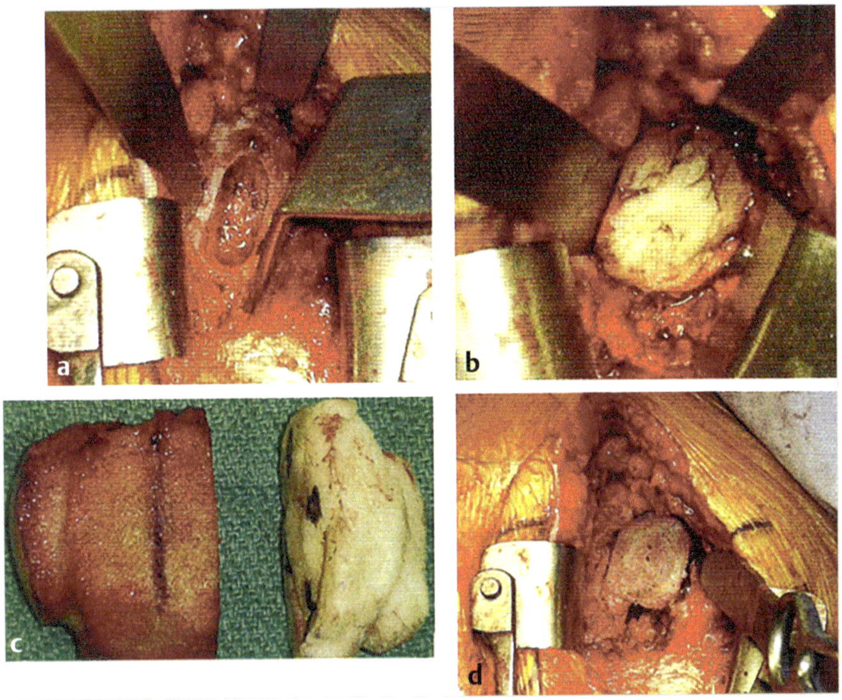

Fig. 47.6 Treatment of severe cavitary glenoid defects with a shape allograft. (a) Intraoperative example of a severe cavitary lesion. (b) Cement sizer/spacer placement into lesion. (c) Shape allograft created from the cement model. (d) Final placement of allograft for humeral head articulation.

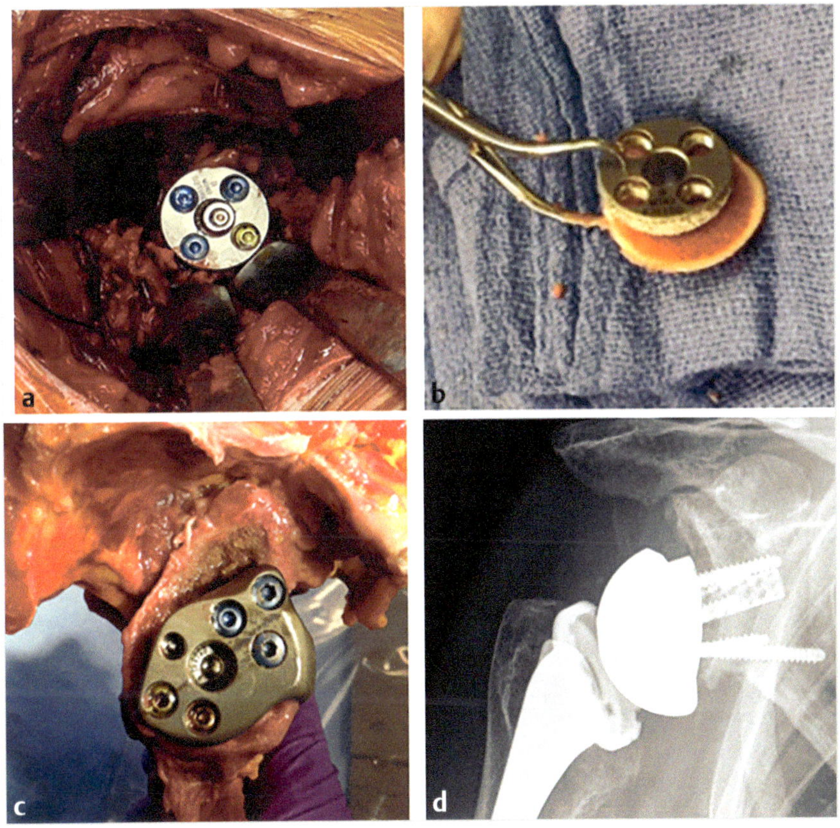

Fig. 47.7 Glenoid bone stock deficiency additional treatment options. (a) Reverse total shoulder arthroplasty (RTSA) plus eccentric reaming. (b) TSA plus bone graft. (c) RTSA with augmented baseplate. (d) Patient-specific RTSA implant.

Suggested Readings

Hasan SS, Leith JM, Campbell B, Kapil R, Smith KL, Matsen FA III. Characteristics of unsatisfactory shoulder arthroplasties. J Shoulder Elbow Surg 2002;11(5):431–441

Hill JM, Norris TR. Long-term results of total shoulder arthroplasty following bone-grafting of the glenoid. J Bone Joint Surg Am 2001;83-A(6):877–883

Levine WN, Djurasovic M, Glasson JM, Pollock RG, Flatow EL, Bigliani LU. Hemiarthroplasty for glenohumeral osteoarthritis: results correlated to degree of glenoid wear. J Shoulder Elbow Surg 1997;6(5):449–454

Steinmann SP, Cofield RH. Bone grafting for glenoid deficiency in total shoulder replacement. J Shoulder Elbow Surg 2000;9(5):361–367

Walch G, Badet R, Boulahia A, Khoury A. Morphologic study of the glenoid in primary glenohumeral osteoarthritis. J Arthroplasty 1999;14(6):756–760

Hsu JE, Ricchetti ET, Huffman GR, Iannotti JP, Glaser DL. Addressing glenoid bone deficiency and asymmetric posterior erosion in shoulder arthroplasty. J Shoulder Elbow Surg 2013;22(9):1298–1308

Chan K, Knowles NK, Chaoui J, et al. Characterization of the Walch B3 glenoid in primary osteoarthritis. J Shoulder Elbow Surg 2017;26(5):909–914

Bercik MJ, Kruse K II, Yalizis M, Gauci MO, Chaoui J, Walch G. A modification to the Walch classification of the glenoid in primary glenohumeral osteoarthritis using three-dimensional imaging. J Shoulder Elbow Surg 2016;25(10):1601–1606

Sears BW, Johnston PS, Ramsey ML, Williams GR. Glenoid bone loss in primary total shoulder arthroplasty: evaluation and management. J Am Acad Orthop Surg 2012;20(9):604–613

48 Convertible Components in Shoulder Arthroplasty

David M. Dines, Philippe Valenti, and Joshua S. Dines

Abstract

Glenoid loosening is the weak link of anatomic total shoulder arthroplasty. Hemiarthroplasty failure (resorption of the great tuberosity, glenoiditis) for complex fracture is much too frequent and a difficult revision is mandatory for painful shoulder. So revision procedures that require removal of well-fixed humeral or glenoid components are difficult and have an increased risk of complications including intraoperative fracture of the humerus, radial nerve palsy, extensive glenoid bone lesion, more extensive soft-tissue damage, increased blood loss, and surgical time. To decrease the rate of complications and to facilitate the revision, many implant designs are now convertible especially on the humeral side (unipolar convertibility) and more unusual on both the humerus and the glenoid (bipolar convertibility).

Keywords: *anatomic shoulder arthroplasty, reverse shoulder arthroplasty, platform system, convertible components, hemiarthroplasty*

48.1 Introduction

The number of primary shoulder arthroplasties being performed throughout the world increases exponentially every year. Many of these procedures are now indicated for younger, more high-demand patients who want to continue their activities. In addition, with increasing life expectancies, we can expect more primary and, ultimately, even more revision procedures of all types in the future. The most common indications for revision shoulder arthroplasty include glenoid component loosening, rotator cuff failure, subscapularis failure after instability, and infection.[1]

Revision procedures that require removal of well-fixed humeral or glenoid components are difficult and have an increased risk of complications including intraoperative fractures, more extensive soft-tissue damage, increased blood loss, and surgical time.[2] In an effort to diminish these risks, many implant designs are now convertible especially on the humeral side (unipolar convertibility; **Fig. 48.1**). Some systems are convertible on both the humerus and the glenoid (bipolar convertibility; **Fig. 48.2**).

48.2 Goals of Procedure

Convertible shoulder arthroplasty components facilitate revision surgery when used in the index arthroplasty procedure. Convertible-type implants can be unipolar (platform stem on the humeral side) or bipolar (convertible components on the humeral and glenoid side). Most of the present-day third- and fourth-generation shoulder arthroplasty systems consist of humeral platform stems of all types and lengths that are adaptable to anatomic or reverse components.

Several present-day shoulder arthroplasty systems have both convertible humeral components and metal-backed glenoid components that can also be adapted for use as an anatomic glenoid component or a glenosphere for use in reverse shoulder arthroplasty (RSA). Implant systems like these can be used to carry out primary hemiarthroplasty (HA) or anatomic shoulder arthroplasty successfully and can be revised to RSA if needed in the future.

48.3 Advantages

The advantage of these convertible component systems is the fact the revision cases can be made much easier because in most cases the well-fixed humeral stem does not need to be removed. Removing a well-fixed stem can be difficult and can result in intraoperative humeral fractures and increased blood loss and surgical time.

In cases of bipolar convertible systems, the glenoid component can be exchanged without removing the well-fixed metal baseplate in most cases. This is extremely helpful in that it reduces the risk of glenoid bone deformity and/or loss that would require possible bone graft or even patient-specific implants during the revision procedure.

48.4 Indications

In patients who are indicated for anatomic shoulder arthroplasty for glenohumeral osteoarthritis, HA for acute trauma, avascular necrosis, or any other primary arthritic condition, surgeons should consider using implant systems that are convertible. This convertibility gives the surgeon an important advantage in any revision procedures that may be necessary in the future. This is especially important as younger, more active patients are now being indicated for anatomic shoulder arthroplasty or HA. These patients are at risk for revision surgery in the future, and convertible implants may be particularly beneficial in these clinical situations.

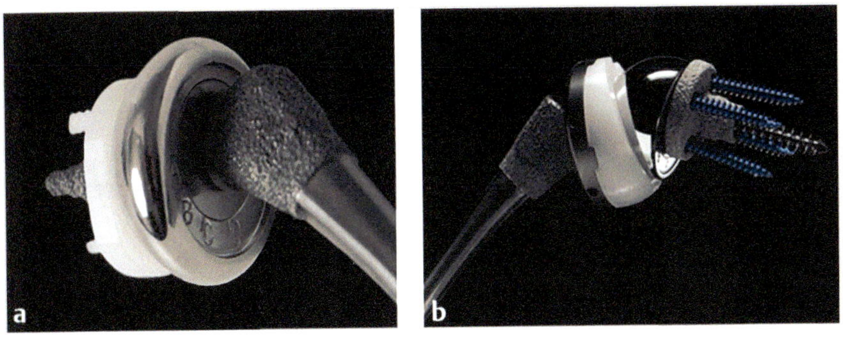

Fig. 48.1 (a,b) The convertible-platform humeral stem articulates with humeral head component for anatomic shoulder arthroplasty or onlay humeral tray and liner for reverse shoulder arthroplasty.

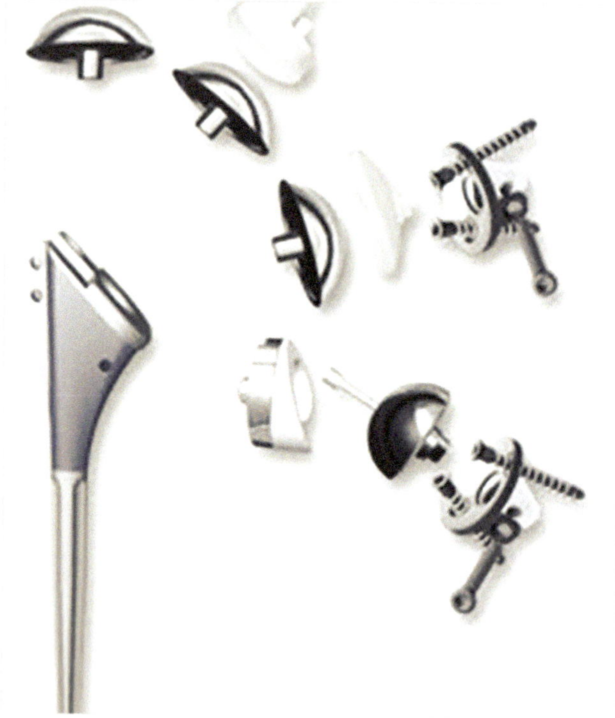

Fig. 48.2 Bipolar convertible-platform implant systems allow revision on both the humeral and the glenoid sides without removing well-fixed implants in some revisions to reverse shoulder arthroplasty.

48.5 Contraindications

There are no absolute contraindications to usage of convertible implants; however, the surgeon should never compromise the index procedure for the sake of a convertible situation. In all orthopaedic procedures, the first procedure is the best opportunity for success, so humeral stem and glenoid baseplate positioning should not be altered from what is best in the index procedure in order to create a more convertible situation. Placing the glenoid baseplate in a bipolar convertible system in an excessive superior or inferior position or with excessive tilt may compromise the outcome of the primary procedure and any subsequent revision procedure. Similarly, placing a platform humeral stem in an abnormal height or version to accommodate a later convertible revision should not be done.

48.6 Preoperative Preparation/ Positioning

Convertible implants are utilized in the standard way that all previous anatomic total shoulder arthroplasties and HAs are carried out. In fact, they are the standard for almost all present-day implant systems. For this reason, preoperative planning including appropriate imaging described in previous chapters should be carried out in all patients to ensure best possible surgical outcomes. Plain X-rays and advanced imaging in conjunction with present-day

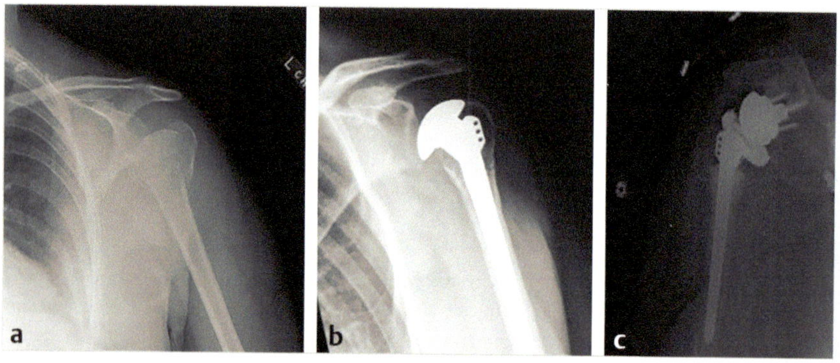

Fig. 48.3 Humeral platform fracture stem converted to reverse shoulder arthroplasty without removing a cemented platform fracture stem.

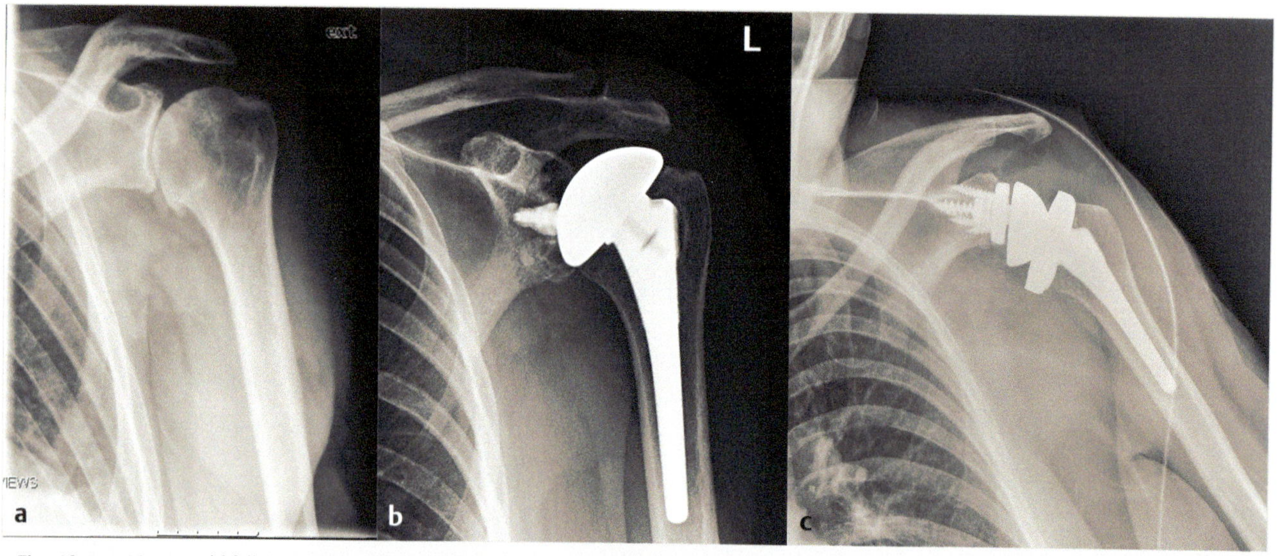

Fig. 48.4 A 72-year-old fell and suffered a total shoulder arthroplasty dislocation with subscapularis rupture. He failed primary repair at 6 weeks, which was revised to reverse shoulder.

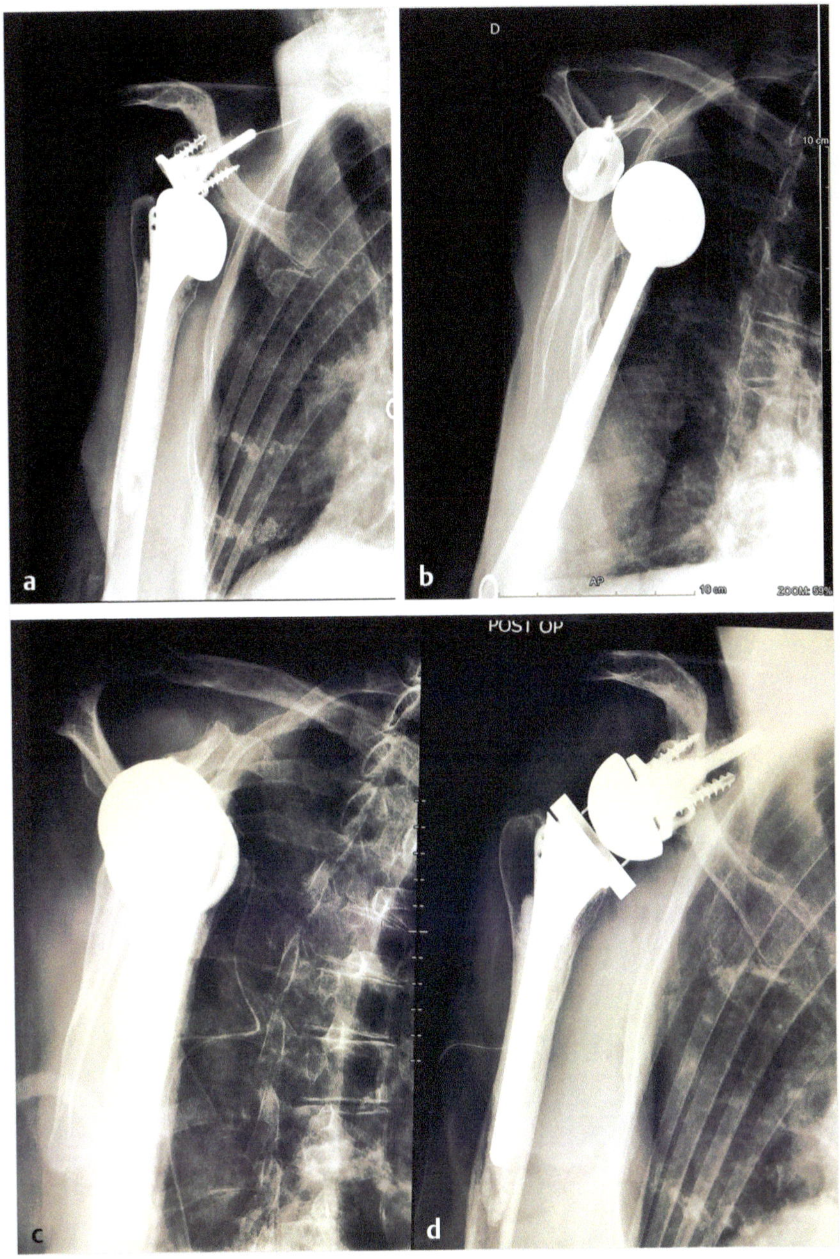

Fig. 48.5 Anterior dislocated anatomic total shoulder arthroplasty (TSA) after trauma with subscapularis rupture. The cemented humeral component is convertible **(a,b)**. Anatomic TSA revised to reverse shoulder arthroplasty without removing the humeral or the glenoid platform **(c,d)**. (Reproduced with permission of Thieme Medical Publishers Inc.)

shoulder arthroplasty planning tools and instrumentation should be considered in cases deemed necessary.

In revision cases, proper workup for infection and soft-tissue insufficiency are critical for best outcomes.

48.7 Technique

The techniques for HA and anatomic shoulder replacement are the same as those described in previous chapters and do not need to be repeated here. Suffice to say that the use of any convertible unipolar or bipolar implants should be carried out in such a way that the implants are positioned in the most ideal position in the index procedure to ensure the most successful outcome.

When carrying out a revision of the primary HA or a total shoulder arthroplasty (TSA), it is critical to have all necessary implants, and equipment in cases where the convertible implants are not acceptable due to primary placement or orientation.

The key to revision procedures utilizing a platform-type convertible implant is proper exposure through an appropriate deltopectoral surgical approach. It is critical to remove all subdeltoid adhesions completely, exposing the conjoint tendon as surgical landmark. Care is taken to recognize the location of the musculocutaneous and axillary nerves.

Next, the subscapularis tendon is released by tenotomy, peel, or tuberosity osteotomy as per the anatomy and/or surgeon's choice.

At this point, the humeral head component is removed with appropriate instrumentation based upon the implant system, which was utilized during the index procedure. Multiple soft-tissue biopsies can be taken for culture and sensitivity to rule out deep infection especially for Propionibacterium acnes. These cultures should be observed for at least 2 weeks, as this is a very indolent organism with a predilection for shoulder joint interventions.

With head component removed, an extensive soft-tissue release of anterior and inferior scar and ligament labral complex exposes the glenoid. If a unipolar convertible system is utilized, then care should be taken to remove the existing glenoid component as described in previous chapters. In these cases or in cases of revision of HA, the chosen glenoid component can be placed without the necessity to remove the well-fixed humeral stem, saving time and limiting blood loss and possible complications stemming from removal of a well-fixed implant (**Figs. 48.3, 48.4**).

In cases of bipolar convertible systems, the polyethylene liner can be removed and the existing metal baseplate platform then utilized to fix a convertible glenosphere component. In many cases, a more lateralized glenosphere component is chosen to ensure stability.

Next, the onlay humeral tray and liner trial component can be used for a trial reduction to demonstrate stability without impingement in order to choose the proper size for the real implant. Once chosen, the real humeral tray and liner are placed (**Fig. 48.5**).

At this point, the subscapularis tendon may be repaired appropriately.

48.8 Tips and Pearls/Expert Suggestions

The primary key to success in the use of a convertible platform system, which is either unipolar (humeral component) or bipolar (humeral and glenoid baseplate platform), is proper component placement at the index procedure without regard for any ultimate revision procedure. The second key is that in some cases (~ 20%) the original convertible implant will not be amenable to simple conversion due to original component placement. Humeral components that are too high or in excessive version would compromise revision component position. On the glenoid side, placing a baseplate too superiorly on the glenoid or with too much superior tilt might create impingement, instability, or scapular notching. In these cases, removal of the well-fixed implant is the better choice for successful revision.

48.8.1 What to Avoid

When using a bipolar-type convertible shoulder system, the surgeon must place the implants in the ideal position for the index procedure. Placing the glenoid baseplate in a bipolar convertible system in too low a position or with inferior tilt may compromise the outcome of the primary procedure. Similarly, placing a platform humeral stem (unipolar or bipolar systems) in an abnormal height or version to accommodate a later convertible revision should not be done.

48.9 Complications/Bailout/Salvage

The simple bailout for convertible implant systems that are not amenable to conversion is to abort that type of revision and be prepared to remove the index components as necessary to proceed with the standard revision.

48.10 Postoperative Care

Postoperative care is similar to that described in other chapters for the index arthroplasty procedure; however, in the revision setting the postoperative care will need to be individualized for each patient based upon the status of the soft tissues and any fixation issues of the replaced components.

48.11 Discussion

There are many options in treating glenoid loosening including component resection, one- or two-stage revision, and revision to RSA. Due to substantial glenoid bone loss, revision to anatomic shoulder is often compromised and results have been overall only fair in many studies where bone graft was used to revise the index arthroplasty to RSA.[3-7] Flury et al[8] and Ortmaier et al[9] reported high complication rates related to component removal.

The use of a convertible platform system has been documented to decrease risks of humeral and glenoid fracture, thereby reducing operative time, soft-tissue dissection, and bleeding. Castagna et al,[10] Valenti et al,[11] and Weber-Spickschen et al[12] have all reported excellent pain relief, improvement in function, and reduced rate of complications utilizing a bipolar convertible-platform system in revision of an anatomical TSA to RSA.

Even with all this said, conversion was only possible in 75% of cases due to the position of platform components in the index procedure. These series had no controls and were relatively short in follow-up time; however, they do demonstrate that in proper situations convertible-platform systems can be very beneficial in reducing risks, blood loss, and operating time in revision situations.

48.12 Conclusion

With expected increases in revision shoulder arthroplasty discussed earlier, convertible-platform shoulder arthroplasty systems will offer a much easier option in those cases where conversion is possible. Many present late-generation implant systems have convertible-platform humeral components, and a few systems have convertible glenoid baseplates with more expected.

These implant systems facilitate the conversion of HA or anatomical TSA to RSA with good results in terms of pain relief and improved function. These platform systems reduce operating time, bleeding, and the risk of humeral or glenoid fractures in these convertible revision techniques.

References

1. Chin PY, Sperling JW, Cofield RH, Schleck C. Complications of total shoulder arthroplasty: are they fewer or different? J Shoulder Elbow Surg 2006;15(1):19–22
2. Sperling JW, Cofield RH. Humeral windows in revision shoulder arthroplasty. J Shoulder Elbow Surg 2005;14(3):258–263

3. Neyton L, Walch G, Nové-Josserand L, Edwards TB. Glenoid corticocancellous bone grafting after glenoid component removal in the treatment of glenoid loosening. J Shoulder Elbow Surg 2006;15(2):173–179
4. Bonnevialle N, Melis B, Neyton L, et al. Aseptic glenoid loosening or failure in total shoulder arthroplasty: revision with glenoid reimplantation. J Shoulder Elbow Surg 2013;22(6):745–751
5. Melis B, Bonnevialle N, Neyton L, et al. Glenoid loosening and failure in anatomical total shoulder arthroplasty: is revision with a reverse shoulder arthroplasty a reliable option? J Shoulder Elbow Surg 2012;21(3):342–349
6. Cofield RH, Edgerton BC. Total shoulder arthroplasty: complications and revision surgery. Instr Course Lect 1990;39:449–462
7. Iannotti JP, Frangiamore SJ. Fate of large structural allograft for treatment of severe uncontained glenoid bone deficiency. J Shoulder Elbow Surg 2012;21(6):765–771
8. Flury MP, Frey P, Goldhahn J, Schwyzer HK, Simmen BR. Reverse shoulder arthroplasty as a salvage procedure for failed conventional shoulder replacement due to cuff failure--midterm results. Int Orthop 2011;35(1):53–60
9. Ortmaier R, Resch H, Matis N, et al. Reverse shoulder arthroplasty in revision of failed shoulder arthroplasty-outcome and follow-up. Int Orthop 2013;37(1):67–75
10. Castagna A, Delcogliano M, de Caro F, et al. Conversion of shoulder arthroplasty to reverse implants: clinical and radiological results using a modular system. Int Orthop 2013;37(7):1297–1305
11. Valenti P, Katz D, Kany JThe use of convertible glenoid component makes revision to reverse total shoulder arthroplasty easier. In: Dines D, Dines J, Edwards TB, eds. Reverse Shoulder Arthroplasty: A Practical Approach. New York, NY: Thieme Medical Publishers Inc.; 2017
12. Weber-Spickschen TS, Alfke D, Agneskirchner JD. The use of a modular system to convert an anatomical total shoulder arthroplasty to a reverse shoulder arthroplasty: Clinical and radiological results. Bone Joint J 2015;97-B(12):1662–1667

49 Superior Approach to the Shoulder

Victor A. Olujimi, Paul J. Cagle Jr., and Evan L. Flatow

Abstract

The deltopectoral approach is a commonly used surgical approach when performing shoulder arthroplasty. The superior approach can be used as an alternative approach when implanting a reverse total shoulder arthroplasty. This approach can be especially useful in cases with proximal migration of the humeral head. Our technique, instrumentation details, and key points to consider will be outlined.

Keywords: *shoulder arthroplasty, superior approach, rotator cuff arthropathy, reverse shoulder arthroplasty*

49.1 Goals of Procedure

- Present an alternative surgical exposure for shoulder arthroplasty that maintains adequate exposure of the humeral head and visualization of the glenoid.
- Techniques to guide dissection and protection of the deltoid and axillary nerve.
- Demonstrate how, via this approach, to accurately place both the humeral and the glenoid components in a reverse total shoulder arthroplasty.
  - A superior approach may be used for standard/anatomic and reverse total shoulder arthroplasty based on surgeon preference or to accommodate for a prior incision or specific patient requirement.
  - The approach is thought to allow improved "straight on" visualization of the glenoid surface.

49.2 Advantages

- Direct visualization of the glenoid surface.
- Minimal or partial release of the subscapularis.
- Decreases risk of injury to the cephalic vein.
- Avoids retractor traction on anterior deltoid.
- Lower rate of instability and dislocations.
- Allows for prior incision to be used for a patient who had previously undergone an approach through the deltoid.

49.3 Indications

- Total shoulder arthroplasty, both standard/anatomic and reverse.
- Shoulder arthroplasty for proximal humerus fractures.
- Reverse total shoulder for rotator cuff arthropathy.
- Open reduction and internal fixation for proximal humerus fractures.
- Open rotator cuff repair.

49.4 Contraindications (Relative)

- Poor preoperative range of motion.
- Shoulder dysplasia.
- Extensive osteophyte formation.
- Axillary nerve injury.

49.5 Preoperative Preparation

49.5.1 Imaging

X-rays

- Anteroposterior (AP), true AP of the glenohumeral joint, scapular Y, and axillary views.

CT Scan and MRI (Noncontrast)

1. Allows for evaluation of glenoid version, bone stock, and rotator cuff muscle–tendon unit integrity.
2. Evaluation of osteophyte size and location:
   a. Extensive osteophyte formation along the inferior humeral head may be difficult to visualize and address from the superior approach.
   b. If there is any suspicion for infection, preoperative labs should be obtained:
      i. Complete blood count (CBC).
      ii. Erythrocyte sedimentation rate (ESR).
      iii. C-reactive protein (CRP).
   c. If there is high suspicion clinically with inconclusive laboratory findings, then proceed to perform an arthrocentesis or arthroscopic biopsy sent for the following:
      i. Cell count.
      ii. Gram stain.
      iii. Culture (aerobe and anaerobe): cultures should be held for at least 14 days to allow adequate culture time for *Propionibacterium acnes.*

Instruments (Fig. 49.1)

1. Positioning:
   a. Anesthesia: general or laryngeal mask airway.

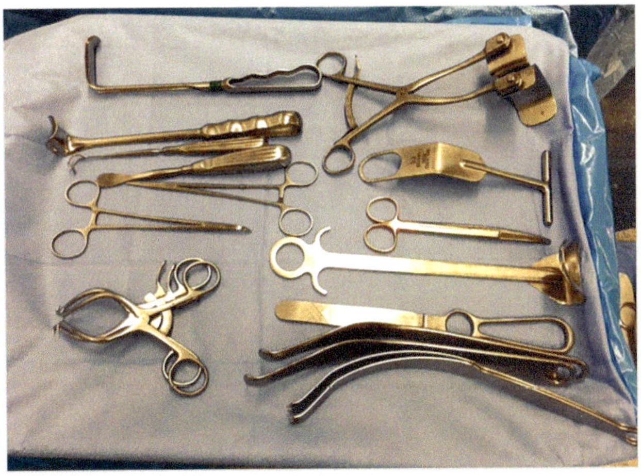

Fig. 49.1 Example of instruments used for shoulder arthroplasty.

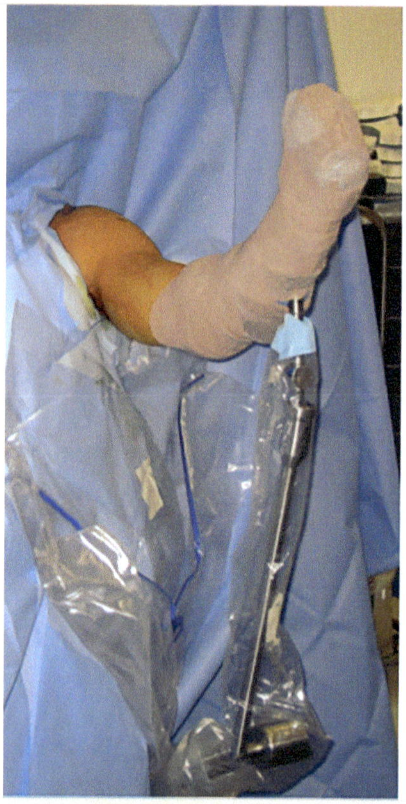

Fig. 49.2 Attachable limb positioner can be used to assist with holding and manipulating the shoulder throughout the procedure.

b. Preoperative regional anesthesia via an interscalene injection or catheter is used adjunctively for pain management.
c. Patient is placed in a semi-beach-chair position (~ 45 degrees of hip flexion and 30 degrees of knee flexion):
    i. The head is secured in a padded holder with the neck in a neutral position.
d. The operative arm is secured in a pneumatic arm holder (**Fig. 49.2**).
   Important: Take the operative arm through the range of motion to ensure unimpeded motion especially adduction and extension.
    i. The contralateral arm is secured across the body or with a well-padded arm holder.
    ii. Venodynes (sequential compression devices) are placed on the calves to decrease the incidence of deep venous thrombosis.
e. Prep and drape:
    i. The authors' preference is for a chlorhexidine scrub, followed by chlorhexidine prep.
    ii. Drape as medial on the scapula as possible.
    iii. Use of a bump placed under the scapula may direct the glenoid surface forward and assist in visualization.

49.6 Operative Technique

49.6.1 Incision

1. Mark any prior incisions and determine the utility of the planned incision or if a separate surgical approach is necessary.

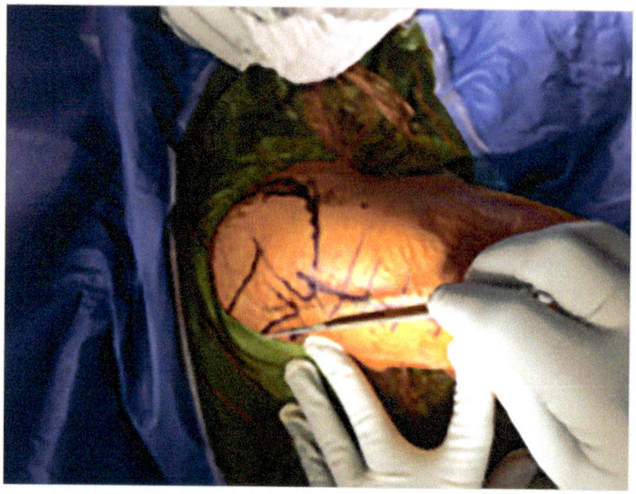

Fig. 49.3 Location of incision over anterolateral acromion.

2. Standard landmarks are outlined on the shoulder:
   a. The anterior, lateral, and posterior borders of the acromion, the acromioclavicular joint, the clavicle, and the coracoid process.
3. Anterosuperior incision (**Fig. 49.3**):
   a. Vertical incision marked a few centimeters above the anterolateral edge of the acromion extending distally along the anterolateral edge of the acromion for 4 to 6 cm.
   Important: keep incision relatively parallel to a standard deltopectoral incision.

49.6.2 Exposure

Anterosuperior Approach

1. Superficial exposure:
   a. Subcutaneous skin flaps are raised using sharp dissection or electrocautery.
   b. Deltoid fascia is visualized and the raphe between the anterior and middle head of deltoid is identified.
   Important: Anterolateral acromion can be used to help identify the interval.
   c. A stay stitch is placed with nonabsorbable suture along the distal extent of the raphe between the anterior and middle head of the deltoid (about 3.5 cm distal to greater tuberosity) to prevent distal propagation potentially injuring the axillary nerve (**Fig. 49.4**).
   d. Starting a few millimeters posterior to the anterolateral edge of the acromion, incise the raphe with electrocautery along the interval extending distally for 3 to 4 cm (**Video 49.2**).
   e. Extend incision a few millimeters posterior to the anterolateral edge of acromion incorporating the coracoacromial ligament into the release:
      i. Provides stout tissue for final repair of deltoid, which allows for distal clavicle excision as well (**Fig. 49.5**).
   f. Continue release of subacromial, further releasing the coracoacromial ligament with the anterior deltoid.

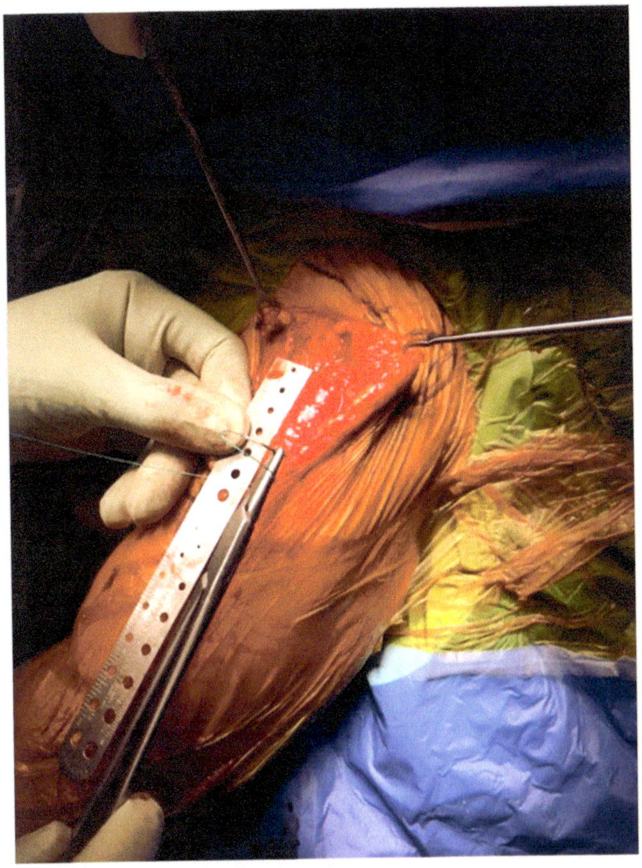

Fig. 49.4 Placement of stay stitch 4 to 6 cm from lateral acromion to prevent distal propagation of dissection through anterior and middle heads of the deltoid. Excessive distal propagation can result in axillary nerve injury.

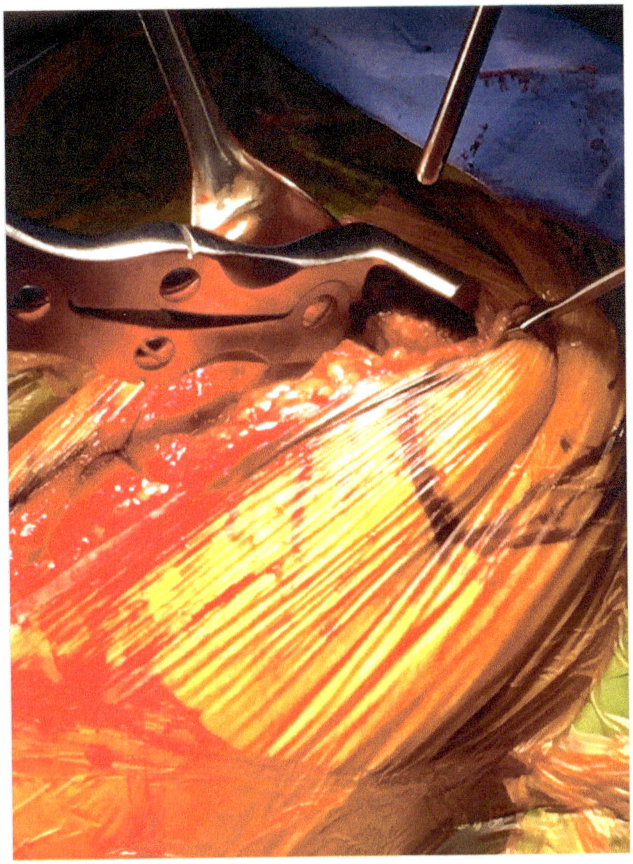

Fig. 49.5 Distal clavicle resection performed through the same incision for preoperative acromioclavicular joint pain.

Deep Exposure

1. The long head of the biceps is identified within the bicipital groove and
   a. Followed proximally, releasing the transverse humeral ligament.
   b. A tenotomy is performed near the supraglenoid tubercle and a tenodesis performed to the upper border of the pectorals major with a heavy suture (i.e., 0 Ethibond).
2. The subscapularis is visualized and released sharply or with electrocautery from the lesser tuberosity (**Video 49.3**):
   a. The upper one-half to two-thirds portion of the tendon can be released leaving a portion intact distally:
      i. In some cases, it is possible to leave the entire subscapularis tendon intact.
      ii. The anterior circumflex vessels can be avoided by limiting or not performing a complete subscapularis release. **Important:** Injury to the vessels may cause bleeding that is difficult to control due to the exposure.
3. Heavy traction sutures are placed within the subscapularis tendon (if released fully or partially).
4. Capsular release and capsulectomy is performed deep to subscapularis to further mobilize the tendon.
   Important: Palpate and identify axillary nerve to avoid inadvertent injury during subscapularis release (especially along inferior portion).
   a. Capsular release is extended distally on the humeral shaft if the entire subscapularis tendon is released.

Humeral Head Exposure and Preparation

1. Applying superior force to the humerus, the humeral head is presented through the split in the deltoid muscle (**Video 49.4**):
   Important: Extension, external rotation, of superiorly directed force helps facilitate head exposure.
2. Darrach retractors are placed to help with humeral head exposure and soft-tissue retraction.
3. Identify a point posterior and medial from the superior portion of the biceps groove (reference entry point for reamers; **Fig. 49.6**).
4. Sequential reamers are placed until contact with the endosteum is obtained:
   a. Cementation of the humeral component is preferred; therefore, the final implant will be 1 to 1.5 mm smaller to allow for an adequate surrounding cement mantle.
5. A cutting guide with version rods attached to the intramedullary reamer are assembled (**Fig. 49.7**):
   a. Rotate cutting guide to align version rods at a retroversion angle between 0 and 20 degrees (the authors' preference is 20 degrees of retroversion).
   b. The guide is pinned into place and the intramedullary reamer is removed.

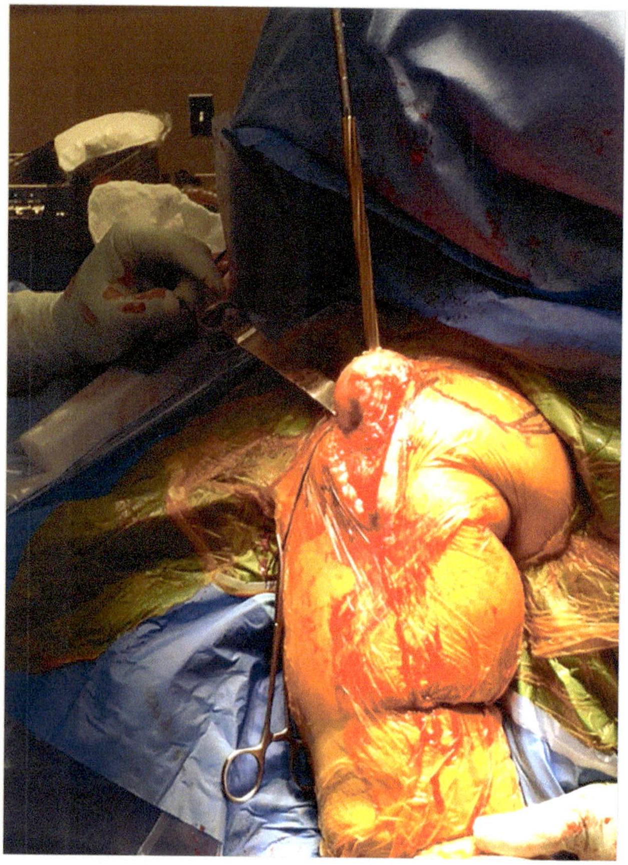

Fig. 49.6 Proximal presentation of the humeral head through superior incision with retractors placed along the medial calcar allowing for adequate exposure.

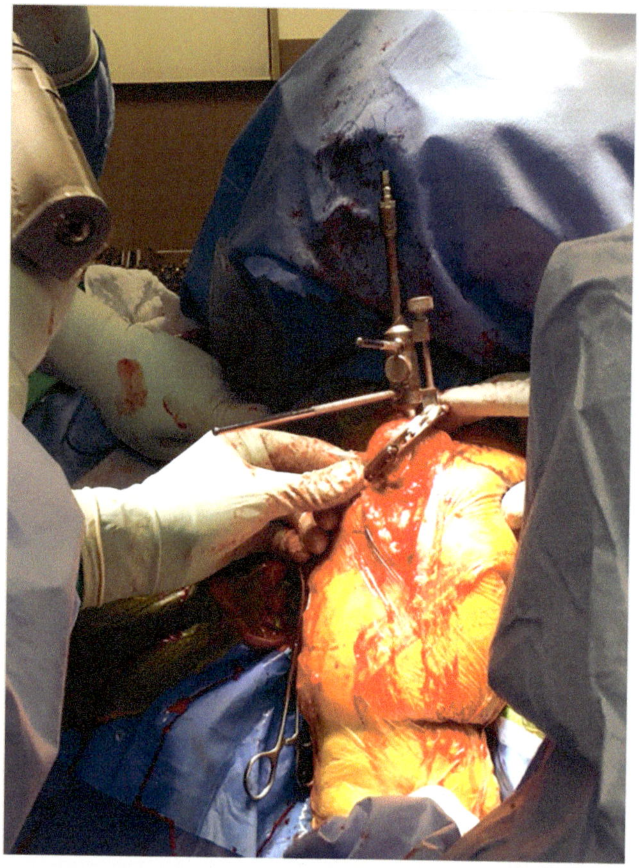

Fig. 49.7 Following intramedullary reaming, the humeral head cutting guide is assembled with version rod in place.

6. The humeral head osteotomy is performed with an oscillating saw.
7. A secondary conical hand reamer with version rods is placed into the humeral shaft and reamed until flush with humeral cut (**Fig. 49.8**).
   Important: Maintain orientation with version rods while ensuring conical reamer remains parallel with the humeral cut.

A humeral trial can be inserted to assess the preparation and may be left in place to protect the proximal humerus during glenoid preparation (**Figs. 49.9, 49.10**).

Glenoid Exposure and Preparation

1. For adequate glenoid exposure, the humeral head needs to be able to translate inferiorly. A lack of motion preoperatively may suggest a limitation during this step, which may lead to the inability to properly visualize the glenoid.
2. Retractor placement:
   a. Fukuda retractor: inferior glenoid neck.
   b. Large Kolbel glenoid retractor: anterior glenoid neck (deep to subscapularis).
   c. Small Kolbel glenoid retractor: posterior superior glenoid (**Fig. 49.11**).
3. Perform circumferential lobectomy:
   a. Inferior capsular release:
      i. Using digital protection or a blunt retractor placed along the inferior glenoid neck allows protection of the axillary nerve.
      ii. Carefully resect the inferior labrum with care to protect the axillary nerve.
      iii. Perform a subperiosteal release along the glenoid. from the 3 o'clock to the 9 o'clock position. A small amount of triceps insertion can be safely released. A Cobb elevator can be used for further release from the medial glenoid neck.
   Important: Inferior capsular release must be carefully performed as direct or thermal injury can harm the axillary nerve as it courses along the inferior glenoid neck.
4. Glenoid prosthesis:
   a. Appropriate-sized glenoid guide is used to direct the guide pin through the center of the glenoid vault (**Figs. 49.12, 49.13**).
   Important: The glenoid guide should be seated on the inferior glenoid rim and can be kept in a neutral position or tilted inferiorly 5 to 10 degrees to reduce the incidence of scapular notching
   b. The cannulated drill for the peg hole is placed over guide pin and drilled.
   c. The guide pin is removed and secondary reamer is used to remove the overlying cartilage and prepare a bleeding bone surface on the glenoid (**Fig. 49.14**).
   Important: Periodically inspect glenoid face to avoid excessive reaming and disruption of subchondral bone.

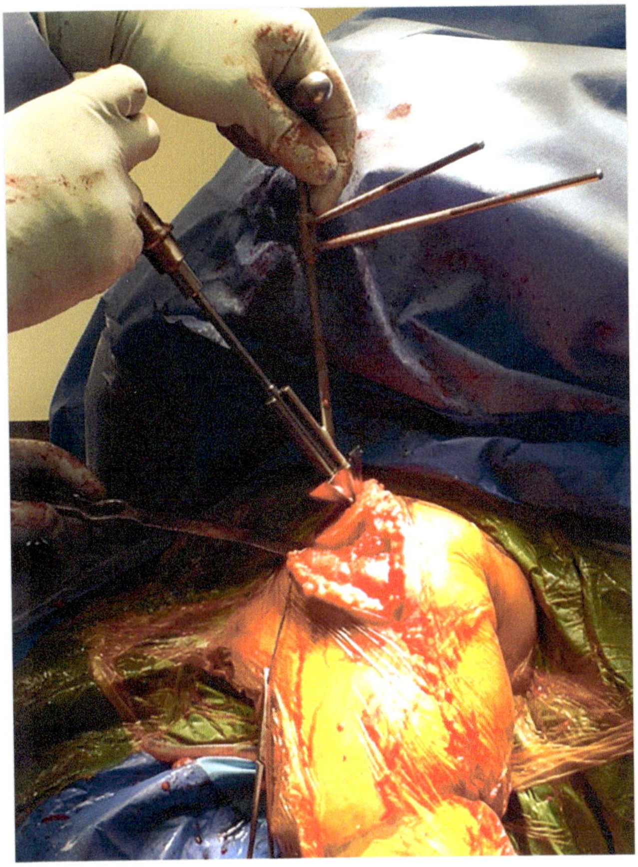

Fig. 49.8 Secondary conical reamer being used to prepare proximal humerus with version rods to maintain orientation.

d. A peripheral reamer can be used to remove peripheral bone:
   i. Removing peripheral bone ensures an unimpeded articulation between the glenosphere and the baseplate.

   Important: If unable to use the peripheral reamer due to exposure limitations, then a burr can be used.

e. Additional preparation is performed based on implant design requirements.
f. Baseplate is impacted into place.
g. Screws are placed into the baseplate (**Fig. 49.15**):
   i. The preference of the senior author is to use superior and inferior screws with locking caps for added fixation.

   Important: The superior screw is aimed toward the base of the coracoid and the inferior screw is directed horizontally for maximal screw length.

h. The glenosphere is implanted.

5. Humeral prosthesis:
   a. Retractors are placed and the humeral head is translated superiorly through the deltoid.
   b. The trial stem is inserted with a polyethylene insert:
      i. Trial reductions with differing size polyethylene may be necessary.
      ii. Important: Evaluate arm motion in all positions. (i.e., contralateral axilla, adduction and external rotation, forward elevation).

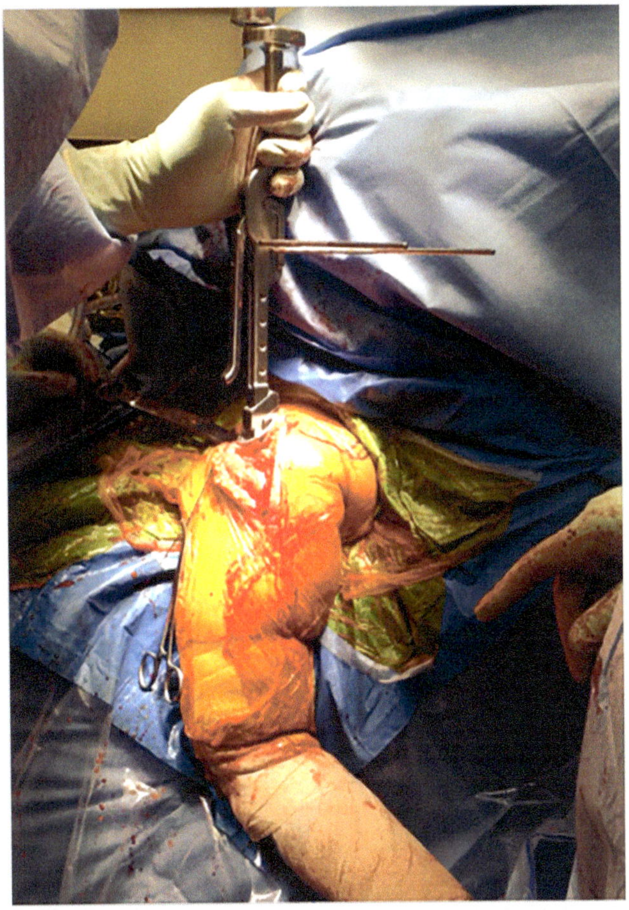

Fig. 49.9 Broaches being used to prepare proximal humerus with version rods to maintain orientation.

6. Humeral prep and implantation:
   a. The humeral component may be press fitted or cemented into place (the senior author's preference is to use cement).
   b. The final prosthesis is inserted with the assistance of retroversion rods.
   c. Repeat trial reduction is performed with polyethylene insert.
   d. The joint is reduced and taken through full range of motion again (**Fig. 49.16, Video 49.6**).
7. Closure:
   a. The wound is thoroughly irrigated.
   b. The subscapularis is repaired.
      i. The authors prefer the Krackow and Masson–Allen stitch through the subscapularis tied over the transosseous tunnels in the lesser tuberosity.
   c. Heavy nonabsorbable sutures are used to place a Mason–Allen stitch to the anterior deltoid and secured through bone tunnels within the acromion.
   d. The intervals between the anterior deltoid and middle deltoid are sutured together (**Fig. 49.17**).
   e. A drain is placed laterally within the shoulder.
   f. Monofilament sutures are used to close deep dermal and subcuticular layers.

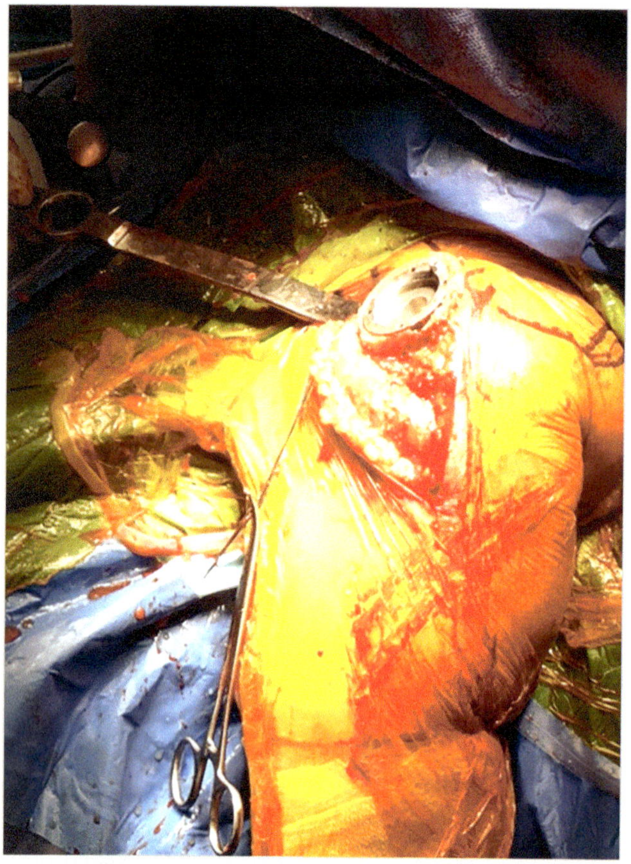

Fig. 49.10 Impacted trial implant in place.

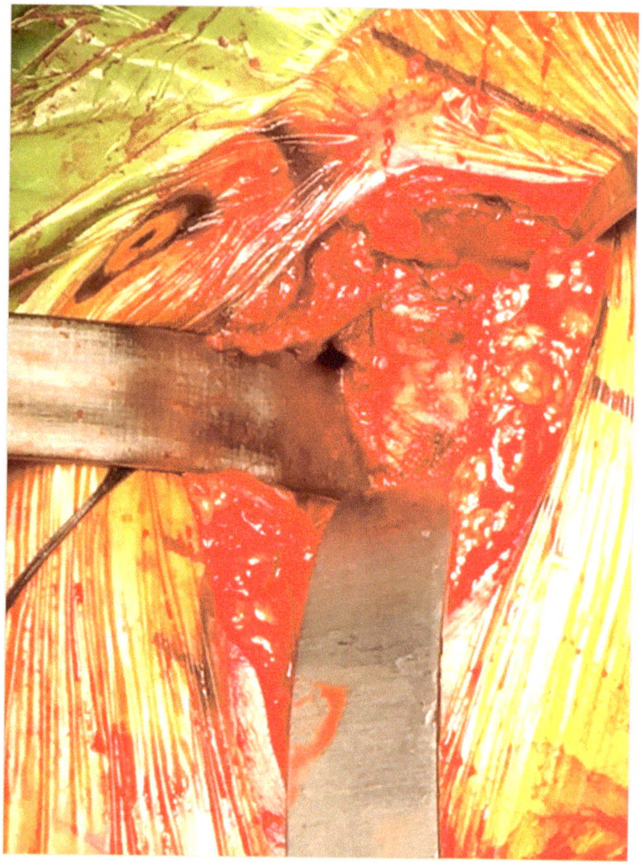

Fig. 49.11 Glenoid retractors placed with en face view of glenoid surface.

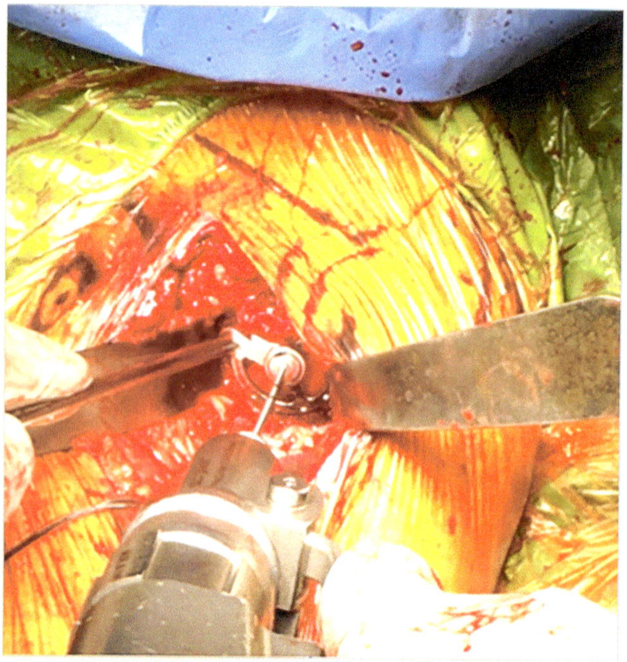

Fig. 49.12 Allowing for proper placement and orientation of guide and guide pin.

49.7 Tips and Pearls/Expert Suggestions

1. Adequate translation of the shoulder is necessary for glenoid exposure. If superior translation of the humeral head is present, we prefer to examine the patient under anesthesia to assess the ability for the head to translate inferiorly. An examination demonstrating stiffness in inferior translation is an indication for the authors to go to a deltopectoral approach. Lack of appropriate inferior translation can limit glenoid visualization.
2. Inferior humeral head osteophyte should be assessed carefully. The typical osteophyte associated with glenohumeral arthritis can be difficult to visualize along the inferior and medial humeral neck.
3. Once an opening in the deltoid is created, placed a finger through the approach to palpate the axillary nerve.
4. A benefit of this approach is the ability to maintain all or part of the subscapularis insertion. If release of the subscapularis is required, begin by releasing only the superior one-third and reassess.
5. A stitch placed at the bottom of the deltoid split may assist in inadvertently placing traction on the axillary nerve by preventing unintended extension of the approach.

6. A risk with difficulty in translating the humeral head is glenoid component malalignment. Complete release of the subscapularis and anterior translation may assist in improving visualization.

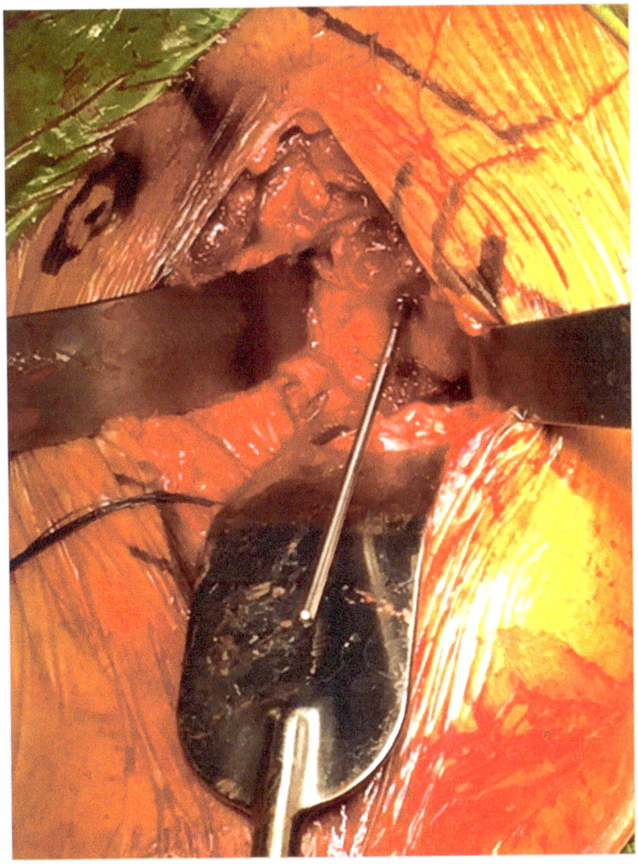

Fig. 49.13 Direct view of guide pin placement.

49.8 What to Avoid

1. Monitor distal extension of split between anterior and middle deltoid to avoid injury to axillary nerve.
2. Transmuscular release of the anterior deltoid from the acromion. If this is done, it can result in difficult repair and subsequent anterior deltoid dysfunction.

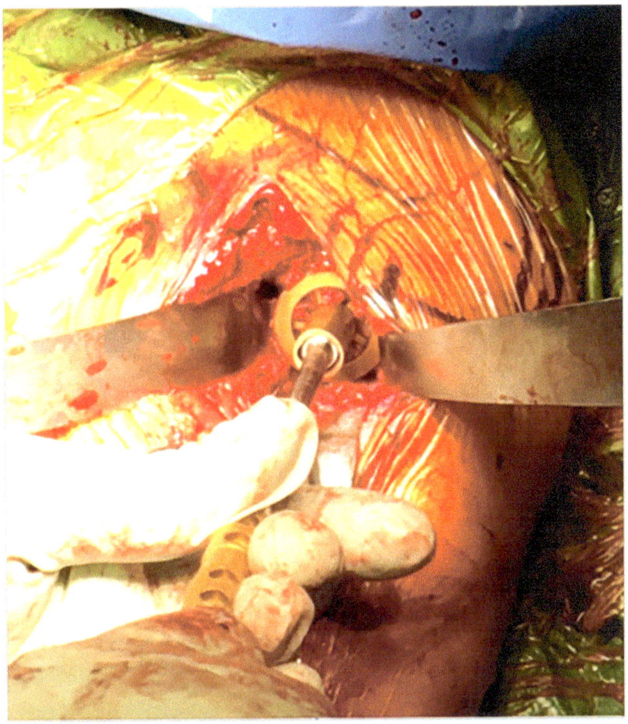

Fig. 49.14 Unobstructed ability to perform glenoid reaming.

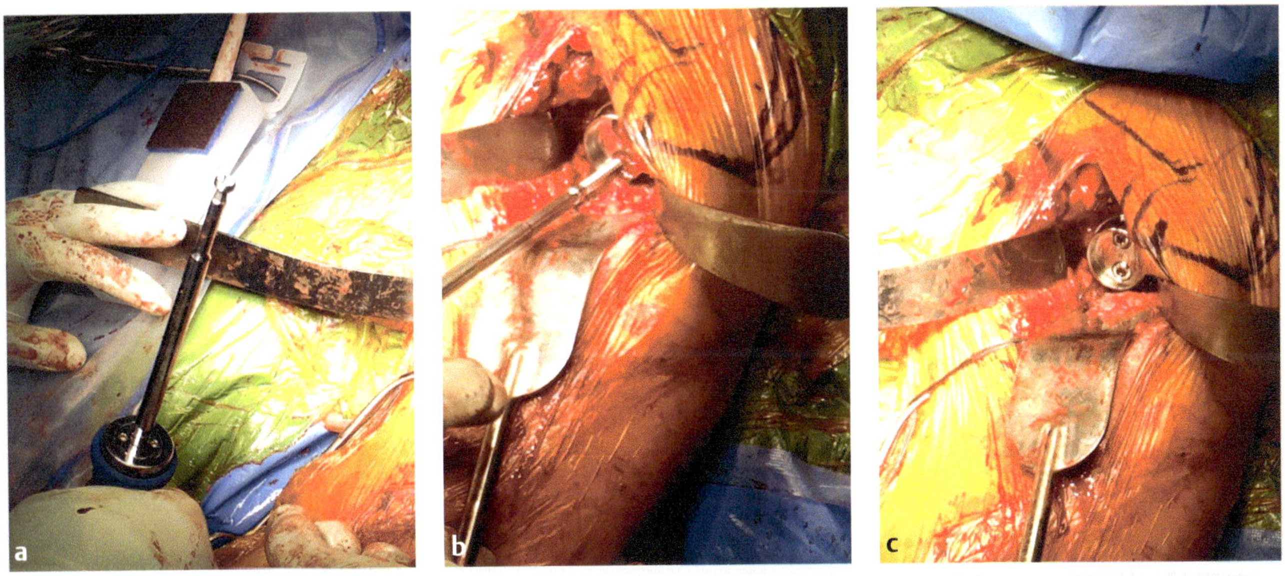

Fig. 49.15 Glenoid baseplate in place with placement of proximal and distal compression screws **(a)** and placement of locking caps **(b,c)**.

3. Superior angulation of glenoid component:
   a. If necessary, use intraoperative fluoroscopic imaging to assess position of pin within scapula.
4. Overtensioning prosthesis:
   a. Assess soft-tissue tensioning of the deltoid, conjoint tendon, and axillary nerve prior to inserting final humeral polyethylene liner.

49.9 Complications/Bailout/ Salvage

Nerve injury:
   a. Iatrogenic.
   b. Traction.

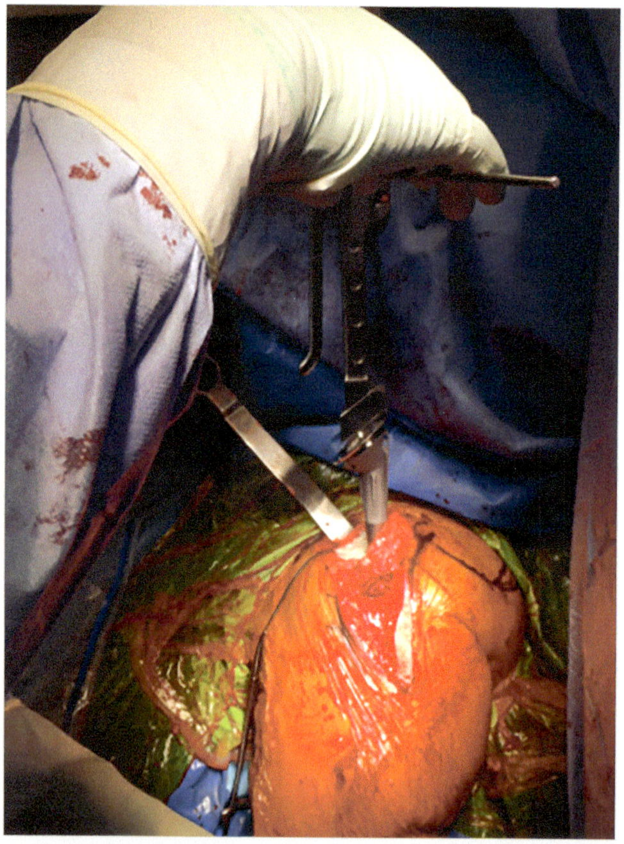

Fig. 49.16 Direct view of the final humeral implant placement.

49.9.1 Bailout

1. Nerve stimulator to determine nerve integrity.
2. If intact but diminished response:
   a. Downsize polyethylene liner to reduce any excess tension without compromising stability.
   b. Reevaluate postoperatively.
   c. Nerve conduction velocity (NCV)/electromyography (EMG) at 6 to 8 weeks.
3. If lacerated:
   a. Perform primary repair and neurolysis.
   b. Nerve conduit or grafting.

49.9.2 Deltoid Dysfunction

1. Excessive traction causing distal propagation of deltoid split into circumflex nerve.
2. Place stay stitch at the distal extent of the split.
3. Minimize excessive distraction with retractors.
4. Slightly posterior release of the anterior deltoid off the acromion.

Bailout

1. Tendon/muscle suture placement and transosseous-based repair.
2. Prolonged immobilization in abduction pillow.

49.10 Postoperative Care

1. Sling immobilization for 4 to 6 weeks. Abduction pillow can be utilized to minimize tension on deltoid repair.
2. Weeks 1 to 6: early passive range of motion, pendulum, and pulleys, and hand, wrist, and elbow motion within the sling.
3. Weeks 7 to 12: discontinue sling; progress to active range of motion; okay to use for activities of daily living and isometric strengthening; continue stretching and range-of-motion exercises, periscapular strengthening, and postural mechanics.
4. Weeks 12 to 18: light resistive exercises and resistive exercise bands for external/internal rotators, and deltoid.

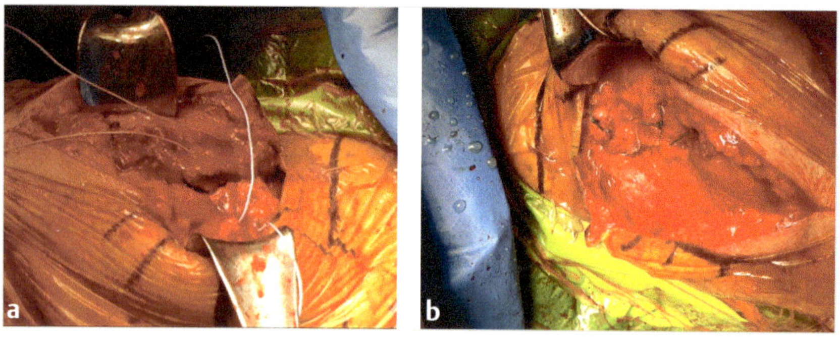

Fig. 49.17 Final closure of the deltoid interval with closure of the deltotrapezial fascia over the acromioclavicular joint resection.

50 Reverse Shoulder Arthroplasty

Dave R. Shukla and John W. Sperling

Abstract

Reverse shoulder arthroplasty is being performed with increasing frequency for a wider range of indications than for which it was previously intended. Given its versatility, it can reliably restore function, reduce pain and significantly improve a patient's ability to return to activity. This chapter reviews essential considerations in the perioperative phases specific to reverse shoulder arthroplasty, while emphasizing critical technical points that will help the surgeon optimize outcomes and avoid complications.

Keywords: *reverse shoulder replacement, rotator cuff tear arthropathy, shoulder arthroplasty, shoulder arthritis*

50.1 Goals of Procedure

The goals of reverse shoulder arthroplasty (RSA) are to restore function and minimize pain related to arthritic change of the glenohumeral joint. While originally found to be most advantageous for shoulders with deficient rotator cuffs, the procedure's indications and use have expanded dramatically in the past decade. An additional goal of the procedure is to provide a stable joint that can restore function with a reasonable degree of longevity.

50.2 Advantages

There are several advantages to using reverse shoulder prosthesis. The most widely accepted advantage is restoration of the ability to raise the arm in those with a massive, irreparable rotator cuff tear and chronic loss of elevation. This procedure has demonstrated promising results in those with rotator cuff-tear arthropathy (CTA), as well as in those with irreparable rotator cuffs and little or no glenohumeral arthritis. Another advantage is that because the glenoid component relies on secure screw fixation to the scapula, this prosthesis can be used in the setting of altered glenoid anatomy, such as in patients with glenoid version abnormalities or bone loss. As such, it is also ideal for revision shoulder arthroplasty, such as in cases of failed anatomic shoulder implants in which the glenoid bone stock has been eroded. A third advantage of the RSA is its versatility as an excellent option for proximal humerus fractures. Recent data have demonstrated promising outcomes when a reverse implant is used to treat unfixable acute proximal humerus fractures as well as proximal humeral nonunions. Anatomic shoulder implants and hemiarthroplasties function poorly when the tuberosities fail to heal, and as the reverse implant is not reliant on healed tuberosities or a functional rotator cuff, the reverse has demonstrated superior results in these clinical scenarios. With similar consideration, the reverse implant can be used in patients with intact but degenerated rotator cuffs, in whom an anatomic replacement may function well temporarily but will eventually fail as the rotator cuff quality deteriorates.

50.3 Indications

The original and most commonly applied indication for RSA remains for CTA with glenohumeral arthritis. The indications are expanding, and though there are many favorable studies that incorporate heterogeneous indications, the outcomes for this indication have demonstrated reliable results.[1–4] As discussed earlier, the reverse prosthesis has also been reported to be used successfully in patients with an intact rotator cuff, particularly those with glenoid version abnormalities or bone loss, those with proximal humeral malunions, or those with at-risk rotator cuffs including those with degenerated or thin cuffs and those with inflammatory arthropathy (i.e., rheumatoid arthritis). An additional indication for this implant is for complex or comminuted proximal humerus fractures that are unfixable or in which the tuberosities would be at risk for nonhealing if a hemiarthroplasty were to be used, as the outcomes of hemiarthroplasties are dependent on tuberosity healing. The reverse prosthesis can also be used to treat patients with preoperative deltoid impairment, and while there is some improvement in pain and function, the results remain inferior to those with unimpaired deltoid muscles. The RSA has also been used successfully in managing patients with significant proximal humeral bone loss, and in those cases of failed hemiarthroplasty.

50.4 Contraindications

One of the primary contraindications to the RSA is the absence of a functional deltoid muscle, secondary to any cause (i.e., permanent axillary nerve dysfunction, failure to heal following prior surgery). Another contraindication would be any limitation of mental capacity, such as severe dementia, that would preclude appropriate adherence to postoperative restrictions. Patients who are unable to comply with the critical portions of the postoperative protocol are at high risk of complications. An additional general contraindication to any sort of arthroplasty would be the presence of medical comorbidities that might place the patient's life at risk should he or she undergo anesthesia.

The presence of a local or systemic infection precludes the implantation of an RSA, and the infection should be confirmed to be eradicated prior to placement of any prosthesis. Finally, inadequate glenoid bone stock precludes placement of the glenosphere portion of the RSA, and in these cases, we would typically utilize a hemiarthroplasty.

50.5 Preoperative Preparation/ Positioning

Preoperative preparation begins with a thorough history and physical examination of the patient. Particular attention is given toward portions of the history that might elucidate whether one of the above-mentioned contraindications is present, as well as if the patient is taking any medications that may affect surgery such as anticoagulants or disease-modifying antirheumatic drugs (DMARDs) in rheumatoid patients. Standard radiographs of the shoulder are obtained, with the two most useful views being the anteroposterior (AP) view in external rotation and the axillary view. Though CT scan is obtained as well, we find that the axillary radiograph provides a more general picture of humeral head subluxation relative to the glenoid. The gravity-assisted (i.e., standing) AP radiograph is useful to appreciate the superior migration that is typical of patients with CTA, as well as to obtain a general sense of medialization of the center of rotation (COR).

The CT scan is critical for preoperative planning, and we routinely obtain this on almost every patient, unless the patient is unable to undergo this imaging study. We utilize the Walch classification[5] to evaluate the glenoid morphology. On an axial view that is representative of the center of the glenoid, Friedman's line[6] is used to evaluate the glenoid version. The coronal views are used to assess glenoid inclination.

The patient is secured comfortably in the beach-chair position, with the backrest inclined to roughly 60 degrees. The torso is angled roughly 20 to 30 degrees off the backrest to ensure that the entire scapula is free. This modified lateralized position allows for adduction and extension of the humerus. Great care is taken during this portion to ensure that the head and neck are safely positioned without tension on the brachial plexus. The knees are bent slightly, and all bony prominences are well padded. We do not use a pneumatic arm holder, but rather a well-padded Mayo stand. The entire upper extremity is draped freely and prepared in a sterile manner.

50.6 Operative Technique

A long deltopectoral approach is used to approach the glenohumeral joint. The clavicle, acromion, and coracoid are marked with a sterile surgical marker. The incision begins at the distal edge of the clavicle, directed roughly 1 cm lateral to the coracoid toward the junction of the medial and middle third of the humerus. The skin and subcutaneous fat are incised using a no. 10 scalpel. The fasciocutaneous flap is elevated proximomedially until the infraclavicular fat triangle is visualized. The cephalic vein is typically identified and dissected free, with care to cauterize the typically present large branches to the deltoid. This is accomplished with the help of a band retractor deep to the proximal deltoid and gentle countertraction on the vein. Once the vein has been mobilized, it can be retracted medially within the exposure.

Electrocautery is then used to incise the clavipectoral fascia. This fascia is released from the lateral edge of the conjoined tendon proximally to the clavicle. A portion of the coracohumeral ligament can be released to improve exposure. A thin Richardson retractor, or something similar, can then be placed deep to the proximal conjoined tendon just distal to the coracoid, with care not to inadvertently retract the axillary and musculocutaneous nerves distally.

The arm is then abducted, which relaxes the deltoid muscle. The interval between the deltoid and proximal humerus is then entered by incising the subdeltoid fascia. The subdeltoid space is bluntly cleared of bursae using a Darrach retractor or with two fingers. A deltoid retractor is placed deep to the deltoid.

The arm can then be slightly externally rotated, and the subscapularis is then on slight tension. If external rotation is less than 30 degrees, a subscapularis peel is performed. Otherwise, a tenotomy through the tendon substance roughly 1 cm medial to the lateral edge of the lesser tuberosity (i.e., medial edge of the bicipital groove) is performed. For every 1 cm that the subscapularis is advanced medially, one gains approximately 20 to 30 degrees of external rotation. The rotator interval is then incised. This release is continued through the subscapularis tendon and distally to release the inferior capsule directly off the humeral neck. The biceps tendon is tenodesed proximally in the groove. The biceps is then tenotomized proximal to the level of the tenodesis. Tagging sutures are placed in the proximal and distal corners of the subscapularis tendon. During the inferior capsular release, the arm is gradually externally rotated as the electrocautery remains directly on the bone, which will minimize the risk to the axillary nerve.

Following capsular release, a Darrach retractor is placed between the glenoid and the humeral head as the head is dislocated with progressive external rotation and delivered out of the joint.

50.6.1 Humeral Preparation

A burr is used to create a large entry hole that is collinear with the humeral shaft, 1 cm posterior to the bicipital groove and 1 cm medial to it. A sharp awl is used to obtain canal access, and then preparation with hand reamers begins. Reamer size is increased by 2-mm increments until firm resistance is encountered. At this point, the reamer is left in place, the handle is removed, and a cutting jig is placed.

We routinely cut the humeral head in 30 degrees of retroversion for standard primary RSA, unless patient anatomy dictates otherwise. Such situations include those with significant posterior subluxation and glenoid wear, in which cases less than 30 degrees of retroversion may be selected. A version rod on the cutting jig is set to 30 degrees, adjusted so that it is collinear with the forearm, and the jig height is then set such that the saw blade will exit at the margin of the native rotator cuff insertion. Depending on the difficulty of the glenoid exposure, additional head may need to be resected. Darrach retractors are placed posterior to the head to protect the soft tissues during this portion. The head is cut and the canal is then broached to one size below the final reamer size, for our system.

A critical next step is to adequately remove peripheral osteophytes with a rongeur, as this will facilitate glenoid exposure. Additionally, any remaining posteroinferior capsule can be released at this stage. As the RSA is a constrained implant, this release can be carried circumferentially because of the implant's inherent stability, whereas such an extensive release is sometimes not performed when implanting an anatomic arthroplasty. The trial broach is left in place.

50.6.2 Glenoid Exposure

The arm is placed in roughly 70 degrees of abduction and slight flexion. A Fukuda or double-pronged retractor is placed over the posterior lip of the glenoid to then retract the cut humeral neck posteriorly. It is critical to remember that this is the portion of the procedure in which the brachial plexus is under the greatest degree of tension, so effort should be made to minimize the time and extent of traction. The space between the subscapularis and anterior labrum is developed and a smaller double-pronged retractor is placed there. At this point, the labrum is meticulously debrided circumferentially, as it is critical that the entire glenoid is visualized. This is particularly important inferiorly, as determination of the true inferior rim is of utmost importance to avoid placing the glenosphere superiorly. To achieve this, we use a Darrach retractor to protect the axillary nerve while releasing the inferior capsule with electrocautery.

The CT scan is then re-reviewed to confirm the glenoid version and true anatomic center of the glenoid. An awl or burr can be used to create a centering hole. Trial glenoid baseplates are used to determine the appropriate size. A 3.2-mm Steinmann guide pin is inserted using a power driver, with sufficient depth that the medial cortex is captured. A cannulated baseplate reamer is then used to ream the cartilage and subchondral bone such that roughly 80% of the baseplate will be in contact with the bleeding bone. Based on the information from the CT scan, one can preferentially ream away more bone in certain quadrants to maximize the likelihood that the baseplate will sit flat against the glenoid. For example, if there is posterior glenoid wear, one should ream more of the anterior glenoid. A glenoid planer can then be used to flatten the face of the glenoid and remove any overhanging bone that may prevent complete seating of the component.

Once the centering hole has been drilled and the baseplate has been placed, the next priority is to strive to achieve bicortical purchase with the 6.5-mm central screw. The central screw hole is drilled, measured, and placed. Then, the superior, inferior, anterior, and posterior screws are placed. Depending on where on the glenoid the baseplate is resting, and if the system allows for modularity, eccentricity and laterality can be incorporated into the final construct, and the glenosphere is then impacted onto the baseplate.

50.6.3 Final Component Position

Once the glenosphere has been placed, a trial tray can be placed onto the broach that was left in the humerus. The trial reduction should ensure that there is no impingement during full range of motion. After reduction, there should be roughly 2 mm of opening with longitudinal traction applied to the arm to ensure that the articulation is not overtightened.

50.6.4 Closure

The subscapularis is repaired using drill holes either to the proximal humerus (lesser tuberosity) if a peel was performed or to the remaining lateral tendon stump if a tenotomy was performed. The deltopectoral interval is approximated and the subcutaneous layer and skin are closed in the standard fashion.

50.7 Tips and Pearls/Expert Suggestions

50.7.1 Preoperatively

- Carefully evaluate the glenoid version based on the CT scan. Intraoperatively, the position of the scapula may be deceiving, so the CT measurements should be used in conjunction.

50.7.2 Intraoperatively

- During humeral preparation, ensure that a sufficiently large entry hole is created in the articular surface so that the instruments are free to find the canal, and not forced into the wrong trajectory.
- Pearls for obtaining glenoid exposure: if it is difficult to obtain adequate exposure, one can usually return to address one or all of four key aspects:
  - Deltoid mobilization.
  - Adequate humeral head cut.
  - Humeral osteophyte removal.
  - Sufficient capsular release.
- Strive for bicortical central screw purchase to maximize the chance of glenosphere fixation and longevity.
- Minimize operative time with the wound open to decrease the risk of infection.

50.8 What to Avoid

- Avoid prolonged retraction of the humeral head in excessive extension, as this increases the risk of iatrogenic brachial plexus injury.
- Avoid performing an inadequate capsulolabral release. If the inferior edge of the glenoid is not visualized, this could lead to glenoid malposition.
- Avoid placing too much stress on the final glenoid by forceful dislocation and relocation during humeral trialing. This could lead to pullout of the baseplate intraoperatively.

50.9 Complications/Bailout/Salvage

50.9.1 Complications

There are several complications to be aware of after RSA, some that are unique to this procedure and some that simply occur with a higher frequency versus other procedures. Scapular notching, as graded using the system of Sirveaux et al,[4] has been reported with a wide range of incidences, though its true significance is somewhat unclear. Strategies that have been shown to minimize the risk of notching include using an implant with an increased humeral neck shaft angle, incorporating some inferior tilt (10–20 degrees) of the glenoid component, lateralizing the component's COR, and inferiorly translating the glenosphere such that there is up to 5 mm of overhang of the baseplate. While early literature reported a rate of up to 96%,[7] later reports demonstrated much lower incidences of notching when the above measures where employed.

Infection following RSA typically occurs secondary to *Propionibacterium acnes*, *Staphylococcus aureus*, or *S. epidermidis*. Our preferred method to maximize the chance of eradication is to perform a two-stage revision, with placement of an antibiotic-impregnated dynamic spacer for roughly 2 months between stages. Following the 2 months, the final implantation of another prosthesis can be carried out if laboratory testing confirms the absence of infection.

An acromion fracture is a complication unique to RSA, and the surgeon should consider this in a patient who initially is progressing well and then presents with the acute onset of pain or dysfunction, in the absence of other implant-related issues. A CT scan is typically required to detect this entity, and the majority are managed nonoperatively.

Success of the RSA is dependent on secure fixation of the glenosphere. One scenario in which a bailout may be necessary is typically found in the case of revision surgery for a failed anatomic RSA, during which it is noticed that there is insufficient glenoid bone stock to support the glenosphere. In this case, the surgeon may opt to implant a hemiarthroplasty. This is a more effective solution if there is a contained defect of the glenoid into which the hemiarthroplasty can articulate. Should all other implantation options fail, one can consider resection arthroplasty.

50.10 Postoperative Care

Postoperatively, all patients are immobilized in a shoulder sling. For 6 weeks, they are typically allowed only very gentle passive range of motion with limited forward elevation and external rotation. The exercises, which are demonstrated prior to surgery, are reiterated to the patients by physical therapists on the morning following surgery. The simple early exercises are done by the patients for the first 6 weeks without formal physical therapy. Progressive strengthening is then initiated.

References

1. Frankle M, Levy JC, Pupello D, et al. The reverse shoulder prosthesis for glenohumeral arthritis associated with severe rotator cuff deficiency. a minimum two-year follow-up study of sixty patients surgical technique. J Bone Joint Surg Am 2006;88(Suppl 1, Pt 2):178–190
2. Naveed MA, Kitson J, Bunker TD. The Delta III reverse shoulder replacement for cuff tear arthropathy: a single-centre study of 50 consecutive procedures. J Bone Joint Surg Br 2011;93(1):57–61
3. Nolan BM, Ankerson E, Wiater JM. Reverse total shoulder arthroplasty improves function in cuff tear arthropathy. Clin Orthop Relat Res 2011;469(9):2476–2482
4. Sirveaux F, Favard L, Oudet D, Huquet D, Walch G, Molé D. Grammont inverted total shoulder arthroplasty in the treatment of glenohumeral osteoarthritis with massive rupture of the cuff. Results of a multicentre study of 80 shoulders. J Bone Joint Surg Br 2004;86(3):388–395
5. Walch G, Badet R, Boulahia A, Khoury A. Morphologic study of the glenoid in primary glenohumeral osteoarthritis. J Arthroplasty 1999;14(6):756–760
6. Friedman RJ, Hawthorne KB, Genez BM. The use of computerized tomography in the measurement of glenoid version. J Bone Joint Surg Am 1992;74(7):1032–1037
7. Nicholson GP, Strauss EJ, Sherman SL. Scapular notching: Recognition and strategies to minimize clinical impact. Clin Orthop Relat Res 2011;469(9):2521–2530

51 Reverse Shoulder Arthroplasty with a Shaped Humeral Head Autograft for B2/B3 and C Glenoids

Samuel M. Harmsen and Tom Norris

Abstract

Glenoid bone loss and altered glenoid morphology can present a difficult challenge when considering shoulder replacement surgery. As a consequence, results with anatomic hemi and total shoulder arthroplasty are unpredictable and are associated with higher complication and failure rates. Reverse shoulder arthroplasty has gained favor in these difficult patients. In this chapter, we present a technique utilizing a shaped humeral head autograft with reverse shoulder arthroplasty that can be used to treat primary glenohumeral osteoarthritis with significant glenoid bone loss, with or without an intact rotator cuff. This technique is associated with excellent and predictable clinical and radiographic outcomes and a low complication profile in these demanding cases.

Keywords: *shaped humeral head autograft, posterior glenoid bone loss, glenoid retroversion, reverse shoulder arthroplasty, glenohumeral arthritis*

51.1 Goals of Procedure

The goals of the procedure are to achieve predictable stable fixation of the glenoid component, restore glenoid version and bone stock, and obtain predictable clinical outcomes while limiting complications and failure.

Posterior glenoid bone loss (PGBL) can present a difficult challenge when considering shoulder replacement for the treatment of primary glenohumeral osteoarthritis. As described by Neer and Friedman, and later classified by Walch, glenoid morphology can change with the progression of the arthritic process. Advanced osteoarthritis can result in glenoid bone loss, retroversion of the glenoid, loss of normal glenoid vault anatomy, and posterior subluxation of the humeral head. When altered glenoid morphology corresponding with Walch's classification of B2, B3 or C is present, results with anatomic shoulder replacement surgery can be unpredictable and have been associated with high complication profile.[1-3] The use of eccentric reaming, glenoid bone grafting, augmented glenoids, and reverse shoulder arthroplasty (RSA) has been described. When correction of glenoid version and recentralization of the humeral head are achieved, satisfactory results can be obtained. However, this can prove to be a surgical challenge. Compared to total shoulder arthroplasty (TSA) in patients without significant PGBL, decreased functional results, increased pain levels, and higher rates of glenoid loosening and complications have been reported.[4-13]

When PGBL and retroversion exceed the boundaries of safe eccentric reaming or there is insufficient bone for glenoid fixation, structural support using bone graft or other material has been attempted with TSA. The use of bone grafting is generally associated with a high percentage of radiolucency, glenoid component failure, graft failures, and instability.[2,3] The senior author reported on 17 patients who underwent bone grafting.[5] Despite average correction of retroversion to 4 degrees, 29% required revision surgery for fixation failure and 47% unsatisfactory results. This experience led to the development and use of RSA with a shaped humeral head autograft to the glenoid in these difficult patients.

51.2 Advantages

Grafting the glenoid with a shaped humeral head autograft allows restoration of glenoid bone stock and version. RSA allows for stable graft fixation with the baseplate and avoids recurrent posterior instability associated with anatomic shoulder arthroplasty.

51.3 Indications

This technique is considered for patients with glenohumeral arthritis associated with significant glenoid bone loss. Though described for PGBL, this technique can also be predictably used in patients with anterior, superior, or central glenoid bone loss as well.

51.4 Contraindications

Contraindications to shoulder arthroplasty include active infection, significant medical comorbidity, Charcot's arthropathy, and severe neurologic pathologies. Contraindications for RSA also include axillary nerve palsy and deltoid dysfunction. Finally, if glenoid bone stock is severely limited and/or the bone quality is inadequate for stable baseplate fixation, we would recommend against this procedure.

51.5 Preoperative Preparation/ Positioning

Preoperative evaluation should always emphasize the patient's history of disease, any prior treatment, and medical comorbidities. Physical examination should assess motion, strength, deformity, cervical disease, and neurologic function. Preoperative radiographs should include internal and external rotation Grashey, scapular Y, and axillary views. Advanced imaging should include at minimum a 2D CT scan. We recommend obtaining a 3D reconstruction CT scan with minimum 1-mm thin cuts. An MRI is not felt to be necessary. The surgeon should assess the glenoid morphology, bone loss, retroversion, inclination, and subluxation of the humeral head in relation to the glenoid. The use of imaging software capable of appropriately setting the axis of rotation along the scapular line can help enable better understanding of glenoid morphology. This information will be used to help plan the appropriate starting point and trajectory for guide pin placement. Recently, 3D planning software and patient specific guides have become more available and can be utilized to improve guide pin placement if desired.

The patient is positioned in the beach-chair position. We prefer the head of bed to be at roughly 35 degrees. A towel or small bump is placed just medial to the medial border of the scapular in order to rotate the scapula anteriorly. This helps deliver the glenoid anterior, providing better exposure to the posterior glenoid neck. We prefer using an arm holder; however, use of a padded Mayo stand is also an option. We prefer utilizing both a regional interscalene nerve block and general anesthesia.

51.6 Operative Technique

The surgical techniques for RSA have been well described.[14,15] The majority of this procedure follow these techniques, with variations in the harvesting of the humeral head autograft, glenoid preparation, and shaping of the humeral head autograft. We prefer to use a long post baseplate (Tornier, Edina, MN), two peripheral compression screws, and two peripheral locking screws; however, other baseplate designs can also be used.

Using a standard deltopectoral approach, the proximal humerus is exposed and prepared using the standard technique. The long head of the biceps tendon is tenodesed to the superior border of the pectoralis major insertion. The subscapularis tendon is released using the surgeon's preferred technique, and the humeral head is dislocated and delivered through the deltopectoral interval. A 2.5-mm guide wire is placed in the center of the humeral head perpendicular to the planned humeral head cut and driven through the lateral humeral cortex for stabilization. Using a cannulated system, the glenoid reamer is used to flatten the humeral head just beyond the articular surface. A 29-mm hole saw with a central 8-mm cannulated drill (**Fig. 51.1a**) is then passed along the wire to obtain a deep cylinder graft and a central hole (**Fig. 51.1b**). The guide wire is removed and the humeral head cut is made to the desired depth of the graft. We prefer starting with at least a 15-mm graft. The donut-shaped graft is removed (**Fig. 51.1c**) placed in a saline-soaked sponge and saved on the back table. The remaining humeral preparations can be completed now or after the glenoid has been addressed.

51.6.1 Glenoid Preparation

The glenoid is exposed and cleared of all remaining cartilage and soft tissue. A complete capsular release is performed and the subscapularis is elevated off the anterior glenoid neck (**Fig. 51.2**). The glenoid centering point is palpated anteriorly and used to determine the correct orientation and version of the central guidewire.[16] The guide wire is placed in this version, 0 to 10 degrees of inferior tilt, and approximately 14 mm superior to the inferior border of the glenoid. When a significantly altered glenoid morphology is present, these measurements may be difficult to achieve. Imaging software and patient-specific guides can also be used to achieve appropriate placement of the guide wire. Once the guide wire is placed, the glenoid is reamed using a cannulated glenoid reamer until the anterior glenoid is flat to the level of the guide wire. This results in a flat anterior surface with the neoglenoid extending beyond the guide wire posteriorly (**Fig. 51.2b**). The neoglenoid is trephinated and decorticated to promote bleeding and

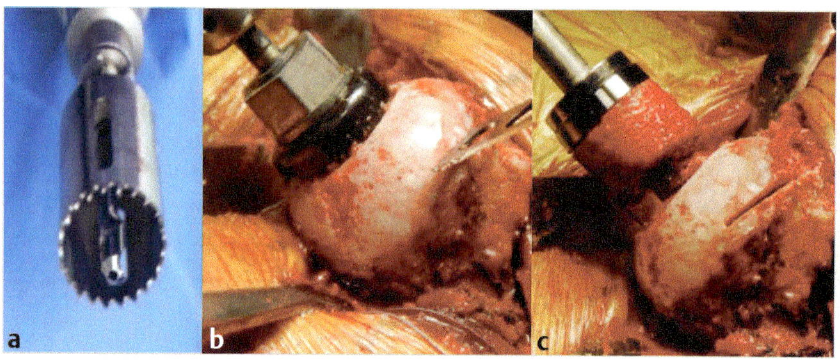

Fig. 51.1 Shaped humeral head autograft harvesting. (a) A 29-mm hole saw with 8-mm central cannulated drill. (b) Use of a 29-mm cannulated hole saw to obtain a deep cylindrical autograft. (c) Harvested humeral head autograft. The baseplate can be used to safely remove the graft from the humeral head if needed.

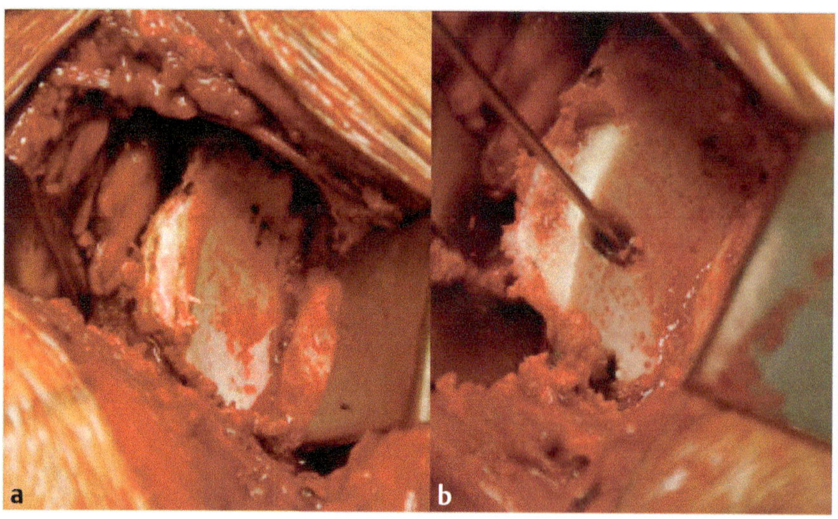

Fig. 51.2 Glenoid preparation. (a) Glenoid exposure with complete, circumferential capsular release. (b) Prepared glenoid after reaming the anterior glenoid flat to the level of the guide wire, drilling of the central hole, and trephination/decortication of the neoglenoid completed.

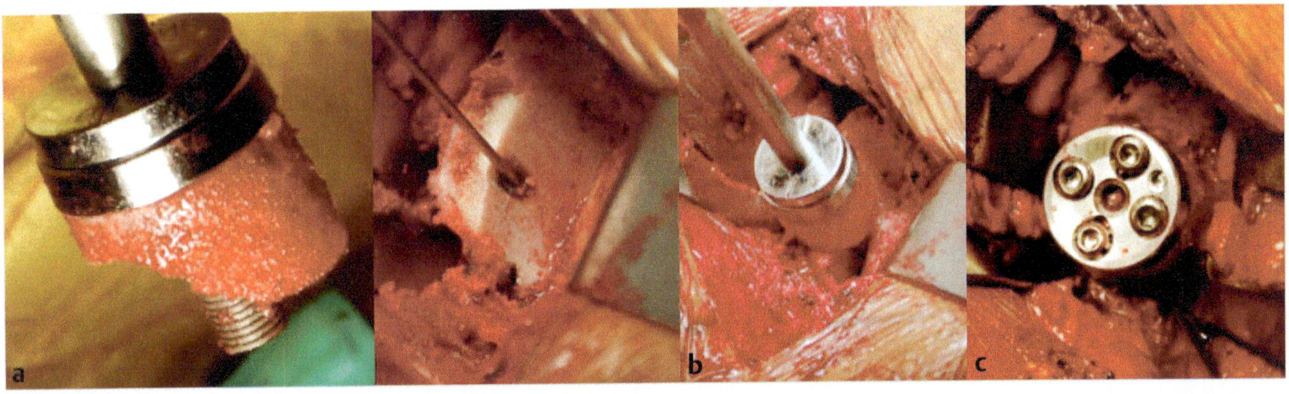

Fig. 51.3 Shaped humeral head graft preparation and implantation. **(a)** The prepared "shaped" graft/baseplate construct ready for implantation (left) onto the prepared glenoid (right). **(b)** Impaction of the graft/baseplate complex onto the prepared glenoid with the "shaped" graft in matching orientation. **(c)** The graft/baseplate complex has been compressed and locked into place on the glenoid.

autograft incorporation. The center hole is then drilled using a cannulated drill per implant technique.

51.6.2 Graft Preparation and Implantation

The humeral head autograft is then "shaped" on the back table to match the prepared glenoid. Using a microsagittal saw, the anterior portion of the graft is flattened to the level of the midline of central hole, preserving the thickness of graft to achieve desired lateralization. We generally preserve 6- to 8-mm graft thickness anteriorly; however, a thicker graft may be used if needed. This also allows for a portion of the graft to be compressed directly perpendicular to the glenoid, optimizing graft compression and incorporation. The posterior portion of the graft is then shaped to match the retroversion of the remaining neoglenoid and placed onto a long post baseplate (**Fig. 51.3a**). The graft/baseplate complex is then impacted or secured, depending on the type of baseplate used, onto the glenoid in the correct orientation (**Fig. 51.3b**). Further graft compression and secure baseplate fixation is achieved by placing the peripheral screws (**Fig. 51.3c**) and the glenosphere is impacted onto the baseplate.

51.7 Tips and Pearls/Expert Suggestions

This technique can be utilized using other baseplate designs. During graft preparation, the appropriate central-hole drill and glenoid reamer should be used to ensure adequate baseplate/graft apposition. When using a screw-in-type baseplate, the graft will rotate when advancing the baseplate. We recommend either securing the graft to the glenoid with angled peripheral k-wires prior to advancing the baseplate or using a towel or bone clamp to secure the graft and preventing graft rotation while advancing the baseplate.

If the graft is too thin or the angle is cut too far anteriorly, it will have a tendency to break at the apex of the "shape." We prefer at minimum a 6-mm-thick graft anteriorly. This helps avoid graft fracture as well as provides lateralization of the center of rotation. We also recommend placing the apex of the "shape" at or short of the middle of the central peg hole, which also helps avoid graft fracture.

If visualization and/or access to the glenoid is compromised, we recommend taking the time to improve access to allow in-line placement of the graft/baseplate complex.

51.8 What to Avoid

If the humeral head graft quality is poor, or solid baseplate fixation beyond the graft cannot be obtained at time of implantation, we do not recommend using this technique. As mentioned earlier, take care to avoid graft fracture and failure at the time of implantation. As with all RSA, avoid placing the baseplate in superior inclination and ensure that the baseplate is fully seated prior to placing peripheral screws and the glenosphere.

51.9 Complications/Bailout/Salvage

If the graft fractures, the posterior portion of the autograft can be used alone as a wedge allograft, advancing the baseplate to the native glenoid anteriorly. Further preparation of the glenoid may be necessary in order to do so. In this situation, we recommend use of a lateralized glenosphere in order to optimize center of rotation.

If the graft is not salvageable, or the quality is poor, the distal clavicle is an easily accessible option that has had some success. Alternatively, a tricortical iliac crest autograft can also be utilized. Other options include humeral or femoral head allografts. These can be prepared in similar fashion to the shaped humeral head autograft. Some implant systems also have metal augmentation options available.

In cases where the bone loss is so severe that baseplate fixation cannot be achieved, the surgeon can consider a staged procedure, autografting the glenoid at the index procedure, and returning once the graft has incorporated for definitive surgery. We recommend the use of a tricortical iliac crest autograft in these situations. Alternatively, a hemiarthroplasty with more limited goals can be performed.

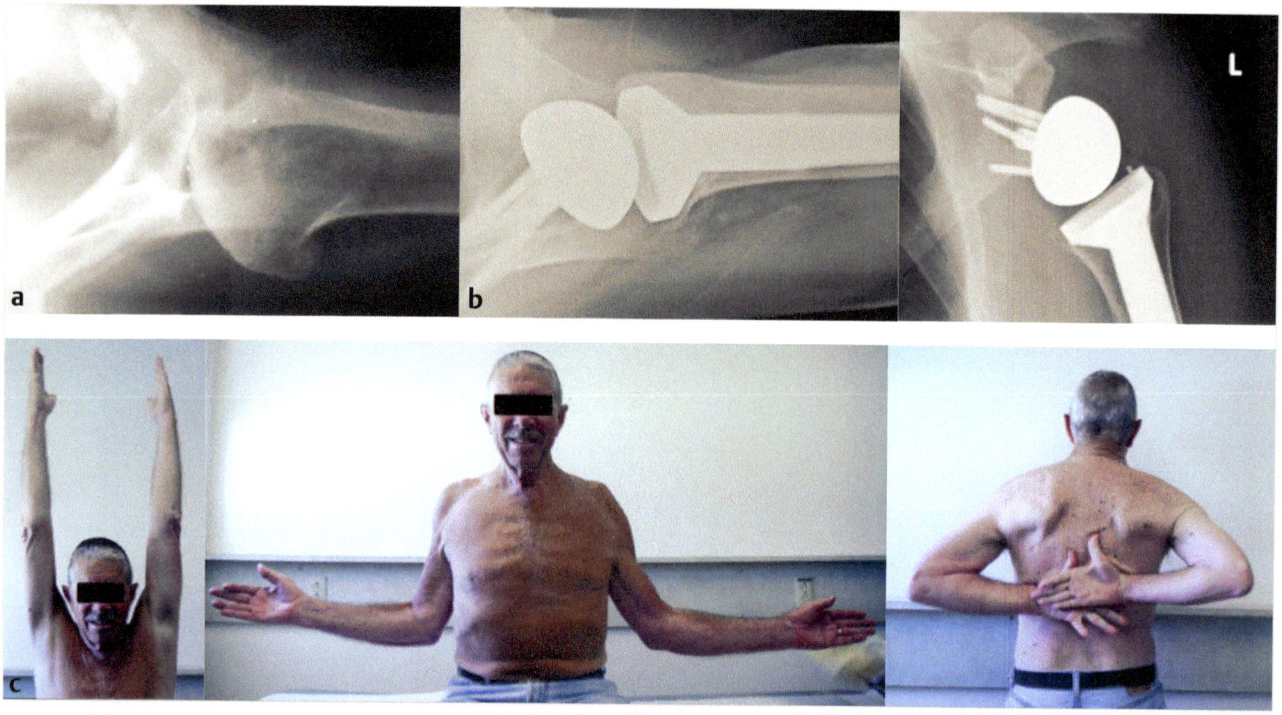

Fig. 51.4 Case example. (a) Preoperative digital axial radiograph of a 66-year-old male with primary glenohumeral osteoarthritis with significant posterior glenoid bone loss, retroversion, and posterior humeral subluxation (B2 glenoid). (b) Axial and anteroposterior digital radiographs 5 years after surgery. (c) Clinical images obtained at 5-year follow-up.

51.10 Postoperative Care

No special consideration is given to RSA with humeral head autograft. We recommend standard RSA postoperative protocol in these patients. In our practice, patients are in a simple sling for 3 to 4 weeks, coming out of the sling three to four times per day for pendulum, elbow, wrist, and hand exercises. Patients are also allowed to come out of the sling for hygiene. Simple tasks are allowed with the operative hand; however, no active lifting is recommended. After 3 to 4 weeks, the sling is removed and progression of light activities of daily living as tolerated is allowed. Passive, active-assisted, and active range of motion exercises are initiated, and, if necessary, physical therapy is recommended. Return to full activity is permitted at 10 to 12 weeks postoperatively.

Excellent long-term results can be obtained using this technique in patients with significant glenoid bone loss (**Fig. 51.4a–c**).

References

1. Denard PJ, Walch G. Current concepts in the surgical management of primary glenohumeral arthritis with a biconcave glenoid. J Shoulder Elbow Surg 2013;22(11):1589–1598
2. Stephens SP, Paisley KC, Jeng J, Dutta AK, Wirth MA. Shoulder arthroplasty in the presence of posterior glenoid bone loss. J Bone Joint Surg Am 2015;97(3):251–259
3. Sears BW, Johnston PS, Ramsey ML, Williams GR. Glenoid bone loss in primary total shoulder arthroplasty: evaluation and management. J Am Acad Orthop Surg 2012;20(9):604–613
4. Habermeyer P, Magosch P, Lichtenberg S. Recentering the humeral head for glenoid deficiency in total shoulder arthroplasty. Clin Orthop Relat Res 2007;457(457):124–132
5. Hill JM, Norris TR. Long-term results of total shoulder arthroplasty following bone-grafting of the glenoid. J Bone Joint Surg Am 2001;83-A(6):877–883
6. Sabesan V, Callanan M, Ho J, Iannotti JP. Clinical and radiographic outcomes of total shoulder arthroplasty with bone graft for osteoarthritis with severe glenoid bone loss. J Bone Joint Surg Am 2013;95(14):1290–1296
7. Friedman RJ, Hawthorne KB, Genez BM. Glenoid augmentation for total shoulder arthroplasty. Orthop Trans 1992;16:66
8. Iannotti JP, Frangiamore SJ. Fate of large structural allograft for treatment of severe uncontained glenoid bone deficiency. J Shoulder Elbow Surg 2012;21(6):765–771
9. Neer CS II, Morrison DS. Glenoid bone-grafting in total shoulder arthroplasty. J Bone Joint Surg Am 1988;70(8):1154–1162
10. Steinmann SP, Cofield RH. Bone grafting for glenoid deficiency in total shoulder replacement. J Shoulder Elbow Surg 2000;9(5):361–367
11. Rice RS, Sperling JW, Miletti J, Schleck C, Cofield RH. Augmented glenoid component for bone deficiency in shoulder arthroplasty. Clin Orthop Relat Res 2008;466(3):579–583
12. Sabesan V, Callanan M, Sharma V, Iannotti JP. Correction of acquired glenoid bone loss in osteoarthritis with a standard versus an augmented glenoid component. J Shoulder Elbow Surg 2014;23(7):964–973

13. Walch G, Young AA, Boileau P, Loew M, Gazielly D, Mole D. Patterns of loosening of polyethylene keeled glenoid components after shoulder arthroplasty for primary osteoarthritis. J Bone Joint Surg Am 2012;94(2):145–150
14. Hatzidakis AM, Norris TR, Boileau P. Reverse shoulder arthroplasty indications, technique, and results. Tech Shoulder Elbow Surg 2005;6(3):135–149
15. Wall B, Nové-Josserand L, O'Connor DP, Edwards TB, Walch G. Reverse total shoulder arthroplasty: a review of results according to etiology. J Bone Joint Surg Am 2007;89(7): 1476–1485
16. Matsen FA. Practical evaluation and management of the shoulder. Philadelphia, PA: WB Saunders; 1994

52 Patient-Specific Instrumentation for Severe Deformity in Reverse Shoulder Arthroplasty

Prem N. Ramkumar, Jared M. Mahylis, Eric T. Ricchetti, and Joseph P. Iannotti

Abstract
In cases of severe glenoid bone loss and other deformity managed with reverse shoulder arthroplasty, we discuss in this chapter how patient-specific surgical planning software and instrumentation can be used as a critical preoperative planning tool as it relates to implant sizing, positioning, and graft use.

Keywords: *deformity, patient-specific instrumentation*

52.1 Goals of Procedure

Reverse shoulder arthroplasty (RSA) can provide excellent function to patients with a spectrum of glenohumeral pathology. Implant selection and positioning, however, remains a potential challenge of this nonanatomic prosthesis, especially in cases of significant glenoid bone loss. Patient-specific preoperative planning using 3D CT can allow for selection of optimal implant size and position in these cases of severe deformity, including allowing the surgeon to decide whether bone graft is needed. The use of patient-specific instrumentation (PSI) provides the surgeon with tools to transfer information from the preoperative planning software to the surgical site. The focus of this chapter will be on the techniques for utilization of patient-specific surgical planning software and instrumentation for surgical treatment using RSA in cases of severe glenoid bone loss.

52.2 Advantages

The glenosphere and baseplate may be defined by their superoinferior (SI), anteroposterior (AP), and mediolateral (ML) positions, or by their orientation relative to the glenoid and scapular planes (inclination, version, and rotation). The position and orientation of the glenosphere directly influence glenohumeral range of motion, stability, implant impingement, and scapular notching. Ideal glenosphere placement is in a location that maximizes impingement-free range of motion and stability while avoiding notching. Multiple studies have shown lateral offset and inferior placement of the glenosphere results in increased range of motion and reduced scapular notching,[1–5] while neutral or slight inferior tilt of the glenosphere limits the risk of decreased postoperative range of motion.[4,6–9] Despite our understanding of appropriate implant position, execution of correct glenosphere placement still remains a challenge. Verborgt et al showed standard instrumentation without advanced imaging resulted in an error range of 16 degrees for glenosphere inclination and 12 degrees for glenosphere version.[9] This finding supports the value of 3D templating to determine the optimal location of the implant. Virtual 3D implant templating has been shown to improve the accuracy of guide pin position and orientation when using standard instrumentation or PSI when compared to 2D imaging and use of standard instrumentation, both in a preclinical sawbones study and in a prospective clinical trial.[10,11] In the preclinical sawbones study, PSI provided additional accuracy for guide pin placement when used in combination with 3D preoperative planning, while in the clinical trial, PSI tools were not of further benefit in guide pin accuracy compared to 3D preoperative planning alone.[10,11]

52.3 Indications

The use of RSA has expanded since its inception. Indications for RSA include rotator cuff-tear arthropathy (CTA) with or without glenoid bone loss,[12] massive irreparable rotator cuff tear, primary osteoarthritis (OA) with rotator cuff tear, primary OA with an intact rotator cuff but with severe glenoid bone loss, posttraumatic arthritis with glenoid bone loss with or without malunion, failed hemiarthroplasty with glenoid bone loss and/or rotator cuff deficiency, and failed total shoulder arthroplasty (TSA) with bone loss and/or rotator cuff deficiency. The use of RSA for primary OA with severe glenoid bone loss or deformity has increased in the recent years, due to the worse clinical outcomes that have been reported in this setting with anatomic TSA using a standard nonaugmented glenoid component.[13] Walch et al originally reported on glenoid bone loss in OA and defined three fundamental types of glenoid morphology patterns, type A, B, and C glenoids,[14] with worse clinical outcomes reported in B2 glenoids when using an anatomic TSA with a nonaugmented glenoid component. More recent studies of primary OA using 3D CT reconstructions have defined additional patterns of glenoid pathoanatomy that have modified the original Walch classification[15,16] and further differentiated more severe forms of glenoid bone loss and deformity that may not perform well with an anatomic TSA. Glenoid bone loss remains a significant challenge in all cases of shoulder arthroplasty and is not isolated to primary OA. Severe superior glenoid bone loss can occur in CTA, and large contained or uncontained defects are often present in revision TSA. Despite the presence of glenoid bone loss in these different clinical settings, RSA offers the potential for stable fixation into the glenoid because of the locking screw construct of the glenoid baseplate that can incorporate a bone graft into the glenoid construct. Patient-specific tools can increase the ability to place the glenoid component in optimal position to maximize patient function and implant fixation, and to determine the optimal location for bone graft placement, if needed.

52.4 Contraindication

There are several relative and absolute contraindications to RSA, which include severe deltoid deficiency or dysfunction that cannot be reconstructed, axillary nerve injury with severe loss of deltoid function, severe near total loss of glenoid bone that prevents placement of a stable glenoid baseplate even with bone grafting, active infection, neurological conditions such as syringomyelia, Charcot's arthropathy, and patients with medical comorbidities that prevent surgical treatment. 3D preoperative planning tools can be particularly helpful to determine if the amount of glenoid bone loss is severe enough to not allow for stable fixation of the glenoid baseplate or if the risk of baseplate failure will be high due to inadequate glenoid bone stock.

52.5 Preoperative Planning/ Positioning

52.5.1 History and Physical Examination

As in all patients who are evaluated for shoulder pathology, a detailed history taking and physical examination are performed.

52.5.2 Imaging and Patient-Specific Presurgical Planning

Standard 2D CT scans can be helpful to assess glenoid pathology, including glenoid retroversion and bone loss, but are limited by the ability to acquire imaging planes perpendicular to the plane of the scapula resulting in inaccurate measurements of glenoid version and inclination. However, 3D CT imaging and implant templating provide superior accuracy over 2D CT imaging for quantifying glenoid bone loss and guiding surgical decision-making.[17,18] 3D planning with a CT scan should include the entire scapula with 1 mm or thinner slices imported within a software application that allows for both 3D and reconstructed 2D imaging in planes orthogonal to the plane of the scapula. Modern 3D surgical planning applications also include methods to define glenoid bone loss, glenoid version, and inclination, and allow placement and manipulation of a desired implant system. The plane of the scapula can be defined by the inferior angle of the scapula, the center of the glenoid, and the scapula trigonum, which is defined as the confluence of the scapular body and spine at the medial border. The plane of the glenoid is defined by three points on the glenoid surface that generally represent the surface of the glenoid on coronal and axial 2D imaging (**Fig. 52.1a**).

The glenoid vault model has been used as a research tool to define the premorbid anatomy from the pathologic state. Although the authors have used this tool for surgical planning, this tool is not commercially available in any Food and Drug Administration (FDA) approved software. The vault model is the 3D shape of the normal glenoid vault[10,19] and can be used with 3D planning to estimate native glenoid version, inclination, and joint line position in the setting of glenoid bone loss.[19–22] When the vault model is positioned correctly, its anterior and medial portion will closely follow the preserved 3D internal architecture of the patient's anterior glenoid (**Fig. 52.1b**). In pathologic shoulders, the lateral surface of the vault model represents the premorbid glenoid version, inclination, and joint line (**Fig. 52.1c, d**). By this method, the bone loss associated with the patient's pathology can be defined. The senior authors have used the vault model for surgical planning in the selection of implant type and its placement for both anatomic and reverse TSA, as well as to define the size and location of bone graft needed. After placement of the glenoid vault model and the desired implant, simulated bone reaming is defined as well as the location and orientation of the glenoid guide pin (**Fig. 52.1e**). The location of the guide pin in relation to the glenoid bone landmarks can then be replicated at the time of surgery using standard or patient-specific instrumentation (**Fig. 52.1f**).[23,24] Bone loss can be accurately visualized (**Fig. 52.1g, h**) and may be addressed by bone grafting the glenoid or selecting an implant system with a lateralized glenosphere design. Patients with a pathologic or a short native scapular neck may be another indication to bone graft the glenoid or select an implant system with a lateralized glenosphere design to avoid bony impingement and scapular notching. Paisley et al suggested lateralizing the glenosphere in patients with a scapular neck length less than 9 mm measured on a true anteroposterior radiograph.[24]

Once the desired implant and its location are chosen with the 3D preoperative templating, the implant can be placed intraoperatively using PSI tools or standard instrumentation used in a patient-specific way based on the 3D preoperative plan.

52.5.3 Positioning

General anesthesia is administered to all patients and we advocate use of regional anesthesia (e.g., interscalene block). Patients are positioned in a 45-degree beach-chair position. The head is secured to the table and all bony prominences are well padded. The surgical limb is draped free and positioned to allow maximal adduction and hyperextension, which will permit insertion of the humeral stem and glenoid exposure. The limb is prepped with chlorhexidine gluconate and sealed off with an iodophor plastic barrier.

52.6 Operative Technique

52.6.1 Approach

The standard deltopectoral approach that is described elsewhere in this volume is utilized to perform the procedure; however, surgeons should be familiar with an extended approach to facilitate appropriate surgical exposure. For RSA, it is our preference to perform a subperiosteal peel of the subscapularis tendon from the lesser tuberosity to expose the humeral head prior to osteotomy. This technique maximizes subscapularis tendon length to allow for repair at the end of surgery. Humeral-sided releases of the inferior capsule as posterior as possible during subscapularis peel are also important for increased glenoid exposure, as they allow for increased posterior retraction of the humerus.

52.6.2 Humeral Head Osteotomy

Once an unobstructed view of the humeral head is obtained, osteophytes should be removed along the humeral neck and head to define the margins of the articular surface. An oscillating saw is then used to osteotomize the humeral head in approximately 20 to 30 degrees of retroversion. The angle of the osteotomy varies depending on the implant used and should be made according to the recommended surgical technique. Following the osteotomy, we routinely place a humeral cut protector over the osteotomy surface and proceed to glenoid exposure and preparation prior to completing the humeral implantation.

52.6.3 Glenoid Exposure

In all cases of RSA, appropriate glenoid exposure is key to achieving optimal placement of the glenoid baseplate and glenosphere. A posterior glenoid retractor is placed along the posteroinferior

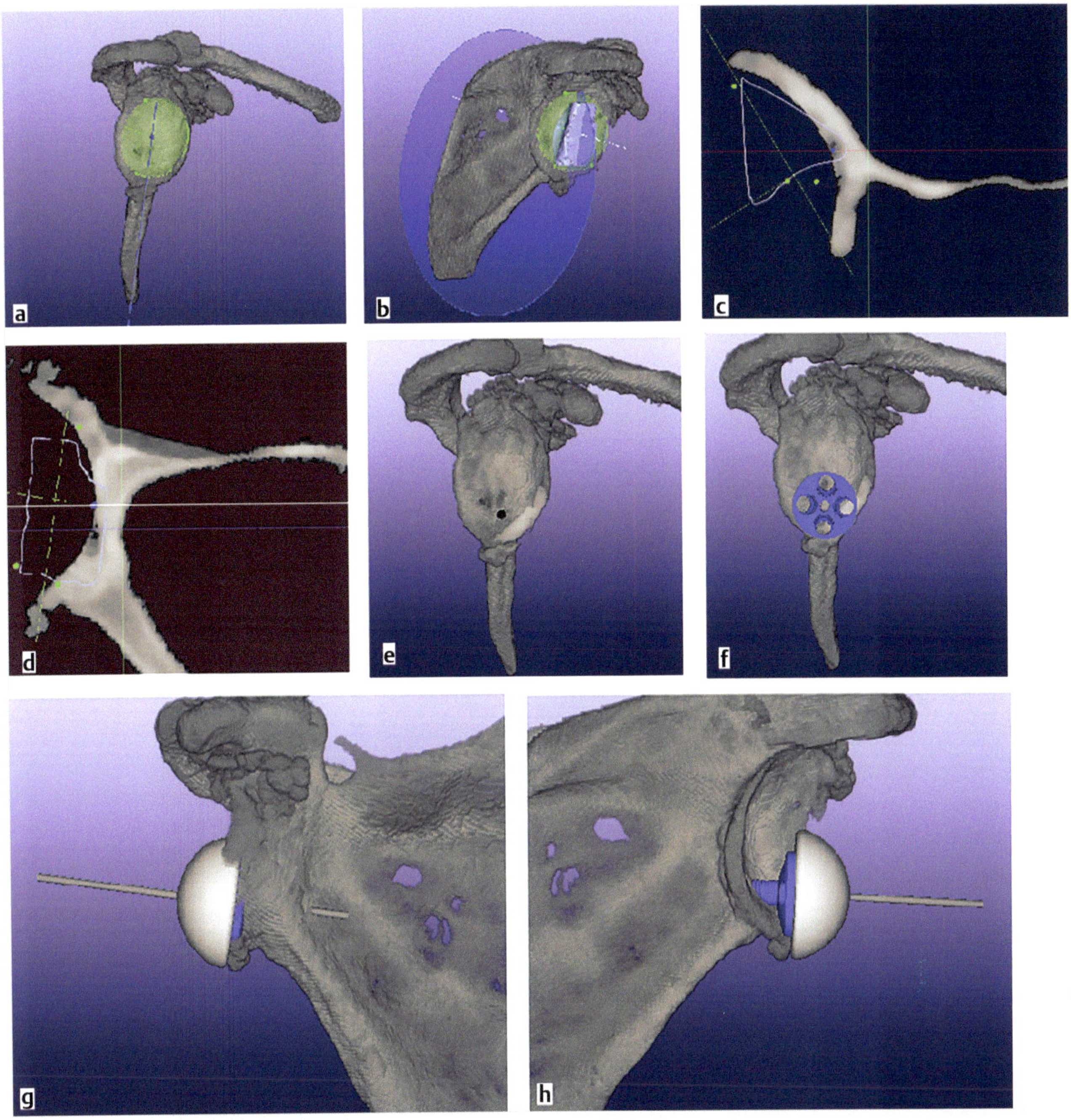

Fig. 52.1 OrthoVis preoperative planning software from OrthoVis Research (Cleveland Clinic; Cleveland, OH). **(a)** Three points on the glenoid and scapula are selected to determine the planes of the glenoid (*green*) and scapula (*blue*). The software uses this information to automatically calculate glenoid version (–31.4 degrees) and inclination (8.6 degrees). **(b)** The vault model (*purple*) has been positioned and sized to match the inner cortex of the glenoid in the axial and coronal planes. **(c, d)** The lateral extent of the vault model represents the premorbid joint line. **(e)** The guide pin (*black dot*) has been positioned based on vault model and area of simulated reaming is shown (*white*). **(f)** The location of the baseplate (*blue*) shown following simulated reaming. **(g)** Anterior and **(h)** posterior 3D reconstructed views showing the significant bone loss with unsupported baseplate. Consequently, the surgeon plans for selective inferior reaming and posterior glenoid bone grafting.

border of the glenoid to displace the humerus posteriorly out of the visual field. A Bankart or Hohmann retractor is placed anteriorly for exposure of the anterior glenoid rim and to protect the axillary nerve. We routinely perform a resection of the anterior and inferior joint capsule to maximize glenoid exposure (**Fig. 52.2a**). The anteroinferior capsule is first separated from the subscapularis tendon and then resected off its glenoid attachment. This procedure can be performed without concern for injury to the axillary nerve with appropriate identification of the nerve and protection with retractors. Further subperiosteal release of the superior and posterior portions of the capsule from the glenoid rim is performed. A reverse Hohmann retractor is then placed over the superior glenoid to achieve 360-degree visualization of the glenoid face (**Fig. 52.2b**).

52.6.4 Patient-Specific Implantation

Once the glenoid is fully exposed, the patient-specific preoperative plan is utilized to achieve optimal position of the glenosphere baseplate. A standard drill guide that has the size and shape of the eventual glenoid component can be used to place a guide pin or drill the center hole in a patient-specific manner when referencing 2D and 3D views within the 3D preoperative plan. Alternatively, reusable and adjustable PSI or single-use PSI tools can be used for this step. To replicate the preoperative plan intraoperatively, the surgeon should reference the local anatomy of the glenoid fossa. Areas of small indentation, biconcavity, or osteophytes on the periphery help guide the trajectory and location of the guide pin relative to the glenoid surface based on the patient-specific 3D template. It is essential to expose and visualize the entire glenoid rim to accurately represent the bony anatomy that is found on the preoperative plan. Once placed, the intraoperative position of the guide pin should be compared against the guide pin position on the preoperative plan for accuracy (**Fig. 52.3a, b**). Utilization of the template helps optimize the position of the guide pin and ultimately the baseplate, as acquired glenoid bone loss, posterior erosion, and significant osteophyte formation may skew the surgeon's perceptions of the true face of the glenoid. However, with use of a 3D preoperative plan, cases of advanced bone loss or deformity may have multiple different bony landmarks on the glenoid that can help with guide pin placement at the time of surgery.

Many commercially available PSIs are single use and made by the manufacturer based on either CT or MRI and a preoperative plan (**Fig. 52.4**). Additional forms of PSI include adjustable and reusable guides that can be set based on the preoperative plan (**Fig. 52.5**). Surgeons should know if the imaging source used to generate the PSI was created from bony anatomy (CT scan) or from bony *and* cartilaginous anatomy (MRI). If the CT scan is use to create the PSI template, surgeons should carefully remove any remaining cartilage or capsulolabral tissue from the glenoid fossa. Osteophytes should be preserved to provide the best fit of the PSI, as most of these tools are often created from images that include the osteophytes. The surgeon should routinely reference images from the 3D preoperative

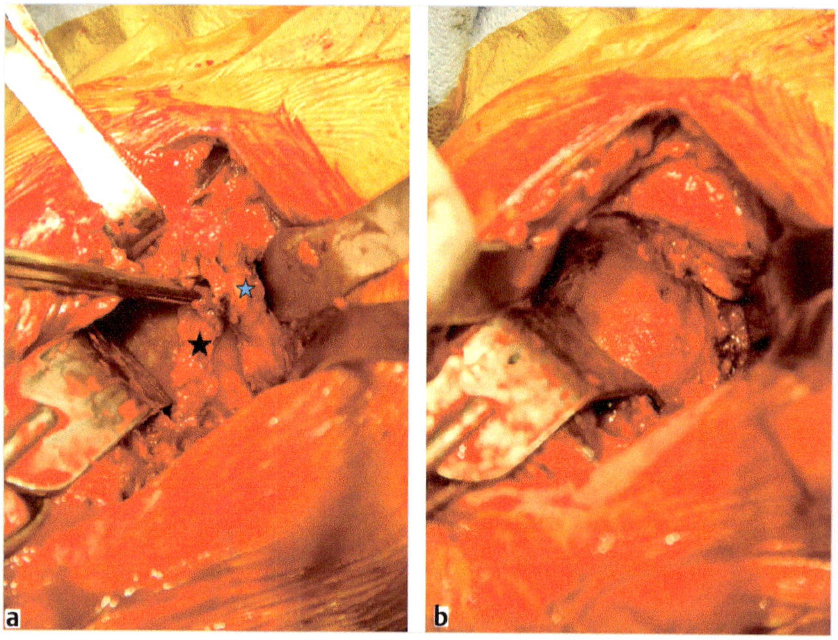

Fig. 52.2 Intraoperative pictures of dissection for glenoid exposure. **(a)** Isolated anterior and inferior glenohumeral capsule (*black star*) and subscapularis tendon (*blue star*). **(b)** Glenoid exposure following resection of anterior and inferior glenohumeral capsule and superior and posterior capsular release.

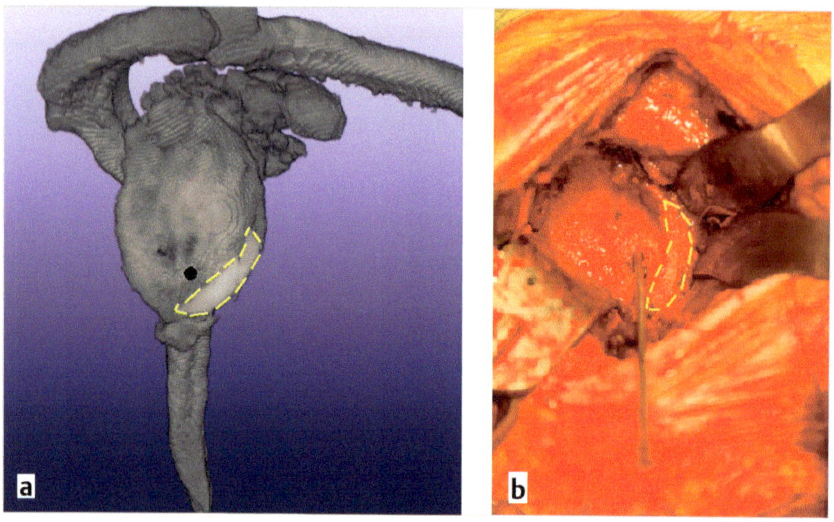

Fig. 52.3 **(a)** Comparison of guide pin placement (*black dot*) for the preoperative 3D patient-specific surgical plan to **(b)** intraoperative guide pin placement prior to glenoid reaming (*dotted yellow area*) and drilling for baseplate central peg.

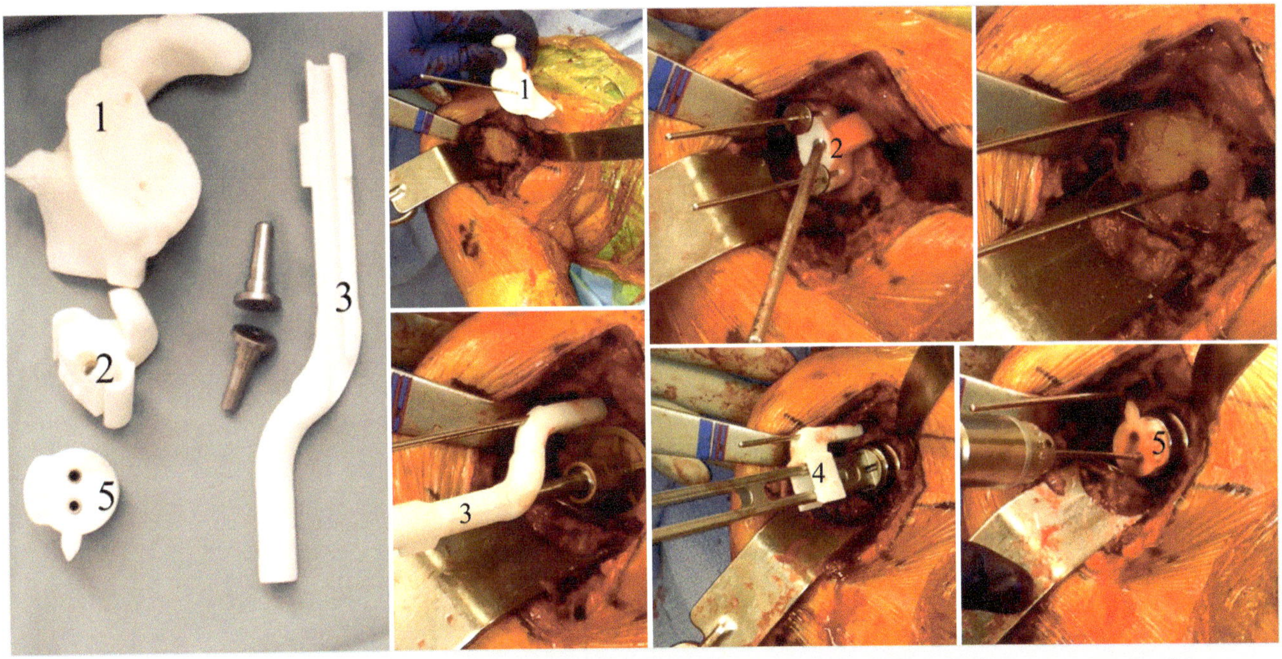

Fig. 52.4 Zimmer patient-specific instrumentation for Trabecular Metal Reverse Glenoid System (Zimmer Biomet; Warsaw, IN). The patient-specific guides and bone model are shown (*left*). The bone model (1) is generated from a 3D reconstruction of the patient's glenoid and comes with two predrilled holes and an engraved outline of the pin guide to help the surgeon orient the guide on the patient's glenoid. The pin guide (2) is placed flush on the glenoid with the hook referencing the anterosuperior quadrant. The guide is then secured with two 2.5-mm pins. A 6-mm cannulated drill bit is placed over the inferior pin to create a pilot hole for the glenoid reamer. The cannulated reamer is then placed over the inferior pin and the ream guide (3) is attached to the superior pin. After reaming, the inferior pin is removed and the pilot hole is overdrilled with a 7.5-mm drill bit to accommodate the baseplate post (not shown). The baseplate is then inserted with the roll guide (4) attached to the insertion handle and superior pin. The screw guide (5) is placed in the cavity of the baseplate with the arrow pointing toward the superior pin. After drilling pilot holes for the two baseplate screws, the guide is removed and a depth gauge is used to confirm screw length.

plan to ensure the PSI fits the glenoid as intended. Again, it is essential to expose and visualize the entire glenoid rim to accurately represent the bony anatomy that is found on the preoperative plan and to allow the PSI tool to rest on the glenoid as planned. Once the PSI is correctly positioned and stable, the guide pin is inserted. Again, guide pin placement should be compared to the preoperative plan for accuracy to allow for any adjustments to be made before proceeding with further glenoid instrumentation.

Should glenoid bone graft be required to address bone loss and obtain appropriate implant offset and backside bony support, both autograph and allograft may serve as appropriate options. Our preference is to use autologous graft when available to improve potential for integration. In primary RSA cases with severe glenoid bone loss that requires grafting, our preference is to use the resected humeral head. The glenoid defect is measured and the humeral head is contoured to the necessary dimensions (**Fig. 52.6a, b**). The articular surface of the humeral head graft can be placed against the glenoid defect for a matched fit (**Fig. 52.6c**). Both sites should be burred back to bone to create optimal surfaces for integration. The central peg or screw hole for the baseplate should be drilled prior to graft fixation, and a corresponding hole should be made in the graft if the central peg or screw will pass through it (**Fig. 52.7a, b**). The graft is then provisionally secured at its periphery to the native glenoid using Kirschner's wires. In cases of revision surgery with glenoid bone loss, alternative graft options include iliac crest or structural allograft (e.g., femoral head). Gentle reaming of the graft and native glenoid surface may be performed to create a uniform surface for the baseplate. The baseplate is then inserted and secured using locking screw with or without compression screws (**Fig. 52.8a**). We prefer initial compression of the baseplate against the bone graft through center screw for compression, followed by locking of the peripheral screws. Kirschner's wires are removed once all screws have been placed and the bone graft can be further contoured, in situ, if needed prior to final glenosphere placement (**Fig. 52.8b, c**).

52.6.5 Humeral Implantation

Completion of the humeral component implantation is performed according to the appropriate technique of the selected implant and is described in detail in the preceding chapters.

52.7 Surgical Pearls

The key to using advanced tools and PSI for glenoid placement is recognizing the need to do so. In cases without bone loss or deformity, implant placement can be accurately performed without need for preoperative or intraoperative patient-specific tools. However, when correcting more severe pathology, surgeons can be inaccurate with standard imaging and instrumentation. In this setting, 3D templating and/or PSI tools have been

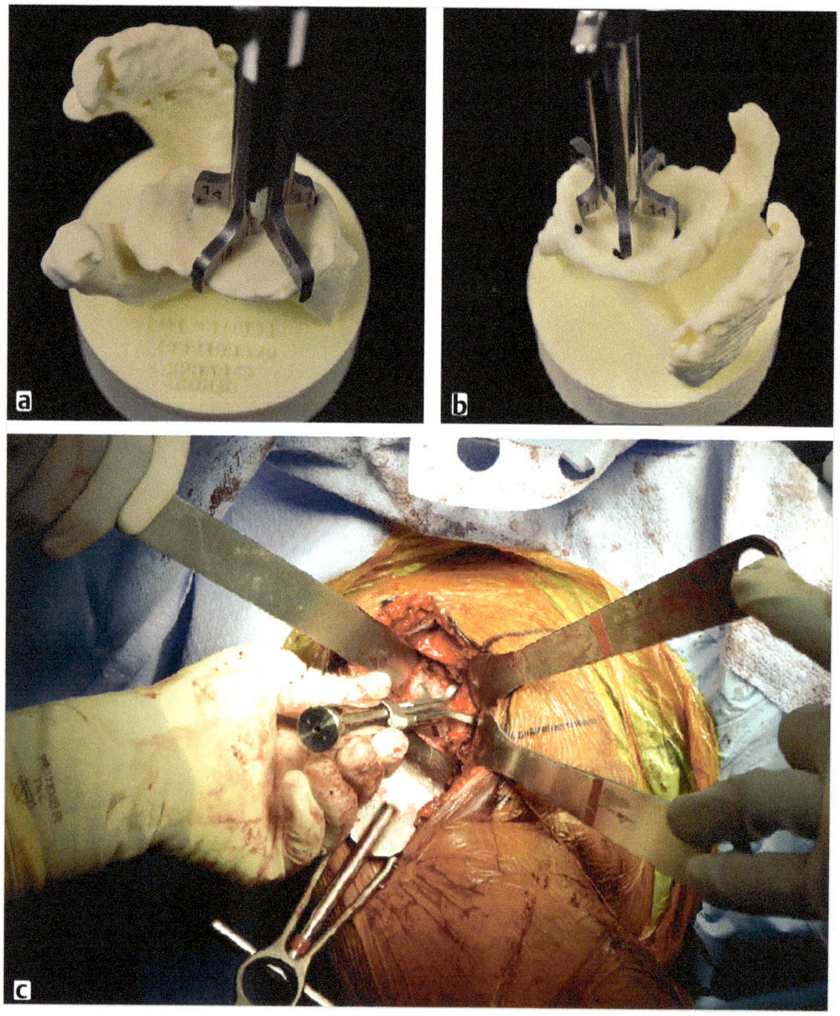

Fig. 52.5 Intelligent Reusable Instrument (IRI; Custom Orthopaedic Solutions; Cleveland, OH). (a,b) A bone model is generated from the 3D preoperative planning software with a hole showing the guide pin position based on planned version, and inclination of the implant. A guide pin can be placed in the bone model hole and the IRI guide placed over the pin, with the five interchangeable feet of the IRI guide adjusted to match the surface anatomy of the glenoid bone model and then set. (c) The IRI guide can then be transferred to the patient and once correctly positioned and stable, the guide pin is inserted through it. The IRI guide position intraoperatively can be compared to its position on the bone model and the 3D preoperative plan for accuracy.

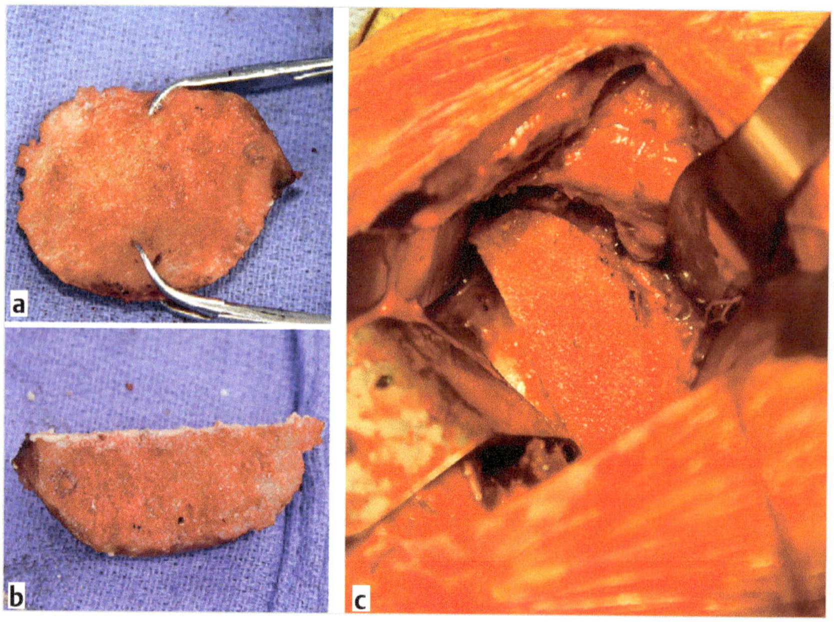

Fig. 52.6 Humeral head bone graft. (a) Prior to implantation of baseplate, autologous humeral head bone graft is sized and (b) cut to shape. (c) The graft is then matched to the glenoid surface intraoperatively to ensure proper contour and fit.

shown to improve the surgeon's ability to achieve the desired implant location.

Obtaining proper exposure of the glenoid prior to using any PSI device is critical to ensuring the device correctly fits the patient's anatomy, thus allowing improvement in the accuracy of implant placement. This includes proper retractor placement and appropriate capsular releases off the humerus and glenoid. We advocate resection of the anterior and inferior capsule to

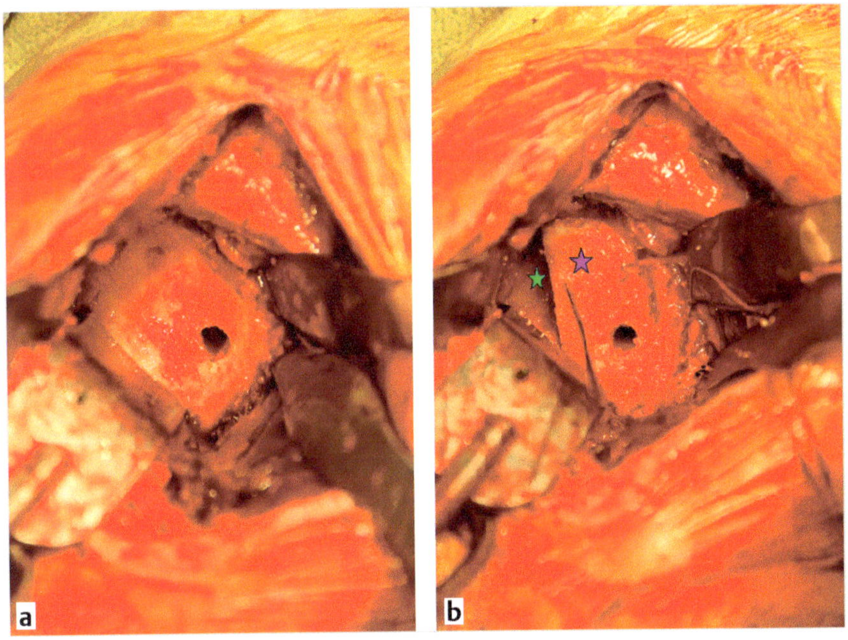

Fig. 52.7 (a) The central hole for the baseplate peg is drilled over the guide wire that was placed based on the 3D preoperative surgical plan. (b) The glenoid bone graft (*purple star*) is provisionally secured to native glenoid and the central hole for baseplate peg is created in the graft and connected to the central hole for the baseplate that was created in the native glenoid (*green star*).

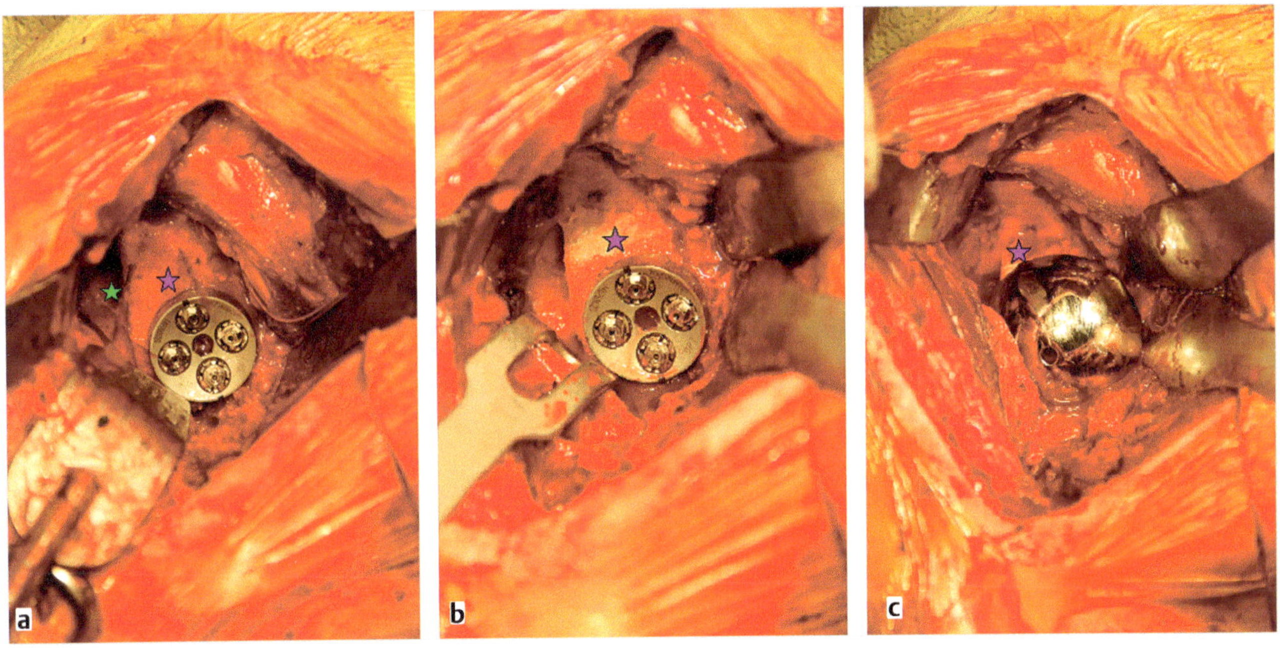

Fig. 52.8 Intraoperative photographs of glenoid implantation. (a) Placement of glenoid baseplate through autologous humeral head bone graft (*purple star*) into native glenoid (*green star*). (b) Final glenoid baseplate secured through bone graft (*purple star*) with contouring of graft to allow for placement of glenosphere. (c) Final glenosphere with contoured posterior glenoid bone graft (*purple star*).

ensure maximal glenoid exposure and allow for unhindered use of standard or PSI tools. This is especially important for the majority of severe pathologic cases when exposure is more challenging. Inadequate exposure may lead to poor seating of the PSI and subsequent inaccurate guide pin placement. Even if standard instrumentation is used, it is essential to expose and visualize the entire glenoid rim to accurately represent the bony anatomy that is found on a 3D preoperative plan. Whether PSI or standard instruments are used, the intraoperative position of the guide pin once placed should always be compared against the preoperative plan for accuracy.

52.8 What to Avoid

Surgeons must be mindful of the method used to create the 3D preoperative plan and PSI tools, and if the surgical technique calls for maintenance of the osteophytes or cartilage to appropriately fit the PSI to the glenoid surface. Care should be taken not to remove peripheral osteophytes for CT-based PSI, while excessive cartilage and soft-tissue removal should be avoided for MRI-based PSI.

After guide pin placement, the surgeon must avoid excessive reaming and remove bone in a controlled manner based on the patient's specific preoperative plan. Aggressive reaming risks joint line medialization and removal of subchondral bone weakening the support for the final implant, which may lead to eventual loosening.

It is essential to remember that the PSI tool does not define the optimum implant placement. Rather, it only provides the ability to accurately reproduce the planned position of the implant. The surgeon must still use judgment in deciding what implant to use and where to place it for each patient.

52.9 Complications/Bailout/ Salvage

We are not aware of any reported complications resulting from use of PSI. However, possible risks include increased operative time and/or exposure. In most studies, use of PSI has not been shown to increase operative time. If the 3D preoperative plan or PSI tools are not correctly utilized and inaccurate or excessive glenoid reaming occurs, loss of adequate glenoid bone stock for stable placement of a glenoid baseplate may occur in the setting of severe glenoid bone loss or deformity. In this scenario, hemiarthroplasty is a salvage option. Hemiarthroplasty is also a salvage option in instances of intraoperative fracture or insufficient native bone to permit placement of a glenoid baseplate even with bone grafting.

52.10 Postoperative Care

Our postoperative care remains the same following use of PSI for severe deformity. We advocate use of indwelling peripheral nerve catheters (i.e., interscalene nerve catheter) for pain control over the first 3 to 4 postoperative days to facilitate immediate range of motion. A shoulder immobilizer or sling is used in the first few days, due to weakness associated with use of the nerve catheter, but its use can be discontinued once muscle function has returned. The patient begins supine passive forward elevation to 120 degrees and external rotation to 30 degrees for approximately 5 to 10 minutes, five times per day, using their contralateral hand to perform the exercises. This progresses from supine to sitting passive exercises. At 4 to 6 weeks, we begin scapular strengthening, active-assisted motion, and closed chain and isometric exercises.

References

1. Nyffeler RW, Werner CM, Gerber C. Biomechanical relevance of glenoid component positioning in the reverse Delta III total shoulder prosthesis. J Shoulder Elbow Surg 2005;14(5):524–528
2. Gutiérrez S, Comiskey CA IV, Luo ZP, Pupello DR, Frankle MA. Range of impingement-free abduction and adduction deficit after reverse shoulder arthroplasty. Hierarchy of surgical and implant-design-related factors. J Bone Joint Surg Am 2008;90(12):2606–2615
3. Simovitch RW, Zumstein MA, Lohri E, Helmy N, Gerber C. Predictors of scapular notching in patients managed with the Delta III reverse total shoulder replacement. J Bone Joint Surg Am 2007;89(3):588–600
4. Li X, Knutson Z, Choi D, et al. Effects of glenosphere positioning on impingement-free internal and external rotation after reverse total shoulder arthroplasty. J Shoulder Elbow Surg 2013;22(6):807–813
5. Poon PC, Chou J, Young SW, Astley T. A comparison of concentric and eccentric glenospheres in reverse shoulder arthroplasty: a randomized controlled trial. J Bone Joint Surg Am 2014;96(16):e138
6. Heylen S, Van Haver A, Vuylsteke K, Declercq G, Verborgt O. Patient-specific instrument guidance of glenoid component implantation reduces inclination variability in total and reverse shoulder arthroplasty. J Shoulder Elbow Surg 2016;25(2):186–192
7. Randelli P, Randelli F, Arrigoni P, et al. Optimal glenoid component inclination in reverse shoulder arthroplasty. How to improve implant stability. Musculoskelet Surg 2014;98(Suppl 1):15–18
8. Subramanya SHJ. Reverse shoulder arthroplasty with patient-specific glenoid implant positioning guides. Tech Shoulder Elbow Surg 2014;15(4):122–129
9. Verborgt O, De Smedt T, Vanhees M, Clockaerts S, Parizel PM, Van Glabbeek F. Accuracy of placement of the glenoid component in reversed shoulder arthroplasty with and without navigation. J Shoulder Elbow Surg 2011;20(1):21–26
10. Iannotti J, Baker J, Rodriguez E, et al. Three-dimensional preoperative planning software and a novel information transfer technology improve glenoid component positioning. J Bone Joint Surg Am 2014;96(9):e71
11. Iannotti JP, Weiner S, Rodriguez E, et al. Three-dimensional imaging and templating improve glenoid implant positioning. J Bone Joint Surg Am 2015;97(8):651–658
12. Sirveaux F, Favard L, Oudet D, Huquet D, Walch G, Molé D. Grammont inverted total shoulder arthroplasty in the treatment of glenohumeral osteoarthritis with massive rupture of the cuff. Results of a multicentre study of 80 shoulders. J Bone Joint Surg Br 2004;86(3):388–395
13. Walch G, Moraga C, Young A, Castellanos-Rosas J. Results of anatomic nonconstrained prosthesis in primary osteoarthritis with biconcave glenoid. J Shoulder Elbow Surg 2012;21(11):1526–1533
14. Walch G, Badet R, Boulahia A, Khoury A. Morphologic study of the glenoid in primary glenohumeral osteoarthritis. J Arthroplasty 1999;14(6):756–760
15. Bercik MJ, Kruse K II, Yalizis M, Gauci MO, Chaoui J, Walch G. A modification to the Walch classification of the glenoid in primary glenohumeral osteoarthritis using three-dimensional imaging. J Shoulder Elbow Surg 2016;25(10):1601–1606
16. Iannotti JP, Jun BJ, Patterson TE, Ricchetti ET. Quantitative measurements of bony pathology in advanced osteoarthritis. J Bone Joint Surg Am
17. Scalise JJ, Codsi MJ, Bryan J, Brems JJ, Iannotti JP. The influence of three-dimensional computed tomography images of the shoulder in preoperative planning for total shoulder arthroplasty. J Bone Joint Surg Am 2008;90(11):2438–2445
18. Codsi MJ, Bennetts C, Gordiev K, et al. Normal glenoid vault anatomy and validation of a novel glenoid implant shape. J Shoulder Elbow Surg 2008;17(3):471–478

19. Scalise JJ, Codsi MJ, Bryan J, Iannotti JP. The three-dimensional glenoid vault model can estimate normal glenoid version in osteoarthritis. J Shoulder Elbow Surg 2008;17(3):487–491
20. Ganapathi A, McCarron JA, Chen X, Iannotti JP. Predicting normal glenoid version from the pathologic scapula: a comparison of 4 methods in 2- and 3-dimensional models. J Shoulder Elbow Surg 2011;20(2):234–244
21. Ricchetti ET, Hendel MD, Collins DN, Iannotti JP. Is premorbid glenoid anatomy altered in patients with glenohumeral osteoarthritis? Clin Orthop Relat Res 2013;471(9): 2932–2939
22. Ho JC, Sabesan VJ, Iannotti JP. Glenoid component retroversion is associated with osteolysis. J Bone Joint Surg Am 2013;95(12):e82
23 Iannotti JP, Greeson C, Downing D, Sabesan V, Bryan JA. Effect of glenoid deformity on glenoid component placement in primary shoulder arthroplasty. J Shoulder Elbow Surg 2012;21(1):48–55
24. Paisley KC, Kraeutler MJ, Lazarus MD, Ramsey ML, Williams GR, Smith MJ. Relationship of scapular neck length to scapular notching after reverse total shoulder arthroplasty by use of plain radiographs. J Shoulder Elbow Surg 2014;23(6):882–887

53 Internal Latissimus Transfer for Reverse Shoulder Arthroplasty

Seth Gamradt and Frank Russo

Abstract

This chapter describes the anatomy and technique of a combined reverse total shoulder arthroplasty (TSA) and latissimus dorsi/teres major (LD/TM) transfer for those patients with combined pseudoparesis and loss of external rotation. Massive tearing of the rotator cuff results in active motion loss and is a debilitating condition that often warrants surgery as definitive treatment. Boileau et al have described two patterns of motion loss in patients with massive rotator cuff tears and subsequent cuff arthropathy. These authors describe the dysfunction in patients who exhibit both absent forward elevation (pseudoparesis) and absent active external rotation as combined loss of elevation and external rotation (CLEER). Retensioning the deltoid with a constrained, reversed prosthesis predictably restores forward elevation. However, lack of external rotation can persist after reverse TSA in patients with massive tears of both the infraspinatus and the teres minor. The L'Episcopo transfer was first described in 1934 for obstetric palsy. Using this technique, the LD and TM tendons are transferred posteriorly and laterally on the humerus, such that the function of the transferred muscles changes from internal rotation to external rotation.[3] In their study of 17 patients who underwent reverse TSA with LD/TM transfer, Boileau et al reported significant improvement in subjective and objective results with restoration of active forward elevation and external rotation in patients with CLEER. This procedure restores control of the shoulder in both the coronal and the sagittal planes, thereby improving spatial control of the hand to facilitate activities of daily living.

Keywords: *reverse total shoulder arthroplasty, combined latissimus dorsi transfer, external rotation*

53.1 Goals of Procedure

- To restore forward elevation and external rotation in those patients with combined coronal and sagittal muscle imbalances secondary to rotator cuff arthropathy.

53.2 Advantages

- As opposed to a reverse arthroplasty alone, the latissimus dorsi/teres major (LD/TM) transfer combined with reverse arthroplasty can improve active external rotation in the appropriately selected patient.

53.3 Indications

- Rotator cuff arthropathy with combined loss of forward elevation and external rotation.
- Failed rotator cuff repair with anterior superior escape.
- Failed conventional shoulder arthroplasty.
- Nonunion or malunion of failed three- or four-part proximal humerus fractures.

53.4 Contraindications

- Axillary nerve palsy.
- Previous surgery that would make dissection of the area difficult.
- Infection.
- Patients who are able to maintain the arm in a minimal of neutral external rotation may not need the tendon transfer in combination with the reverse.

53.5 Anatomy

The LD acts to adduct and internally rotate the humerus. The muscle has a broad origin, from the sacrum, iliac wing, ribs 9 to 12, spinous processes of T7–T12, and inferior border of scapula. The average width of the LD tendon at its insertion measures 3.1 cm × 8.4 cm on the posterior lip of the intertubercular groove just medial to the pectoralis major and anterior to TM insertions. Given up to 30% of patients have conjoined LD and TM tendons, these tendons are often transferred together (**Fig. 53.1**).[4]

The neurovascular pedicle of the LD includes the thoracodorsal artery and nerve, which insert into the anterior muscle belly roughly 13.1 cm medial from its humeral insertion.[4]

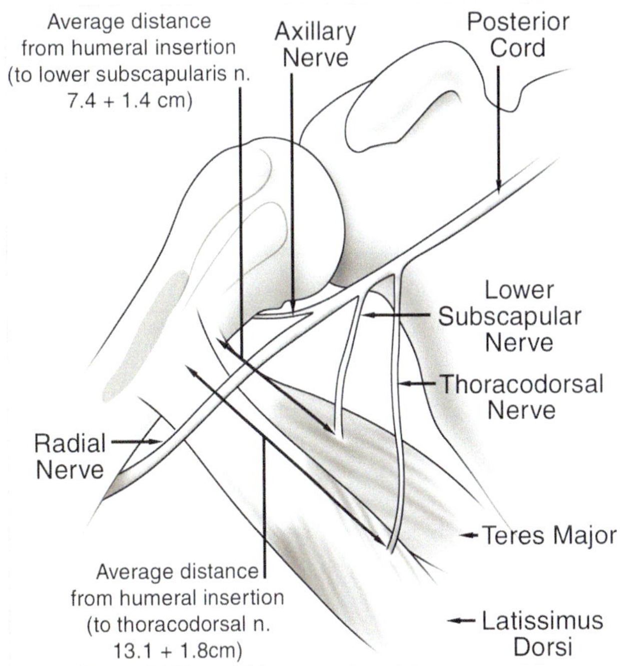

Fig. 53.1 Anterior shoulder depicting the respective lengths of the tendon insertion sites with their respective neurovascular pedicles.
Used with permission from Pearle AD, Kelly BT, Voos JE, Chehab EL, Warren RF. Surgical technique and the anatomic study of latissumus dorsi and teres major transfers. J Bone and Joint Surg Am. 2006; 88: 1524–1531.

A corresponding branch of the lower subscapular nerve inserts into the anterior muscle belly of the TM approximately 7.4 cm medial from its humeral insertion.[4] Each of these nerves branch from the posterior cord of the brachial plexus, and measure 13.5 and 9.3 cm in length to their respective insertions.[4]

Structures at risk during a deltopectoral approach include the radial and axillary nerves. The radial nerve branches from the posterior cord of the brachial plexus and courses medial to the coracobrachialis and anterior to the latissimus tendon, roughly 2.4 cm medial to the humeral shaft in neutral.[5] This distance is variable with positioning of the humerus, measuring up to 4 cm from the insertion in 90 degrees of abduction and 45 degrees of external rotation.[5] Superiorly, the axillary nerve branches and wraps posteriorly around the humerus before exiting via the quadrangular space. With the arm at its side, the axillary nerve travels 1.9 cm above the superior boarder of the latissimus tendon.[5] However, this relationship changes similarly as above with the position of the humerus, increasing to 3.6 cm in 90 degrees of external rotation and 45 degrees of abduction (**Fig. 53.2a–c**).[5]

53.6 Preoperative Preparation

For the combined LD transfer to be effective, patient selection is critical. Indications include primary and revision total shoulder arthroplasty (TSA) in the setting of pseudoparalysis and loss of external rotation. Physical examination in a candidate for combined reverse TSA and latissimus transfer will demonstrate what Bolieau et al termed combined loss of elevation and external rotation, or CLEER.[4,5] a nonfunctional deltoid is a contraindication for reverse TSA. In addition to deficient elevation, the patient will exhibit difficulty in maintaining the arm in neutral or, to a greater extent, external rotation. The Hornblower sign is a tendency for the hand to drift toward the mouth with attempted elevation due to the absence of active external rotation. The external rotation lag sign is typically present; this can be tested by passive external rotation of the shoulder with the arm at the side. A positive test is evident when the arm drifts back into internal rotation, thereby indicating a nonfunctional posterior rotator cuff.

As a means of preoperative planning, we prefer standard radiographs of the involved shoulder, MRI to assess the rotator cuff and soft tissues, and CT scan to evaluate glenohumeral bone stock and glenoid wear/version.

53.7 Positioning

- For a combined reverse TSA and LD transfer, we use the 45-degree beach-chair position.
- A limb positioner allows for ease of patient positioning during the procedure.

53.8 Operative Technique

The deltopectoral approach is utilized with an incision just lateral to coracoid extending distal near the deltoid insertion. The incision is longer than typically utilized for an isolated reverse TSA, as a more distal exposure of the humerus is required.

After placing a self-retaining retractor beneath the conjoined tendon and deltoid, the subscapularis (if present) is taken down. The biceps is cut for later tenodesis. The humerus is dislocated with extension and external rotation. The proximal humerus is cut in 20 to 30 degrees of retroversion and broached in standard fashion, with the final broach left in place for trialing. Glenoid exposure is undertaken and the definitive glenoid baseplate and sphere are implanted. If a trial reduction is successful, the definitive humeral stem is placed. Once we have chosen the proper size polyethylene humeral bearing, we turn our attention to performing the latissimus transfer.

There are two major differences in a combined LD transfer and reverse TSA in comparison to an isolated latissimus transfer for massive cuff tear. First, when performing the transfer in the

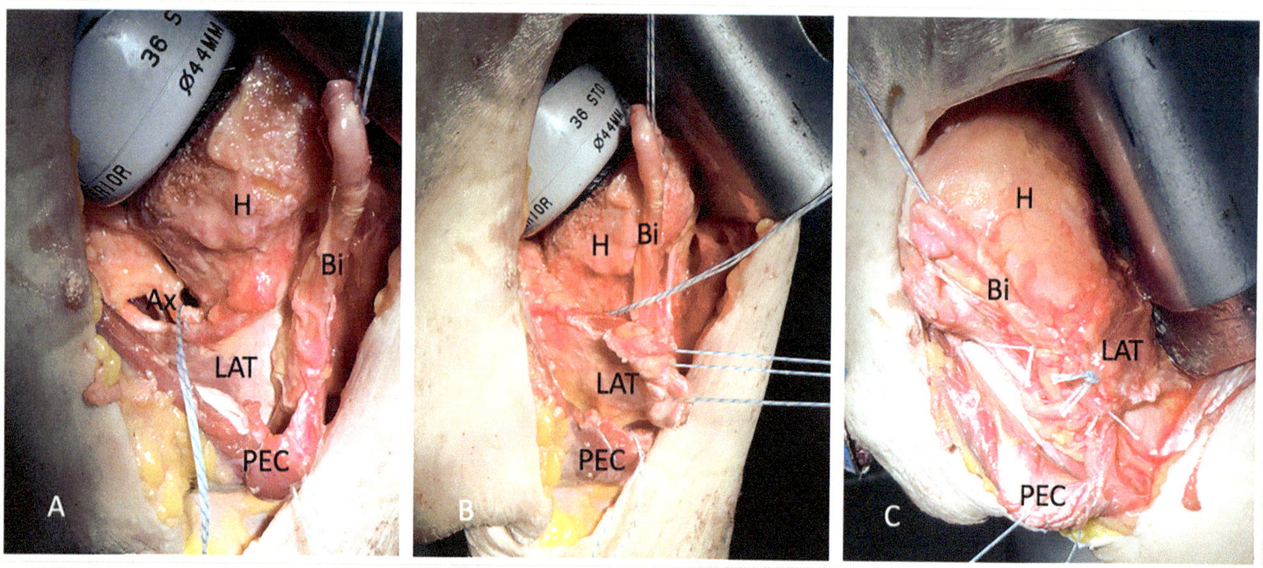

Fig. 53.2 (a) Deltopectoral view of reverse shoulder arthroplasty with trial components in place. External rotation facilitates identification of the latissimus tendon (LAT), medial to the biceps tendon (Bi) and pectoralis major (PEC). The axillary nerve (Ax) is found just superior to the latissimus tendon. **(b)** After detachment of latissimus (LAT). **(c)** After passage of the tendon posterior to the humerus (H) and securing the tendon to the humerus lateral to the biceps groove so it can act as an external rotator.

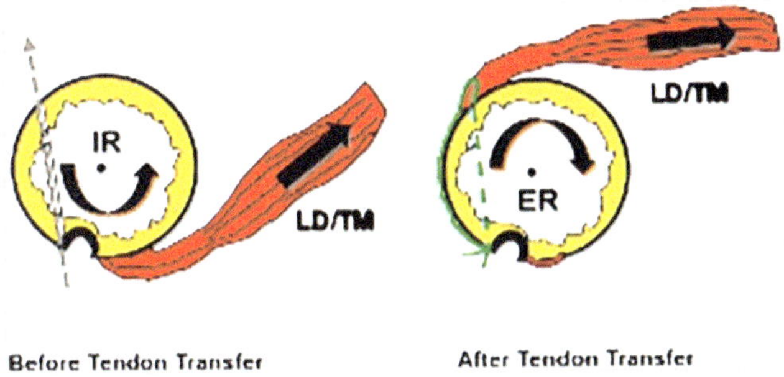

Fig. 53.3 A cross-sectional image of the proximal humerus at the level of the teres major and latissimus insertions. *Left:* The native anatomy of both tendons, and the ideal placement of the transosseous sutures. *Right:* Illustration of both tendons following transfer to their new position posteriorly, which is directly opposite their original insertion site.

setting of a massive rotator cuff tear, the LD is commonly transferred with a dual-incision approach, first to harvest the tendon posteriorly and then shuttling it to a second incision.[4] In a combined LD transfer and reverse TSA, the tendon is located and transferred through the anterior incision as a distal extension of the deltopectoral interval. Second, instead of attaching the LD superiorly to the greater tuberosity, the LD is simply transferred from the anterior humerus posteriorly so that it can become an external rotator without changing the height of the tendon insertion on the humerus (**Fig. 54.3**).

The LD and TM tendon is identified with the arm in external rotation medial to the pectoralis and distal biceps groove. Electrocautery or sharp dissection is used to detach the tendon from the humerus; the tendon is then tagged with multiple heavy sutures.

Next, blunt dissection is utilized to create a free space for tendon passage posterior to the humerus. A Hewson suture passer is used to pass suture from lateral to medial along the posterior humerus and the tendon is shuttled to the posterolateral humeral shaft at the same level as the original insertion of the LD tendon.

Transosseous drilling using three or four drill holes for heavy nonabsorbable suture is used to secure the tendon to the bone posterolateral with the arm in internal rotation. Once the transfer is secured, the definitive polyethylene component is implanted.

53.9 Tips and Pearls/Expert Suggestions

- Appropriate preoperative imaging and physical examination to identify the appropriate candidate with combined loss of shoulder forward elevation and external rotation.
- Externally rotating the arm will help identify the LD on the opposite side of the biceps groove from the pectoralis and releasing pectoralis can aid in exposure in this step.
- Identify and protect the radial nerve and axillary nerve when detaching the LD and transferring it anteriorly on the humerus.
- Transosseous drilling can be challenging around a definitive humeral stem; new all-suture anchors can be used but add cost to the procedure.
- We prefer to implant final components and choose a definitive polyethylene prior to the transfer so that repeated trialing and reinstrumenting of the humerus does not damage the newly transferred tendon.

53.10 What to Avoid

- A dual-incision approach has been classically described; however, this approach is more difficult and not necessary when performing a combine reverse arthroplasty and tendon transfer.[6]

53.11 Complications/Bailout/Salvage

- It is inexcusable to end up with a radial nerve injury or a axillary nerve injury due to this procedure, so if the anatomy is difficult to ascertain, history of prior surgery, and/or postsurgical scarring prevents a simple transfer, the procedure should be avoided and only reverse arthroplasty should be performed in isolation.

53.12 Postoperative Care

Elbow, wrist, and hand range of motion is permitted immediately. A gunslinger-type external rotation sling is used for 6 weeks. Progressive active-assisted range of motion continues for 2 months, followed by light supervised strengthening with the physical therapist for a further 6 weeks. Patients will continue to show functional improvements up to 1 year postsurgery.

References

1. L'Episcopo JB. Tendon transplantation in obstetrical paralysis. Am J Surg 1934;25:122–125
2. Pearle AD, Kelly BT, Voos JE, Chehab EL, Warren RF. Surgical technique and anatomic study of latissimus dorsi and teres major transfers. J Bone Joint Surg Am 2006;88(7):1524–1531
3. Cleeman E, Hazrati Y, Auerbach JD, Shubin Stein K, Hausman M, Flatow EL. Latissimus dorsi tendon transfer for massive rotator cuff tears: a cadaveric study. J Shoulder Elbow Surg 2003;12(6):539–543
4. Boileau P, Chuinard C, Balg F, Trojani C. Modified latissimus dorsi and teres major transfer through a single deltopectoral approach for loss of external rotation: as an isolated procedure or with reverse arthroplasty. J Shoulder Elbow Surg 2007;16:671–682
5. Boileau P, Rumian AP, Zumstein MA. Reversed shoulder arthroplasty with modified L'Episcopo for combined loss of active elevation and external rotation. J Shoulder Elbow Surg 2010;19(2, Suppl):20–30
6. Strecker WB, McAllister JW, Manske PR, Schoenecker PL, Dailey LA. Sever-L'Episcopo transfers in obstetrical palsy: a retrospective review of twenty cases. J Pediatr Orthop 1990;10(4):442–444

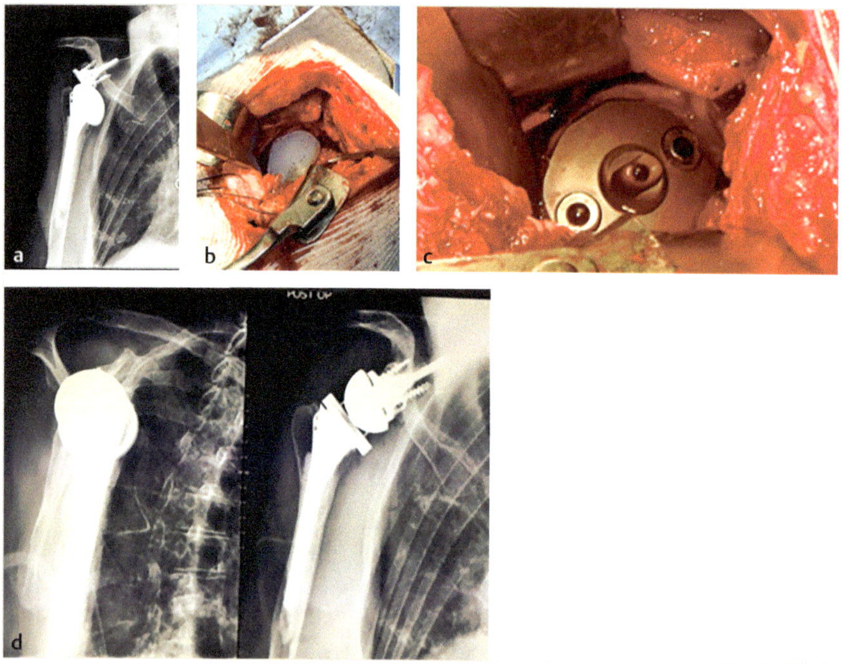

Fig. 54.6 **(a)** Unstable total shoulder arthroplasty with fully convertible implants. **(b)** Revised to reverse shoulder arthroplasty without removal of well-fixed metal-backed glenoid baseplate platform **(c)** and humeral platform stem component **(d)** X-ray of revision. (Reproduced with permission of Thieme Inc.)

and ROM. The University of Cambridge, Los Angeles (UCLA) Score averaged 26/30 and the simple shoulder test (SST) score was 9.1/12. In each case, the failures were in patients who had attempted the repair more than 12 weeks after index TSA. One patient, because of his age and activity demand, underwent a second attempted repair that yielded only a fair result. The other two of these patients who failed primary repair ultimately underwent revision to RSA, while eight other patients underwent revision to RSA as index treatment of this complication. In the 10 patients who underwent revision to RSA, the average UCLA score was 24.6/30 and the SST score was 8.9/12. There were no surgical complications in any of these patients and all were satisfied or very satisfied after revision.

Clearly, subscapularis failure is a very significant postoperative complication of anatomic TSA. The results of our small patient group indicate that primary repair can considered early (<12 weeks) after the index TSA. In situations where the failure occurs later, revision to RSA can be successful; however, the patient expectations and activity may be less than expected with the primary TSA.

54.12 Conclusion

There are very few reports discussing treatment of acute and chronic subscapularis failure in anatomic total shoulder replacement. With primary repair of the subscapularis tendon failure after index shoulder replacement, we have had mixed results in our own series of 15 patients. Those younger patients with early-onset subscapularis failure for less than 3 months had best results with repair at the revision procedure. Older patients and those with late-onset injury with muscle atrophy did best with RSA. Therefore, repair should be considered only in early-onset and in younger patients. Older patients do well with revision to reverse shoulder replacement especially in cases where convertible implants have been used in the index arthroplasty since the revision is easier and faster with less blood loss in cases where a well-fixed humeral component does not have to be removed. Functional results are also better in reverse shoulder replacement in those cases with a well-functioning infraspinatus and supraspinatus as seen in these revision situations.

References

1. Miller SL, Hazrati Y, Klepps S, Chiang A, Flatow EL. Loss of subscapularis function after total shoulder replacement: a seldom recognized problem. J Shoulder Elbow Surg 2003;12(1):29–34
2. Caplan JL, Whitfield B, Neviaser RJ. Subscapularis function after primary tendon to tendon repair in patients after replacement arthroplasty of the shoulder. J Shoulder Elbow Surg 2009;18(2):193–196, discussion 197–198
3. Gerber C, Yian EH, Pfirrmann CA, Zumstein MA, Werner CM. Subscapularis muscle function and structure after total shoulder replacement with lesser tuberosity osteotomy and repair. J Bone Joint Surg Am 2005;87(8):1739–1745
4. Scalise JJ, Ciccone J, Iannotti JP. Clinical, radiographic, and ultrasonographic comparison of subscapularis tenotomy and lesser tuberosity osteotomy for total shoulder arthroplasty. J Bone Joint Surg Am 2010;92(7):1627–1634
5. Giusefi SA, Wongtriratanachai P, Omae H, et al. Biomechanical comparison of lesser tuberosity osteotomy versus subscapularis tenotomy in total shoulder arthroplasty. JSES 2012;21(8):1087–1095

55 Arthroscopic Glenoid Removal and Bone Grafting

Tyler J. Brolin and Mark D. Lazarus

Abstract

Arthroscopic glenoid component removal is an attractive technique of converting a symptomatic total shoulder arthroplasty to a hemiarthroplasty for patients with aseptic glenoid loosening that are not candidates or are unwilling to have an open revision procedure. There are multiple advantages over the open technique, but it is primarily focused on avoiding another violation of the subscapularis tendon. It also has the potential to decrease postoperative pain and expedite the postoperative rehabilitation process. The arthroscopic approach allows the surgeon to easily perform additional procedures such as obtaining intraoperative cultures, synovectomy, capsular release, rotator cuff repair, etc. When necessary, bone grafting of any residual contained glenoid bone defects is easily accomplished as well. In our experience, we have found this arthroscopic technique extremely beneficial in our patients with aseptic glenoid loosening who are not candidates for an open revision surgery.

Keywords: *glenoid loosening, glenoid component failure, conversion of total shoulder arthroplasty to hemiarthroplasty, arthroscopic glenoid removal, arthroscopic glenoid bone grafting*

55.1 Goals of Procedure

The primary goal of this procedure is to relieve shoulder pain and dysfunction attributed to glenoid loosening after a total shoulder arthroplasty in a minimally invasive fashion that allows removal of the glenoid component in a way that is atraumatic to the subscapularis tendon. Previous literature has shown good outcomes after glenoid component removal for aseptic loosening in total shoulder arthroplasty.[1] Although this approach is intended for cases of presumed glenoid loosening, previous literature has shown the difficulty in diagnosing low-grade chronic shoulder infections such as those with *Propionibacterium acnes*. Clinical signs and symptoms, inflammatory markers, diagnostic imaging, and shoulder aspiration lack sensitivity and specificity to accurately diagnose periprosthetic shoulder infections, and the gold standard remains multiple intraoperative cultures and biopsies.[2] This arthroscopic approach allows the surgeon to easily assess the glenohumeral joint and take multiple cultures and biopsies from multiple locations with minimal morbidity if warranted. These results can then be used to guide further treatment if necessary.

A secondary goal of this procedure is to restore glenoid bone stock after component removal. Many times, there remains a contained cavitary defect around the central peg. The following technique describes a simple way of preparing and bone grafting contained lesions arthroscopically. This can be performed in the hope to prevent excessive medialization of the glenohumeral joint line after glenoid removal and subsequent conversion to hemiarthroplasty.[3] We have not and do not recommend arthroscopically bone grafting uncontained glenoid bone defects.

55.2 Advantages

The main advantages of the arthroscopic technique over an open technique revolve around preservation of the subscapularis tendon attachment. This prevents the complications associated with detaching the subscapularis tendon whether it be with a lesser tuberosity osteotomy, peel, or tenotomy. This advantage also translates to easier postoperative rehabilitation since protecting the subscapularis repair is not necessary. Other advantages include less intraoperative blood loss, decreased postoperative pain, and the ability to easily perform other indicated procedures such as synovectomy, capsular release, and rotator cuff repair.

55.3 Indications

The primary indication for arthroscopic glenoid component removal and glenoid bone grafting is a painful total shoulder arthroplasty with radiographic evidence of glenoid loosening in a patient who is not a candidate or willing to undergo glenoid component revision. The presumed diagnosis should be aseptic glenoid loosening and as such all preoperative infection workup should be negative for any obvious periprosthetic shoulder infection. Occasionally, the glenoid component has become dislodged from the glenoid cavity and this can also be an indication to retrieve the glenoid component arthroscopically.

55.4 Contraindications

Contraindications include any patient who is a candidate and willing to undergo open revision of the glenoid component. Active, ongoing infection is another contraindication to arthroscopic management. Finally, any contraindication related to the use of a hemiarthroplasty such as component instability or massive rotator cuff tears where the patient may be best suited for a reverse shoulder arthroplasty is a contraindication for this procedure.

55.5 Preoperative Preparation/Positioning

A standard radiographic examination of the shoulder is necessary to make the diagnosis of a loose glenoid component. The appearance of circumferential radiolucent lines or a change in glenoid implant position leads to diagnosis.[4] CT aids in the ability to gauge the size and extent of any associated glenoid bone loss. As with any planned revision shoulder arthroplasty or painful shoulder arthroplasty, a standardized approach to assess for the presence of a periprosthetic shoulder infection is imperative.

We prefer the beach-chair position and utilization of general anesthesia with an interscalene block for postoperative pain control. Standard prepping and draping occurs. If intraoperative cultures or biopsies are planned, preoperative antibiotics are held until after these have been taken.

55.6 Operative Technique

A standard posterior portal is placed in the soft spot generally at the midglenoid level. Prior to insufflation of the glenohumeral joint with fluid, the 30-degree arthroscope is placed to ensure that the trocar is within the joint. Multiple cultures can be taken from the joint fluid and deep tissues. Preoperative antibiotics are then given. Inflow is then established along with a standard anterior portal within the rotator interval. A thorough diagnostic evaluation is performed of the glenohumeral joint looking for any concomitant pathology, paying special attention to the status of the humeral head component and rotator cuff. A probe is inserted and is used to palpate the glenoid prosthesis–bone interface to evaluate for loosening. It is easiest to assess for loosening by trying to lift or pry the prosthetic glenoid from the bone with the probe (**Fig. 55.1**). Any gross movement away from bone confirms the diagnosis. A motorized shaver may be used to debride any soft tissue around the component edge prior to adequate assessment.

Once the diagnosis has been confirmed, the anterior portal and skin incision are enlarged to accommodate a 0.25-inch osteotome. First, the osteotome is used to "osteotomize" the superior portion of the prosthetic glenoid that includes the superior peg. This is then removed through the enlarged rotator interval portal using a Kocher clamp, making sure that a firm grasp is on the prosthesis as to not lose this within the soft tissues. Next, the inferior portion is "osteotomized," that includes the inferior two pegs and this is removed as well using the technique described above. This leaves the middle portion of the glenoid prosthesis with the central peg remaining. If this is able to be easily manipulated from the glenoid bone, it is taken out similarly with a Kocher clamp. If difficulty is encountered, one trick is to "osteotomize" the remaining articular portion from the central peg and carefully remove this first. Attention is then focused on removing the remaining central peg, especially if prominent. A small osteotome can be used to gently try and disengage the central peg from the surrounding bone interface. A small curette may aid in this process as well. Once the central peg is loose, it can easily be removed with an arthroscopic grasper or a Kocher clamp (**Fig. 55.2**).

After the glenoid prosthesis has been removed, curettes are used to thoroughly debride the central and peripheral peg holes. A motorized shaver is also used to thoroughly debride the remaining glenoid surface (**Fig. 55.3**). If any additional procedures such as synovectomy or capsular release are indicated, they are performed now with the combination of a motorized shaver and arthroscopic electrocautery. The glenohumeral joint is copiously irrigated and if glenoid bone grafting is planned, all arthroscopy fluid is evacuated.

Glenoid bone grafting can be accomplished using a long cannula or trephine placed through the anterior portal. Cancellous allograft chips can then be inserted directly into the central portion of the glenoid bone defect. Using a tamp or the back of a reverse curette, the bone graft can be gently impacted into place and the process is repeated until the defect has been adequately filled. Once complete, final images are taken and the arthroscopic instruments are removed and portal sites closed with interrupted Nylon sutures.

55.7 Tips and Pearls/Expert Suggestions

As with most arthroscopic procedures, adequate visualization is key to this technique. The metallic surface of the humeral head may cause the so-called mirror effect and taking a couple extra moments to orient the arthroscope may be needed (**Fig. 55.4**). This can be mitigated by orientating the camera away from the humeral head with the 30-degree arthroscope to minimize the disorientation from the "mirror effect."

The second pearl is the way in which the glenoid component is divided, which allows for easy removal. A couple of techniques have been described, but what has worked best for us is dividing the glenoid component into thirds with each section containing at least one peripheral or central peg.[3,5,6] The first cut is made superiorly and allows easy removal of the superior portion along with the superior peripheral peg. The second cut

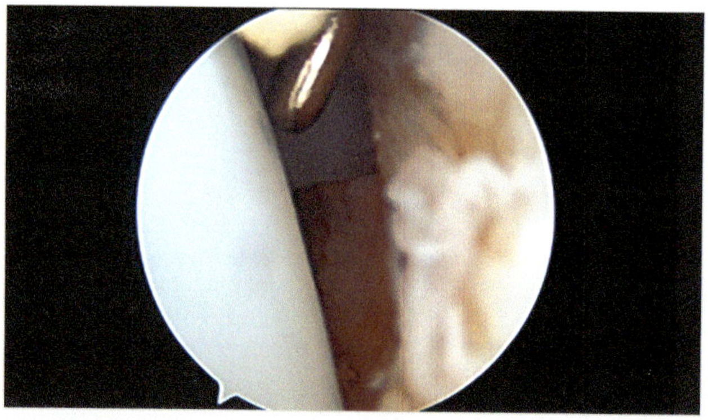

Fig. 55.1 An arthroscopic probe is inserted from the anterior portal and used to lift the glenoid component away from the bony glenoid surface confirming the diagnosis of component loosening.

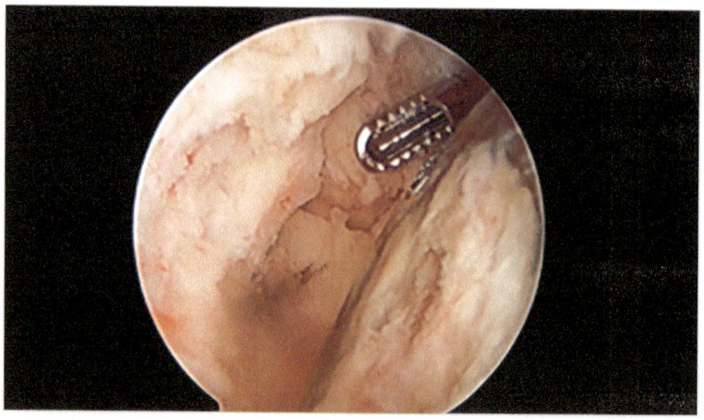

Fig. 55.2 Removal of each "osteotomized" component piece is done with a Kocher clamp through the anterior portal.

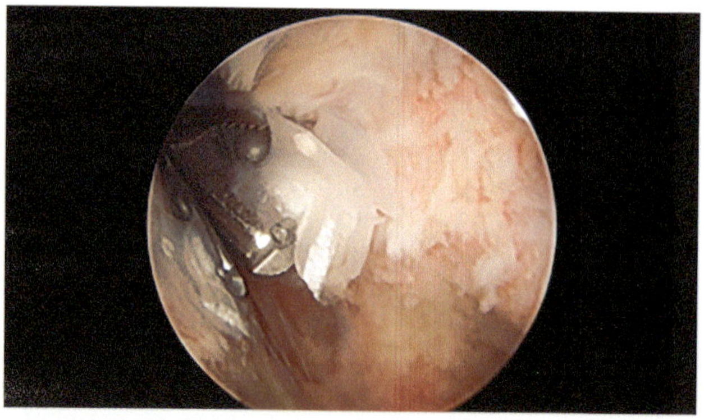

Fig. 55.3 A motorized shaver is used to debride the remaining glenoid surface after glenoid component removal.

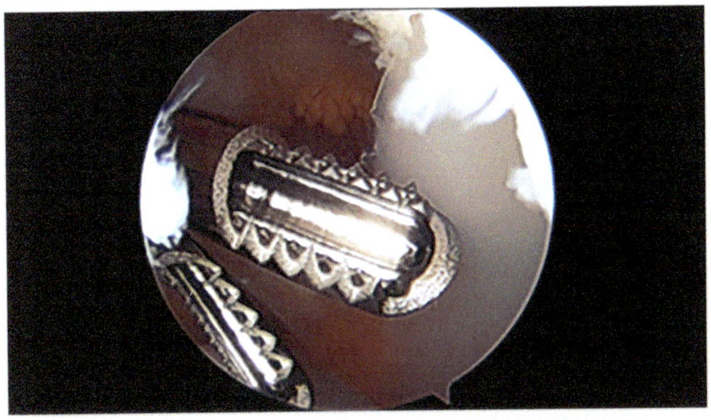

Fig. 55.4 Demonstration of the "mirror effect" and the need to orient the camera away from the humeral head to avoid disorientation.

allows removal of the inferior portion that has the inferior two peripheral pegs. This allows easier visualization of the middle portion that contains the central peg, which from our experience can be the most challenging portion to remove. When grasping each section of the glenoid for removal, the surgeon must ensure that a secure grasp with a Kocher clamp is obtained so the piece does not get lost in soft tissues. If a piece gets caught in the soft tissues, one trick is to try and push it back into the joint; if this is unsuccessful, enlarging the portal incision is helpful.

Care should be taken to protect the humeral head from inadvertent scratching from the introduction or removal of arthroscopic instrumentation. When inserting the trocar from the posterior portal, gentle lateral traction on the humeral head can aid in opening up the glenohumeral space and avoid unintended damage to the articular surface.

Finally, if the glenoid component has become completely dislodged from the glenoid, it can be challenging to remove it in a piecemeal fashion. The easiest solution is to use a probe and manipulate the component anterior to the humeral head. This can be challenging especially if the component is located posterior to the glenoid. Once the prosthesis is anterior to humeral head, it can easily be taken out through the rotator interval incision or the surgeon can utilize the superior extent of a previous deltopectoral incision. Removing the component anteriorly avoids dissection through the posterior rotator cuff muscle bellies.

55.8 What to Avoid

It is important to try and avoid damaging the prosthetic humeral head in the process. As previously discussed, this can be avoided with careful attention to the introduction and removal of all instruments and using lateral pressure when entering the glenohumeral joint with the trocar. Care is also needed when "osteotomizing" the glenoid prosthesis; if this step is too vigorous, a glenoid fracture may result, especially if the glenoid has thinned due to osteolysis. Remove each piece of the component after it has been "osteotomized" to avoid inadvertently dislodging the component prematurely and leading to more difficult removal.

55.9 Complications/Bailout/Salvage

If difficulty is encountered using the osteotome to divide the component and the surgeon is worried about the potential for a glenoid fracture, a motorized shaver can be used to divide the component. However, this does have the potential to generate more polyethylene debris within the shoulder. Also, if a glenoid fracture occurs and needs to be repaired, arthroscopically assisted fixation can be performed using percutaneous incisions for screw placement. The salvage operation, if the component cannot be removed arthroscopically, is to perform open glenoid component removal utilizing the previous deltopectoral incision.

55.10 Postoperative Care

The patient is placed in a sling and passive range of motion exercises are started immediately after surgery. If glenoid bone grafting was performed, active, active-assisted range of motion, and strengthening exercises are withheld until 6 weeks postoperatively to help with graft incorporation. If glenoid bone grafting has not been performed, there are no restrictions on motion or strengthening.

References

1. Aibinder WR, Schoch B, Schleck C, Sperling JW, Cofield RH. Revisions for aseptic glenoid component loosening after anatomic shoulder arthroplasty. J Shoulder Elbow Surg 2017;26(3):443–449
2. Updegrove GF, Armstrong AD, Kim HM. Preoperative and intraoperative infection workup in apparently aseptic revision shoulder arthroplasty. J Shoulder Elbow Surg 2015;24(3):491–500
3. O'Driscoll SW, Petrie RS, Torchia ME. Arthroscopic removal of the glenoid component for failed total shoulder arthroplasty. A report of five cases. J Bone Joint Surg Am 2005;87(4):858–863
4. Throckmorton TW, Zarkadas PC, Sperling JW, Cofield RH. Pegged versus keeled glenoid components in total shoulder arthroplasty. J Shoulder Elbow Surg 2010;19(5):726–733
5. Namdari S, Glaser D. Arthroscopically assisted conversion of total shoulder arthroplasty to hemiarthroplasty with glenoid bone grafting. Orthopedics 2011;34(11):862–865
6. Venjakob AJ, Reichwein F, Nebelung W. Arthroscopic removal of a polyethylene glenoid component in total shoulder arthroplasty. Arthrosc Tech 2015;4(2):e149–e152

56 Conversion of Failed Hemiarthroplasty to Reverse Shoulder Arthroplasty

Brandon Horn and Jonathan C. Levy

Abstract
Revision of failed hemiarthroplasty to reverse shoulder arthroplasty most commonly occurs when hemiarthroplasty has been used to treat proximal humerus fractures, cuff tear arthropathy, and end stage arthritis. Each of these common indications presents unique challenges in managing the presenting pathology. Failed hemairthroplasty for proximal humerus fractures often have significant proximal humeral bone loss. Failed hemiarthroplasty for cuff tear arthropathy and osteoarthritis often have significant glenoid bone loss. While many currently available implants offer the opportunity to convert the hemiarthroplasty to a reverse humeral component, removal of the humeral stem is often necessary to create proper soft-tissue balancing.

Keywords: *hemiarthroplasty, glenoid bone loss, proximal humeral bone loss, convertible shoulder arthroplasty*

56.1 Introduction

The clinical success of total shoulder arthroplasty (TSA) for patients with osteoarthritis together with the recent success of reverse shoulder arthroplasty (RSA) in managing rotator cuff-tear arthropathy (CTA) and fractures not amenable to osteosynthesis has resulted in a decline in the utilization of hemiarthroplasty. Nonetheless, shoulder surgeons are often faced with the need to revise a patient previously treated with a shoulder hemiarthroplasty. There are three common clinical scenarios where a shoulder hemiarthroplasty may have failed and a reverse shoulder replacement is selected as a revision. These include hemiarthroplasties used in treating proximal humerus fractures, those used to treat CTA, and those used to treat various forms of end-stage arthritis. While RSA has demonstrated versatility in managing the complex pathology associated with various hemiarthroplasty cases, each clinical scenario presents its own challenges. Over the course of this chapter, we will outline these three common clinical scenarios in which we employ a reverse shoulder prosthesis (RSP) in a revision setting and present algorithms that can be utilized to address challenging problems that can be encountered.

Common to all clinical scenarios is the need to remove the humeral stem. While many of the more modern humeral components have the ability to be converted to a reverse shoulder replacement, previous generations of implants do not. We will address convertibility of stems in the final section of this chapter. In the setting of uncemented humeral stems, standard stem extraction techniques are utilized. Stem extraction begins by disrupting the prosthetic–bone or prosthetic–cement interface of the proximal body and fins of the stem. This is typically performed using flexible osteotomes and/or a high-speed pencil-tip burr. It is important to obtain clear visualization of all fins to avoid fracture of the tuberosities during stem extraction. A first attempt at stem removal is then performed by either backslapping (using company-specific instrumentation) or utilizing a retrograde impaction at the medial neck junction of the stem with a carbide tip punch (**Fig. 56.1**). In the setting of a cemented humeral stem, the stem is removed with similar extraction techniques. After the stem is removed, the cement mantle is addressed to determine if it is well fixed or loose. In a well-fixed cement mantle, new stems can be cemented into the prior mantle. If the new stem is too long to fit into the previous cement mantle, it can be modified and shortened using a carbide wheel burr. Additionally, smaller diameter stems are often utilized to fit within the previous cement mantle, especially if the previous hemiarthroplasty had flutes that make the minimum diameter of the cement mantle smaller. In a loose cement mantle, the old cement can be removed via osteotome, episiotomy, cortical window, or intramedullary cement extraction technique (**Box Text 1**).

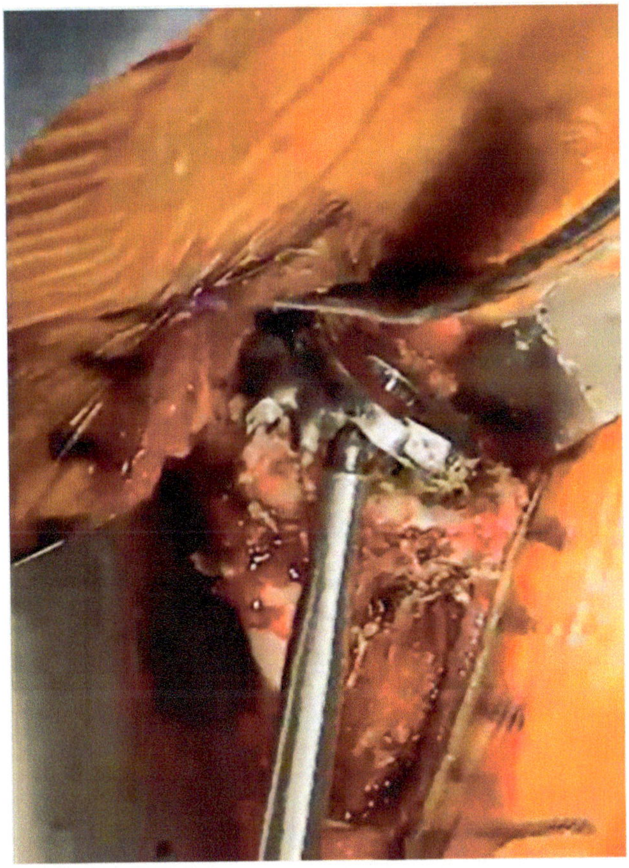

Fig. 56.1 Intraoperative photograph of carbide tip punch (Innomed, Savannah, GA) placed at the medial neck of the humeral stem for retrograde extraction.

Technical Tip I: Cement Extraction

1. Acquire appropriate equipment:
   a. A 2.8-mm threaded guide wire (cannulated screw set).
   b. A 5.0-mm threaded cannulated drill bit (cannulated screw set).
   c. A 6.5-mm cannulated tap (cannulated screw set).
   d. Vice grip pliers.
   e. A mallet.
2. Under fluoroscopic guidance, advance a 2.8-mm threaded guide wire into the cement mantle, ensuring pin placement is center-center to allow appropriate drilling and tap placement to avoid humerus breakthrough.
3. Advance a 5.0-mm threaded cannulated drill bit over guide wire; confirm on fluoroscopy that placement is center-center.
4. Advance a 6.5-mm cannulated tap 2 to 3 cm over the guide wire. Advance to ensure snug fit in the cement mantle.
5. Place the vice grip pliers on cannulated tap as far from humerus as possible to allow strong decisive blows with the mallet to disimpact cement from the cement–bone interface:
   a. Strikes with the mallet should be in line with the cannulated tap to maximize force and prevent iatrogenic damage to the proximal humerus.
6. Repeat steps, confirming center-center placement of the 2.8-mm threaded guide wire, 5.0-mm threaded cannulated drill bit, and snug fit in the cement mantle with 6.5-mm cannulated tap.
7. Loose pieces can be removed with pituitary rongeurs and extended pickups.

56.2 Failed Hemiarthroplasty for Fracture

Primary hemiarthroplasty for comminuted proximal humerus fracture remains one of the most challenging surgical procedures for a busy shoulder surgeon. The procedure is not only technically demanding, but also quite unforgiving. The procedure requires that several technical steps be performed accurately to ensure optimal functional outcomes. Accurate stem height, humeral retroversion, and anatomic reduction and secure fixation of the greater and lesser tuberosities are critical to achieve restoration of shoulder function. Tuberosity failure can result from resorption, nonunion, or malunion of the tuberosities following the index procedure, and can be quite common in older patients. Tuberosity failure mimics rotator cuff deficiency, and many of these patients not only lose function, but also often complain of pain. In this setting, revision shoulder arthroplasty is often considered.

When planning a conversion of a failed hemiarthroplasty for fracture to a reverse shoulder replacement, the challenging pathology relates to the humerus. These cases are commonly associated with various forms of proximal humeral bone loss from tuberosity resorption, nonunion, or malunion, and are approached using the algorithm detailed in **Fig. 56.2**. Appreciation of proximal humeral bone deficiency is critical, as restoring appropriate soft-tissue tension can be challenging in the setting of proximal humeral bone loss. Levy et al[1] first reported higher rates of humeral-sided complications of RSA performed in the setting of proximal humeral bone loss. The additional stress placed across reverse shoulder humeral stem modular junctions in the setting of proximal humeral bone loss can result in modular segment failure. This was confirmed in a mechanical testing

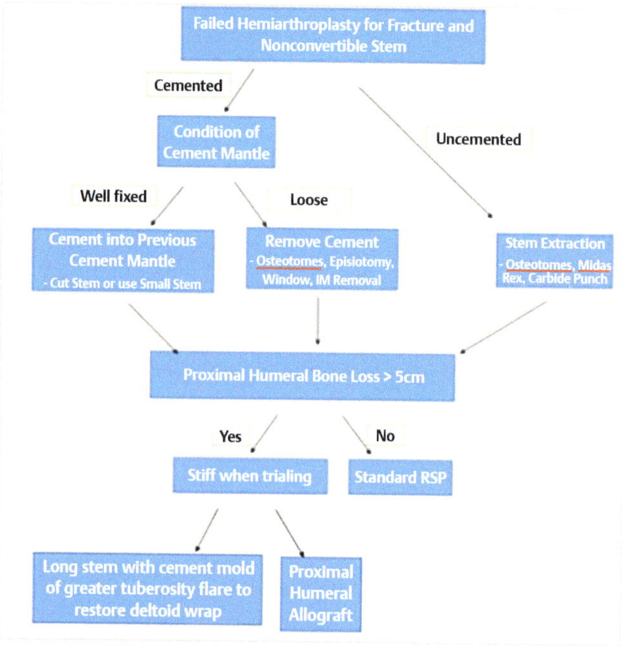

Fig. 56.2 Algorithm for management of humeral stem in failed nonconvertible shoulder hemiarthroplasty.

model of proximal humeral bone loss by Cuff et al.[2] In an effort to avoid humeral-sided complications and to restore the pulley effect of the deltoid,[3] a bulk proximal humeral allograft is often utilized (**Box Text 2**). When the proximal humeral bone was restored using a bulk proximal humeral allograft, humeral-sided complications such as dissociations or dislocations were found to be significantly lower.[4] The decision of when to use a proximal humeral allograft relates to the amount of proximal humeral bone loss as well as the overall flexibility of the shoulder joint.

Technical Tip II: Proximal Humeral Allograft Technical Tip

1. A fresh-frozen proximal humeral allograft with tendon attachments is selected matching the side of the operative shoulder.
2. All soft tissue is removed, with the exception of the subscapularis tendon.
3. The allograft's humeral head is resected at the anatomic neck.
4. All of the cancellous allograft bone is removed from the intramedullary canal.
5. An oscillating saw is then used to create a step cut of the metaphyseal bone such that 5 cm of bone remained laterally and 1 to 2 cm of bone remained medially, resulting in a lateral plate (**Fig. 56.6**).
6. The allograft tendon attachment is later used for repair of the subscapularis.[4]

As Chacon et al noted proximal humeral allografts are typically used when bone loss is greater than 5 cm.[5] In these cases, a trial of the appropriate-sized components is performed. Once soft-tissue balancing is obtained and the appropriate height of the prosthesis is noted, the amount of bone loss is estimated. In cases where dynamic instability has been present and the deltoid has become compliant, a proximal humeral allograft can be used to help restore bone loss, stability, and the deltoid pulley. The additional bone provides further rotational support for the humeral stem (**Fig. 56.3**).

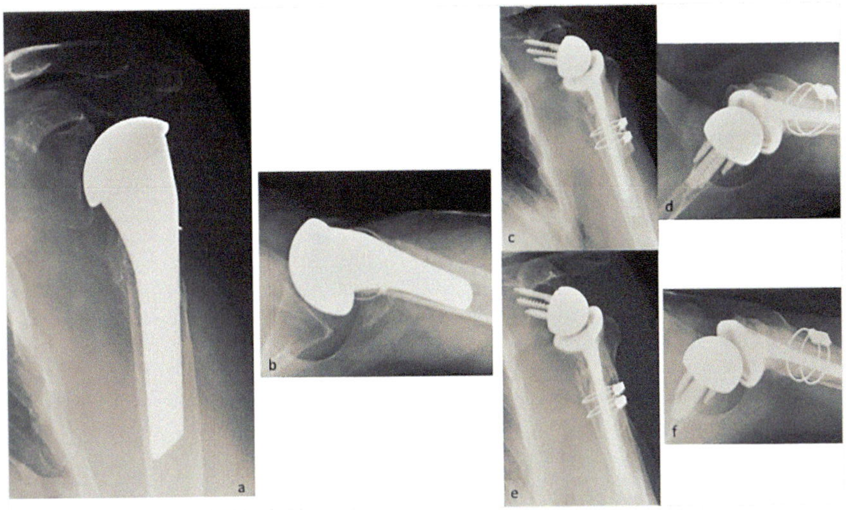

Fig. 56.3 Anteroposterior (a) and axillary lateral (b) radiographs of failed hemiarthroplasty performed for fracture with proximal humeral bone loss greater than 5 cm. Anteroposterior (c) and axillary lateral (d) radiographs following revision reverse shoulder prosthesis with proximal humerus allograft secured with cables. Anteroposterior (e) and axillary lateral (f) radiographs demonstrate 2-year follow-up after revision with incorporation of proximal humeral allograft.

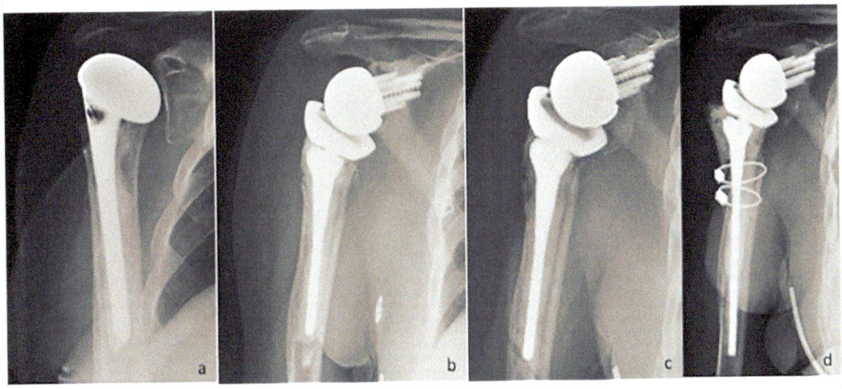

Fig. 56.4 Series of anteroposterior radiographs demonstrating early stem loosening following revision of a failed hemiarthroplasty for fracture with greater than 5 cm of proximal humeral bone loss. (a) Failed hemiarthroplasty for fracture with 5-cm proximal humeral bone loss. (b) Revision to reverse shoulder prosthesis (RSP) with greater than 5 cm proximal humeral bone loss where stem was cemented into previous cement mantle. (c) Two-year follow-up showing loosening around the humeral cement mantle. (d) Two-year follow-up after subsequent revision to long stem humeral component RSP with healed proximal humeral allograft secured with cables.

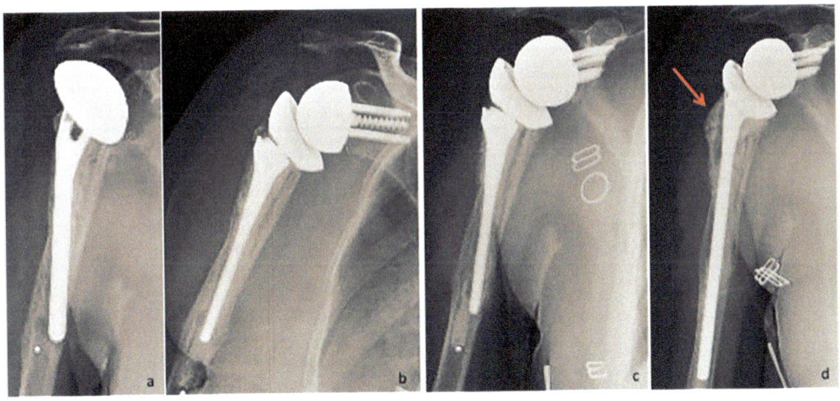

Fig. 56.5 Series of anteroposterior radiographs demonstrating early stem loosening following revision of a failed hemiarthroplasty for fracture with greater than 5cm of proximal humeral bone loss. (a) Failed hemiarthroplasty for fracture with 5-cm proximal humeral bone loss and loose stem. (b) Revision to reverse shoulder prosthesis (RSP) with greater than 5 cm proximal humeral bone loss where stem was cemented into the previous cement mantle. (c) Two-year follow-up showing loosening around the humeral cement mantle with shift in the position of the humeral stem. (d) One-year follow-up after subsequent revision to long stem humeral component RSP with cement reconstruction of proximal humeral bone loss (*arrow*).

If, however, the shoulder soft-tissue envelope is poorly compliant and shoulder motion is limited, there is often insufficient room for a proximal humeral allograft, even in the setting of more than 5 cm of proximal humeral bone loss. In this scenario, a long stem is selected, and cement is used to create a mold of the greater tuberosity flare to restore deltoid wrap. Selection of a long stem humeral component in cases of proximal humeral bone loss helps distribute the rotational forces further down the implant to prevent early loosening. **Fig. 56.4** and **Fig. 56.5** demonstrate two similar cases where a failed hemiarthroplasty with 5 cm of proximal humeral bone loss was revised to a reverse shoulder replacement without a bulk proximal humeral allograft, using a standard length stem. The stem loosened within 2 years and required revision to a long stem implant.

56.3 Failed Hemiarthroplasty for Cuff-Tear Arthropathy

Prior to the release of RSA, patients with CTA were often treated with hemiarthroplasty. Many of these patients had already developed significant glenoid wear, with superior glenoid bone

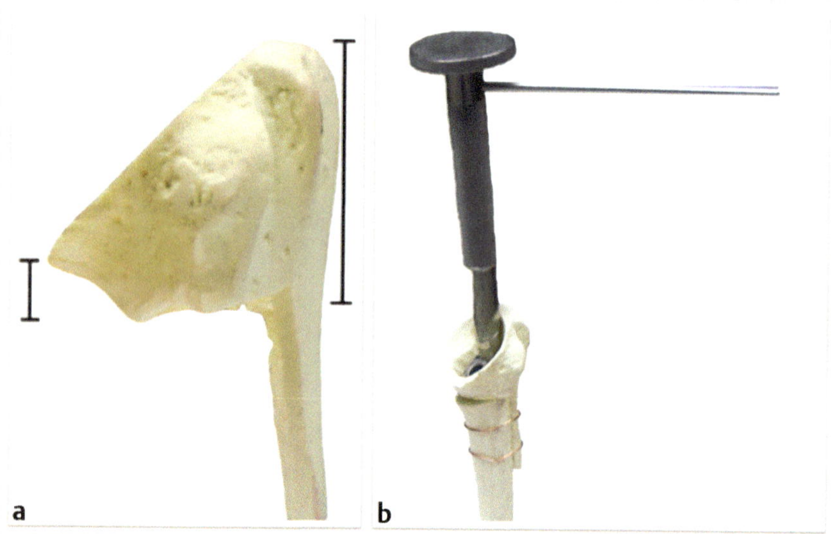

Fig. 56.6 Preparation of proximal humeral allograft. **(a)** A sawbones model of the prepared proximal humeral allograft, illustrating the height of the medial calcar determined during trial reduction as well as the lateral bone plate created by a step cut on the lateral aspect of the graft. **(b)** A sawbones model demonstrating how the proximal humeral allograft is secured to the humeral shaft with use of cables. A version guide is used to ensure placement of the humeral stem in 30 degrees of retroversion. The bicipital groove can often be used to align the allograft anatomically. (Adapted from Chacon et al.[5])

loss and medialization of the superior glenoid due to wear. When treated with the hemiarthroplasty, this bone loss often was accelerated. It is not surprising that the challenges related to revision of a hemiarthroplasty originally performed for CTA relates to managing glenoid bone loss. This was first appreciated by Levy et al[1] as higher rates of glenoid-sided failures were observed in this cohort of patients.

In preparation for a revision to RSA, the pattern of bone loss must be recognized, as it will guide the proper placement of the glenosphere baseplate during revision to RSP, and will help define the need for glenoid bone grafting. CT scans have become critical in recognizing glenoid wear patterns and areas of glenoid deficiencies. Furthermore, metal suppression software, now available as a software upgrade for many CT scans, can dramatically improve the visualization of the glenoid and facilitate surgical planning. The humeral component is addressed in a similar fashion to failed hemiarthroplasty for fracture as described earlier. In this setting, humeral-sided bone loss is rare, even when an extended hood humeral head (CTA Head, Depuy, Warsaw, IN) has been utilized.

Glenoid-sided bone loss is characterized on the preoperative CT scan. When glenoid bone loss is substantial, we typically utilize allograft bone grafting techniques with an allograft femoral head (**Box Text 3**). In these challenging cases, priority is focused on achieving maximal purchase on the central axis of the baseplate. When using a central-screw-type baseplate (DJO RSP, Austin, TX), this can often be identified using the column of bone in the scapula where the base of the scapular spine joins the base of the coracoid. This alternative scapular spine center line[6] intentionally anteverts the baseplate in an effort to maximize fixation into the best bone available.

Once the trajectory of the baseplate has been decided, preliminary reaming will help estimate the amount of bone that needs to be grafted. We previously evaluated the DJO RSP Baseplate in a glenoid bone loss saw bone model and determined that when 25% of the baseplate was supported by native glenoid, there was significantly greater motion at the fixation interface. There was no difference between 50, 75, and 100% baseplate-glenoid-bone coverage.[7] Thus, when preparing the glenoid when glenoid bone loss is present, we typically will ream the native glenoid to a point where 50% of the native glenoid bone has been prepared by the reamer (**Fig. 56.7**). The remaining 50% will be grafted. Other options for addressing glenoid bone deficiency include iliac crest autograft,[8] and custom metal baseplates (see **Fig. 56.8**) or augmented baseplates (Exactech, Gainesville, FL).

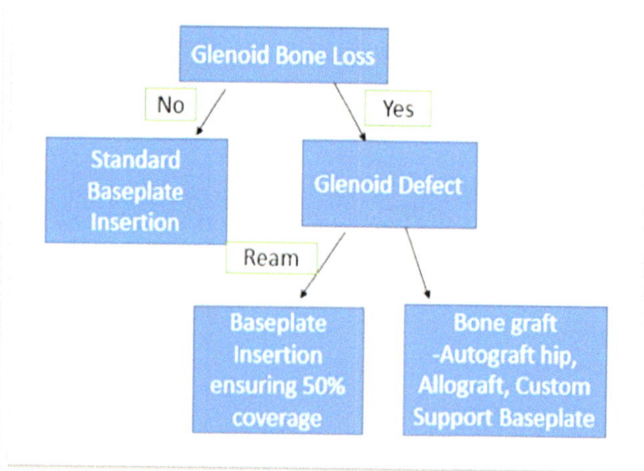

Fig. 56.7 Algorithm for management of glenoid bone loss.

Technical Tip III: Glenoid Bone Grafting (Using the DJO RSP Baseplate)

1. Use a 3.5-mm drill to define the axis for the baseplate.
2. Place a tap, which serves as guide for cannulated reamers.
3. Use the first reamer and advance down to appropriate depth.
4. Create a lemon wedge bone graft and placed along the unreamed glenoid bone surface.
5. Temporary pin placement in graft outside of the diameter of the second reamer.
6. Final reaming.
7. Implant with two screws placed through the bone graft.
8. Remove K-wires.
9. Use a burr to remove any extraneous bone graft.

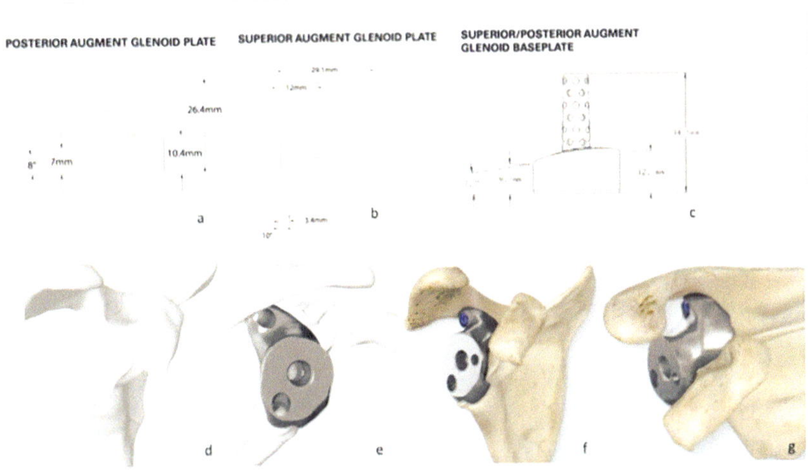

Fig. 56.8 Augmented baseplates. **(a–c)** Various augmented baseplate options available with the Exactech Equinoxe Reverse System (from Operative Technique Addendum); **(d–g)** Zimmer-Biomet Comprehensive Vault Reconstruction System used to manage significant glenoid bone loss (from "Comprehensive Vault Reconstruction System Featuring Dr. Dines; VuMedi).

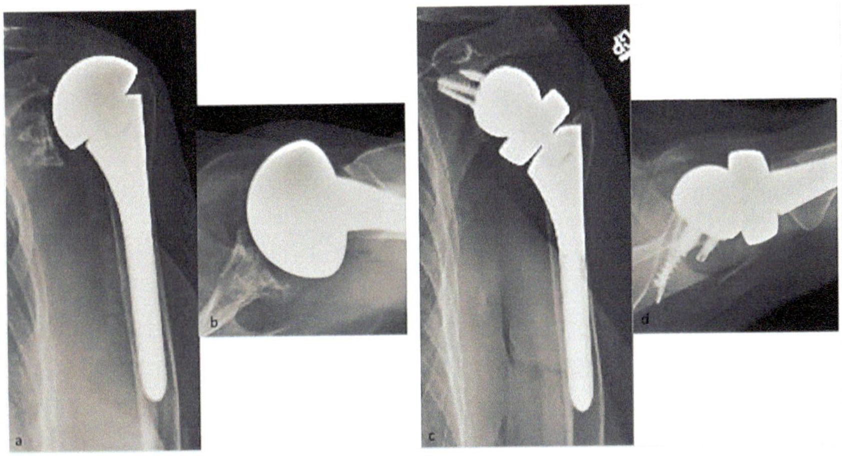

Fig. 56.9 Anteroposterior **(a)** and axillary lateral **(b)** radiographs of failed hemiarthroplasty performed for avascular necrosis using large-diameter humeral stem with superior migration of the humeral head suggesting rotator cuff failure. Anteroposterior **(c)** and axillary lateral **(d)** radiographs 2 years following conversion of hemiarthroplasty to reverse shoulder prosthesis using platform humeral stem. In this case, the revision overstuffed the joint with excessive humeral lengthening resulting in limited postoperative motion and function.

56.4 Failed Hemiarthroplasty for Osteoarthritis

The two most common reasons a hemiarthroplasty performed for arthritis fails are rotator cuff tears and glenoid wear. Postoperative tears of the rotator cuff include failed subscapularis repairs (or lesser tuberosity osteotomy) from the index primary arthroplasty, as well as subsequent tears of the other rotator cuff tendons. Subscapularis failures can relate to overstuffing of the hemiarthroplasty, poor tendon quality, previous surgery, aggressive postoperative rehabilitation, or failure to adhere to postoperative restrictions. Patients with subscapularis insufficiency typically have excessive passive external rotation, loss of internal rotation strength and functions, and/or a positive belly-press or lift-off tests. Radiographs often reveal anterior or anterosuperior subluxation, and displaced lesser tuberosity osteotomies are best seen displaced inferomedially on the Grashey view. A deficient rotator cuff is associated with loss of strength and function, as well as radiographic superior migration. When substantial, it is often associated with dynamic instability and pseudoparesis.

Glenoid wear in the setting of a failed hemiarthroplasty for osteoarthritis is often present. When the pattern of wear is central and erosion is minimal, bone grafting is not typically necessary. However, in cases of eccentric glenoid wear patterns, bone grafting techniques can be utilized. It is conceivable that a painful hemiarthroplasty due to glenoid wear alone could be converted to an anatomic TSA rather than an RSA. Factors that will predict the success of conversion to a TSA most commonly relate to the condition of the subscapularis and the patient's ability to adhere to the postoperative protocols necessary to facilitate subscapularis healing. If the condition of the subscapularis is in question or the glenoid wear pattern is such that placement of an anatomic glenoid component could be compromised, revision of a hemiarthroplasty to an RSA is appropriate.

56.5 Conversion of Platform Stem and Hybrid Constructs

To this point, the discussion has not considered convertible humeral stem options. Recently, the concept of a platform stem has allowed modularity to facilitate conversion of an anatomic humeral head to an RSA humeral component. Numerous implants are now available with this modular feature that has the capacity of revision without the need to remove the humeral stem. In making the decision of whether to utilize the conversion feature, it is critical to assess the soft-tissue tension and soft-tissue balancing during the trialing phase. This typically occurs in the later parts of the case. We prefer to remove the humeral head as an initial step. Attention is turned to the glenoid with the humeral stem left in place to maintain stability and prevent fracture of the humerus during implantation of the glenoid. Once the glenoid is finalized, a trial of the modular conversion is attempted. If good motion is maintained, the conversion option can be utilized (**Figs. 56.9, 56.10**). If, however, the reduction is tight, motion is limited, the

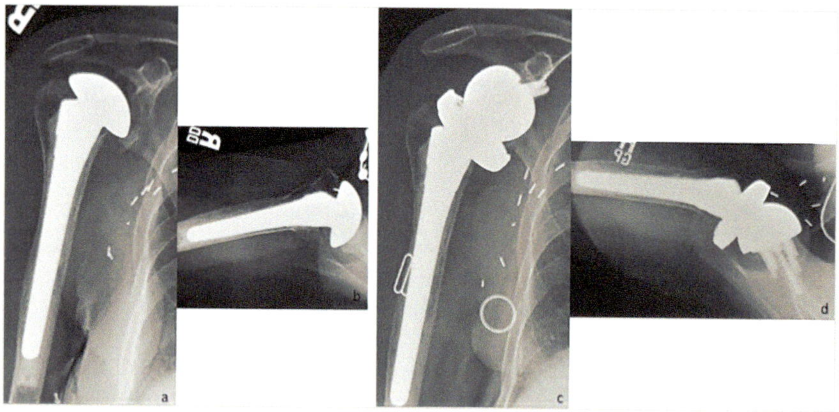

Fig. 56.10 Anteroposterior (a) and axillary lateral (b) radiographs of failed hemiarthroplasty performed for osteoarthritis using cemented large-diameter humeral stem with painful glenoid wear. Anteroposterior (c) and axillary lateral (d) radiographs 2 years following conversion of hemiarthroplasty to reverse shoulder prosthesis using platform humeral stem. Of note, minimal humeral lengthening was performed and postoperative motion and function were excellent.

conjoined tendon becomes a tight bowstring, and/or the axillary nerve becomes taut, we remove the humeral component. One may be tempted to continue to release the remaining rotator cuff as well as additional humeral attachments of the pectoralis major, latissimus dorsi, and teres major in an effort to facilitate motion and not remove the humeral stem. However, this has the potential of weakening the shoulder and creating additional dead space cavities. Furthermore, accepting a tight reduction often results in overlengthening of the shoulder and a poor functional outcome.

56.6 Conclusion

Failed hemiarthroplasty is a complicated problem faced by shoulder surgeons. We have identified three common clinical scenarios where a shoulder hemiarthroplasty may have failed and a reverse shoulder replacement is selected as a revision. These include hemiarthroplasties used in treating proximal humerus fractures, those used to treat CTA, and those used to treat various forms of end-stage arthritis. The need to remove humeral stem and address proximal humeral bone loss and address glenoid-sided bone loss are common issues in these clinical scenarios. We have outlined a systematic approach to handing each of these issues that we believe will lead to successful outcomes with revision RSP.

References

1. Levy JC, Virani N, Pupello D, Frankle M. Use of the reverse shoulder prosthesis for the treatment of failed hemiarthroplasty in patients with glenohumeral arthritis and rotator cuff deficiency. J Bone Joint Surg Br 2007;89(2):189–195
2. Cuff D, Levy JC, Gutiérrez S, Frankle MA. Torsional stability of modular and non-modular reverse shoulder humeral components in a proximal humeral bone loss model. J Shoulder Elbow Surg 2011;20(4):646–651
3. Gagey O, Hue E. Mechanics of the deltoid muscle. A new approach. Clin Orthop Relat Res 2000(375):250–257
4. Levy J, Frankle M, Mighell M, Pupello D. The use of the reverse shoulder prosthesis for the treatment of failed hemiarthroplasty for proximal humeral fracture. J Bone Joint Surg Am 2007;89(2):292–300
5. Chacon A, Virani N, Shannon R, Levy JC, Pupello D, Frankle M. Revision arthroplasty with use of a reverse shoulder prosthesis-allograft composite. J Bone Joint Surg Am 2009;91(1):119–127
6. Klein SM, Dunning P, Mulieri P, Pupello D, Downes K, Frankle MA. Effects of acquired glenoid bone defects on surgical technique and clinical outcomes in reverse shoulder arthroplasty. J Bone Joint Surg Am 2010;92(5):1144–1154
7. Formaini NT, Everding NG, Levy JC, Rosas S. Tuberosity healing after reverse shoulder arthroplasty for acute proximal humerus fractures: the "black and tan" technique. J Shoulder Elbow Surg 2015;24(11):e299–e306
8. Norris TR, Kelly JD, Humphrey CS. Management of glenoid bone defects in revision shoulder Arthroplasty. Tech Shoulder Elbow Surg 2007;8(1):37–46

57 Surgical Technique for Converting a Failed Total Shoulder Arthroplasty to Reverse Shoulder Arthroplasty

Derek Cuff

Abstract

Complications after anatomic total shoulder arthroplasty can lead to failure of this procedure resulting in poor function and pain for the patient. Reverse shoulder arthroplasty has become a reliable salvage operation to treat a failed anatomic total shoulder operation. In this chapter, we discuss the preoperative considerations, surgical exposure, techniques for implant removal, techniques for reconstruction, and the postoperative care associated with this operation. Understanding these techniques and potential surgical pitfalls can allow for successful conversion of a failed anatomical total shoulder arthroplasty to a reverse shoulder arthroplasty in an effort to improve the patient's function and surgical outcome.

Keywords: *total shoulder arthroplasty, reverse shoulder arthroplasty, revision*

57.1 Goals of Procedure

The indications for reverse shoulder arthroplasty (RSA) have expanded significantly since its introduction as a treatment for advanced cuff-tear arthropathy. One of those expanded indications is the use of RSA as a salvage treatment for a failed anatomic total shoulder arthroplasty (TSA).[1] The goal of this procedure is to revise a failed TSA to an RSA in an effort to provide implant stability, decreased pain, and improved function for the patient and will be described in detail in this chapter.

57.2 Indications/Contraindications

There are both early- and late-failure mechanisms that can occur after anatomic TSA, necessitating the need for revision to RSA. Early failures may occur due to complications related to the rotator cuff and the subscapularis repair that is routinely done at the completion of the index TSA. Failure of the repair can lead to subscapularis insufficiency, which results in anterior instability with recurrent subluxations or dislocations of the implant markedly affecting the patient's function in the months or early years following surgery. Instability secondary to a failed TSA in an anterior or posterior direction is an indication for revision to RSA to provide stability and improved function.

A more delayed failure mechanism requiring revision of TSA to RSA can occur in a subset of patients who develop large degenerative rotator cuff tears as they age, eventually leading to poor function and failure of their index arthroplasty after many years (**Fig. 57.1**). Loosening of the glenoid component is another delayed failure mechanism that can occur after anatomic TSA necessitating revision to RSA. Failure of the glenoid–cement or bone–cement interface over time can lead to loosening of the glenoid component, affecting the patient's function and level of pain. In these cases, there may be bone loss on the glenoid side making it difficult to place a new polyethylene glenoid component. RSA offers strong and more reliable glenoid fixation in these glenoid bone loss cases and is a good indication for this difficult problem.

RSA requires an intact and firing deltoid muscle to power the implant. A contraindication to revising a TSA to an RSA would include some type of axillary nerve injury that occurred at the index TSA resulting in permanent nerve injury. Careful assessment of the neurologic status of the operative arm with respect to the axillary nerve and deltoid function should be evaluated on physical examination prior to indicating a patient for revision of the TSA to RSA.

57.3 Preoperative Preparation

Prior to performing the surgical procedure, there are several factors that must be considered. Gathering information about the index TSA is important and obtaining the patient's prior operative report can aid in surgical planning. Understanding which company's product was used, and any specifics in regard to that implant can be valuable as manufactures may have extraction instruments specific to that implant, which may aid in the removal of the components at the time of surgery. The

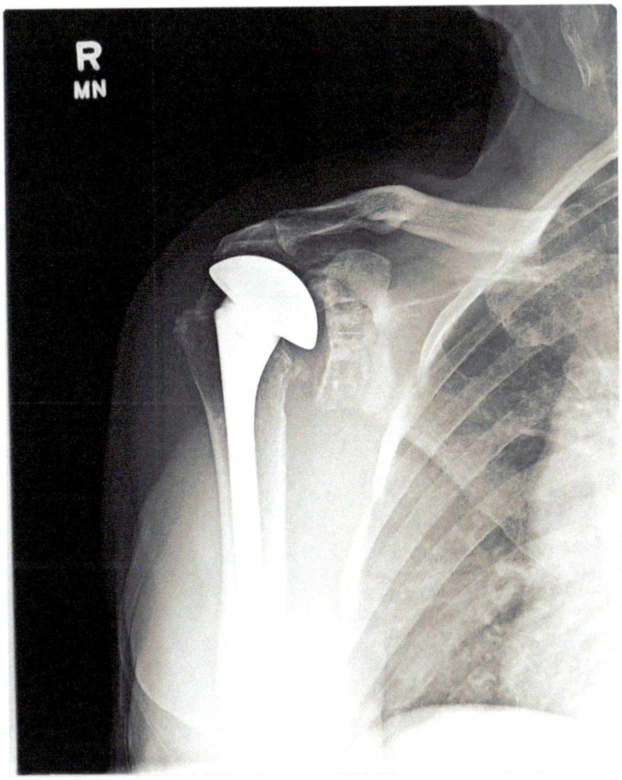

Fig. 57.1 A total shoulder arthroplasty 8 years out from the index procedure. This implant was implanted slightly proud, which most likely led to progressive cuff failure and proximal migration of the humeral component.

prior operative report also allows for the review of the previous surgical technique and any difficulties or complications that may have occurred during the prior surgery.

There is specific instrumentation we have available for all revision of TSA to RSA cases that may be utilized on both the humeral side and the glenoid side of this revision. For the humerus, we have a set of flexible osteotomes available as these may be used to free the proximal portion of the implant from bony ingrowth or cement around the stem. A forked skid instrument is typically used to remove the modular head of the TSA and is on the field. A high-speed burr is available to remove proximal bone around a collared stem if necessary. A carbide-tip punch (Smith & Nephew, Memphis, TN) is on the field as this instrument is often used to disimpact the humeral stem. Finally, a microsagittal saw is available in case a humeral episiotomy is required in effort to split the humerus to remove a well-fixed stem, and cables are available as well to repair this humeral split.

On the glenoid side, a set of solid curved osteotomes are available to assist in removing a polyethylene pegged or keeled glenoid. In these cases, bone graft may be needed if large glenoid defects are encountered and a femoral head allograft is available on all cases if structural grafting is required. Smaller contained glenoid defects may be packed with cancellous allograft chips and demineralized bone matrix putty and they are available in case they are required.

57.4 Operative Technique: Tips and Pearls

57.4.1 Exposure

The patient is placed under general anesthesia and fully paralyzed for the duration of the procedure. The patient is placed in the beach-chair position with the operative extremity draped free and a padded Mayo stand placed under the elbow to support the arm and assist with arm positioning during the case. A deltopectoral approach is used for this procedure. An attempt is made to incorporate or utilize the patient's previous incision; however, if the old incision is not appropriately positioned over the deltopectoral interval, we will not let it define our approach and will create a new incision centered directly over the interval.

A no. 10 blade is used for the surgical incision and electrocautery is used to dissect through the subcutaneous tissue. In these revision cases due to previous dissection and scar tissue, it can be difficult to identify the deltopectoral interval. At the superior aspect of the interval, there predictably is a proximal fat triangle defining the interval with the pectoralis major medially and the anterior deltoid laterally. The interval can be identified here, and as the interval is developed, the cephalic vein can be taken in either the medial or the lateral direction when encountered.

After the interval is developed, it is critical to free up the subdeltoid, subacromial, and subcoracoid spaces to mobilize the shoulder and release adhesions that may have formed from the previous surgery. The deltoid may be scarred onto the lateral humerus and dissection is started distally just above the deltoid insertion on the deltoid tuberosity and moves proximally to mobilize the deltoid off the lateral humerus in an effort to develop the subdeltoid space. The subacromial space is then developed and a Cobb elevator can assist in releasing adhesions in this area. The subcoracoid space must then be defined and this is done by identifying the conjoint tendon and then carefully releasing adhesion underneath the conjoint tendon and typically this is done with careful spreading using a tonsil along with a combination of blunt finger dissection.

At this point, the anterosuperior rotator cuff can be visualized. If the revision surgery is being done secondary to subscapularis failure and anterosuperior rotator cuff tearing after the index TSA, then with the simple release of the anterior capsular scar tissue the humeral head will be visualized. If it is a revision in which the subscapularis is still intact, then a subscapularis peel technique is utilized. The subscapularis is released using electrocautery directly off the lesser tuberosity, and with gentle external rotation of the shoulder with the elbow adducted against the body, the shoulder will be atraumatically dislocated and the humeral head of the implant is exposed.

57.4.2 Humeral Removal

At this point, the humeral head can be removed. The majority of implants developed in the last two decades have modular humeral head and can be disassociated from the humeral stem. A forked skid type retractor can be utilized to disengage the humeral head from the stem of most implant systems (**Fig. 57.2**). Next, the humeral stem needs to be freed up from the surrounding humerus. If this is a press-fit stem or a cemented stem, the technique remains the same and a flexible osteotome is the preferred instrument for stem removal. The flexible osteotome is used to hug the implant and impacting distally to debond the stem from either the implant–bone interface in the press-fit scenario or the implant–cement interface if cemented (**Fig. 57.3**). Care must be taken to stay directly in contact with the humeral implant to not breach or violate the humeral cortex with the osteotome as it is impacted distally and done so repeatedly and circumferentially around the implant to free it.

The humeral component of many TSA systems has a collar on the stem, which can be used to help disimpact the stem from the humeral canal after the osteotomes have been used to circumferentially free the stem. A high-speed burr is used to remove some proximal bone around the anterior collar to expose it. A carbide-tip punch (Smith & Nephew) is an excellent instrument to place on the collar to serve as the punch that will help extract the stem (**Fig. 57.4**). If the stem does not have a collar, then the high-speed burr can be used to burr directly into the metal of the proximal portion of the implant to create a small trough to place the tip of the carbide punch to serve as a stable site to disimpact the stem. Sequential blows to the punch with a heavy mallet can then be used to extract the stem.

In certain cases with extensive porous coating of the implant or a fully cemented stem, it may not be possible to extract the stem with these techniques. In those cases, a humeral episiotomy can be used to split the humerus. A microsagittal saw is used to create the humeral split and this is done longitudinally along the length of the humerus just medial to the bicipital groove. The split is carried distally but is stopped about 2 to 3 cm proximal to the level of the deltoid tuberosity. Straight osteotomes are used to "book open" the humerus just slightly

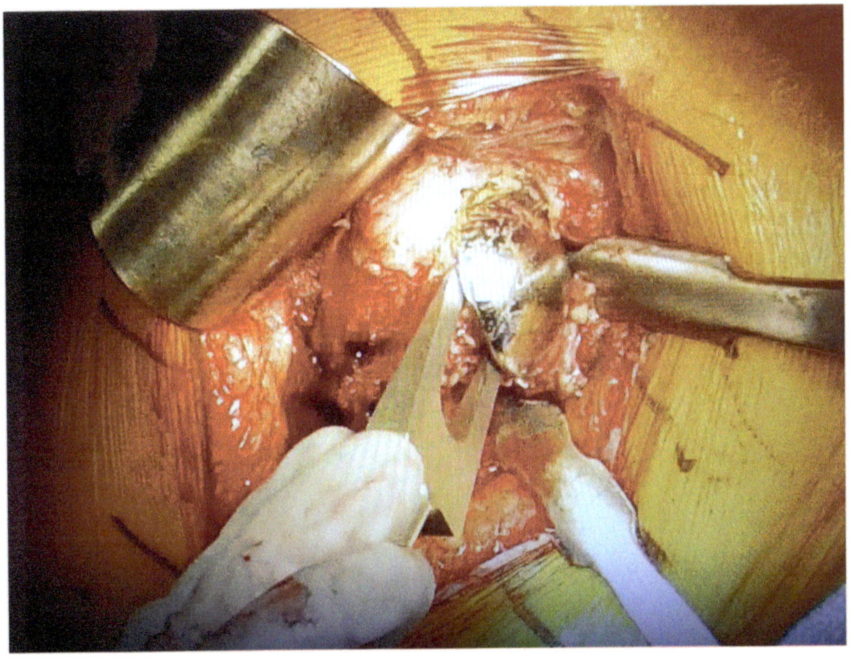

Fig. 57.2 A forked skid instrument can be used to remove a modular humeral head.

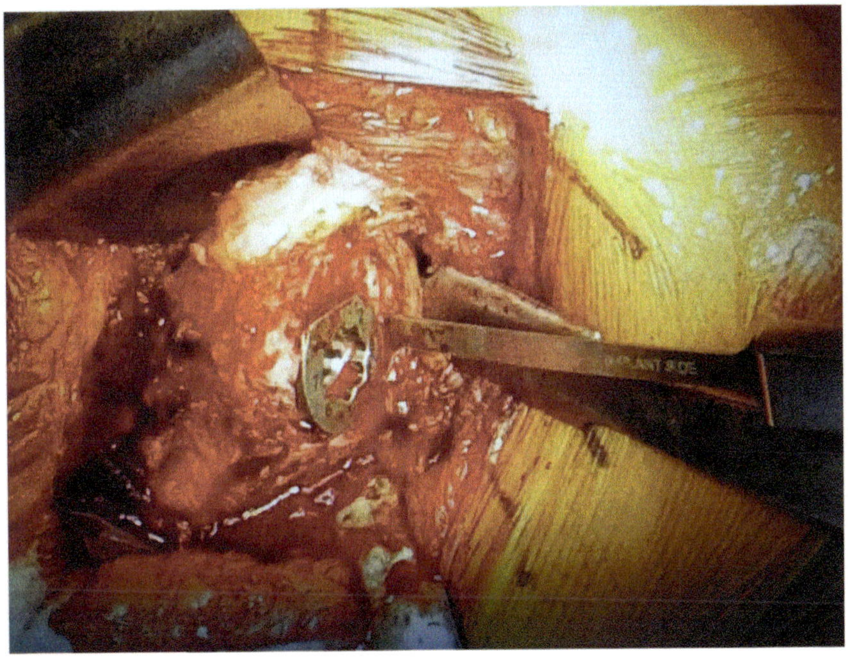

Fig. 57.3 A flexible osteotome is used to circumferentially loosen the proximal portion of the humeral component from surrounding bone or cement.

to release the hoop stresses around the implant. At this point, the stem should be able to be extracted via impaction with the carbide-tip punch. Two or three cables can be used around the humerus to repair this at the end of the case prior to inserting the final RSA stem to complete the case.

57.4.3 Glenoid Removal

The arm is then abducted to 90 degrees on the Mayo stand in order to expose the glenoid. A posterior glenoid retractor is used to visualize the glenoid. If the subscapularis remains and is potentially repairable, then it is tagged with a suture. It is released anteriorly and posteriorly of any adhesions and capsule while the axillary nerve is protected inferiorly with the index finger. The superior border of the subscapularis is released to the base of the coracoid to fully mobilize it. An anterior Hohmann retractor is then placed along the anterior glenoid neck just posterior to the subscapularis and another Hohmann is placed over the superior glenoid to expose the glenoid component. At this point, it is important to remove any residual anteroinferior scar or residual capsule to help with exposure.

The most common glenoid component that is encountered in these revision cases is an all-polyethylene cemented component that is either a pegged or a keeled component. Our goal in removal of these components is to simply shear the face of the glenoid component off the pegs or keel with use of an osteotome (**Fig. 57.5**). A curved 0.75-inch osteotome is placed along the anterior edge of the glenoid component and impacted from

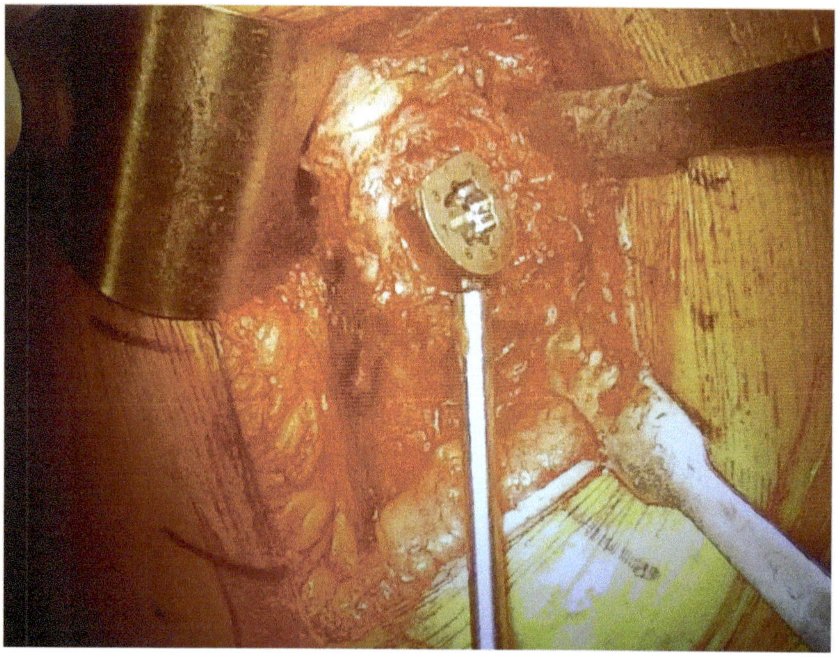

Fig. 57.4 A carbide-tip punch is placed on the collar and utilized to help extract the stem once it has been freed from surrounding bone or cement.

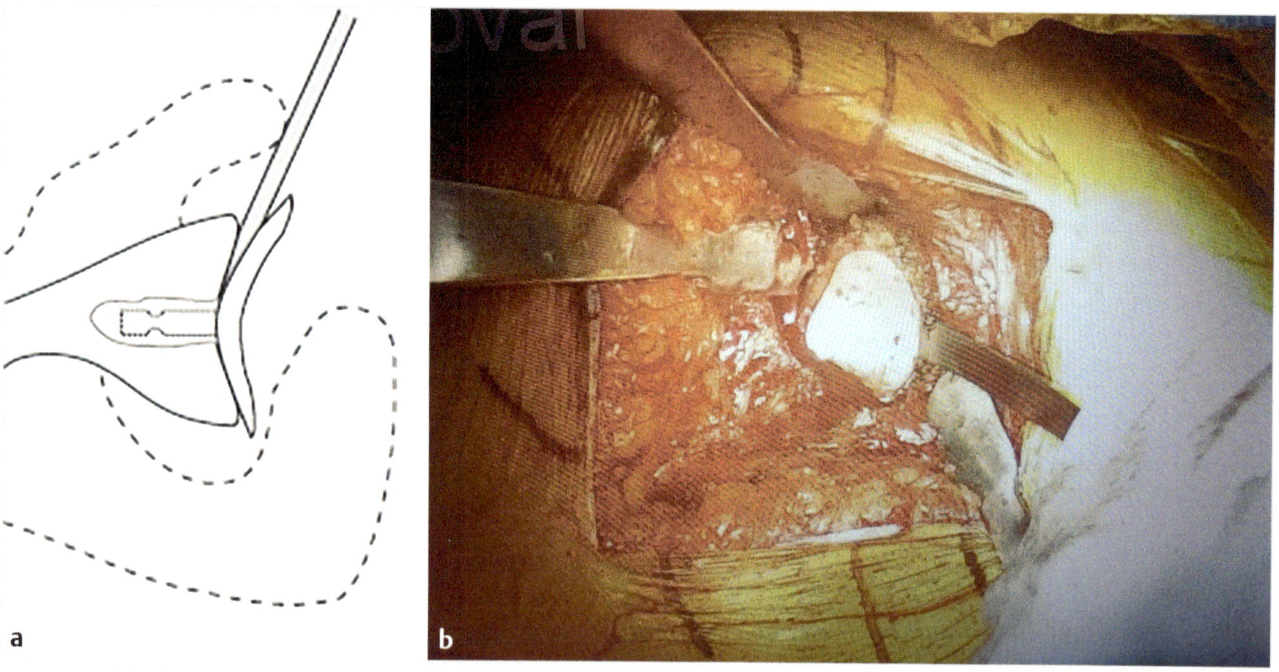

Fig. 57.5 (a) Schematic demonstrating how an osteotome can be used to shear the pegs from the face of the implant. (b) Intraoperative photo showing a 0.75-inch curved osteotome being used to sheer the polyethylene pegs from the face of the component.

and anterior to posterior direction to shear off the pegs or keel. The pegs or keel can then be removed from the glenoid vault with a tonsil. We do not take time to meticulously remove the glenoid cement as this can serve as a good substrate for screw purchase when the RSA baseplate is placed. Other glenoid components such as older metal-back glenoids, or newer hybrid fixation glenoids, may have manufacturer-specific instruments to help remove them. This is where the prior operative report and understanding the implant that was previously utilized as noted earlier in the chapter are important with respect to the removal of the glenoid component.

57.4.4 Glenosphere Placement

At this point if there is minimal glenoid bone loss, then placement of the RSA baseplate and glenosphere proceeds in the standard fashion. The author uses an implant with a center screw for RSA cases. In this system, a 10-degree inferiorly tilted drill guide is used to drill along the glenoid center line exiting out the anterior glenoid neck at a depth of typically 26 to 30 mm. A tap is then placed along that pilot drill hole to check for purchase. The tap is then over-reamed to prepare the glenoid. The tap is then removed and the baseplate inserted. Four peripheral 5.0-mm locking screws are inserted to augment the glenoid fixation. Care is then taken to remove any tissue around the periphery of the baseplate and then the glenosphere is inserted. In an effort to avoid any potential chance of a glenosphere dissociation, a special instrument that screws into the glenosphere is used to perform a glenosphere "tug test" to make sure the taper between the baseplate and glenosphere is fully engaged and solid to complete the glenoid portion of the case (**Fig. 57.6**). There are special circumstances that may be encountered on the glenoid side that the surgeon must be prepared to address. In certain cases after component removal, there may be a contained defect in the glenoid vault. In these cases of glenoid bone loss, the baseplate technique may need to be altered in an effort to get a stable fixation of the RSA. In a standard RSA case with no glenoid bone loss, the center screw or post of the baseplate is placed along the glenoid center line. However, in a glenoid bone loss case there may not be enough bone to anchor that center screw or post before exiting out the anterior glenoid neck. In glenoid bone loss cases, we prefer a center screw baseplate and orient it along the alternate scapular line as described by Klein et al (**Fig. 57.7**).[2]

The alternate scapular line engages a dense pillar of bone where the scapular spine meets the scapular body and is present even in the worse glenoid bone loss cases. This bone can be accessed by orienting the pilot drill hole posteriorly by anteverting the drill about 15 degrees and maintaining a 10-degree inferior tilt of the drill. Using the drill as a sound as it is advanced will give tactile feedback to determine if that dense pillar of bone along the alternate scapular line was fully engaged. The tap can then be placed over that pilot drill hole to check for bony purchase to ensure that

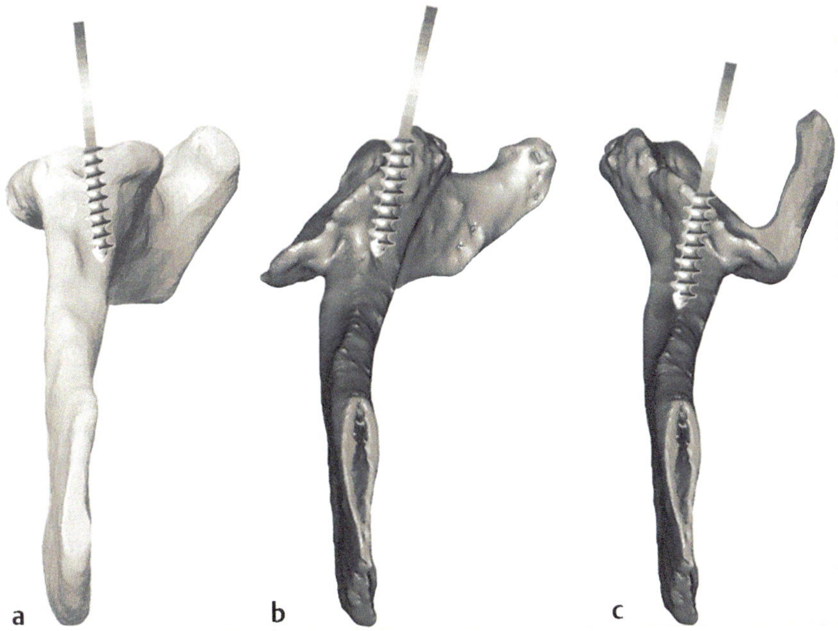

Fig. 57.6 **(a)** Schematic demonstrating the standard alignment of the tap along the glenoid center line in a case with no glenoid bone loss. **(b, c)** The alignment of the tap along the alternate scapular line to orient the baseplate in this dense pillar of bone in cases with posterior or anterior bone loss.

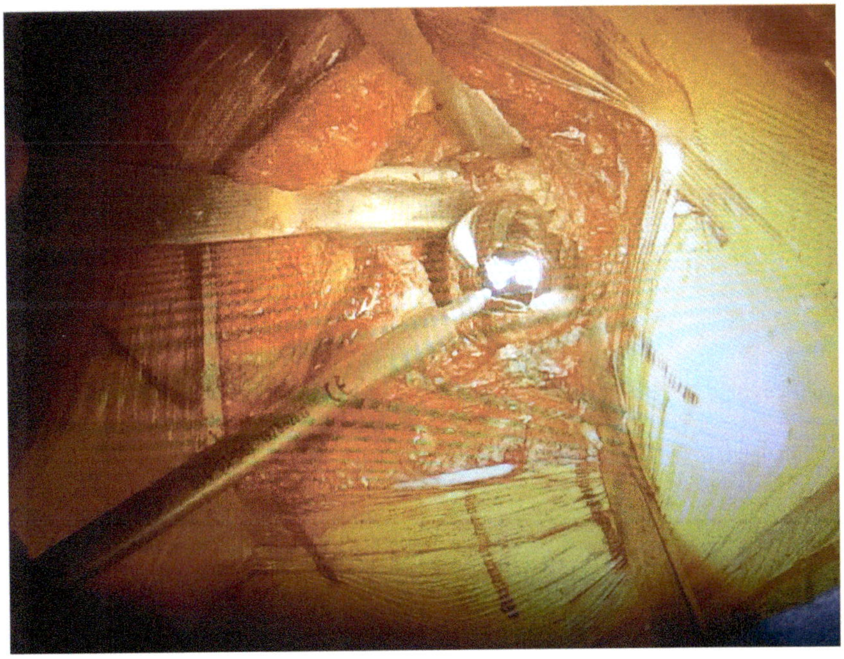

Fig. 57.7 Glenosphere placement with instrument threaded in to allow for a "tug test" to check for engagement of the glenosphere-baseplate taper.

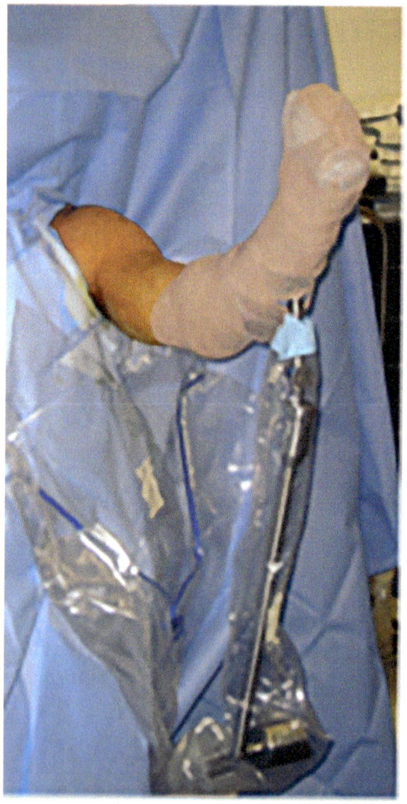

Fig. 58.2 Contralateral arm is secured to the body or with a well-padded arm holder.

ii. Drape as medial to the scapula as possible.
iii. Expose distal humerus to allow for extension of prior incision for humeral exposure as needed.

- Operative technique:
  - Incision:
    i. Standard landmarks are outlined on the shoulder:
      a. The anterior, lateral, and posterior border of the acromion, the acromioclavicular joint, the clavicle, and the coracoid process.
    ii. Mark prior incision extending it distal and lateral if extensile approach is needed.
  - Instruments:
    i. Implant-specific extraction system.
    ii. Osteotome (flexible or Lambotte osteotomes).
    iii. Burr (narrow tip).
    iv. Sagittal saw.
    v. Curettes.
    vi. Cerclage wires.
    vii. Wire cutters.
    viii. Strut allograft (available).
    ix. Nerve stimulator.
    x. Ultrasound cement remover.
    xi. Fluoroscopy.
- Operative technique:
  - The patient is placed in the semi-beach-chair position with the operative arm in a pneumatic holder:
  - Incision:
    i. Mark prior incisions and determine the utility of the incision or if a separate one is necessary.
    ii. Preference: extensile deltopectoral incision (deltopectoral approach with distal extension to an anterolateral humeral incision as needed).
  - Exposure:
    i. Deltopectoral approach:
      a. In revision cases, deltopectoral interval can be obscured by scarring/adhesions:
        - Important:
          - Coracoid is an important marker to avoid excessive medial dissection.
          - Start proximally to identify the triangular space formed by the superior medial portion of the deltoid and the superior medial portion of the pectoralis major muscle.
          - Nerve stimulator is useful to guide dissection when muscle planes appear confluent.
      b. Continue dissection to the distal extent of the stem:
        - Native tissue may be defined easier by exposing distally beyond prior surgical field.
        - Soft-tissue attachments should be maintained, but release may be required to improve visualization (i.e., pectoralis major and latissimus dorsi).
        - Deep cultures:
          - Taken along the stem–bone interface.
    ii. Once the interval is defined:
      a. It is important to develop submuscular spaces:
        - Subdeltoid:
          - Subperiosteally elevate the anterior deltoid with a Cobb elevator:
            - **Important:** Aberrant dissection of the anterior deltoid off the humerus can denervate the muscle.
            - **Tip:** Start distally in native tissue and continue proximally.
            - **Important:** As the anterior deltoid is released distally, watch for bridging vessels.
          - Subdeltoid adhesions can be extensive and a clear space should be developed to the posterior rotator cuff.
        - Subacromial:
          - Often subacromial space can be difficult to enter due to scar tissue:
            - Place axial traction on the arm maximizing subacromial space.
            - A Cobb elevator or a no. 15 blade placed parallel to acromion can be used to open space allowing further blunt finger dissection.
        - Subcoracoid:
          - Often scarred in as well:
            - Identifying the proximal musculature of the short head of the biceps can help define the lateral-most extent of the conjoined tendon.
            - Sharp and blunt dissection can help open a space deep to the conjoint tendon allowing retractor placement and continued dissection.
    iii. Perform the tug test (evaluates continuity of axillary nerve):
      a. Use the index finger to find the axillary nerve medial and deep to the conjoint tendon.
      b. Next, find the circumflex branch along the deep lateral portion of the deltoid.
      c. Apply gentle traction to the medial portion of the nerve. This will transmit across the nerve and should be felt with the contralateral index finger.

- **Important:** In revision cases, scar tissue and adhesions can make identifying the axillary nerve difficult. A nerve stimulator can be especially helpful in isolating the nerve.

iv. Retractors are placed deep to the anterior deltoid and conjoint tendon exposing the proximal humerus:
   a. The rotator cuff tendon can be evaluated at this point.

v. Excise any visible scar tissue.

vi. Rotator interval and biceps release:
   a. The biceps tendon (if present) is identified and the sheath is opened proximally along the bicipital groove.
   b. The biceps can be followed proximally; once the top of the humerus is reached:
      - Identify the coracoid process and the coracoid base.
      - Direct the remainder of the release toward the coracoid base effectively opening the rotator interval.
      - The biceps tendon can be transected as close to its origin on the superior glenoid.
         - **Important:** Avoid continuing release by following the biceps tendon posteriorly as this can cause transecting of the supraspinatus tendon.

vii. Subscapularis tendon release:
   a. Release the subscapularis tendon as far lateral on the lesser tuberosity to preserve as much soft tissue for subsequent repair.
   b. Tag tendon with nonabsorbable sutures (i.e., 0 Ethibond).
   c. Advance soft-tissue release inferiorly along the humeral shaft and continue the capsular release posteromedial along humeral neck.
      - **Important:** Check the location of the axillary nerve as it can often be scarred to the inferior capsule and can be at risk of injury during the medial release.

viii. Dislocate prosthesis:
   a. Extension, adduction, and external rotation will help facilitate and maintain exposure of the humeral head.
   b. Blunt retractors are placed medially and a brown deltoid is used laterally to help retract the deltoid posteriorly.

- Stem removal:

i. Remove the prosthetic head or the polyethylene component with an extraction device or round tamp/osteotome and mallet.

ii. The surrounding soft tissue is removed with a rongeur to clearly visualize the bony margins.

iii. Evaluate the implant fixation.
   a. If grossly unstable, the stem may be removed by hand; if not, an extraction device may be necessary.

iv. Attach an extraction device:
   a. If trial with an extraction device is unsuccessful, then a narrow-tip burr or a thin osteotome can be used to circumferentially interrupt the proximal bone–cement interface with the prosthesis.
      - **Important:** Keep the instrument parallel with the prosthesis to avoid iatrogenic fracture or unwanted bone removal.
   b. **Alternative:** A tamp can be placed along the medial edge of the prosthesis and may dislodge the implant with a mallet.

v. Prosthesis well fixed:
   a. Humeral window:
      - Boundaries of the pectoralis major tendon are identified.
      - A rectangular anterior humeral osteotomy is performed along the proximal, lateral, and distal portion of the pectoralis major tendon.
         - The size of the osteotomy is determined based on the stem length and the ability to reach the proximal and distal portions of the stem.
            - The distal extent of the osteotomy should be carefully planned because if the osteotomy length is too short, it may be difficult to disrupt the bone–cement interface distally.

      Tip: Extending the osteotomy to the tip of the stem may assist in easier removal of the implant especially if the entire cement mantle and cement restrictor require removal.
      - After planning the osteotomy size and location, an osteotome can be used to open the top, lateral, and inferior portions.
      - With the osteotome in the lateral opening, flexing and bending the osteotome will help open the osteotomy along the medial border.

      Tip: A series of drill holes placed medially can help with reducing the risk of fracturing the cortical window (Fig. 58.3).

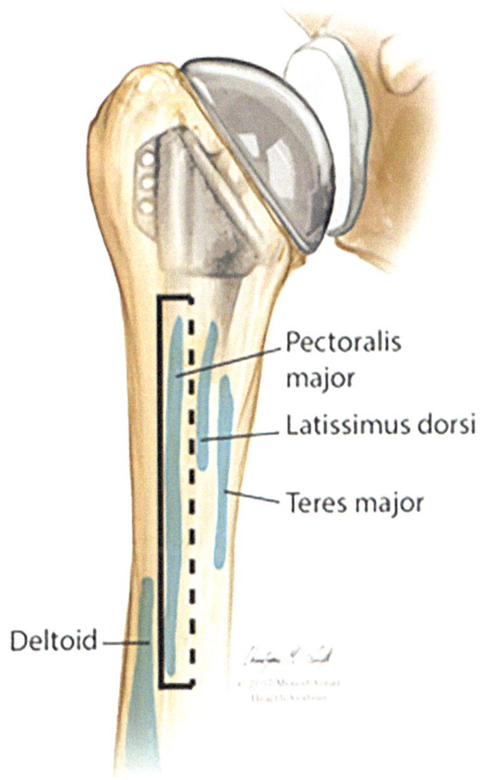

Fig. 58.3 Humeral window osteotomy for stem removal. Used with permission, © Mount Sinai Health System, 2007.

- Once osteotomy is completed, the cortical window is wedged open.
- An osteotome can be used to disrupt the interface with the humeral prosthesis.

b. Longitudinal humeral osteotomy (preferred method):
- Insertion points of the deltoid and the pectoralis major are identified along with the bicipital groove.
- A microsagittal saw is used to score the bone along the length of the bicipital groove continuing medial to deltoid insertion and lateral to pectoralis major insertion.
- Use a narrow osteotome to create a linear osteotomy extending through the cement to prosthesis.
  - Osteotomy is continued distally in small increments while gently attempting to wedge open the osteotomy interrupting bone–implant or cement–implant interface.
- As the osteotomy is continued distally, reassess if the humeral prosthesis has disengaged:
  - Antibiotics stem removal with an extraction device or tamp and mallet.
- A narrow osteotome can be placed carefully within the osteotomy along the implant to help disrupt the interface.
  - **Important:** As the osteotomy is wedged open, monitor for distal progression of the osteotomy and inadvertent fracturing of the osteotomy site (**Fig. 58.4**).

c. Stem removed:
- Revision for aseptic loosening:
  - The cement mantle can be retained and a new prosthesis cemented into it.
- Revision for septic loosening:
  - If cemented, curette out the cement and the membranous tissue with
    - Reverse cutting curettes.
    - Ultrasound cement remover.

d. Osteotomy closure (performed prior to reimplantation):
- Cerclage wires are placed around the humerus:
  - **Important:** Stay along the cortical surface to avoid entrapping any neurovascular structures.
- Drill holes are placed on both sides of the osteotomy and with heavy sutures passed through the holes and tied closing osteotomy:
- Cortical strut graft:
  - If the cortex is relatively thin, with concerns for potential fracture, then the osteotomy can be augmented with a cortical strut graft (i.e., fibula).

58.6 Tips and Pearls/Expert Suggestions

- Once the implant is removed, clear away any surrounding scar tissue to visualize the proximal bone–implant interface.
- Stay in line with prosthesis when working proximally with burr or osteotome.

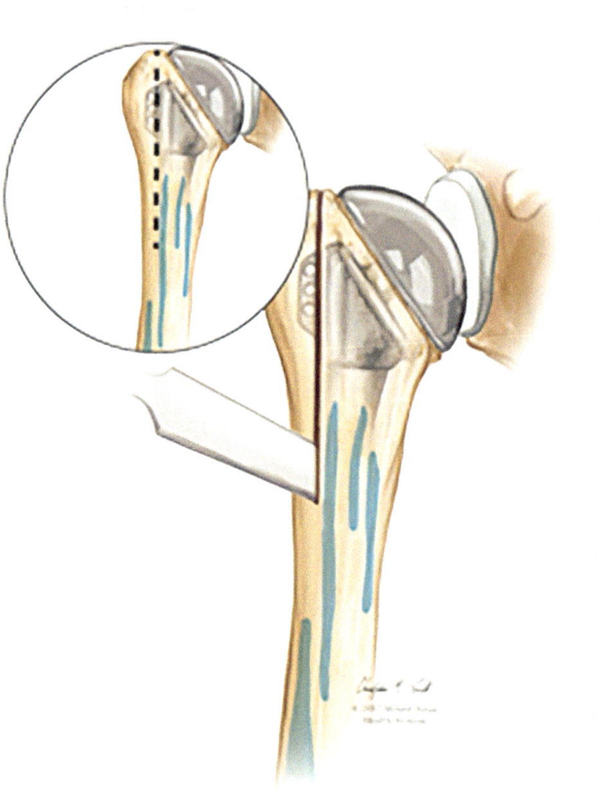

Fig. 58.4 Longitudinal osteotomy for humeral stem removal. Used with permission, © Mount Sinai Health System, 2007.

- During cement removal, ensure the curette is hooked to the cement and not endosteum to prevent fracture or bone loss.
- Check for clear passage of cerclage wires around humerus; subperiosteal release may be necessary.

58.7 What to Avoid

- Iatrogenic fracture with the following:
  - Implant removal.
  - Osteotomy or osteotomy closure:
    - If this occurs:
      i. Extend dissection if needed to evaluate extent of fracture.
      ii. If possible, stabilize with additional cerclage wires.
      iii. Augment with cortical strut graft.
      iv. Consider bypassing with longer cemented prosthesis.
- Thermal injury to soft tissue with ultrasound cement remover:
  - Prevent by periodically irrigating canal with saline.
- If cementing, cement extravasation through bone deficiencies or osteotomy site into surrounding tissues:
  - Place retractors proximal and distal retracting soft tissue away from osteotomy.
  - During cementation, evaluate around osteotomy for visible cement extravasation and quickly remove.
- Poor reduction or fixation following osteotomy:
  - Once osteotomy is closed and secured, reassess reduction and stability with arm motion.

59 Explant/Insertion of Spacer for Infected Shoulder Arthroplasty

Samuel R.H. Steiner and Stephen F. Brockmeier

Abstract
The explant or insertion of an antibiotic spacer in the setting of an infected shoulder arthroplasty can be challenging and fraught with complication, but outcomes can be improved with a methodological approach. Addressing a periprosthetic shoulder infection starts with a thorough workup and identification of the offending organism. Initial debridement and removal of components is of paramount importance for infection eradication. Antibiotic cement spacers can provide local antibiotic delivery while maintaining soft-tissue tension and shoulder function until infection eradication can be achieved. There are a variety of ways to construct a cement spacer. It is to a surgeon's benefit to have these varying techniques in their repertoire. No matter which type is employed, it is imperative to have a primary plan for implantation and removal, followed by sequential backup options should the primary plan not work.

Keywords: *antibiotic spacer, shoulder arthroplasty, explant, implant, infection*

59.1 Goals of Procedure

59.1.1 Eradication of Infection

The primary goal of management of an infected shoulder arthroplasty is eradication of the infection. Most bacteria have the ability to create a polysaccharide biofilm and adhere to foreign material and devitalized tissue, rendering them impervious to antibiotic therapy alone. Clearance of a chronic periprosthetic joint infection can only be successful with removal of all implants and debridement of devitalized tissue. An antibiotic spacer is then inserted and used for local delivery of antibiotics in conjunction with systemic intravenous antibiotics.

59.1.2 Improvement in Pain

One of the most consistent findings in any periprosthetic joint infection is the subjective symptom of pain. The range of severity can vary from minor to debilitating. Control of the infection is the only means by which to improve a patient's pain. Removal of the compromised prosthesis without placement of another implant or spacer compromises joint function and can lead to persistent pain.

59.1.3 Maintenance of Function

In addition to local delivery of antibiotics, a spacer can provide a means of articulation, thus providing glenohumeral mobility and extremity function. It also functions to preserve the soft-tissue envelope and prevent significant contractures, thereby maintaining tissue planes and improving the feasibility of a second-stage reimplantation.

59.2 Advantages

59.2.1 Local Antibiotic Delivery

Following a thorough debridement, insertion of an antibiotic spacer provides local delivery of antibiotics and time for infection clearance. Certain antibiotics, such as gentamicin, have a better bony penetrance via dissolution from a spacer than they do systemically. The delivery of high doses of antibiotics from a spacer directly to the site of infection can achieve concentrations higher than those reached with systemic antibiotics alone, while at the same time avoiding the potential systemic toxicity that can arise from high-dose intravenous use.

59.2.2 Pathogen Identification

The reported sensitivity of joint aspiration in diagnosing a prosthetic joint infection ranges from 12 to 100%, with the majority of studies demonstrating a sensitivity between 45 and 75%.[1,2] When a pathogen cannot be identified via a preoperative aspirate, performing a two-stage procedure allows for deep tissue cultures to be obtained, and antibiotics to be tailored to sensitivities of bacterial cultures prior to reimplantation of hardware.

59.2.3 Single- versus Two-Stage Reconstruction

The current gold standard for treatment of chronic infections of the hip and knee is a two-stage revision. This has also shown favorable results in the shoulder.[3,4] This includes removal of the prosthesis and all hardware, a thorough debridement of all devitalized tissue, insertion of an antibiotic-impregnated cement spacer, followed by at least 6 weeks of intravenous antibiotics with assurance of infection eradication prior to second-stage revision, and reimplantation of components.

59.3 Indications

Implantation of an antibiotic cement spacer is performed in cases of documented or highly suspected chronic prosthetic joint infection. The removal of a spacer is performed when there is reason to believe the infection has been eradicated. We allow at least 6 weeks' duration of systemic antibiotic therapy, followed by a 4- to 6-week antibiotic holiday. If subjective symptoms and serologic markers (erythrocyte sedimentation rate [ESR], C-reactive protein [CRP], or interleukin-6 [IL-6]) remain normal, the patient is sent for a guided aspiration of the joint (with cultures held for 14 days) to confirm the absence of persistent infection. If this aspiration is negative, then the second-stage procedure can be undertaken.

59.4 Contraindications

Implanting or explanting an antibiotic spacer should not be undertaken if a patient is medically unfit for surgery. In the case of a periprosthetic joint infection, if the patient is relatively asymptomatic or is elderly, frail, or has an unacceptable level of medical risk to undergo another surgical procedure, chronic suppressive antibiotic therapy alone with retention of the implanted prosthesis is an option. In the setting of an acute prosthetic infection with a typical bacterial pathogen, irrigation and debridement with polyethylene exchange and retention of components is currently considered the standard of care. For patients who have already undergone stage I with implantation of an articulating spacer, retention of the spacer as definitive treatment can be an alternative to second-stage reimplantation.[4–8] This is typically seen in patients who are low demand, have severe medical comorbidities, or who decline a second-stage reimplantation due to satisfactory symptoms and/or function with their retained spacer.

59.5 Preoperative Preparation/ Positioning

59.5.1 Infectious Workup

Wound Appearance

The surgical wound is evaluated for signs of infection including erythema, warmth, delayed closure with drainage, fistula formation, or subcutaneous fluid collection. The location of the prior incision can have ramifications with regard to surgical planning and the approach for explantation and spacer placement.

Imaging

Standard shoulder radiographs consisting of a true anteroposterior (AP; Grashey) view and axillary lateral view are obtained and evaluated for signs of humeral or glenoid component loosening. Further imaging workup in these cases often includes CT scan with or without intra-articular contrast to assess the soft-tissue envelope, glenoid and humeral bone stock, and prosthetic positioning and version, and to plan extraction of the current implant.

Labs

Blood laboratory values are obtained evaluating for leukocyte count, ESR, and CRP. If hematogenous origin is suspected, blood cultures can also be obtained.

Aspirate

We prefer to perform a radiographic-guided aspirate of the glenohumeral joint in order to reliably obtain an intra-articular fluid sample.

Scope Biopsy

If an aspirate is unable to identify a pathogen, an arthroscopic exploration and biopsy can be performed. A tissue sample can be obtained, the joint thoroughly irrigated, and any adhesions released.

59.5.2 Current Implants

Prior to starting any revision arthroplasty, it is imperative to know the current implants and how best to remove them. This information can be gleaned most commonly from the prior operative dictation. In a circumstance where this is not available, there are web-based sites that can be helpful in identifying unknown implants. Device-specific extraction tools and techniques should be employed to most safely and effectively remove the prior implant.

59.5.3 Positioning

With a preoperative regional block and under general anesthesia, the patient is positioned in the beach-chair position (**Fig. 59.1**). The operative arm is held securely in a pneumatic articulating device. This allows for the arm to be adjusted and held in position during implant removal and insertion, thus freeing up an assistant. Protective eyewear is applied to the patient to protect against iatrogenic injury, especially during implant removal.

59.6 Operative Technique

59.6.1 Approach

Perioperative antibiotics are held until cultures are obtained. The previous skin incision is used and extended if necessary. If the wound developed a fistula, this should be excised and the tract followed. Prior nonabsorbable sutures in the deltopectoral interval, if placed by the previous surgeon, can be helpful to reidentify the deltopectoral interval as this can be less distinct in revision procedures. Once the interval has been identified, meticulous care is taken to develop tissue planes, identify pertinent anatomic structures, and release adhesions.

59.6.2 Debridement

When implanting an antibiotic spacer, the first step requires successful removal of all previous hardware. If the previous humeral stem implant was cemented into place, it is not necessary to remove all previous cement. Doing so may lead to removing bone and compromising proximal humeral osseous integrity. Maintaining proximal humerus bone stock is vital. All devitalized tissue needs to be debrided as this provides a nidus for persistent infection. Multiple deep tissue samples are obtained and sent for culture. We prefer to send five deep tissue samples from distinct locations to optimize organism identification while limiting false-positive findings. If there is still question about the presence of infection intraoperatively, a tissue sample can be sent to pathology to quantify the number of neutrophils per high-powered field. Once all samples are obtained, perioperative antibiotics are initiated. This is followed by a thorough irrigation of the entire wound. Our preferred technique involves pulse lavage irrigation with 3 L of Betadine-infused saline, followed by 3 L of bacitracin-infused saline, and completed with 3 L of additional normal saline.

59.6.3 Spacer Implantation

Sizing

Once the debridement has been completed, preparation for the cement spacer is performed. When possible, we prefer to use a

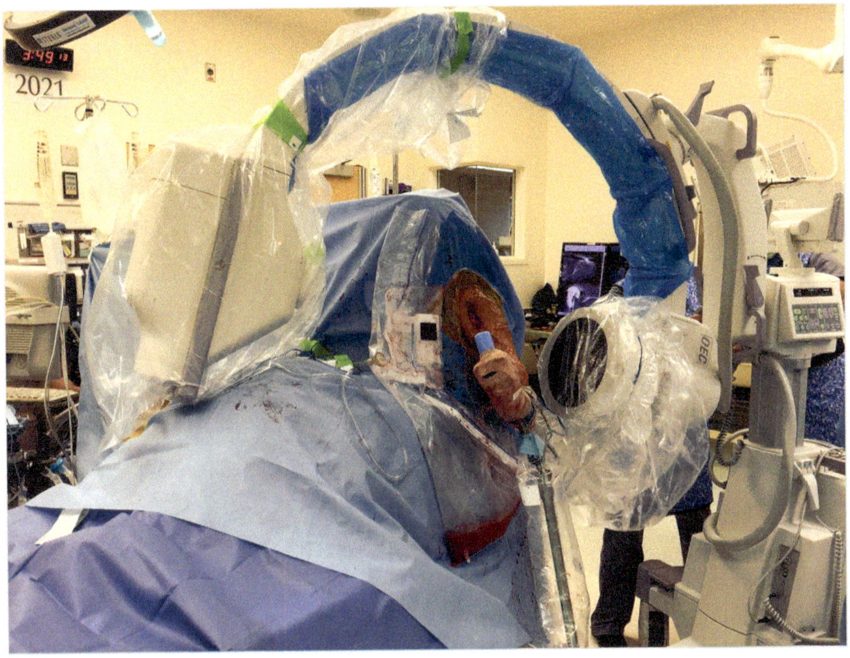

Fig. 59.1 Patient positioned in the beach-chair position. Intraoperative fluoroscopy can be used should the situation warrant.

prefabricated mold to create a spacer as will be discussed below. To prepare for this, the humeral canal is hand reamed and then trialed. The proximal humerus is gently broached, starting with the previous sized implant and sequentially increasing until a snug fit is achieved; typically, this is the size of the reamer. When malleting, use gentle strikes so as to avoid iatrogenic fracture. Beware not to remove too much proximal bone during this process.

Fabrication

Articulating or nonarticulating spacers can be placed. There are several ways to construct an articulating spacer, ranging from placing cement around the stem of a hemiarthroplasty prosthesis to hand-molding a head and stem.[2,5,9] We prefer to use a commercially available prefabricated mold (**Fig. 59.2**) to construct a uniform hemispacer constructed with antibiotic-impregnated cement with or without a central metal rebar. Antibiotic-containing methyl methacrylate cement loaded with 40 g of gentamicin is used. To this we typically add 1 to 2 g of vancomycin per 40-g polymer packet. Ideally, the choice of antibiotics is tailored to sensitivities of bacterial culture. There are, however, several limiting factors. The antibiotic must be in powdered form. Liquid antibiotics can alter the integrity of cement. It also must be heat resistant due to the exothermic reaction of polymethyl methacrylate polymerization. The cement is hand mixed as vacuum mixing can decrease the porosity of cement, which decreases the rate of antibiotic elution.[10] The powdered polymer and liquid monomer are combined and mixed, followed by the addition of powdered antibiotics. Mixing in this order increases the elution of the antibiotic.[11] If the cement is not dyed, methylene blue can be added in order to aid in removal during reimplantation (**Fig. 59.3**).

Insertion

Once the antibiotic spacer is constructed, it is time to insert. For a nonmolded spacer, it is gently hand pressed into the canal after the cement becomes firm but still moldable. This allows for the spacer to conform to the proximal humerus but decreases interdigitation

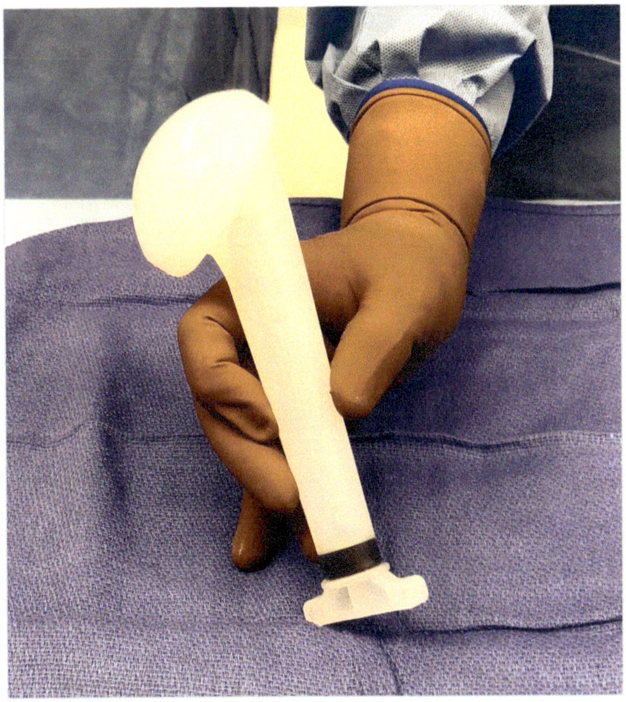

Fig. 59.2 A commercially available prefabricated mold used to construct an antibiotic cement spacer.

in order to facilitate with extraction during second-stage reimplantation. For molded spacers, we recommend allowing the cement to completely cure. In patients with good bone quality and an appropriately sized spacer, no further cement is warranted as long as a snug fit is achieved. The stem fit should be snug enough to prevent gross motion, but loose enough to allow removal at a later time. If a snug fit cannot be achieved or if the patient has poor bone quality, the cement spacer can be cemented into place. Antibiotic cement is placed around the collar of the spacer to secure it proximally, which allows for less trauma to the remaining humeral bone during second-stage spacer removal.

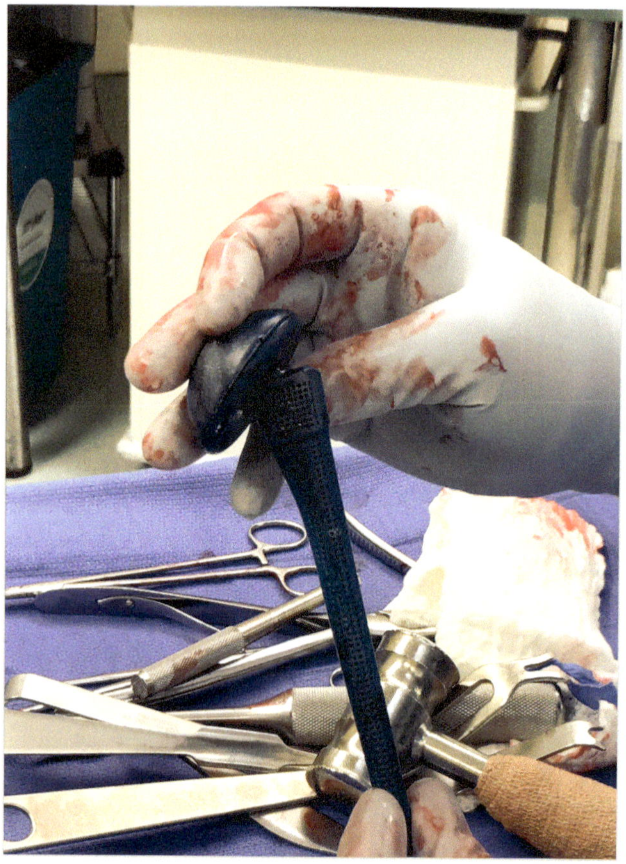

Fig. 59.3 A recently explanted antibiotic cement spacer. Note the blue coloring. This was due to methylene blue that was added during the fabrication process.

Proper positioning of an articulating spacer is imperative. If there is proximal bone loss, then the spacer should be left proud in order to provide proper soft-tissue tension. The head of the spacer should be centered and with proper version to optimize glenohumeral stability.

Closure

Typical soft-tissue closure is undertaken. If a total shoulder prosthesis was previously in place and the supraspinatus and subscapularis are intact, these should be repaired. The deltopectoral interval is closed with dyed monofilament suture in order to aid in identification during reimplantation.

59.6.4 Extraction

If the infection is believed to have been successfully eradicated and reimplantation desired, or if a revision antibiotic spacer is needed to be performed, the same approach as the initial implantation is undertaken. If the initial implantation was performed correctly, the antibiotic spacer should be able to be removed with little difficulty. If simply pulling on it is unsuccessful, several gentle taps with a tamp and mallet on the undersurface of the head should be able to dislodge it. If this is still unsuccessful, then the cement–component interface will need to be disrupted. Once the spacer has been removed, we thoroughly irrigate the joint space and remove all cement particulate.

59.7 Tips and Pearls

- When cementing in a nonmolded spacer, allow the cement to become firm but not completely hard before insertion. This will aid in later extraction.
- Maintain proper soft-tissue tension after spacer implantation.
- Have a plan for reimplantation components during the initial debridement and spacer placement. This will effect rotator cuff preservation.

59.8 What to Avoid

- If removing a cemented component, it may be necessary to leave cement in place in order to avoid removing excess bone.
- When cementing in the spacer only apply cement to the undersurface of the head.
- Avoid cementing down the canal as this will hinder extraction.
- Hand place a molded cement spacer. Do not impact it into place as this may cause fracture of the spacer.

59.9 Complications/Bailout/Salvage

59.9.1 Complications

Loss of Proximal Bone

Greater and lesser tuberosity avulsion fractures are a common complication with shoulder arthroplasty revision surgery. In the setting of revision arthroplasty, patients with intact tuberosities will have superior postoperative function.

Failure to Eradicate Infection

Even with bacterial identification, antibiotic spacer placement, and systemic antibiotic therapy, eradication of infection is not assured. If sufficient time has passed without successful infection clearance, a repeat debridement and spacer exchange may need to be performed.

Humeral Canal Perforation or Iatrogenic Fracture

If the canal is perforated or the humeral shaft fractured, this needs to be addressed at the time of spacer implant or explant. Wires rather than braided cable are used in addition to a long stemmed humeral component.

Nerve Injury

Though all peripheral nerves are at risk with shoulder arthroplasty, the axillary and radial nerves are at greatest risk due to their close proximity. The radial nerve is especially at risk with proximal humeral bone loss. Careful attention must be paid to identify and protect these nerves throughout the case.

59.9.2 Bailout/Salvage

Single Stage

If a patient cannot medically tolerate a staged reimplantation, or if an antibiotic spacer cannot be implanted, a single-stage procedure is an alternative.

Resection Arthroplasty

Resection arthroplasty has been shown to provide excellent infection control but at the expense of shoulder function.[12,13] This can be an option for patients who are medically unfit for multiple surgeries, or who have failed all other surgical options for infection eradication.

59.10 Postoperative Care

Patients are given the same postoperative rehabilitation protocol whether they have undergone insertion of an antibiotic spacer or removal of one proceeded by insertion of a final component. For the first 2 weeks, an ultrasling is maintained at all times until they are seen for their first postoperative clinic visit and their wound is assessed. They may come out of this for bathing purposes but are not to begin any passive motion exercises. For weeks 2 to 6, supervised physical therapy is initiated with the goal of two to three therapy sessions per week. Under the guidance of a therapist, passive forward flexion and external rotation exercises are initiated. These are limited to 130 and 25 degrees, respectively, for 2 weeks and then advanced as tolerated. For weeks 6 to 12, the sling may be discontinued gradually and active motion in all planes is initiated. During this time, light resistive exercises are begun. For weeks 12 and beyond, patients are encouraged to continue with flexibility exercises and begin working with light weights.

References

1. Fink B, Makowiak C, Fuerst M, Berger I, Schäfer P, Frommelt L. The value of synovial biopsy, joint aspiration and C-reactive protein in the diagnosis of late peri-prosthetic infection of total knee replacements. J Bone Joint Surg Br 2008;90(7):874–878
2. Coste JS, Reig S, Trojani C, Berg M, Walch G, Boileau P. The management of infection in arthroplasty of the shoulder. J Bone Joint Surg Br 2004;86(1):65–69
3. Sperling JW, Kozak TK, Hanssen AD, Cofield RH. Infection after shoulder arthroplasty. Clin Orthop Relat Res 2001(382):206–216
4. Stine IA, Lee B, Zalavras CG, Hatch G III, Itamura JM. Management of chronic shoulder infections utilizing a fixed articulating antibiotic-loaded spacer. J Shoulder Elbow Surg 2010;19(5):739–748
5. Levy JC, Triplet J, Everding N. Use of a functional antibiotic spacer in treating infected shoulder arthroplasty. Orthopedics 2015;38(6):e512–e519
6. Proubasta IR, Itarte JP, Lamas CG, Escribá IU. Permanent articulated antibiotic-impregnated cement spacer in septic shoulder arthroplasty: a case report. J Orthop Trauma 2005;19(9):666–668
7. Haddad S, Corona PS, Reverté MM, Amat C, Flores X. Antibiotic-impregnated cement spacer as a definitive treatment for post-arthroscopy shoulder destructive osteomyelitis: case report and review of literature. Strateg Trauma Limb Reconstr 2013;8(3):199–205
8. Themistocleous G, Zalavras C, Stine I, Zachos V, Itamura J. Prolonged implantation of an antibiotic cement spacer for management of shoulder sepsis in compromised patients. J Shoulder Elbow Surg 2007;16(6):701–705
9. Mahure SA, Mollon B, Yu S, Kwon YW, Zuckerman JD. Definitive treatment of infected shoulder arthroplasty with a cement spacer. Orthopedics 2016;39(5):e924–e930
10. Meyer J, Piller G, Spiegel CA, Hetzel S, Squire M. Vacuum-mixing significantly changes antibiotic elution characteristics of commercially available antibiotic-impregnated bone cements. J Bone Joint Surg Am 2011;93(22):2049–2056
11. Pithankuakul K, Samranvedhya W, Visutipol B, Rojviroj S. The effects of different mixing speeds on the elution and strength of high-dose antibiotic-loaded bone cement created with the hand-mixed technique. J Arthroplasty 2015;30(5):858–863
12. Verhelst L, Stuyck J, Bellemans J, Debeer P. Resection arthroplasty of the shoulder as a salvage procedure for deep shoulder infection: does the use of a cement spacer improve outcome? J Shoulder Elbow Surg 2011;20(8):1224–1233
13. Weber P, Utzschneider S, Sadoghi P, Andress HJ, Jansson V, Müller PE. Management of the infected shoulder prosthesis: a retrospective analysis and review of the literature. Int Orthop 2011;35(3):365–373

Table 60.1 Types of platform shoulder arthroplasty systems commercially available

In-side or Inlay	On-top or Onlay
Depuy Global Unite (Warsaw, IN) Integra Titan (Plainsboro, NJ) Smith & Nephew PROMOS (Cordova, TN) SMR Lima (Arlington, TX)	Tornier Aequalis Ascend Flex (Stafford, TX) Zimmer-Biomet Comprehensive (Warsaw, IN)[a] Exactech Equinoxe (Gainesville, FL) Lavender Medical UNIC Evolutis (Briennon, France) DJO Turon (Austin, TX) Stryker ReUnion (Mahwah, NJ)

[a]Also has a humeral tray to use in conjunction with a Bio-Modular stem to convert to a reverse total shoulder arthroplasty.

an "In-side" or "Inlay" system or an "On-top" or "Onlay" system. Inlay systems have a modular body that connects to the humeral stem, whereas Onlay systems have no modular component. Rather, the humeral tray connects directly to the stem. Several of the currently available components are listed in **Table 60.1**. The modular body in Inlay systems allows for more flexible optimization of implant height and version. Onlay systems with malpositioned stems (either too proximally or retroverted) may result in unacceptable lengthening of the humerus or persistent instability. Finally, stem retention is obviously contraindicated when the stem is loose or when there is concern for infection.

Contraindications that apply to all revision situations include active infection, axillary nerve deficit, compromised deltoid function, and inadequate glenoid bone stock to support a glenosphere. Indolent infections should always be considered in revision shoulder arthroplasty and unexpected positive cultures frequently occur. *Propionibacterium acnes* is a frequent culprit and presents indolently with pain and may be difficult to culture.

60.5 Preoperative Planning/ Position

60.5.1 History and Physical

Preoperative planning for revision shoulder arthroplasty begins with a detailed history and physical examination. Important aspects of the history address the nature of the patient's symptoms that prompted the initial surgical intervention, postoperative complications (wound issues, dislocation, fracture, etc.), subsequent procedures, and whether a pain-free interval existed postoperatively. Additionally, it is imperative to obtain previous surgical records. This will indicate whether the primary system is convertible and may describe the integrity of the rotator cuff during the index procedure. The presence of inflammatory arthropathy is important to elucidate since this may increase the risk of progressive rotator cuff insufficiency. Physical examination should focus on evaluating for signs of indolent infection, as well as the overall function of the deltoid, with a particular focus on internal and external rotation strength.

60.5.2 Labs and Imaging

Routine labs and imaging studies are part of our standard preoperative evaluation in revision shoulder arthroplasty. A complete blood count (CBC), erythrocyte sedimentation rate (ESR) and C-reactive protein (CRP) are obtained to evaluate for infection. If the ESR and CRP are elevated, we will typically obtain an image-guided shoulder aspiration and culture with a special attention for anaerobic cultures and P. acnes. In addition to a standard shoulder plain film series, CT is often useful to assess the degree of glenoid bone loss, component version, and deformity. The integrity of the glenoid bone stock may influence the type of implant (i.e., augmented baseplate) and the need for bone graft. Metal subtraction MRI sequencing (MARS) can also be obtained to evaluate the integrity of the rotator cuff.

60.5.3 Patient Positioning

We prefer to position patients in the beach-chair position with the back elevated approximately 40 degrees. A wedge pillow placed underneath the thighs helps facilitate the seated position and provide stability. The patient is positioned with the operative extremity over the lateral aspect of the table, which allows for adequate humeral access during adduction and extension of the extremity. We also place a rolled towel behind the medial border of the scapula, which enhances glenoid exposure. It is critical to assure that the arm can be sufficiently extended to allow for humeral canal access and instrumentation free of interference from the patient's head. With the patient positioned, we routinely perform an examination under anesthesia to assess for forward flexion and external rotation. The patient is then prepped and draped to allow maximum exposure of the extremity. We also routinely use a hydraulic mechanical arm holder to aid in positioning of the extremity during the procedure.

60.6 Operative Technique

60.6.1 Approach

We prefer to use a deltopectoral approach as it is extensile and reliably results in excellent visualization. Most patients will have a previous deltopectoral incision, which can often be utilized. The incision is made from just proximal and lateral to the coracoid process extending toward the deltoid tuberosity. This can be extended distally down the anterolateral aspect of the arm to allow for a brachialis split if a larger exposure is needed. The incision is carried deep to the subcutaneous tissue down to but not through the underlying deltopectoral fascia. Care is taken to identify the cephalic vein, which we tend to laterally as this disrupts less tributaries. Scar tissue often distorts the surgical approach, so it is important to reestablish soft-tissue planes through a combination of electrocautery and blunt dissection. Working from normal tissue planes proximal or distal to the previous dissection helps establish the correct intermuscular plane in the scarred regions.

The deltopectoral interval is then developed through blunt dissection. The pectoralis major is retracted medially, while the deltoid is retracted laterally. The subdeltoid space is often firmly adhered to the lateral aspect of the proximal humeral prosthesis. A finger placed deep to the deltoid and lateral to the humeral component can break up adhesive scar tissue. This step is critical to help mobilize the humerus. Next, we identify the lateral border of the conjoined tendon. The tendon of the pectoralis major is often firmly scarred to the conjoined tendon. We develop this interval through blunt dissection with the arm adducted to minimize the risk of neuropraxia to the musculocutaneous nerve. After mobilization of these layers, we retract the conjoined tendon medially to identify the subscapularis. External rotation of the arm brings the subscapularis into the field and farther from the axillary nerve. If the subscapularis is present, it can be detached several ways. In a revision setting, we prefer to peel the subscapularis off the lesser tuberosity subperiosteally while preserving maximum tendon length for eventual repair.

A capsulotomy is made with electrocautery while progressively externally rotating, extending, and adducting the arm. This maneuver allows exposure of the medial and proximal aspects of the humeral component while maximizing the distance between our dissection and the nearby neurovascular structures. We do not routinely dissect out the axillary nerve; however, it is imperative to palpate the nerve and perform a "tug test" throughout the procedure to be cognizant of its location. A circumferential exposure of the proximal humeral component can be obtained by releasing any remaining subscapularis or inferior capsule that precludes adequate external rotation. A circumferential release of the subscapularis tendon is performed by excising the underlying capsule to allow for normal tendon excursion for later repair.

60.6.2 Humeral Exposure and Preparation

Retractors are placed to bring the humeral component anteriorly into the operative field. It is often necessary to remove osteophytes, cement, and surrounding soft tissue to provide adequate exposure of the prosthesis. The humeral head component can be removed at this point using various extraction devices to disengage the head from either the stem (Onlay prosthesis) or the modular body (Inlay prosthesis). Following humeral head removal, we routinely send multiple samples to pathology for intraoperative culture and frozen section. The number of neutrophils per high power field can be assessed on the frozen section and is a reasonable indicator for infection. Any greater than 5 neutrophils per high-power field is a cause for concern and may warrant aborting the conversion in lieu of a resection and antibiotic spacer placement.

Onlay prostheses allow for a more direct conversion from an ATSA to an RTSA. Once the humeral head component is disengaged from the stem, the reverse humeral tray can be inserted directly onto the humeral stem without the need for additional reaming of the proximal humeral metaphysis. Most systems have humeral trays with several different offsets and thicknesses, which can be combined with polyethylene liners of various thicknesses to optimize the stability of the implant while minimizing impingement.

The ability to adjust humeral length and version may be more limited with Onlay components. For humeral stems that are malpositioned too proximally, the resulting humeral length and deltoid tension created by the thickness of the humeral tray and polyethylene may preclude stem retention. Overtensioning the deltoid can have deleterious consequences as this results in increased load on the glenosphere and scapular spine, which potentially may result in glenoid component loosening and fatigue fractures of the acromion/scapular spine. Similarly, the humeral version is dictated by the position of the anatomic stem. Some systems have the capacity to adjust the humeral version to a certain degree by modifying the humeral tray. However, this modest adjustment may not be sufficient in cases of excessive retroversion. If the height or version preclude a simple conversion, the anatomic stem needs to be removed.

Inlay prostheses require additional humeral preparation to convert from an ATSA to an RTSA; however, ultimately they have more versatility compared to Onlay components. After removal of the humeral head, the modular body needs to be removed. We prefer to use a flexible osteotome to separate any bony ingrowth between the body of the humeral stem and the proximal humeral metaphysis. Flexible osteotomes are thinner and more maneuverable, ultimately allowing more of the proximal humeral bone stock to be preserved. This step is critical for cemented as well as uncemented components as circumferential separation of the body from the humerus is necessary for safe component removal.

Following removal of the modular body, the overall position of the humeral component needs to be assessed prior to preparing the proximal humeral metaphysis for the reverse body component. If the humeral component is malpositioned too proximally, one can address this in one of two ways: additional resection of the proximal humerus or by adjusting the height of the modular body component. One of the unique benefits of the Inlay system is that additional humeral resection can be performed without interfering with the well-fixed stem distally.

Another benefit of the Inlay prosthesis is that the modular body for the RTSA can be reoriented and therefore is not limited by the humeral version from the index procedure. Prior to reaming, it is often necessary to remove bone from the proximal lateral metaphysis with a rasp or rongeur to avoid conflict with the reamer guide, which may push the components into varus. During reaming, the guide must be collinear to the axis of the humeral stem. While the typical humeral version for ATSA is between 30 and 40 degrees of retroversion, our goal for RTSA is between neutral and 20 degrees of retroversion. Therefore, it is important to preferentially ream more bone anteriorly to achieve the desired version. Once reaming is complete, it is important to debride between the proximal metaphysis and the humeral stem to remove interposed soft tissue, which may potentially obstruct the Morse taper. After preparation of the proximal humerus is complete, a trial reverse body can be placed on to the well-fixed stem.

60.6.3 Glenoid Revision

Glenoid component revision from an ATSA to an RTSA is largely dependent on the glenoid fixation as well as the initial implants used. Glenoid component loosening is a common indication for revision arthroplasty. In these instances, one may have to address issues pertaining to bone loss and component malposition. Preoperative CT is helpful to assess the location and degree of bony insufficiency. We find this particularly useful as it will often direct the need for bone grafting and may influence our choice in baseplate. Certain platform shoulder systems use metal-backed glenoid components, which allow for a straightforward conversion to a glenosphere. However, it is more common to encounter either loose or well-fixed cemented all-polyethylene glenoids.

60.6.4 Glenoid Exposure and Preparation

Revision of the glenoid component starts with obtaining excellent exposure. The humeral component must be protected as it is mobilized posteriorly. Retractors are placed to expose the glenoid. A thorough circumferential soft-tissue release along the margins of the glenoid is necessary. In particular, a meticulous release of all scar tissue along the anterior and inferior rim of the glenoid is critical to ensure eventual accurate component placement. If the glenoid component is grossly loose, it can often be removed easily along with adherent cement. Well-fixed components can be more challenging; however, the ultimate goal is to remove the component and cement while preserving as much bone as possible.

Removal of the glenoid component is first attempted by separating the component en bloc from the glenoid with an osteotome. It is critical to approach the component parallel to the component–glenoid interface as angulation may result in violation of the glenoid vault and compromise valuable bone stock. If obtaining the ideal starting position is compromised, it is safer to remove the component in a piecemeal fashion. Once the component is removed, the remaining cement can be removed with an osteotome or a rongeur.

It is essential to assess the remaining glenoid bone stock following component and cement removal. The location and degree of bone loss will often dictate further management. Central contained defects are most easily managed with simple bone grafting. These defects do not typically result in problems with fixation since the majority of glenoid baseplates have options for central as well as peripheral fixation. Conversely, large unconstrained defects may require a structural bone graft in order to provide enough mechanical support to allow for adequate baseplate fixation. In these instances, we prefer to use iliac crest bone graft. Finally, for glenoids with asymmetric bone loss, augmented glenoid baseplates provide a good option to optimize fixation and glenosphere position.

The remainder of the glenoid preparation as well as baseplate and glenosphere placement is similar to that of a primary RTSA with a few notable differences. We tend to hand ream the glenoid in order to preserve valuable bone stock. Additionally, for revision situations we are typically more inclined to use a larger central peg with longer peripheral screws for the baseplate and will also frequently use a larger glenosphere. While the use of a larger glenosphere may potentially reduce maximum mobility, it is advantageous for increasing the stability of the prosthesis. We position the glenosphere low on the glenoid with inferior offset and tilt in order optimize function while increasing anterior translation and clearance to prevent notching.

60.6.5 Final Assessment and Closure

Following placement of the final components, it is important to assess overall joint stability, impingement, and range of motion. Joint stability is tested by observing distraction with the shuck test as well as stability throughout the range of motion, particularly with the arm in extension. We evaluate for impingement in abduction and throughout the functional range of motion. The wound is copiously irrigated and closed in a layered fashion. We routinely place a deep drain next to the implant. We also obtain postoperative radiographs of the shoulder and the entire humerus.

60.7 Tips and Pearls/Expert Suggestions

- Preoperative planning is critical, including a thorough history and physical examination.
- Preoperative CT is very useful for detecting and assessing the location and extent of bone loss.
- Routinely send multiple specimens to pathology to evaluate for an unexpected infection. Be prepared to perform a staged resection arthroplasty if the frozen section is suggestive of infection.
- Have a low threshold to remove the humeral stem if retention is not possible without overlengthening the humerus or if there is persistent instability.
- If a cemented stem is loose and needs to be removed, it can be recemented in the previous cement mantle, thereby avoiding the need for complete cement removal.

60.8 What to Avoid

Converting from an ATSA to an RTSA while retaining the humeral stem can be an effective procedure; however, one must be cognizant of its limitations. The main limitation to this procedure is retaining a stem that is malpositioned either proximally or in excessive retroversion. Often this can be corrected to provide a stable joint without overlengthening the humerus. Retaining a well-fixed stem that results in persistent instability or overlengthening of the humerus can have deleterious consequences such as neuropraxia, premature glenoid loosening, and iatrogenic fatigue fracture.

60.9 Complications/Bailout/Salvage

One of the most common situations necessitating a bailout procedure is when the humeral stem cannot be retained due to either unexpected loosening or proximal malposition resulting in overlengthening of the humerus. In both instances, the surgeon must be prepared to extract the stem and perform additional procedures such as a humeral shaft corticotomy if the stem is well fixed and cannot be removed more conservatively. Furthermore, the surgeon must be prepared to deal with intraoperative fracture necessitating fixation and possibly revision with a long humeral stem. Finally, if the intraoperative frozen section is concerning for infection, the surgeon should be prepared to do a staged resection arthroplasty with an antibiotic spacer.

60.10 Postoperative Care

Our postoperative protocol for revision shoulder arthroplasty when using a platform system to convert from an ATSA to an RTSA with retention of the humeral stem is similar to that of a primary RTSA unless it is a complex revision. A deep drain may be left in place for at least 24 hours. We instruct patients to avoid external rotation beyond neutral with their arm at their side. We allow them to perform the Codman pendulum exercises in a sling. By 2 to 3 weeks postoperatively, we allow patients to initiate forward flexion in the scapular plane to approximately 100 degrees.

Part IV

Trauma

61 Open Reduction and Internal Fixation for Proximal Humerus Fracture

Johanna C.E. Donders, Lionel E. Lazaro, Danielle N. Sin, and Dean G. Lorich

Abstract

Proximal humerus fractures are the third most common fracture in the elderly population, and often need operative treatment. Despite improved surgical techniques including locking plates, fixation failure still occurs due to poor bone stock. Modified surgical techniques including enhanced exposure through tenodesis of the long head of the biceps, and the use of intramedullary fibula allograft for augmented construct stability increase successful fracture fixation.

Keywords: *humerus, fracture, ORIF*

61.1 Goals of Procedure

The goal of this procedure is to anatomically restore the proximal humerus, creating a stable enough construct to allow early mobilization and ultimately a return to full function.

61.2 Advantages

Proximal humerus fractures (PHFs) typically occur in patients older than 60 years, often with poor bone quality.[1]

The development of locking plate and angle stable technology counterbalance the effect of poor bone quality on fixation stability, minimizing fixation failure.[2] However, poor outcomes and postoperative complications are relatively common due to poor bone stock in the humeral head. The central portion of the humeral head is often a hollow shell of subchondral bone. Furthermore, the metaphysis is also often devoid of bony trabeculae. To circumvent poor biomechanical fixation due to compromised bone stock, we have successfully used intramedullary augmentation and inferomedial support of the calcar by placing an endosteal fibular allograft. This technique has clearly demonstrated better maintenance of reduction during healing.[2–4] Anatomic restoration of the fracture fragments helps ensure the correct position of the rotator cuff musculature. During the described surgical technique, tenodesis of the long head of the biceps is performed to facilitate fracture reduction, and likely decreases associated symptoms.

61.3 Indications

Indications include unacceptable displacement of the fracture fragments, or fracture patterns too unstable to allow early range of motion. The characteristics of the fracture (i.e., displacement and angulation of the parts more than 1 cm or more than 45 degrees) and the patient are the most important decisive factors on whether to operate or not operate.

61.3.1 Relative Indications[5,6]

- Greater than 5 mm displacement of either one of the tuberosities.
- Marginal articular fracture with greater than 2 mm of displacement.
- Greater than 100% displacement of the surgical neck.

61.4 Contraindications

Patients who are unfit for anesthesia or unable to engage in postoperative rehabilitation protocols are contraindicated for this procedure. The experience has been that these patients due to either physical or mental illness do not receive sufficient benefit from operative treatment.

Other contraindications are the following:

- An unreconstructable humeral head (significant head split, or multiple articular fragments).
- A devascularized humeral head (no soft-tissue attachment to the articular segment, calcar length less than 8 mm, and disruption of the medial hinge).

61.5 Preoperative Preparation/ Positioning

Plain radiographs (including an anteroposterior [AP], scapular Y, and axillary views) and a 3D CT scan should be obtained for each patient prior to surgical intervention and used for planning (**Fig. 61.1a–c**). The condition of the calcar, bone quality, and displacement pattern should be noted. MRI may be useful when rotator cuff tears and labral lesions are suspected.[2,7–9]

The patient is placed in the sloppy lateral position on a radiolucent table, in which patients are angled 30 to 40 degrees above the lateral with assistance of a beanbag (**Fig. 61.2**). With the patient in this position, the surgeon has access to the anterior, posterior, and the lateral aspects of the proximal humerus. It also presents the anterolateral aspect of the shoulder directly to the surgeon. The image intensifier (C arm) is placed on the opposite side of the table and draped into the sterile field. With the C arm rotating between 45 degrees rollback and 45 degrees rollover views, orthogonal fluoroscopic images and scapular Y views are easily obtained with little movement of the arm. Prior to draping the patient, the ability to obtain all intraoperative views with the C arm is checked. We do not use an arm holder.

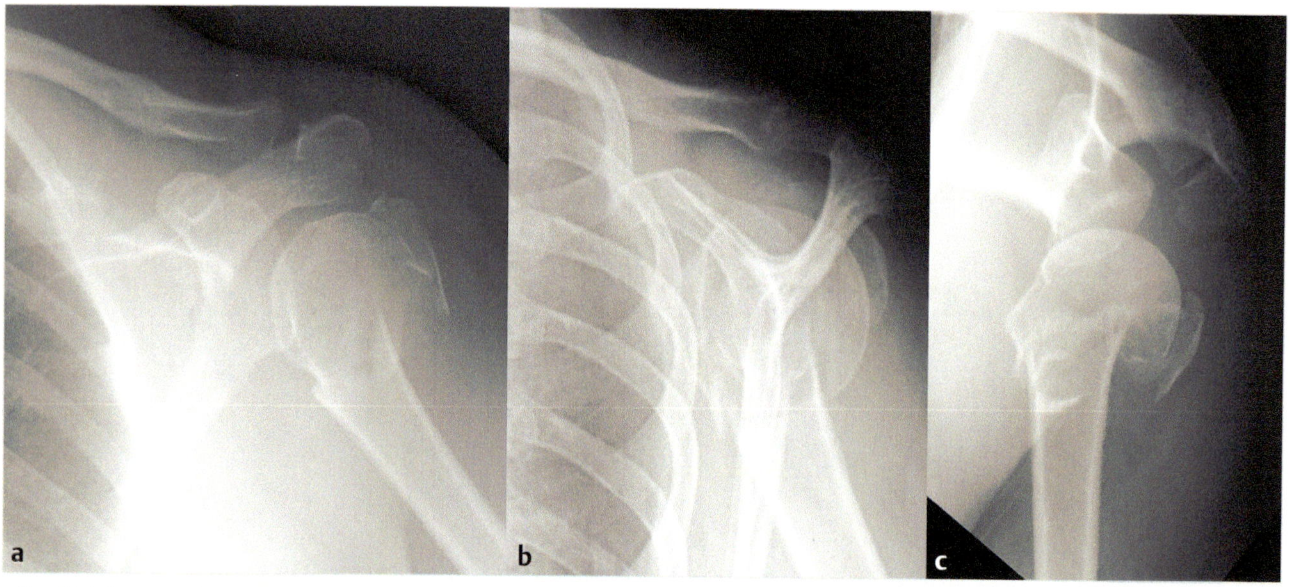

Fig. 61.1 Preoperative preparation. **(a-c)** Plain radiographs in anteroposterior (AP), scapular Y, and axillary views are obtained prior to surgical intervention and used for planning.

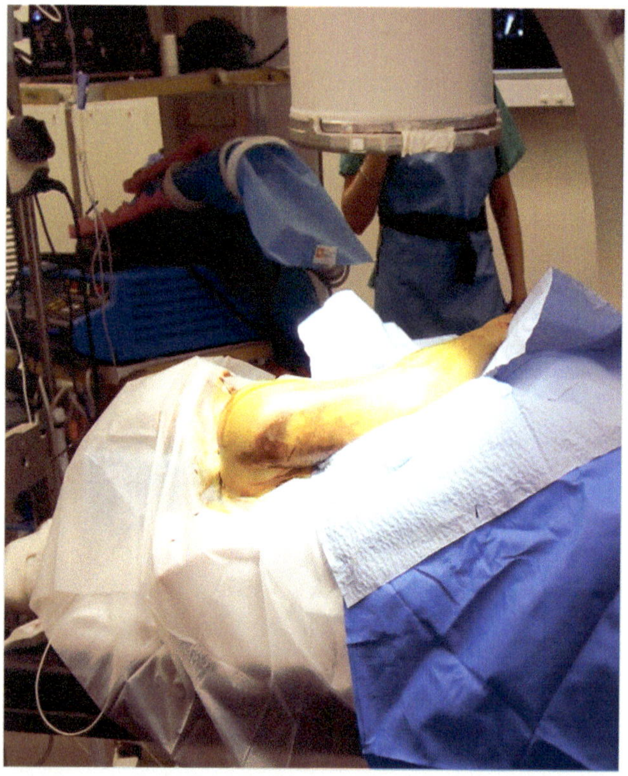

Fig. 61.2 Positioning. The patient is placed on a radiolucent table in the sloppy lateral position in which patients are angled 30 to 40 degrees above the lateral with assistance of a beanbag.

61.5.1 Alternative Procedures

Arthroplasty treatment is reserved for cases where the fracture is unreconstructable (significant head split or multiple articular fragments) or the humeral head is devascularized (no soft-tissue attachment to the articular segment, calcar length less than 8 mm, and disruption of the medial hinge). To date, we cannot accurately predict whether osteonecrosis of the humeral head will develop after a fracture. In addition, studies have suggested that revascularization of the head can occur if anatomic reduction and stable fixation is achieved.[10-13] In young patients, we always err toward a head-preserving reconstruction.

61.6 Operative Technique

Using the extensile anterolateral approach (**Fig. 61.3**), an incision is made between the anterior and middle heads of the deltoid, beginning at the anterolateral corner of the acromion and extending distally enough toward the lateral epicondyle of the humerus. The raphe between the anterior and middle head of the deltoid muscle is identified and carefully opened bluntly in line with the deltoid fibers to obtain an avascular approach (**Fig. 61.4a, b**).[14] The axillary nerve is identified approximately 6.5 cm distally to the acromion and 3.5 cm from the greater tuberosity (**Fig. 61.4c, d**).[2,8,14,15] Neurolysis is performed to mobilize and protect the nerve through the procedure. In order to gain further exposure, without disrupting the soft tissue, the rotator cuff is put into view by incising the subacromial bursa. Nonabsorbable traction sutures are placed into the three heads of the rotator cuff: subscapularis tendon, supraspinatus tendon, and infraspinatus tendon.[16] Care is taken to identify the rolled edge of the subscapularis so sutures are not placed in the rotator interval that may limit motion.

The bicipital groove is exposed and the oblique fascicle is released to expose the long head of the biceps tendon (LBTH; **Fig. 61.5a**). The LBTH is marked with stay sutures and incised at the level of the bicipital groove (**Fig. 61.5b**). The intra-articular segment of the LBTH is incised sharply from the superior labrum (**Fig. 61.5c**).[9,17] This allows much improved visualization of the fractured fragments (**Fig. 61.5d**).

61.6.1 Reduction

The fracture fragments can now be reduced. Using the sutures in the rotator cuff tendons, control of the head and tuberosity

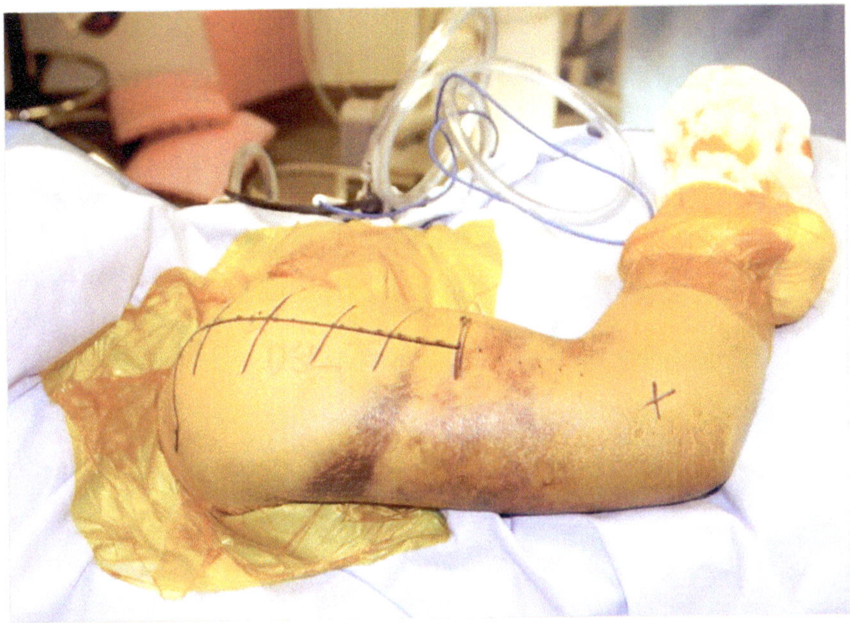

Fig. 61.3 Extensile anterolateral approach.

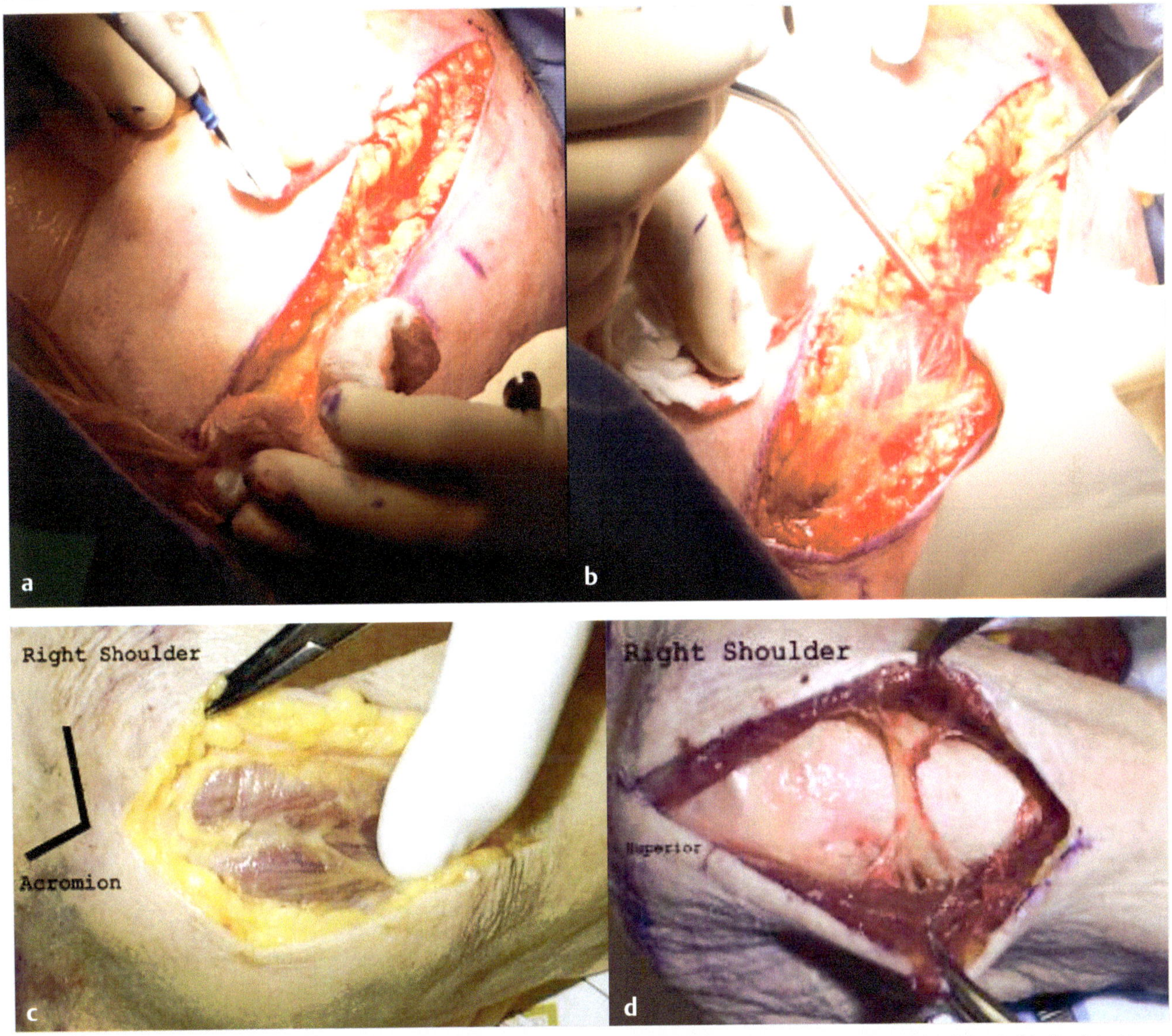

Fig. 61.4 Extensile anterolateral approach. (a) An incision is made between the anterior and middle heads of the deltoid. (b) The deltoid muscle is carefully opened bluntly in line with the muscle fibers. (c, d) The axillary nerve is identified approximately 6.5 cm distally to the acromion and 3.5 cm from the greater tuberosity.

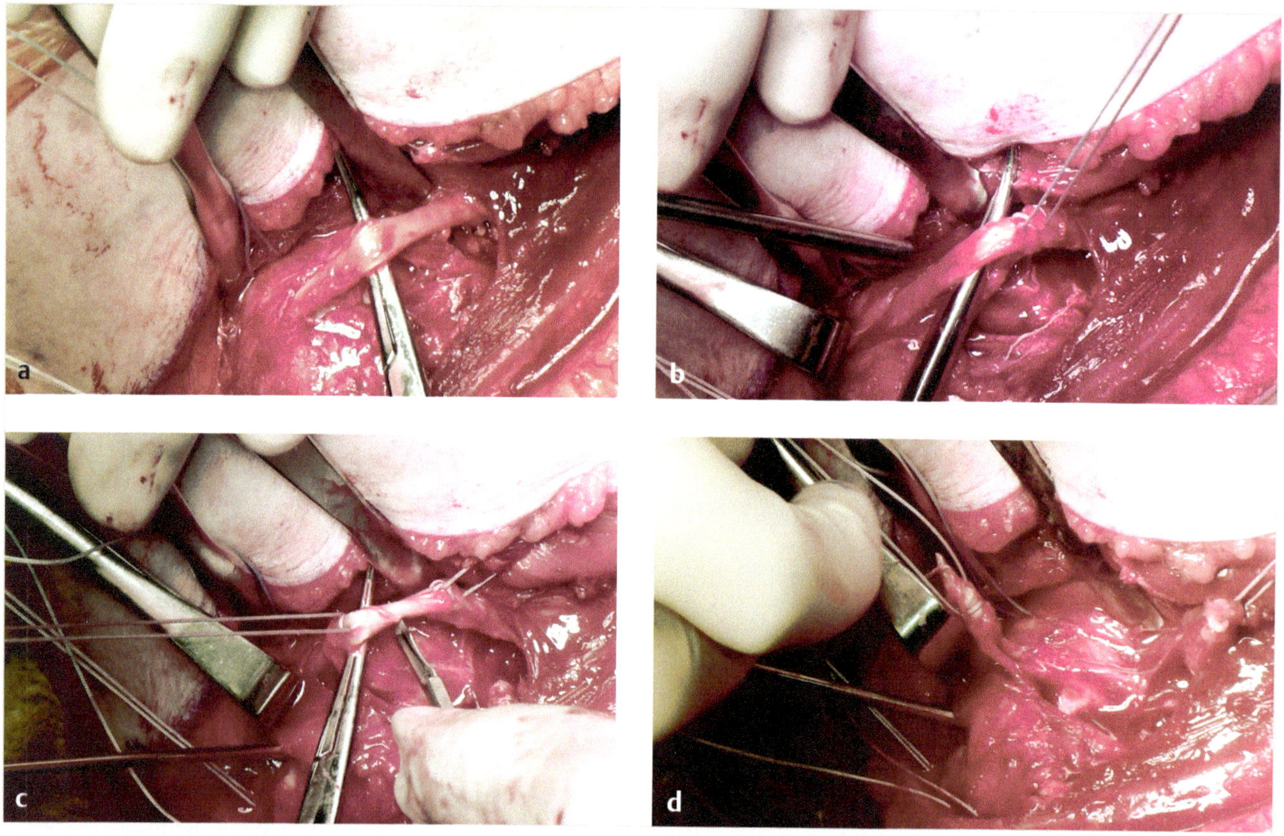

Fig. 61.5 Tenodesis of the long head of the biceps for enhanced exposure and improved fracture reduction. **(a)** The bicipital groove is exposed and the oblique fascicle is released to expose the long head of the biceps tendon. **(b)** The long head of the biceps is marked with stay sutures and incised at the level of the bicipital groove. **(c)** The intra-articular segment of the LBTH is incised sharply from the superior labrum. **(d)** Improved visualization of the fractured fragments after the tenodesis of the long head of the biceps.

fragments is obtained. Additionally, threaded K-wires and 2.5-/4.0-mm Schanz screws can be used as joysticks to assist in the reduction. An Easter plate (DePuy/Johnson & Johnson/ Synthes, Paoli, PA) is cut and prebent to accommodate the proximal humeral anatomy and placed on the bone with attention to the axillary nerve (**Fig. 61.6a**). Positioning should be performed so the distal screws would be in the most inferior aspect of the greater tuberosity into the allograft.[17] Vessels branching from the anterior and posterior circumflex arteries are undisturbed by the plating position.[14] Anterior placement is critical as it avoids vascularity coming into the humeral head. After visual and fluoroscopic confirmation of optimal plate positioning, the plate is distally transfixed with two compression screws (**Fig. 61.6b**).

The plate is now used both as template and as subsequent reduction tool, allowing the diaphyseal and metaphyseal fragments to be reduced to the plate. Using pointed reduction (Weber) clamps, the head is now reduced to the plate. Next, the tuberosities are reduced to the head while fine-tuning the metaphyseal and diaphyseal fragments. Once the plate, humeral head, both tuberosities, and shaft are both visually and fluoroscopically in the correct position (**Fig. 61.6c**), two anterior locking screws subsequently are placed as provisional fixation of the head in anticipation of placement of the fibular allograft.

The fibular allograft is then used as an intramedullary nail that fixates the head to the shaft as well as being a secure reinforcement for screws in the osteoporotic bone.[18] Using a 4.5-mm drill, an entry portal for the fibula allograft is created. The fibula allograft is then gently tamped into the intramedullary canal under fluoroscopy, taking care that the reduced fragments stay in position (**Fig. 61.6d**).

The proximal protruding part of the fibula is removed using an oscillating saw under cooling. The fibula allograft is transfixed to the humeral shaft with a 3.5-mm compression screw, capturing the graft within the canal. After radiographic imaging in the AP and lateral views, locked screws can be placed through the plate to secure the head and pass through the fibular allograft. Medial calcar support is acquired by placing locking screws into the inferomedial aspect of the humeral head fragment.[4]

Proximally, a mixture of locking and standard screws is used to further transfix the head, of which many also capture the fibular allograft. If required, an osteotome can be used to correct calcar alignment during screw fixation (**Fig. 61.6e**).

The rotator cuff sutures are then tied to the plate, thereby fixating the greater and lesser tuberosities. The distal end of the LHBT is secured to the plate as tenodesis. A keyhole is drilled in the bicipital groove using a 4.5-mm drill, and the biceps is tunneled into that hole and pulled up to the plate and fixed intraosseously (**Fig. 61.7**). Wounds are irrigated copiously and the axillary nerve is checked to ensure there is no undue tension. The rotator cuff interval and deltoid interval are closed using absorbable sutures, followed by a meticulous subcutaneous tissue and skin closure.

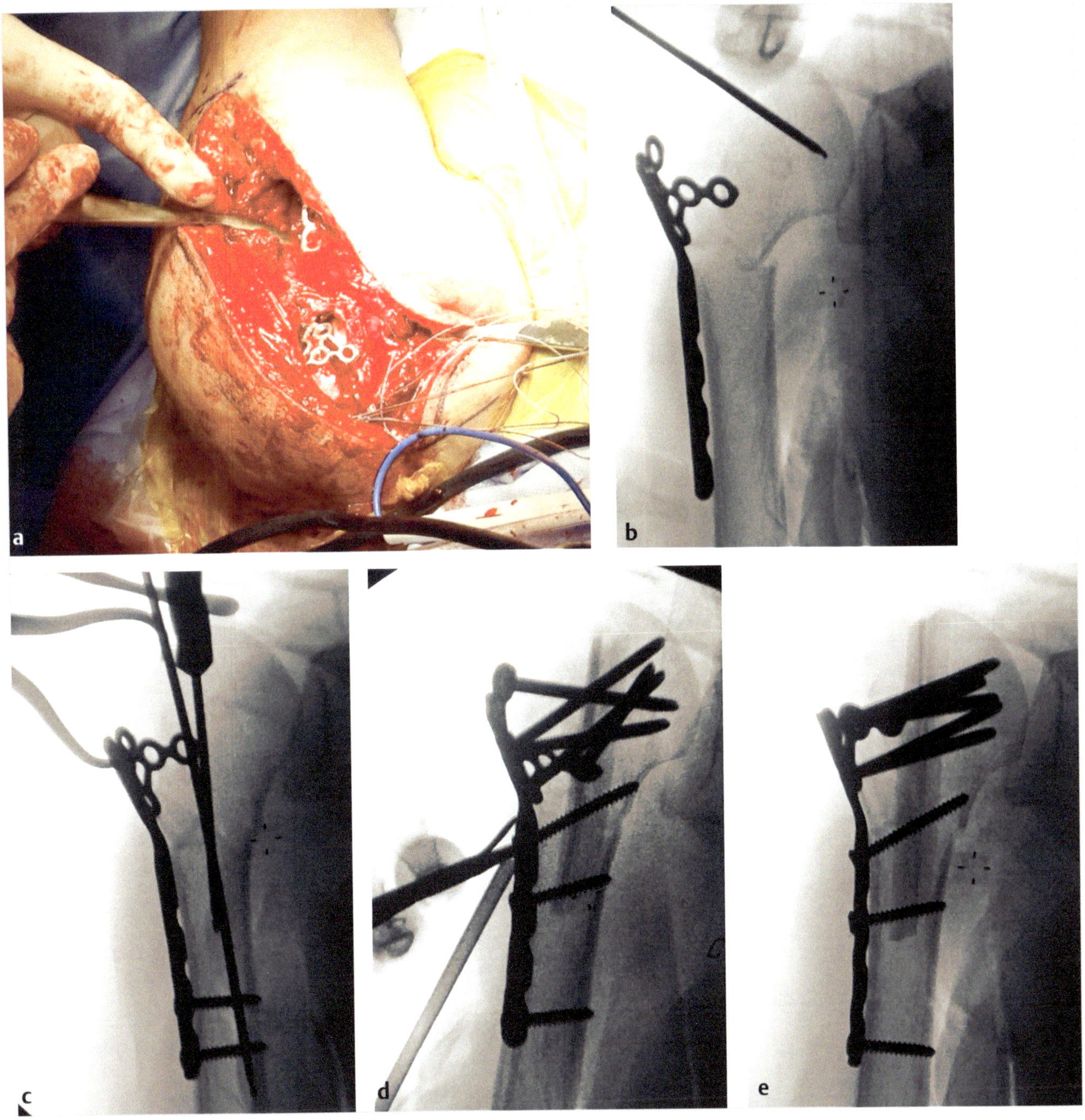

Fig. 61.6 Tenodesis of the long head of the biceps for enhanced exposure and improved fracture reduction. **(a)** The bicipital groove is exposed and the oblique fascicle is released to expose the long head of the biceps tendon. **(b)** The long head of the biceps is marked with stay sutures and incised at the level of the bicipital groove. **(c)** The intra-articular segment of the LBTH is incised sharply from the superior labrum. **(d, e)** Improved visualization of the fractured fragments after the tenodesis of the long head of the biceps.

61.7 Tips and Pearls/Expert Suggestions

Abduction of the shoulder relaxes the deltoid and facilitates exposure and reduction of the fracture.

In order to reduce the greater and lesser tuberosity fracture fragments, the sutures in the rotator cuff are used to manipulate the fragments.

The fibula allograft is shaped into the fitting model (**Fig. 61.7**). The edges of the distal aspect of the fibula are flattened with the shaver, to manipulate and move the fibula allograft and reconstruct the inferomedial calcar.

61.8 What to Avoid

- Axillary nerve damage.
- Poor reduction of the calcar.

61.9 Complications/Bailout/Salvage

Failures typically manifest as varus collapse due to the deforming pull of the rotator cuff and loss of fixation. Studies have consistently shown that reduction and support of the medial

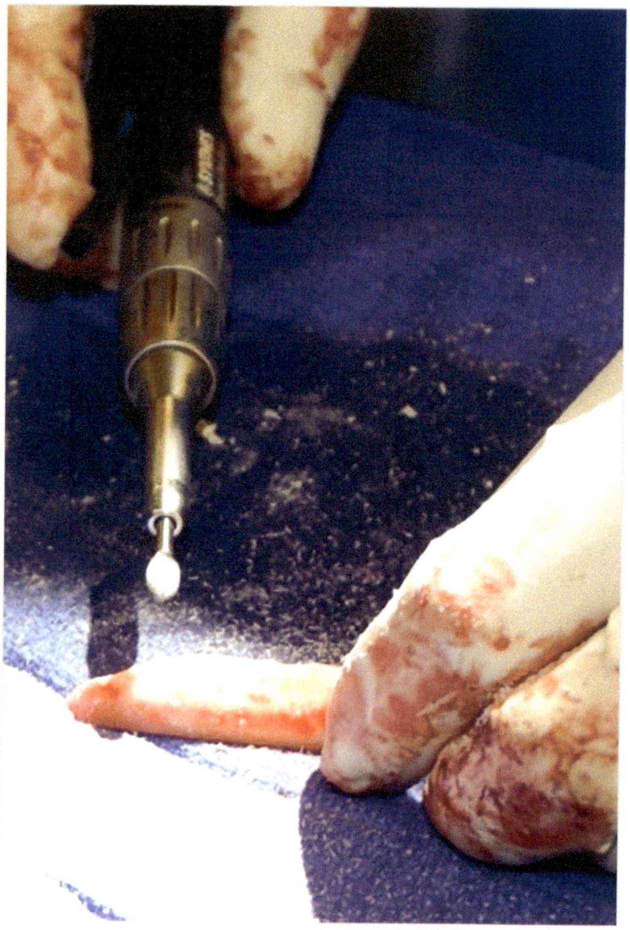

Fig. 61.7 The fibula allograft is shaped into the fitting model. The edges of the distal aspect of the fibula are flattened with the shaver.

calcar can prevent varus collapse and screw cutout. The technique as described earlier, using the allograft endosteal support to augment fixation of a laterally placed locking plate, is more versatile and allows for better screw purchase. Use of this additional augmentation minimizes the risk of postoperative loss of reduction. Avascular necrosis (AVN) is another complication seen in PHF treatment. The AVN can be partial or complete. Risk factors for AVN are fracture type, extensive soft-tissue stripping, surgical approach, and fixation failure. We have demonstrated that the posterior humeral circumflex artery is a significant contributor to the main blood supply to the humeral head. The surgcal technique as described earlier, using the extensile anterolateral approach, does not place this vascularity at increased risk. Even so, the significance of this complication is controversial.

Stiffness: Since our patients are starting with supervised motion on postoperative day 1, we rarely see stiffness in our patients.

Nonunion after a proximal humerus nonunion is uncommon. Revision surgery is compromised by poor bone stock, stiffness, and soft-tissue scarring. In the elderly patient, salvage with prosthesis is a good option. In the younger patient, revision surgery with revision plating, debridement, autologous bone grafting, and adhesiolysis of the subacromial space can be considered.

Literature on the treatment of proximal humerus malunion is even scarcer. Three types of malunions have been categorized by Beredjiklian et al. according to the presence of osseous abnormalities, including malposition of the greater or lesser tuberosity, incongruity of the articular surface, and malalignment of the articular segment.[19] Most often, malunion causes impingement of a malunited greater tuberosity fragment. An osteotomy with distalization of the malunited fragment can alleviate symptoms. With attention to detail, we feel that anatomic restoration is nearly always possible.

61.10 Postoperative Care

Average length of stay in the hospital is 2 to 3 days. Active-assisted and passive-assisted range-of-motion exercises including flexion, extension, and abduction are done twice daily under supervision of an occupational therapist starting the first day after surgery. A continuous passive motion (CPM) machine is used daily for 4 to 6 hours beginning at 45 degrees forward flexion, advancing according to the patient's tolerance. Patients are instructed to continue home stretching exercises upon discharge until their first postoperative appointment at 2 weeks. When not performing exercises, the patient can wear a sling for comfort; however, it is not necessary. The wound should not get wet during hygienic routines.

At the 2-week postoperative appointment, sutures are removed. Radiographic images including AP and lateral views are obtained at 6 weeks, 3 months, 6 months, and 1 year. Active and passive range-of-motion physical therapy is prescribed. Once the bone is fully healed, usually at 3 months, focus should be on strengthening.

61.11 Conclusion

PHFs can be treated successfully using the modified techniques for operative fixation repair that combines the enhanced exposure gained through LHBT release, with the augmented construct stability gained through an intramedullary fibula allograft.

In Memoriam: Dean Gerald Lorich, MD (1963–2017)

This chapter represents Dr. Lorich's innovation, strategy, techniques, and results of proximal humerus fracture treatment and fixation—we were just the scribes. Unfortunately, Dr. Lorich is no longer with us, but his legacy has changed our management of these injuries and will continue to leave a lasting impact on our specialty!

References

1. Berkes MB, Little MTM, Pardee NC, Schottel PC, Lazaro LE, Lorich DG. Outcomes of proximal humerus fracture open reduction internal fixation with concomitant ipsilateral shoulder girdle injuries: a case control study. HSS J 2016;12(2):105–110
2. Berkes MB, Little MTM, Lorich DG. Open reduction internal fixation of proximal humerus fractures. Curr Rev Musculoskelet Med 2013;6(1):47–56
3. Mathison C, Chaudhary R, Beaupre L, Reynolds M, Adeeb S, Bouliane M. Biomechanical analysis of proximal hu-

meral fixation using locking plate fixation with an intramedullary fibular allograft. Clin Biomech (Bristol, Avon) 2010;25(7):642–646
4. Gardner MJ, Weil Y, Barker JU, Kelly BT, Helfet DL, Lorich DG. The importance of medial support in locked plating of proximal humerus fractures. J Orthop Trauma 2007;21(3):185–191
5. Guy P, Slobogean GP, McCormack RG. Treatment preferences for displaced three- and four-part proximal humerus fractures. J Orthop Trauma 2010;24(4):250–254
6. Robinson CM, Amin AK, Godley KC, Murray IR, White TO. Modern perspectives of open reduction and plate fixation of proximal humerus fractures. J Orthop Trauma 2011;25(10):618–629
7. Khmelnitskaya E, Lamont LE, Taylor SA, Lorich DG, Dines DM, Dines JS. Evaluation and management of proximal humerus fractures. Adv Orthop 2012;2012:861598
8. Gardner MJ, Griffith MH, Dines JS, Lorich DG. A minimally invasive approach for plate fixation of the proximal humerus. Bull Hosp Jt Dis 2004;62(1-2):18–23
9. Christ AB, Gausden EB, Warner SJ, Nellestein AM, Thacher RR, Lorich DG. Rotator cuff-sparing approach for antegrade humeral nailing with biceps tenodesis: a technical trick with clinical implications. J Orthop Trauma 2017;31(2):e60–e65
10. Neviaser AS, Hettrich CM, Beamer BS, Dines JS, Lorich DG. Endosteal strut augment reduces complications associated with proximal humeral locking plates. Clin Orthop Relat Res 2011;469(12):3300–3306
11. Neviaser AS, Hettrich CM, Dines JS, Lorich DG. Rate of avascular necrosis following proximal humerus fractures treated with a lateral locking plate and endosteal implant. Arch Orthop Trauma Surg 2011;131(12):1617–1622
12. Crosby LA, Finnan RP, Anderson CG, Gozdanovic J, Miller MW. Tetracycline labeling as a measure of humeral head viability after 3- or 4-part proximal humerus fracture. J Shoulder Elbow Surg 2009;18(6):851–858
13. Bastian JD, Hertel R. Initial post-fracture humeral head ischemia does not predict development of necrosis. J Shoulder Elbow Surg 2008;17(1):2–8
14. Gardner MJ, Boraiah S, Helfet DL, Lorich DG. The anterolateral acromial approach for fractures of the proximal humerus. J Orthop Trauma 2008;22(2):132–137
15. Gardner MJ, Griffith MH, Dines JS, Briggs SM, Weiland AJ, Lorich DG. The extended anterolateral acromial approach allows minimally invasive access to the proximal humerus. Clin Orthop Relat Res 2005(434):123–129
16. Christ AB, Gausden EB, Warner SJ, Nellestein AM, Thacher RR, Lorich DG. Rotator Cuff-Sparing Approach for Antegrade Humeral Nailing With Biceps Tenodesis: A Technical Trick With Clinical Implications. J Orthop Trauma. 2017 Feb;31(2):e60-e65
17. Hettrich CM, Neviaser A, Beamer BS, Paul O, Helfet DL, Lorich DG. Locked plating of the proximal humerus using an endosteal implant. J Orthop Trauma 2012;26(4):212–215
18. Hinds RM, Garner MR, Tran WH, Lazaro LE, Dines JS, Lorich DG. Geriatric proximal humeral fracture patients show similar clinical outcomes to non-geriatric patients after osteosynthesis with endosteal fibular strut allograft augmentation. J Shoulder Elbow Surg 2015;24(6): 889–896
19. Beredjiklian PK, Iannotti JP, Norris TR, Williams G. Operative treatment of malunion of a fracture of the proximal aspect of the humerus. J Bone Joint Surg Am. 1998 Oct;80(10):1484-97

and absence of rotator muscle atrophy are necessary before opting for a hemiarthroplasty procedure.

62.3.4 The Absence of Glenoid Arthrosis

Glenoid arthrosis should be considered in the decision on whether or not to perform a hemiarthroplasty. Glenoid arthrosis is a factor when it comes to choosing between total shoulder arthroplasty and hemiarthroplasty depending on the patient's expectations of return to physical activities.

In older patients who want predictable pain relief and short-term functional outcome, studies show that total shoulder arthroplasty may be a better option. However, in younger patients (<55 years), hemiarthroplasty is a less complicated and faster procedure without the worry of glenoid wear or loosening.[6] Therefore, hemiarthroplasty is generally preferred for younger patients because they tend to expect to return to high-level activities postsurgery, for example, sports, exercise, and other physically demanding activities.[7]

62.4 Contraindications

The contraindications for hemiarthroplasty are the presence of a poor tuberosity bone stock because of a comminuted fracture or osteoporosis, preexisting rotator cuff tear, rotator cuff arthropathy, coracoacromial ligament deficiency, and glenoid arthrosis. Additional contraindications include the presence of other secondary disorders and active infections that may make surgical management a challenge.

Furthermore, candidates for hemiarthroplasty should be able to follow a very demanding rehabilitation protocol, as physical therapy is essential for achieving optimal results.

62.5 Preoperative Preparation/ Positioning

62.5.1 Preoperative Preparation

Preparation for surgery is a very important step in arthroplasty of shoulder fractures. Patient discomfort often limits radiographic analysis. Typically, a true scapular anteroposterior (AP), scapular Y, and axillary lateral radiographs are obtained to evaluate the fracture and to check whether a dislocation is present. Since radiographic images are so important, it is imperative that preparation for surgery includes preoperative radiographic planning.

The principle of restoring the native anatomy is a constant. Two critical evaluations for obtaining optimal results are the correct height and the retroversion of the implant.[8] To evaluate the appropriate humeral height, scaled radiographs of the injured and uninjured arms are necessary. On these radiographs, we should evaluate if the calcar is still present or broken. We can also measure the height of the greater tuberosity and, of course, determine the correct height of the prosthetic implant based on the uninjured arm (**Fig. 62.1**).

In certain instances, a CT scan can be obtained to better understand the fracture pattern and for reference during surgery. CT scans could be very useful for identifying the margins of fracture, as well as the tuberosity fragmentation and displacement.

During the procedure, unless there is a compromise in the vasculature, surgery should not be immediately performed through edematous skin. The best time for surgery is usually 6 to 10 days after injury. From our experience, after 20 days it gets more challenging to mobilize tuberosity fragments because of early fracture healing. If the fracture heals early, this will cause the surgery to be more challenging, requiring a more extensive dissection of both the soft tissue and bone. This extensive dissection may negatively affect the final healing of the tuberosity.

Another important factor to consider during the preoperative planning is the prosthesis design. The traditional humeral prosthesis has not been adapted sufficiently to suit the needs of proximal humerus fracture surgery. The stems can be too bulky and hence prevent anatomic reduction of the tuberosity. In addition, the stems allow only minimal contact between the tuberosity and the diaphysis. Therefore, the probability of bony union is low, and the risk of tuberosity migration and malunion is high.

Specific fracture-dedicated stems consisting of relatively little metal seem to allow unaltered tuberosities to be reduced anatomically, with more space available for bone grafting to further promote healing. Recent studies have shown better results for tuberosity healing using fracture-specific stems as opposed to conventional bulky stems.[4,9] However, other authors disagree with this theory showing only 14% of failure using a large metaphyseal volume hemiprosthesis for complicated fractures of the proximal humerus.[10] Nevertheless, a recent report showed that the use of large metaphyseal volume arthroplasty in complex proximal humerus fracture is correlated with poor results in a large amount of patients, and the tuberosity resorption was observed in 70% of cases.[11] In the light of this controversial issue, we assume that correct indications, appropriate surgical technique, and the correct implant are the mainstays to achieving a satisfactory clinical outcome.

62.5.2 Positioning

During surgery, the patient should be put in the "beach-chair" position, with the scapula supported and all bony projections padded appropriately. The arm should be freely movable. Complete arm extension and adduction should be ensured prior to starting the procedure, to achieve a good access to the medullary canal.

62.6 Operative Technique

62.6.1 Dissection and Identification

A 2.5- to 3-inch incision is placed into the deltopectoral interval. If the incision is placed well in a limited space, and specific retractors are used, this will allow the surgery procedure to go smoothly (**Fig. 62.2**). The deltopectoral interval is dissected with the arm in the abducted position. This allows for an easy identification of the deltopectoral interval. The cephalic vein is identified. We prefer to take the vein medially with the small strip of deltoid. We use the Bovie electrocautery like an elevator to assist in identifying the clavipectoral fascia.

Next, the coracoid process is identified and a small Hohmann retractor is inserted on top of the coracoacromial ligament.

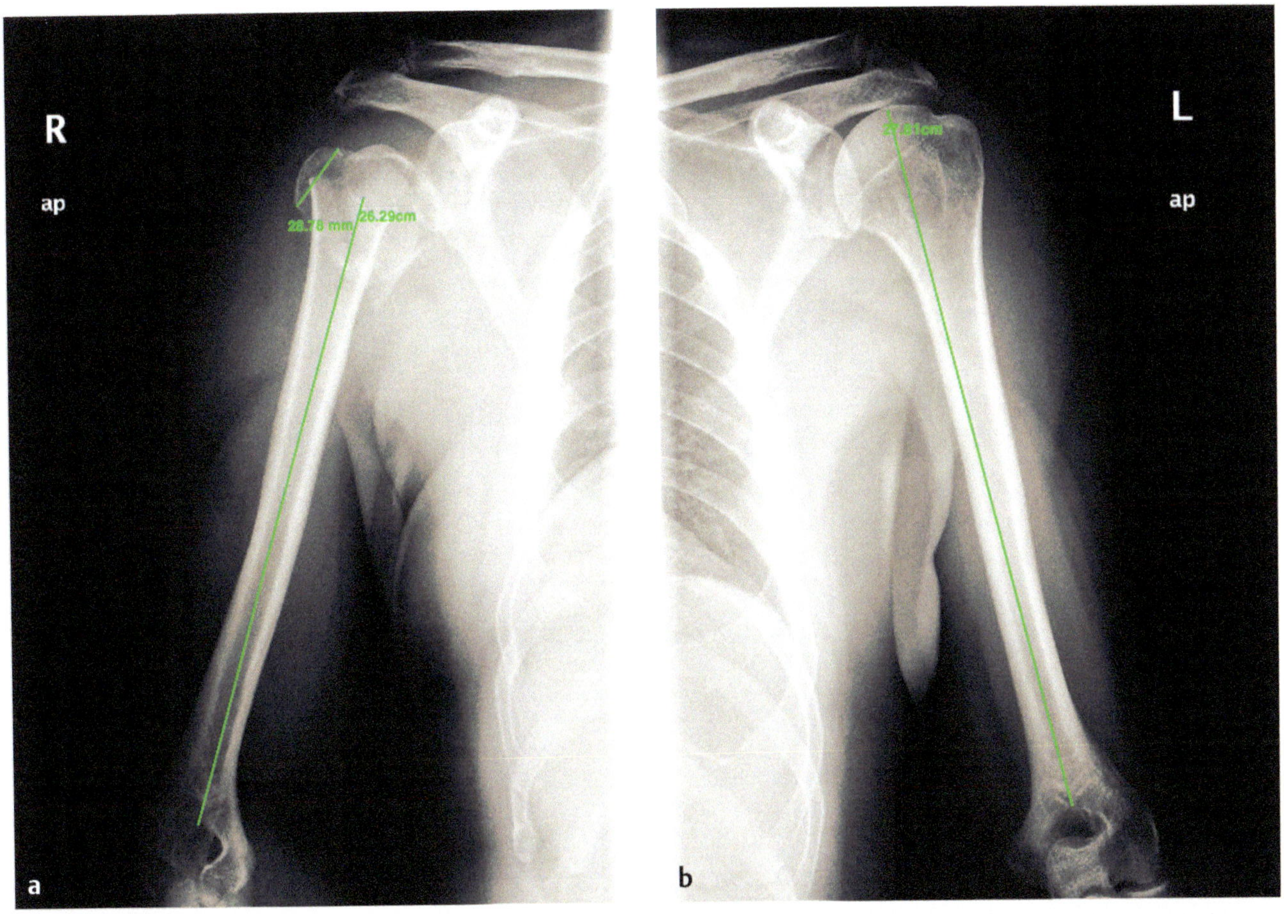

Fig. 62.1 Preoperative scaled X-ray of the fractured humerus **(a)**. Preoperative scaled X-ray of the normal, contralateral humerus. In the case of standard (not electronic) X-ray, magnification with a ruler should be utilized. The greater tuberosity should also be measured **(b)**.

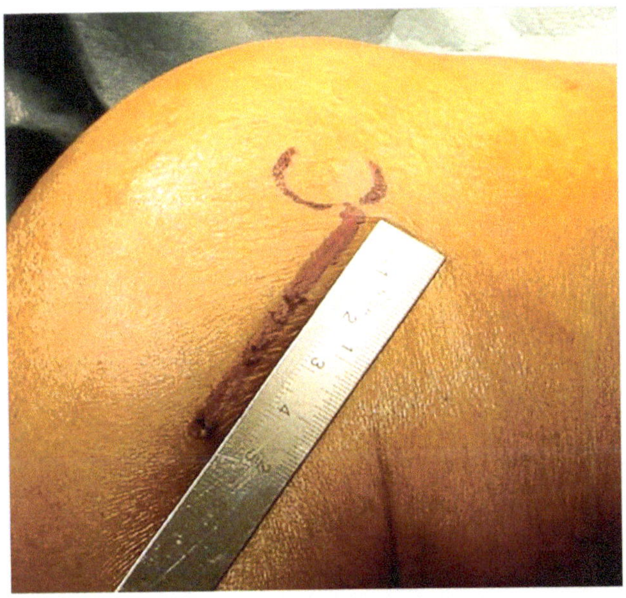

Fig. 62.2 A limited 3-inch incision placed in the deltopectoral interval is used for shoulder fracture arthroplasty.

After elevating, abducting, and internally rotating the arm, we dissect underneath the deltoid shell to identify the acromion. Once the acromion is identified, a curved retractor is inserted on top of the acromion.

With the arm in the neutral position, the conjoint tendon is located and identified. The clavipectoral fascia is cut in a lateral direction to the connected tendon. The arm is moved by slight flexion and a self-retaining retractor is used to hold the deltoid in the lateral position, as well as the conjoint tendon in the medial position.

The superior margin of the pectoral major is identified. According to some authors, this could be an anatomic landmark in verifying the height of the future implant. The arm is moved with slight internal rotation. Next, the long head of the biceps tendon (LHBT) is identified, which serves as a critical landmark for finding the interval between the tuberosities.

The bursa overlying the proximal part of the humerus should be removed. Once the LHBT is identified, it should be tagged with sutures. We perform tenodesis of the LHBT at the end of the procedure. We follow the LHBT through the rotator interval, just to the supraglenoid tubercle, and then a tenotomy is performed. The intra-articular portion of the tendon is removed.

Placing an osteotome or an elevator with a blunt end in between the tuberosities, the line of the fracture can be found. The line of fracture should be followed by going through the rotator cuff's soft tissue. It is better to follow this line instead of making a separate (iatrogenic) fracture line. If bleeding originates from the anterior humeral circumflex artery and/or from any of its supporting vessels, it can be controlled using electrocautery.

To better expose the greater tuberosity, the arm is placed in abduction and internal rotation. The greater tuberosity is gently mobilized. Next, just at the bone–tendon junction, four horizontal heavy no. 5 high-resistance nonabsorbable sutures are positioned around the greater tuberosity; two sutures are planted in the infraspinatus, while the other two sutures are placed in the teres minor (**Fig. 62.3**).

The lesser tuberosity is identified by bringing the arm in flexion and internal rotation. Two stay sutures are placed where the subscapularis meets the bone tendon. The tuberosities are retracted gently and the rotator interval is completely opened along the line of the fracture until the glenoid rim. Preservation of the coracoacromial ligament is advised to maintain the coracoacromial arch.

The humeral head fragment is located, mobilized, and taken out and measured using a caliper. It is important to measure the resected humeral head to decide the corrected size (diameter and height) of the implant. When the size falls between two measures, the smaller one should be selected. This is important to obtain an easy soft-tissue reconstruction and to avoid the chance of using an implant that is too large for the space (overstuffing), which may cause complications like glenoiditis and tendon impingement.

The glenoid surface is evaluated to see if there is some cartilage wear zone or rim fracture. If everything is good, we move on. The humeral shaft is exposed and the arm is placed in extension. Then cylindrical reamers are used to prepare the medullary canal and trial implants are inserted by increasing the diameter. During this preparation, the proximal end of the shaft should be evaluated properly and the calcar checked. If the calcar is broken or fractured, it should be fixed during preparation of the medullary canal. We prefer to fix the calcar using a cerclage technique using a Luque wire (**Fig. 62.4**).

The trial stem is placed such that the stem sits just on the medial calcar so as to restore the so-called gothic arch.[12] After determining the correct trial implant and measuring the head size, retroversion should be selected. The prosthetic head should be turned in the direction facing the glenoid. The forearm should be at the side and in neutral rotation (about 20 inches retroverted in comparison with the elbow's transepicondylar axis). Using an electrocautery or marking pen, place a mark on the lateral cortical humeral shaft. We prefer to use implants that have eccentric head offset. This allows a rotation to the most lateral position. In this position, a minimal "medial overhang" of the humerus head will be observed when the "gothic arch" is being restored.

62.6.2 Determination of Prosthetic Height

Several methods have been proposed for determining the prosthetic height during surgery. Some authors recommend measuring the distance from the superior edge of the pectoralis major to the superior aspect of the humerus head (mean, 5.5 cm).[13,14]

62.6.3 Restoration of the Gothic Arch

A technique we recommend for repairing the anatomy of the proximal humerus is the gothic arch reconstruction. The "gothic arch" forms the core of the anatomy of the proximal part of the shoulder girdle. The arch can be seen on a normal radiograph when the medial edge of the proximal humeral calcar is traced to the articular surface, and then the articular surface is traced to the lateral edge of the scapula. Join these lines together to form the classic "vaulted" or "gothic" arch shape from the medieval period renaissance architecture.

The restoration of the gothic arch requires four steps. Two of these steps are X-ray and the other two are intraoperative. These steps restore the humeral height and consequently the anatomic tuberosity, and they can be reproduced as follows:

- **Step 1**: Use the scaled X-rays of the injured and uninjured arms to allow templating of the appropriate humeral height and humeral head size.
- **Step 2**: Calculate the greater tuberosity length (G) on the computer X-ray; G should be inside the range of 3 to 5 mm of the fracture to the top of the humerus head.
- **Step 3**: Using a metal ruler, measure the actual length of the tuberosity intraoperatively. Compare the actual length to G above; it should be inside the range of 5 mm of G. This is the most important measurement and should supersede the others (if the X-ray measurements are not comparable).

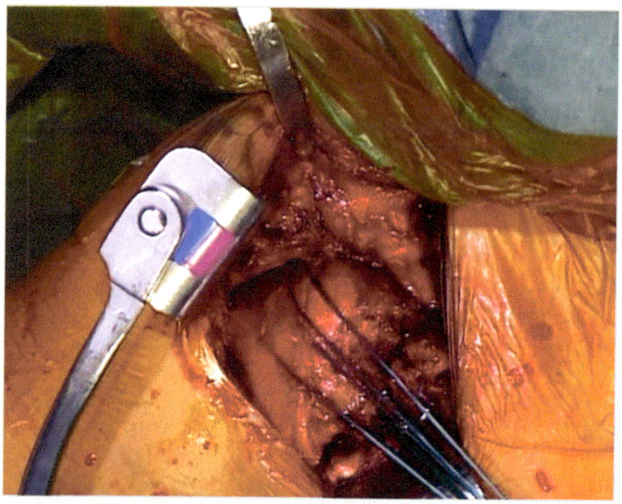

Fig. 62.3 Four heavy nonabsorbable sutures are placed around the greater tuberosity at the bone–tendon junction. The arm is placed in abduction and internal rotation for a better exposure.

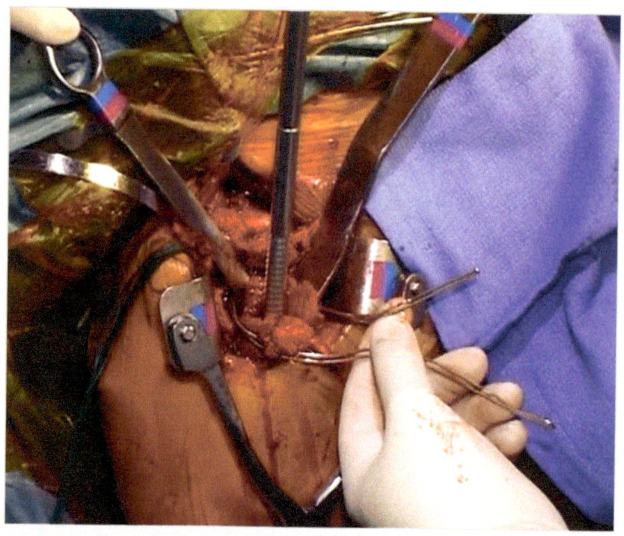

Fig. 62.4 The calcar should be identified and when disrupted should be fixed before the main procedure.

- **Step 4**: Visualize the gothic arch intraoperatively. Once the above measurements are completed and a mark is correctly placed on the prosthetic implant, insert the implant into the humeral shaft with the chosen trial head. Do not disregard the lateral half of the gothic arch that connects the medial calcar of the humerus to the inferior edge of the anatomic neck.

If the arch cannot be seen, then it means that either the prosthetic height is not correct (the most common operational error) or the medial calcar is fractured. It could also be that the head size is either too large or not rotated into the most "lateral" offset position, which can cause medial "overhang" of the inferior portion of the prosthetic head (the next most common operational error; **Fig. 62.5**). At this point, before definitive cementation, we recommend putting the arm in neutral position and either conducting a trial X-ray or producing a fluoroscopic image to show that the gothic arch has been repaired.

62.6.4 Prosthetic Cementation

Before prosthetic cementation, two holes are drilled into the proximal humeral shaft. In a "horizontal mattress fashion," two no. 5 nonabsorbable heavy sutures are inserted into the two holes, respectively. The sutures are used as "tension band" sutures for final tuberosity osteosynthesis. A cement restrictor is then placed and the humeral canal is cleaned and dried. The stem is placed into the minimally cemented, predetermined depth within the humerus.

All of the cement within the proximal 1 to 2 cm of the fracture should be removed. The wedges of bone grafts that were collected from the fractured humeral head should be placed in the following locations:

- Inside the "window" of the prosthesis.
- Under the greater tuberosity at the "lateral" fin of the prosthesis.
- Under the "medial" edge of the prosthetic head, which is between the head and the neck of the implant.

Next, take the four sutures from the greater tuberosity, split them, and then pass the medial sutures around the neck of humeral stem (*lasso maneuver*; **Fig. 62.6**). At this point, reduce the prosthesis into the glenoid vault.

The spaces in between the tuberosities, prosthesis, and shaft should be packed with the autogenous cancellous bone graft from the resected humeral head. Because the healing of the tuberosities strongly affects clinical outcomes, the technique of tuberosity fixation should be as accurate as possible. We use a construct with six sutures (four horizontal and two vertical tension band sutures) to fix the tuberosities to one another as well as the prosthesis and the diaphysis, thereby maximizing interfragmentary stability (**Fig. 62.7**).

The greater tuberosity is reduced anatomically and two of the four sutures are placed rigidly over the bone graft. The remaining two sutures are passed through the subscapularis tendon from the posterior side, and then brought out through the anterior side and sutured rigidly over the medial bone graft.

The transosseous "tension band" sutures can create tension in a vertical direction. The first suture should go from the anterior through the tendons of the subscapularis and the supraspinatus. The second suture should go from the posterior through the tendons of the infraspinatus and the supraspinatus. A tenodesis of the LHBT is performed at a horizontal plane with the tubercle groove (**Fig. 62.8**). The rotator interval is closed with one or two stitches using nonabsorbable sutures with the arm maintained in abduction and 20 to 30 degrees of external rotation. After all sutures are tied, trial motion is tested to ensure stable fixation of the tuberosities of the shaft (no movements are allowed between all the structures). Next, the surgical wound is closed.

62.7 Tips and Pearls/Expert Suggestions

- Reduce and hold the tuberosities anatomically before finalizing suture fixation.

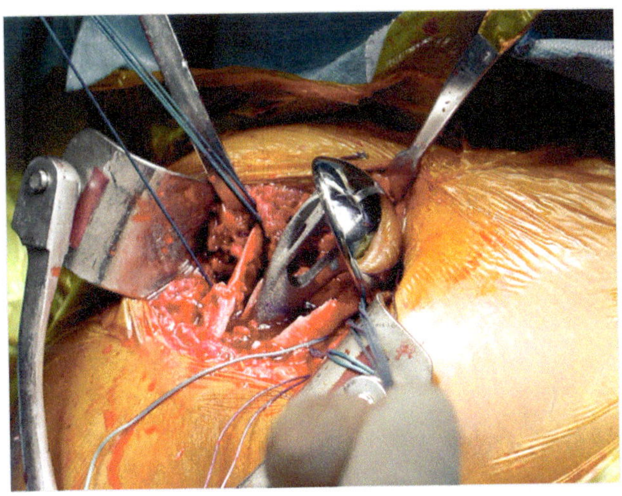

Fig. 62.5 Gothic arch restoration before final implantation is performed intraoperatively. The use of an eccentric head can help restore this arch. A ruler can be used to check the height with respect to the preoperative template and greater tuberosity height.

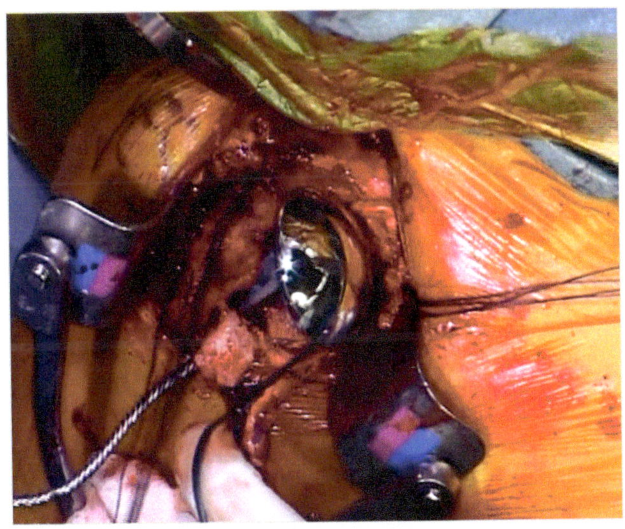

Fig. 62.6 The lasso maneuver. All the medial limbs of the four sutures previously passed through the greater tuberosity are passed around the neck of the stem of the prosthesis.

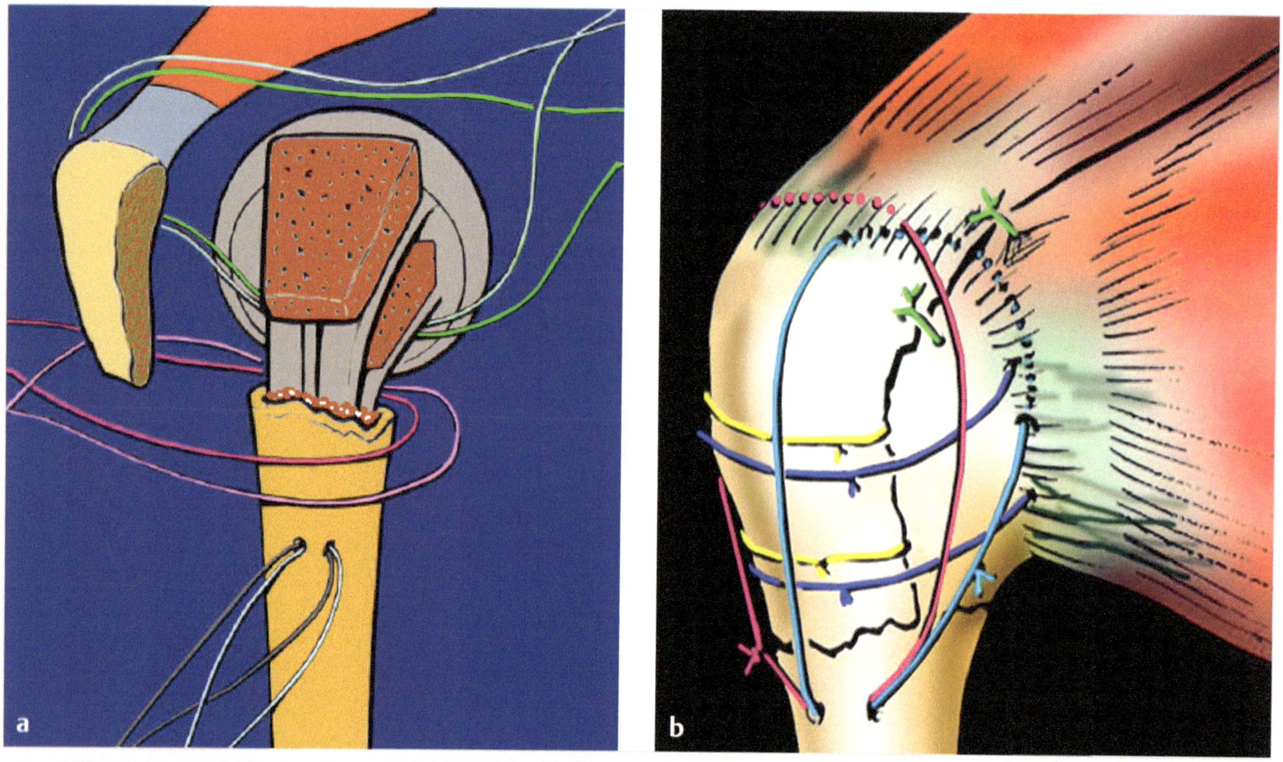

Fig. 62.7 Six-suture configuration for anatomic tuberosity fixation is shown. Four sutures are horizontal and two sutures are directed from the diaphysis and are used as tension bands (a).[12] The final construct is shown (b).[12]

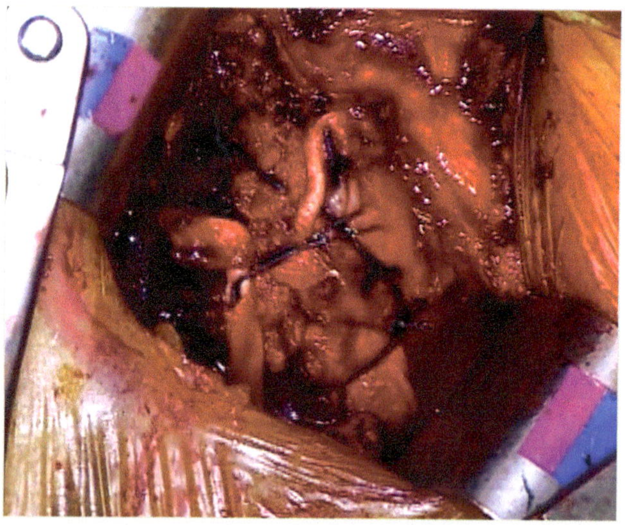

Fig. 62.8 Intraoperative view of soft tissue and long head of the biceps tendon tenodesis final repair construct is shown.

- Abduct when fixing the greater tuberosity and adduct when fixing lesser tuberosity.
- Suture fixation must cerclage the tuberosities (horizontal plane) and attach tuberosities to the shaft (vertical plane).
- Use a suture that will not cut through the bone or tissue.

62.8 What to Avoid

- Over-reduction or under-reduction of the tuberosities.
- Overtension on the sutures during fixation.

62.9 Complications/Bailout/Salvage

62.9.1 Complications

Common complications can include delay in wound healing, infection, periprosthetic fracture, heterotopic bone formation, component loosening, and glenoid erosion.[15] The specific complications related to the hemiarthroplasty used for proximal humeral fracture involve the tuberosities. These complications include migration, malunion, nonunion, and resorption.[16,17]

Another complication can arise from the use of an inappropriate implant. Inappropriate implantation can occur when the stem of the implant is too short or too tall, or when there is excessive anteversion or retroversion. Inappropriate implantation can also be due to a head diameter that is either too large or too small.

For hemiarthroplasty to be successful, the tuberosities need to be fully healed. A successful outcome depends on identifying correct indications, using proper implants, and implementing accurate surgical techniques, especially sutures.

Posttraumatic glenoid bone surface arthritis is also another complication that can reduce patient satisfaction in the long-term and decrease functionality.

62.9.2 Salvage

In the case of a failure, a salvage can be done by a conversion to a reverse shoulder arthroplasty. Therefore, the use of a convertible stem is suitable particularly in these situations because the revision surgery involves less surgical time, less complications of

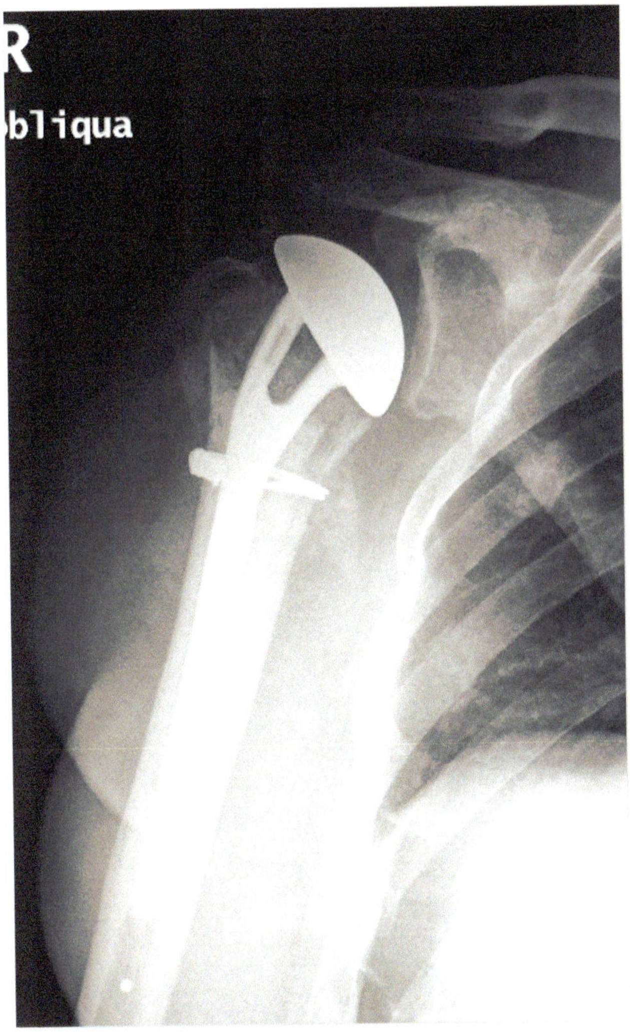

Fig. 62.9 A 1-year X-ray follow-up is shown. The calcar was fixed, and a good restoration of the gothic arch and an anatomic tuberosity osteosynthesis can be observed.

intraoperative humeral fracture, and reduced blood loss.[18] Therefore, it is recommended to have a reverse shoulder arthroplasty in the room in case immediate conversion is necessary.

Nevertheless, to use a convertible stem in the revision setting, the primary implant should be appropriately positioned. Again, the surgical technique should be very accurate and the stem should be placed at the correct height and retroversion to avoid any change of the stem in case of revision surgery.[19]

62.9.3 Management Options for Postfracture Shoulder Arthritis Sequelae

Although a hemiarthroplasty or total shoulder arthroplasty are options for treatment of postfracture shoulder arthritis sequelae, the "ream and run" procedure may be offered to young and very active patients who wish to circumvent any risks of restriction from activities postsurgery and/or other potential risks that can occur after the traditional total shoulder replacement surgery.[20] Studies show that patients with posttraumatic arthritis, osteoarthritis, and arthropathy can benefit from this procedure.[20]

The "ream and run" procedure involves creating an opening in between the deltoid and pectoralis major muscles, and then replacing the sequelae proximal humerus with a hemiarthroplasty instead of a total shoulder arthroplasty.[20] Unlike total shoulder arthroplasty where the humeral head of the prosthesis rubs against the polyethylene material (or the glenoid component) placed on top of the glenoid, in the ream and run procedure the prosthesis comes in direct contact with the glenoid. Therefore, the failure of the glenoid component that occurs in total shoulder arthroplasty has been reported not to occur with this procedure.[20]

The technique involves minimal reaming of the arthritic glenoid joint surface and it requires leaving the reamed glenoid surface for a period to allow the healing to occur. During healing, a fibrocartilaginous layer has been reported to form acting like a biologic glenoid surface.[20]

In the interim period of healing, early motion exercises help mold the new fibrocartilage layer to an optimal position.[20] It is critical that the patient exercise with a continuous passive motion machine and consistent stretching exercises.[20] In order to be successful, the patient has to reach and maintain a forward elevation position of 150 degrees.[20] Three exercises can help the patient to achieve this position: the supine stretch, the forward lean, and the pulley. All rehabilitation exercises must be supervised by an expert physical therapist.

62.10 Postoperative Care

Postoperatively, the arm should be placed in a sling for 6 weeks. Patients are allowed to start immediate gentle, active elbow, wrist, and hand range of motion and scapular stabilization exercise. After 2 weeks, a supine passive elevation to 90 degrees in the scapular plane and only 30 degrees of external rotation with the arm at the side are allowed. After 4 to 6 weeks, patients are advanced to full supine passive elevation and external rotation is progressively increased. After 6 weeks, passive internal rotation is allowed. From the seventh week, active motion is allowed. Resistance isometric exercises for the internal and external rotators are also initiated.

At the postoperative third month, strengthening may be implemented. Maximal motion and function are obtained at about 12 months from surgery (**Fig. 62.9**).

References

1. Neer CS. II. The classic: articular replacement for the humeral head. 1955. Clin Orthop Relat Res 2011;469(9):2409–2421
2. Konrad GG, Mehlhorn A, Kühle J, Strohm PC, Südkamp NP. Proximal humerus fractures - current treatment options. Acta Chir Orthop Traumatol Cech 2008;75(6):413–421
3. Olerud P, Ahrengart L, Ponzer S, Saving J, Tidermark J. Hemiarthroplasty versus nonoperative treatment of displaced 4-part proximal humeral fractures in elderly patients: a randomized controlled trial. J Shoulder Elbow Surg 2011;20(7):1025–1033
4. Boileau P, Winter M, Cikes A, et al. Can surgeons predict what makes a good hemiarthroplasty for fracture? J Shoulder Elbow Surg 2013;22(11):1495–1506

5. Hertel R, Hempfing A, Stiehler M, Leunig M. Predictors of humeral head ischemia after intracapsular fracture of the proximal humerus. J Shoulder Elbow Surg 2004;13(4):427–433
6. Zarkadas PC, Throckmorton TQ, Dahm DL, Sperling J, Schleck CD, Cofield R. Patient reported activities after shoulder replacement: total and hemiarthroplasty. J Shoulder Elbow Surg 2011;20(2):273–280
7. Johnson MH, Paxton ES, Green A. Shoulder arthroplasty options in young (50 years old) patients: review of current concepts. J Shoulder Elbow Surg 2015;24(2):317–325
8. Boileau P, Krishnan SG, Tinsi L, Walch G, Coste JS, Molé D. Tuberosity malposition and migration: reasons for poor outcomes after hemiarthroplasty for displaced fractures of the proximal humerus. J Shoulder Elbow Surg 2002;11(5):401–412
9. Krishnan SG, Reineck JR, Bennion PD, Feher L, Burkhead WZ Jr. Shoulder arthroplasty for fracture: does a fracture-specific stem make a difference? Clin Orthop Relat Res 2011;469(12):3317–3323
10. Fucentese SF, Sutter R, Wolfensperger F, Jost B, Gerber C. Large metaphyseal volume hemiprostheses for complex fractures of the proximal humerus. J Shoulder Elbow Surg 2014;23(3):427–433
11. White JJE, Soothill JR, Morgan M, Clark DI, Espag MP, Tambe AA. Outcomes for a large metaphyseal volume hemiarthroplasty in complex fractures of the proximal humerus. J Shoulder Elbow Surg 2017;26(3):478–483
12. Krishnan SG, Pennington SD, Burkhead WZ, Boileau P. Shoulder arthroplasty for fracture: restoration of the "gothic arch.". Tech Shoulder Elbow Surg 2005;6(2):57–66
13. Murachovsky J, Ikemoto RY, Nascimento LGP, Fujiki EN, Milani C, Warner JJP. Pectoralis major tendon reference (PMT): a new method for accurate restoration of humeral length with hemiarthroplasty for fracture. J Shoulder Elbow Surg 2006;15(6):675–678
14. Torrens C, Corrales M, Melendo E, Solano A, Rodríguez-Baeza A, Cáceres E. The pectoralis major tendon as a reference for restoring humeral length and retroversion with hemiarthroplasty for fracture. J Shoulder Elbow Surg 2008;17(6):947–950
15. Compito CA, Self EB, Bigliani LU. Arthroplasty and acute shoulder trauma. Reasons for success and failure. Clin Orthop Relat Res 1994(307):27–36
16. Liu J, Li S-H, Cai Z-D, et al. Outcomes, and factors affecting outcomes, following shoulder hemiarthroplasty for proximal humeral fracture repair. J Orthop Sci 2011;16(5):565–572
17. Valenti P, Kilinc AS, Sauzières P, Katz D. Results of 30 reverse shoulder prostheses for revision of failed hemi- or total shoulder arthroplasty. Eur J Orthop Surg Traumatol 2014;24(8):1375–1382
18. Werner BC, Dines JS, Dines DM. Platform systems in shoulder arthroplasty. Curr Rev Musculoskelet Med 2016;9(1):49–53
19. Kany J, Amouyel T, Flamand O, Katz D, Valenti P. A convertible shoulder system: is it useful in total shoulder arthroplasty revisions? Int Orthop 2015;39(2):299–304
20. Matsen FA III. The ream and run: not for every patient, every surgeon or every problem. Int Orthop 2015;39(2):255–261

63 Reverse Total Shoulder Arthroplasty for Proximal Humerus Fracture

Matthew P. Noyes and Patrick J. Denard

Abstract

Historically, hemiarthroplasty had led to unpredictable results in the treatment of proximal humerus fractures. Reverse total shoulder arthroplasty (RTSA) has emerged as a reliable treatment option for three- and four-part proximal humerus fractures in older patients. This chapter discusses our surgical technique and pearls for RSTA in the setting of a proximal humerus fracture.

Keywords: *reverse, shoulder, arthroplasty, fracture, tuberosity, technique*

63.1 Goals of Procedure

The primary goal of reverse total shoulder arthroplasty (RTSA) for proximal humerus fractures is to provide pain relief and range of motion sufficient for the performance of activities of daily living. A secondary goal is to perform a reliable procedure with a low chance of a secondary option (i.e., avoid hardware failure or avascular necrosis [AVN] associated with treatment of certain types of proximal humerus fractures).

63.2 Advantages

Multiple recent studies have supported functional advantages for RTSA over hemiarthroplasty in the treatment of three- and four-part proximal humerus fractures. The latter is fraught with a poor potential for tuberosity healing that can lead to substantial compromise in outcome.[1] With RTSA, tuberosity malunion and nonunion are better tolerated by patients because the implant design allows for some preservation of active forward elevation and joint stability.[2] At the same time, RTSA is actually associated with a higher rate of tuberosity healing compared to hemiarthroplasty, likely because of the medialized center of rotation, which decreases tension upon the tuberosity repair.[3] If tuberosity healing occurs, external rotation is usually retained and improves patients' function with activities away from the body.[4]

63.3 Indications

Whenever possible, we believe in joint preservation and aim to treat a proximal humerus fracture with conservative treatment or open reduction and internal fixation (ORIF). RTSA is considered for displaced three- and four-part fractures, head split, and fracture dislocations in patients older than 65 years (**Fig. 63.1**). Several factors are used to determine if the fracture is repairable including bone quality, potential vascularity, and medical comorbidities. Bone quality is estimated based on cortical thickness with less than 4 mm combined proximal diaphyseal thickness corresponding to osteoporosis.[5] While AVN is difficult to predict in the long term, vascularity at the time of injury is likely compromised in the setting of a metaphyseal extension of the humeral head of less than 8 mm and loss of the medial hinge.[6] Finally, we consider medical factors such as smoking status and medical comorbidities. If vascularity is potentially compromised but the patient is in good health and has good bone quality and health, we will consider ORIF. On the other hand, if bone quality is poor and functional demand is low, we proceed with arthroplasty and choose between hemiarthroplasty and RTSA based on age. In general, for patients older than 65 years, we proceed with RTSA and for younger patients we perform hemiarthroplasty (which is rare given that most

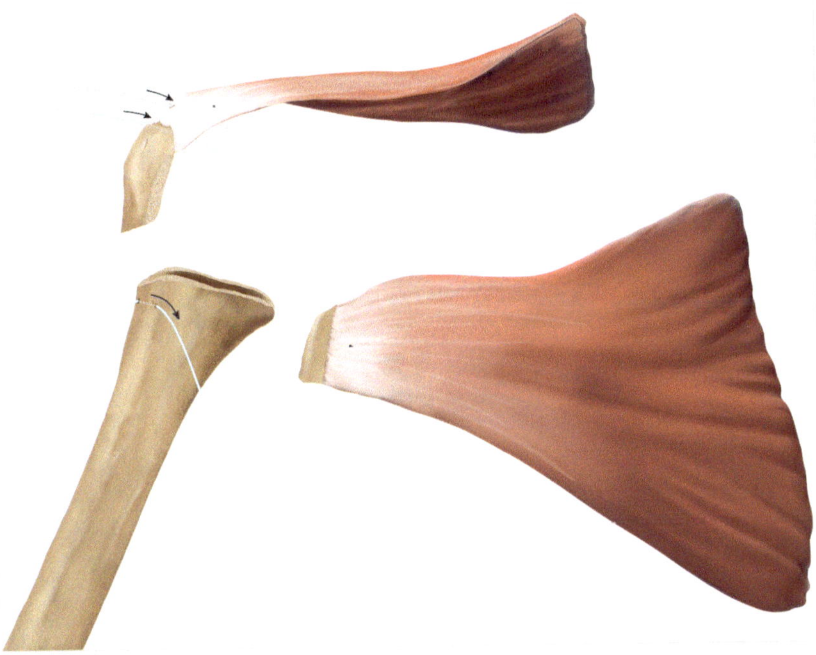

Fig. 63.1 Two no. 5 high-tensile-strength sutures (FiberWire, Arthrex) are passed through the supraspinatus tendon from lateral to medial to tag the tuberosity and for subsequent cerclage. One no. 2 FiberWire is placed through drill holes in the lateral humeral shaft just distal to the fracture edge.

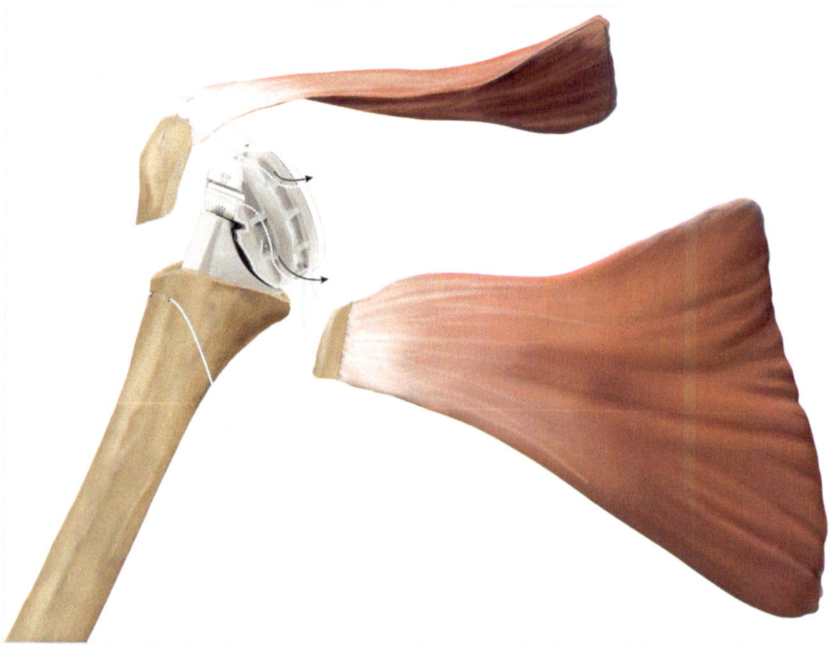

Fig. 63.2 The humeral component is secured in the humeral shaft. The Suture Cup of the prosthesis is preloaded with two no. 2 TigerWire sutures that will be used for tuberosity repair.

younger patients have good bone quality). Tuberosity healing is a critical step to achieve satisfactory outcomes when utilizing either a constrained or an unstrained arthroplasty for treatment of three- and four-part proximal humerus fractures (**Fig. 63.2**).[7]

63.4 Contraindications

Contraindications for RTSA are comparable to unconstrained arthroplasties implanted for fracture cases. Active infection is an absolute contraindication for prosthesis implantation. Young patients with good bone stock, two-part surgical neck fractures, fractures amenable to ORIF, and significant medical morbidities are relative contraindications for RTSA. Furthermore, axillary nerve palsy and acromion fractures are contraindications specific to RTSA.

63.5 Preoperative Preparation/ Positioning

A thorough history and physical examination are essential to determine if the patient is a candidate for RTSA. Information such as previous history of shoulder pain and inability to raise arm overhead before the injury allow the surgeon to discuss potential function postoperatively. Neurovascular assessment is critical, as an axillary nerve palsy in the setting of RTSA could result in prosthetic instability and poor function with forward elevation. Concomitant fractures need to be considered in the preoperative workup. Acromion fractures, either traumatic or pathologic, may have higher chance of developing nonunion after RTSA secondary to lengthening of deltoid and displacement forces placed across fracture site.

Essential radiographic assessment includes true glenohumeral anteroposterior (AP; Grashey's), scapular Y, and axillary views. A CT scan can be obtained to evaluate fracture pattern, bone quality, and rotator cuff fatty infiltration. However, we find that with good-quality radiographs, a CT scan is not necessary in most cases as the comminution and displacement requiring RTSA is usually obvious.

63.6 Operative Technique

A single-shot interscalene block is performed prior to induction of anesthesia. The patient is placed in the beach-chair position on a specialized positioner (Tenet; Smith & Nephew; Memphis, TN) at approximately 45 to 60 degrees upright. The operative side is positioned slightly to edge of the table to allow for full extension and adduction of the humerus. The operative arm is prepped, draped, and placed in a hydraulic arm holder (SPIDER; Smith & Nephew) to facilitate positioning. A Betadine occlusive drape is placed over the surgical site to eliminate the axilla from the operative field.

In displaced fractures and particularly in fracture dislocations, anatomy becomes distorted and the surgeon must search for reliable landmarks. A standard deltopectoral approach is used. The skin incision is 4 to 6 inches in length and extends from the coracoid tip toward the deltoid insertion. The dissection is carried medially to identify the cephalic vein, which is then retracted laterally with the deltoid. Once the deltopectoral interval is opened, the tip of the coracoid is the first crucial landmark that should become apparent. In fact, if one has trouble defining the interval, the coracoid tip is a good guide to finding the interval at the superior aspect of the incision. Dissection then carries lateral to the coracoid. The clavipectoral fascia is incised and the conjoined tendon is lightly retracted medially. The coracoacromial ligament is followed superolaterally to the acromion in order to establish the subdeltoid space and a Browne deltoid retractor is placed here to retract the deltoid laterally.

The next major structure that provides guidance is the biceps tendon, which is easiest to find passing beneath the pectoralis major tendon (PMT). For this reason, the superior border of the PMT is incised for 5 to 10 mm. The biceps tendon is then tenodesed to the lateral segment of the incised PMT with 2–0 Vicryl sutures. Then, the biceps is tenotomized with an electrocautery just above the tenodesis and the biceps sheath is opened to visualize the bicipital groove, which distinguishes the lesser from the greater tuberosity. The biceps release continues proximally with a curved scissors to open the rotator interval by working toward the base of the coracoid (i.e., the supraspinatus tendon is protected by avoiding cutting posteriorly) and the biceps are released from its origin. An inverted mattress suture (FiberWire; Arthrex, Naples, FL) is placed in both the subscapularis and the posterosuperior rotator cuff at the bone–tendon junction. In the setting of a four-part fracture, the tuberosities will be separated. With a three-part fracture, the bicipital groove can be osteotomized with a saw or osteotome to separate the tuberosities. Finally, the humeral head is removed and saved for bone grafting later in the procedure.

Attention is now turned to further securing the greater tuberosity. Two no. 5 FiberWire sutures are passed from outside to in through the bone–tendon interface, one superiorly through the supraspinatus and one more inferiorly through the infraspinatus. As these are to be used as cerclage sutures, the limbs are tagged without removing the needle in order to facilitate for subsequent passage through the subscapularis. Passing sutures and securing control of the tuberosities is much easier if completed prior to component implantation, which decreases the working space.

Glenoid exposure in the fracture setting is usually less challenging because the displaced tuberosity fragments can be retracted. A two-pronged thin glenoid retractor is placed anteriorly along the glenoid neck, a Darrach or Fukuda retractor is placed posteroinferiorly along the glenoid to retract the greater tuberosity and proximal humeral shaft, and a mini-Hohmann retractor is placed superiorly. The remaining proximal biceps stump and the labrum are excised and the cartilage is removed from the glenoid.

Our preferred RTSA implant uses a baseplate with a combination postcentral screw (Univers Revers; Arthrex; **Fig. 63.3**). Preparation of the glenoid is performed in a cannulated fashion. While three baseplate sizes are available (S, M, and L), we nearly always place a small baseplate since this size is adequate for stability and allows for multiple glenosphere size options. Therefore, a small guide is selected, placed at the inferior aspect of the glenoid, and a guide pin is advanced into the glenoid vault. A two-step reaming process is used to create a central bone socket with an inlay to accommodate the baseplate. The baseplate is impacted into place with a cannulated impactor through which a central compression screw is placed. Two polyaxial peripheral locking screws are then placed, one inferiorly and one superiorly. A circumferential reamer is then used over the top of the baseplate to clear bone and soft tissue for the subsequent placement of the glenosphere, which is then impacted into place. Most commonly, a 36-mm glenosphere with 4 mm of lateralized offset is placed in fracture cases. For large males, we occasionally use a 39 + 4 mm glenosphere. For small females older than 80 years, we may use a neutral 36-mm glenosphere as lateralization of the glenosphere increases deltoid force requirements, which may not be ideal in older frail patients.

With the glenosphere implanted, attention is turned to the humerus, which is exposed with extension and external rotation. A Hohmann retractor is placed medially around the shaft of the humerus and a Fukuda retractor is usually used laterally (since the humeral head is absent). The implant system we use has an inlay metaphyseal cup with an option to choose between a 135- or a 155-degree humeral inclination. We routinely use the 135-degree option in order to limit scapular notching. The humerus is sequentially broached. Reaming is not necessary based on the proximal mediolateral fixation design. In approximately two-thirds of cases, the fixation design also allows us to achieve a press-fit fixation. However, if we have concern about bone quality, we place cement in order to avoid iatrogenic fracture of the shaft. Broaching is performed with the arm in approximately 20 degrees of retroversion using the forearm axis as a guide. In addition, the medial flare of the proximal neck provides a reference for version and we seek to match this flare when aiming for press-fit fixation.

Humeral height can be judged based using several factors. First, the excised humeral head can be used as a guide to estimate the amount of missing medial bone. In most cases of RTSA, this should only be a few millimeters and the medial aspect of the inlay cup should sit just above the medial proximal humeral shaft. Second, the PMT can be used as a guide as has

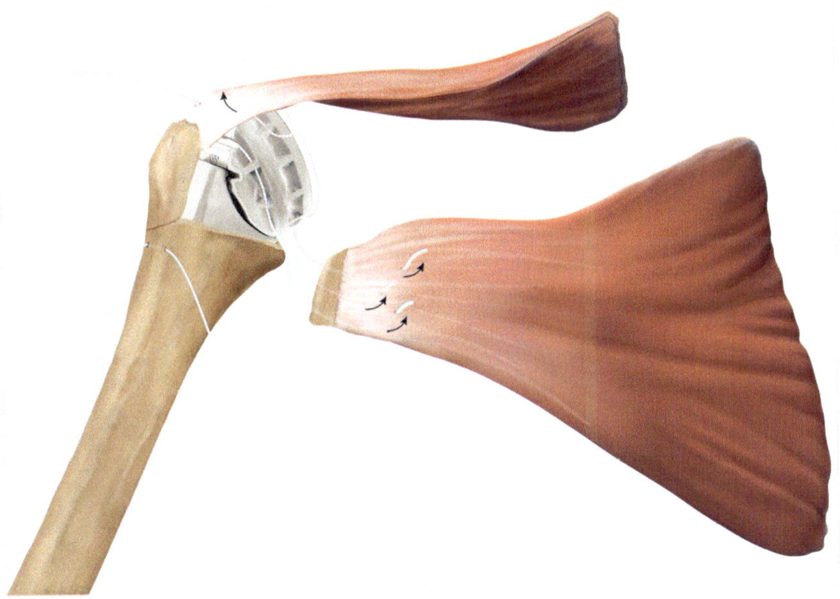

Fig. 63.3 The two no. 5 FiberWire and the inferior no. 2 TigerWire sutures are passed through the subscapularis just medial to the lesser tuberosity. The superior no. 2 TigerWire suture is passed through the supraspinatus tendon just medial to the greater tuberosity.

been reported for hemiarthroplasty.[8] The lateral aspect of the humeral inlay usually sits at the level of the greater tuberosity. Therefore, 5 to 8 mm can be added to this to correspond to the humeral head height used for hemiarthroplasty (5.5 cm).

Once the humerus is prepped, a trial reduction is performed. The tuberosities are reduced to the shaft manually to provide a final confirmation of prosthesis height. It is important to understand that stability in a fracture setting will be slightly compromised until the tuberosities are repaired. In most cases, we use a standard polyethylene (3 or 6 mm) without an additional spacer. Overtensioning by placement of excessive spacers will decrease the chance of tuberosity healing.

Prior to placement of the final humeral component, two holes are placed in the shaft lateral to the bicipital groove with a 2.0-mm drill. A mattress suture is placed with a no. 2 FiberWire such that the suture ends exit the shaft laterally. The no. 5 cerclage sutures are then retrieved and passed around the shaft so that they will surround the humeral component.

The final humeral component is then placed. In the case of cementation, a cement restrictor is placed and a hybrid cementation-impaction grafting technique, called the "black and tan" technique, is utilized.[4] Cement premixed with Gentamicin is prepared and delivered into the humeral diaphysis. Autogenous humeral head cancellous bone graft is used to create an interface between the area of tuberosity repair and proximal cement mantle.

Arguably the most important part of the case is tuberosity repair. Anakwenze et al in a recent meta-analysis compared active range of motion of RTSA with and without greater tuberosity repair in the fracture setting.[9] Both forward elevation (126 vs. 112 degrees, $p < 0.0001$) and external rotation (38 vs. 4 degrees, $p < 0.0001$) were greater with tuberosity repair. First, the two no. 5 cerclage suture ends are passed through the subscapularis just lateral to the lesser tuberosity moving from posterior to anterior. Next, a no. 2 FiberWire suture is passed through the supraspinatus and stem utilizing holes in the metaphyseal component (SutureCup). This suture is tied. This is repeated for the lesser tuberosity. Next, the suture ends from the humeral shaft are passed through the posterosuperior cuff in a figure-of-eight pattern to provide further vertical stability. Finally, the no. 5 cerclage sutures are tied and the tagging sutures for the tuberosities are tied together (**Fig. 63.4**).

63.7 Tips and Pearls/Expert Suggestions

- Place all greater tuberosity sutures before implanting the glenosphere or humeral stem. Ensure that cerclage sutures are passed around the shaft prior to placing the final humeral component as this will facilitate retrieval for passage through the subscapularis.
- With a lateralized 135-degree humeral stem, the baseplate does not have to be placed at the absolute inferior edge of the glenoid. We usually aim for placement 1 to 2 mm above the inferior edge. Placement too low can result in overtensioning and perhaps acromial stress fracture.
- Overstuffing the implant results in tuberosity repair failure, while understuffing leads to deltoid/rotator cuff insufficiency.
- Use the calcar to help restore humeral height by resting the medial portion of the humeral cup on the calcar region (assuming a short metaphyseal segment remaining on the head). In most cases, we reserve use of metallic spacers for cases of proximal bone loss, but it is better to avoid cementing the prosthesis too proud, as excessive tension is much more difficult to deal with than inadequate tension.
- In larger patients, larger diameter glenospheres are favored to ensure stability.

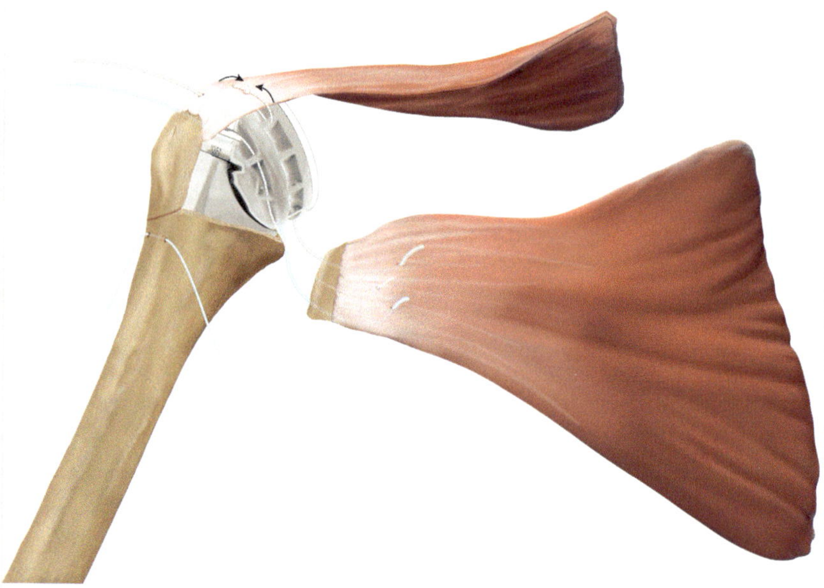

Fig. 63.4 The superior no. 2 TigerWire suture is tied to reduce the greater tuberosity to the prosthesis.

- Use minimal cement in the diaphyseal region and place autogenous bone graft from the humeral head in the proximal portion of the humeral canal after cementing. Place additional bone graft around the stem before tuberosity reconstruction ("black and tan" technique).[4]

63.8 Complications/Bailout/ Salvage

RTSA has been associated with high complication rates in the literature. Complications such as instability (3.5%), acromial fracture (2%), tuberosity nonunion (24%), and neurological injury (5%), along with scapular notching (32%) have been identified in RTSA cases specifically.[9,10] The most frequently reported complication in RTSA is scapular notching, which is the radiographic appearance of reabsorption along the lateral border of the scapula and the inferior neck of the glenoid. While baseplate position has been shown to influence scapular notching,[11,12] its clinical relevance has yet to be determined.[13] A lateralized glenosphere with a more varus humeral inclination prosthesis is less likely to develop scapular notching when compared to a Grammont-style prosthesis.[14] Erickson et al performed a systematic review comparing rates of scapular notching between 135- and 155-degree inclination prostheses.[15] The rate of scapular notching was 2.83% in the 135-degree group and 16.80% in the 155-degree group.

Instability in the setting of RTSA has been reported at 3.5% in a recent meta-analysis with a predominance for the anterior direction.[9] Avoidance of humeral adduction and extension behind the coronal plane of the body is paramount in the early postoperative period. Lack of compressive forces from an insufficient deltoid, surgical approach, quality of subscapularis, and small glenosphere diameter have been associated with increased risk of instability.[16] Intraoperatively, a critical step for the surgeon is ensuring appropriate deltoid tension while trialing implants.[17]

Overlengthening of the extremity could potentially cause two challenging complications: neurological injury and acromion fracture. Excessive tension on the deltoid or conjoined tendon could cause an axillary or musculocutaneous nerve palsy or potentially a diffuse brachial plexopathy. Most of these nerve injuries are neuropraxias that generally resolve over the first 6-month postoperative period.

With overlengthening of the arm, increased tension is applied to the three deltoid heads as it originates from the acromion. A longer lever arm, coupled with a medialized center-of-rotation implant, increases the load on the acromion causing a fracture, especially in the osteoporotic bone. Crosby et al reported on a classification system for acromion fractures in the setting of RTSA; however, this was not specific to proximal humerus fracture cases.[18] While the majority of acromion fractures were treated conservatively, caution is warranted with fractures that extend into the scapular spine. Displacement of fractures in this region may cause significant pain and impairment, requiring ORIF.

63.9 Postoperative Care

Patients are immobilized in a sling for 4 weeks postoperatively. Active hand, elbow, and wrist exercises along with scapular isometrics are started immediately. Passive external rotation with a stick in the supine position is started postoperatively, allowing rotation to neutral. At the 2-week point, table slides to 90 degrees are initiated. Rope and pulley are started at the 6-week

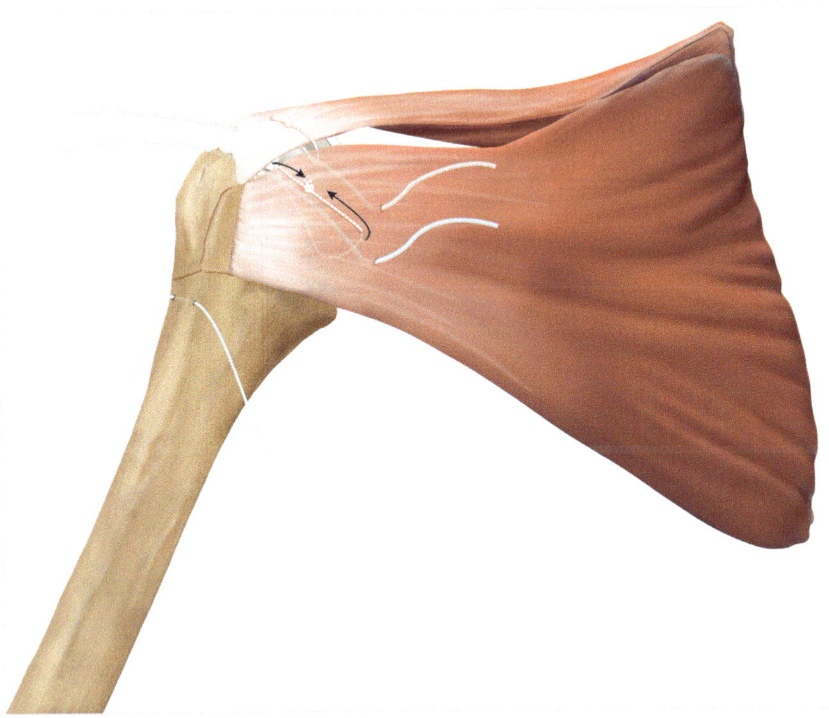

Fig. 63.5 This step is repeated for the lesser tuberosity.

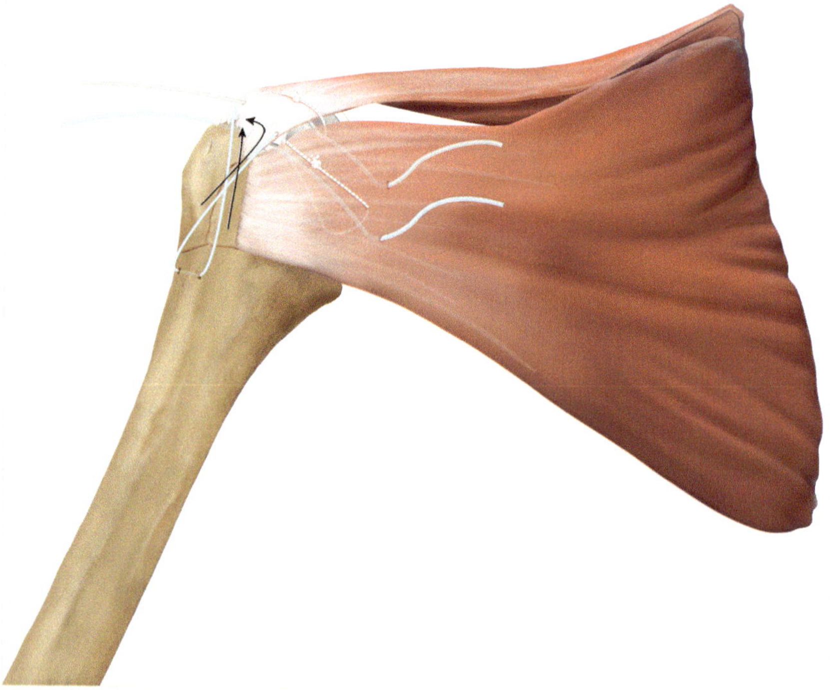

Fig. 63.6 The humeral shaft suture is passed through the posterosuperior rotator cuff as a figure of eight and tied to provide vertical stability.

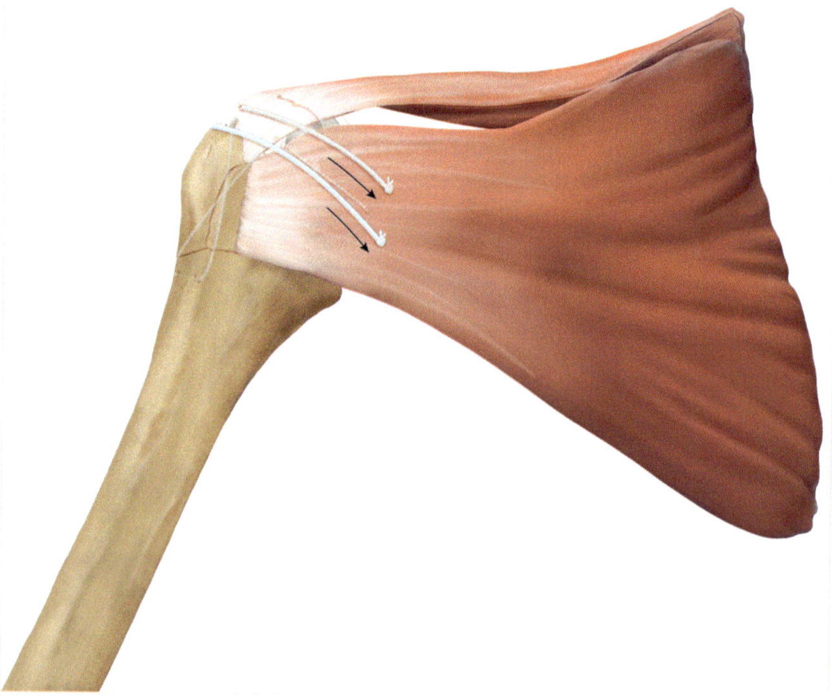

Fig. 63.7 The two no. 5 FiberWire cerclage sutures are tied. SS, supraspinatus; SSc, subscapularis.

follow-up and active range of motion with gentle strengthening is started after 3 months. Recreational activities such as golf and tennis are allowed at 6 months. The position of dislocation is reviewed in detail with the patient, not allowing internal rotation beyond the chest or extension of the arm behind the body until sling is discontinued.

References

1. Noyes MP, Kleinhenz B, Markert RJ, Crosby LA. Functional and radiographic long-term outcomes of hemiarthroplasty for proximal humeral fractures. J Shoulder Elbow Surg 2011;20(3):372–377
2. Bufquin T, Hersan A, Hubert L, Massin P. Reverse shoulder arthroplasty for the treatment of three- and four-part fractures of the proximal humerus in the elderly: a prospective review of 43 cases with a short-term follow-up. J Bone Joint Surg Br 2007;89(4):516–520
3. Cuff DJ, Pupello DR. Comparison of hemiarthroplasty and reverse shoulder arthroplasty for the treatment of proximal humeral fractures in elderly patients. J Bone Joint Surg Am 2013;95(22):2050–2055

4. Formaini NT, Everding NG, Levy JC, Rosas S. Tuberosity healing after reverse shoulder arthroplasty for acute proximal humerus fractures: the "black and tan" technique. J Shoulder Elbow Surg 2015;24(11):e299–e306
5. Tingart MJ, Apreleva M, von Stechow D, Zurakowski D, Warner JJ. The cortical thickness of the proximal humeral diaphysis predicts bone mineral density of the proximal humerus. J Bone Joint Surg Br 2003;85(4):611–617
6. Hertel R, Hempfing A, Stiehler M, Leunig M. Predictors of humeral head ischemia after intracapsular fracture of the proximal humerus. J Shoulder Elbow Surg 2004;13(4):427–433
7. Boileau P, Krishnan SG, Tinsi L, Walch G, Coste JS, Molé D. Tuberosity malposition and migration: reasons for poor outcomes after hemiarthroplasty for displaced fractures of the proximal humerus. J Shoulder Elbow Surg 2002;11(5):401–412
8. Murachovsky J, Ikemoto RY, Nascimento LG, Fujiki EN, Milani C, Warner JJ. Pectoralis major tendon reference (PMT): a new method for accurate restoration of humeral length with hemiarthroplasty for fracture. J Shoulder Elbow Surg 2006;15(6):675–678
9. Anakwenze OA, Zoller S, Ahmad CS, Levine WN. Reverse shoulder arthroplasty for acute proximal humerus fractures: a systematic review. J Shoulder Elbow Surg 2014;23(4):e73–e80
10. Shukla DR, McAnany S, Kim J, Overley S, Parsons BO. Hemiarthroplasty versus reverse shoulder arthroplasty for treatment of proximal humeral fractures: a meta-analysis. J Shoulder Elbow Surg 2016;25(2):330–340
11. Zumstein MA, Pinedo M, Old J, Boileau P. Problems, complications, reoperations, and revisions in reverse total shoulder arthroplasty: a systematic review. J Shoulder Elbow Surg 2011;20(1):146–157
12. Lévigne C, Boileau P, Favard L, et al. Scapular notching in reverse shoulder arthroplasty. J Shoulder Elbow Surg 2008;17(6):925–935
13. Levigine C, Boileau P, Favard LScapular notching. In: Walch G, Boileau P, Mole D, eds. Reverse Shoulder Arthroplasty: Clinical Results, Complications, Revisions. Montpellier: Sauramps Medical; 2006:353–372
14. Gutiérrez S, Levy JC, Frankle MA, et al. Evaluation of abduction range of motion and avoidance of inferior scapular impingement in a reverse shoulder model. J Shoulder Elbow Surg 2008;17(4):608–615
15. Erickson BJ, Frank RM, Harris JD, Mall N, Romeo AA. The influence of humeral head inclination in reverse total shoulder arthroplasty: a systematic review. J Shoulder Elbow Surg 2015;24(6):988–993
16. Wall B, Nové-Josserand L, O'Connor DP, Edwards TB, Walch G. Reverse total shoulder arthroplasty: a review of results according to etiology. J Bone Joint Surg Am 2007;89(7):1476–1485
17. Lädermann A, Williams MD, Melis B, Hoffmeyer P, Walch G. Objective evaluation of lengthening in reverse shoulder arthroplasty. J Shoulder Elbow Surg 2009;18(4):588–595
18. Crosby LA, Hamilton A, Twiss T. Scapula fractures after reverse total shoulder arthroplasty: classification and treatment. Clin Orthop Relat Res 2011;469(9):2544–2549

postoperative stiffness. Weight bearing is restricted for 6 weeks after surgery to prevent postoperative fracture. Full return to activity is permitted 12 weeks postoperatively.

References

1. Dines JS, Hettrich CM, Kelly BT, Savoie FH III, Lorich DG. Arthroscopic removal of proximal humerus locking plates. Knee Surg Sports Traumatol Arthrosc 2010;18(3):409–411
2. Voleti PB, Camp CL, Sinatro AL, Dines JS. Arthroscopic removal of symptomatic proximal humerus locking plates with bone-void filler augmentation. Arthrosc Tech 2016;5(2):e343–e346
3. Beeres FJP, Hallensleben NDL, Rhemrev SJ, et al. Plate fixation of the proximal humerus: an international multicentre comparative study of postoperative complications. Arch Orthop Trauma Surg 2017;137(12):1685–1692
4. Jost B, Spross C, Grehn H, Gerber C. Locking plate fixation of fractures of the proximal humerus: analysis of complications, revision strategies and outcome. J Shoulder Elbow Surg 2013;22(4):542–549
5. Kirchhoff C, Braunstein V, Kirchhoff S, et al. Outcome analysis following removal of locking plate fixation of the proximal humerus. BMC Musculoskelet Disord 2008;9:138
6. Dines JS, Garner MR, Bedi A, Jones K, Lorich DG, Dines DM. Outcomes of arthroscopic hardware removal following locked plating of proximal humerus fractures: a prospective study. J Shoulder Elbow Surg 2015;24(8):e230
7. Maqdes A, Levy B, Klouche S, Hardy P. The feasibility and results of an arthroscopic removal of humeral locking plates and glenohumeral arthrolysis after proximal humeral fractures. Knee Surg Sports Traumatol Arthrosc 2014;22(2):456–461

66 Open Reduction and Internal Fixation Glenoid

Jessica Bear and David S. Wellman

Abstract
Given their complex anatomy, glenoid fractures prove challenging to many orthopaedic surgeons. While historically these fractures have been largely treated with nonoperative management, more recent literature has demonstrated improved functional outcomes in a subset of glenoid fractures. This chapter aims to help guide you in determining your surgical indications, operative planning, and provide you with surgical tips to improve reductions and fixation.

Keywords: *glenoid fractures, glenopolar angle, superior shoulder suspensory complex, Judet approach, Ideberg classification*

66.1 Goals of Procedure

While the majority of scapula fractures can be treated nonoperatively, those involving the glenoid pose a unique set of challenges.[1,2] The primary goals of open reduction and internal fixation (ORIF) of glenoid fractures are to obtain anatomic reduction, restore joint congruency, and obtain/maintain glenohumeral stability.

66.2 Advantages

- Early mobilization.
- Reduced risk of posttraumatic arthritis.
- Improved range of motion.
- Improved function.[3,4]

66.3 Indications

- Intra-articular fractures:[5]
  - Articular step off ≥ 5 mm.[6,7,8]
  - Involvement of ≥ 20% of the glenoid.
  - Failure of the humeral head to remain centered within the glenoid cavity (i.e., glenohumeral instability).
- Extra-articular fractures (**Fig. 66.1**):[5,9,10]
  - Angulation ≥ 45 degrees on the scapular Y view.
  - Glenopolar angle ≤ 20 degrees.[11,12,13]
  - Lateral border offset of ≥ 20 mm.

In the case of multiple disruptions of the superior shoulder suspensory complex (SSSC), each component should be addressed as separate entities, based on specific indication criteria for each individual injury. The presence of double or multiple disruptions of the SSSC is not in itself an indication for fixation of glenoid fractures.

66.4 Contraindications

Although there are no absolute contraindications to glenoid ORIF, severely comminuted fractures and/or poor bone stock may make rigid fixation difficult to achieve, and may be better treated with nonoperative management, followed by shoulder arthroplasty as needed once the acute injury has recovered.

66.5 Preoperative Preparation/ Positioning

Operative planning begins with meticulous evaluation of the fracture. In order to adequately assess the fracture pattern, a true anteroposterior (AP) view of the glenohumeral joint, a true axillary view, and a scapular Y view should be obtained. Furthermore, CT imaging with 3D reconstruction (with humeral and clavicle subtraction) is recommended.[8] This can significantly enhance the surgeon's understanding of both the fracture pattern and the complex anatomy, thereby aiding in choosing surgical approach, and implant positioning.

The choice of approach and positioning is largely influenced by the fracture pattern. The posterior approach is utilized for posterior rim fractures, most glenoid fossa fractures, and glenoid neck fractures, while the anterior approach is useful in the treatment of anterior rim fractures, as well as some fossa fractures (Ideberg III, IV, and Vb).[14]

66.6 Operative Technique

66.6.1 Anterior Approach

This can be done in either the supine or the beach-chair position, and through a vertical incision centered over the glenohumeral joint or a deltopectoral approach. Our preference is a deltopectoral approach, supine, with the arm draped free. In either approach, the deltoid is retracted laterally and the conjoined tendon and pectoralis major retracted medially, to expose the subscapularis. The subscapularis should then be freed from the underlying capsule. The tendon of the subscapularis is then tagged and sharply incised vertically, leaving a cuff for later repair. With the subscapularis reflected medially, the rotator interval and glenohumeral capsule are then sharply incised to expose the glenoid fossa.

66.6.2 Posterior Approach

The patient should be positioned laterally (**Fig. 66.2**) to allow access anteriorly if a counter incision is required, as well as access to the coracoid for manipulation of a cephalad or anteriorly displaced fragment. A Judet or a modified Judet approach can be used depending on the extent of exposure required. An incision is made starting at the posterolateral acromion and extending along the length of the scapular spine, carried distally along the medial border of the scapula. After a full-thickness skin flap is created, the deltoid is detached from the scapular spine and retracted inferiorly, exposing the posterior rotator cuff. The interval between the infraspinatus and teres minor is bluntly developed. With the infraspinatus retracted superiorly, and the teres minor retracted inferiorly, the posterior capsule is exposed and incised (**Fig. 66.3**). If more exposure is required, the infraspinatus can be tagged and released in similar fashion to the subscapularis in the anterior approach.

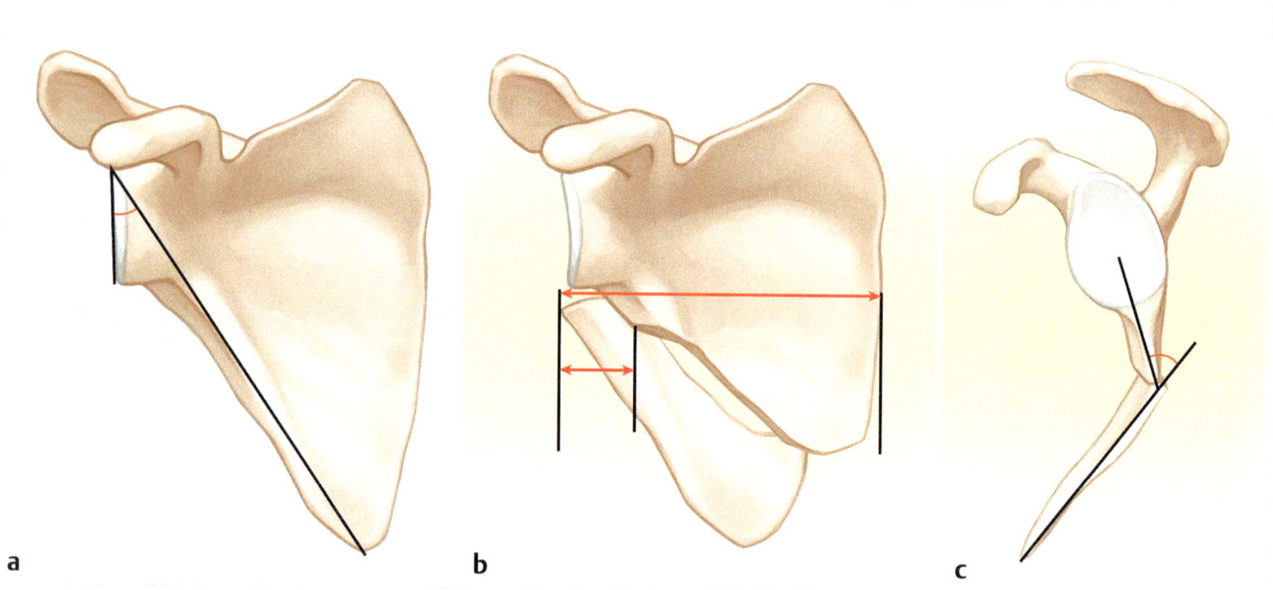

Fig. 66.1 The shaded areas on the image on the left represent the areas with the best bone stock for screw fixation, namely the lateral scapula border, glenoid neck, scapular spine, and coracoid process. The image on the right shows various locations plates can be positioned depending on the fracture pattern.

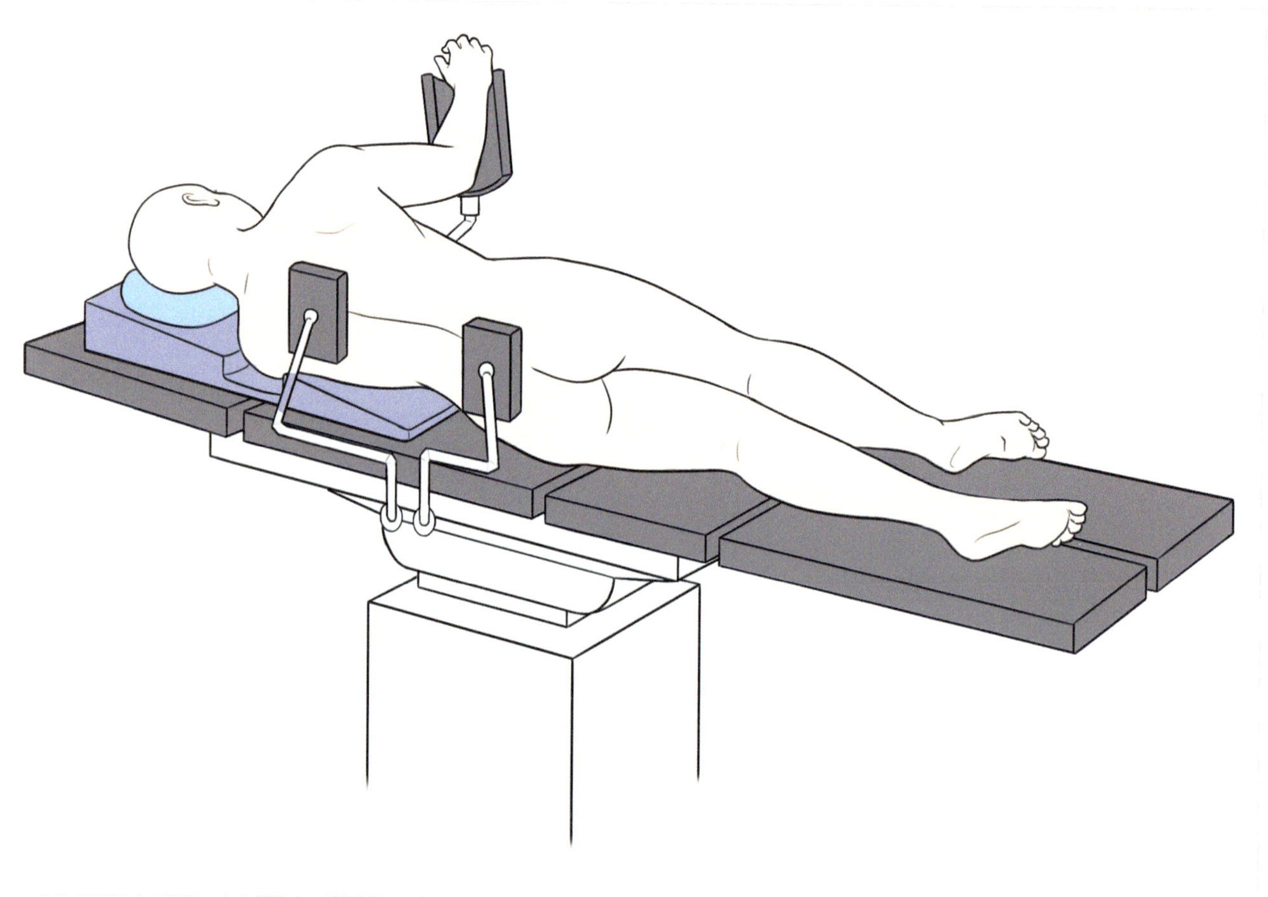

Fig. 66.2 Patient is positioned laterally on a radiolucent table with hip-grips or a bean bag. The operative arm can be placed on a post or draped over a radiolucent bolster. The entire upper extremity should be prepped to allow for easy manipulation and access to the anterior shoulder if a counter incision is needed.

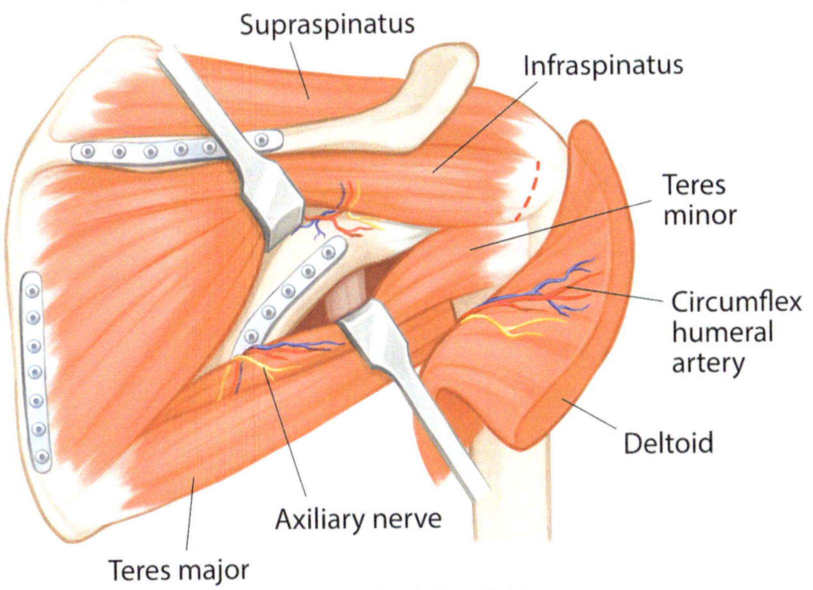

Fig. 66.3 The posterior approach to the scapula. After the deltoid is retracted inferiorly, the interval between the infraspinatus and teres minor is developed to expose the underlying scapula and glenoid. If additional exposure of the glenoid is needed, an infraspinatus tenotomy can be performed (as represented by the red line).

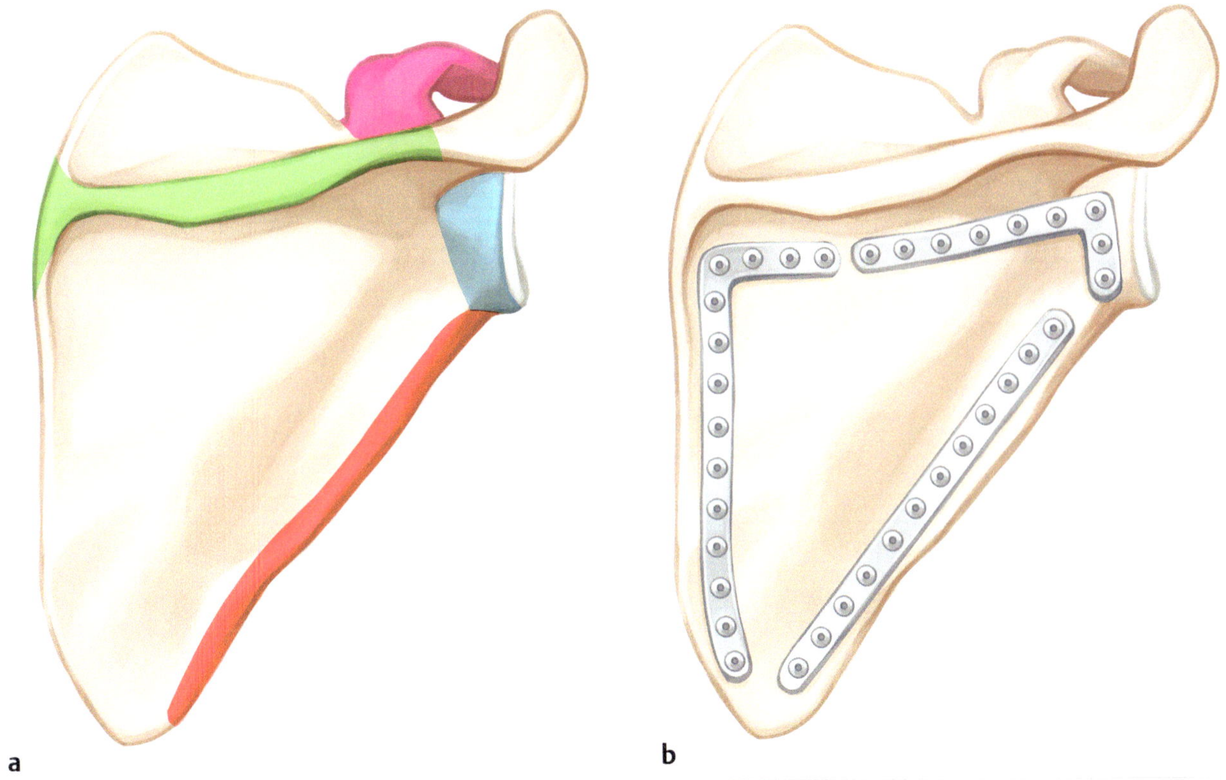

Fig. 66.4 The shaded areas on the image on the left represent the areas with the best bone stock for screw fixation, namely the lateral scapula border, glenoid neck, scapular spine, and coracoid process. The image on the right shows various locations plates can be positioned depending on the fracture pattern.

66.6.3 Reduction/Fixation

Various reduction methods can be utilized as the fracture pattern necessitates. If the fracture pattern allows, pointed reduction clamps can be used to maintain reduction and compress fragments. Kirschner's wires can be used as joysticks to assist with fragment manipulation to achieve reduction. Additionally, Kirschner's wires can be used to keep fragments reduced while applying definitive fixation. We recommend the use of mini-fragment implants (2.7, 2.4, or 2.0 mm), as these can be easily contoured to the shape of the glenoid, while still providing adequate rigidity. Keep in mind that the best bone quality is located at the lateral scapula border, glenoid neck, scapular spine, and coracoid process. An understanding of this is vital when planning hardware position (**Fig. 66.4**).

66.6.4 Closure

A layered closure should be performed, including closure of the capsule, repair of the rotator cuff tendons (if tenotomized), and repair of the deltoid to its attachment bed.

66.7 Tips and Pearls/Expert Suggestions

- When developing the interval between the infraspinatus and teres minor, it is important to remember that the infraspinatus is a bipennate muscle, and the teres minor is unipennate muscle. Take note of the muscle striations to ensure you are in the correct plane.
- The infraspinatus can be completely or partially taken down to improve visualization posteriorly.
- The origin of triceps can also be taken down if you need better exposure to the inferior glenoid.
- Posteriorly based plates on the glenoid neck allow for fixation into the coracoid process.
- Be prepared to encounter the circumflex capsular artery during the posterior approach; ligate the ascending branch if necessary.

66.8 What to Avoid

It is imperative to avoid intra-articular screw penetration. As the 3D anatomy of the glenoid is complicated and the cartilage in this region is thin (~3.8 mm), it is crucial that the articular surface be scrutinized and extra-articular screw placement ensured. This can be done using intraoperative fluoroscopy and direct visualization. If adequate visualization is difficult to obtain, a dental mirror off an ear, nose, and throat (ENT) or oral and maxillofacial surgery (OMFS) tray can be placed within the joint.

Neuropraxias, although rare, are often a result of excessive retraction of the infraspinatus, causing injury to the suprascapular nerve at the spinoglenoid notch. Similarly, injury to the axillary and musculocutaneous nerve can occur via excessive medial retraction when an anterior approach is used. Care should be taken when retracting in these areas.

66.9 Complications/Bailout/Salvage

Complications of glenoid ORIF include infection, stiffness, nerve injury, heterotopic ossification, impingement, and hardware failure; the most common is stiffness. Stiffness is often associated with the presence of concomitant injuries, but may be avoided with early physical therapy. If recalcitrant to guided physical therapy, manipulation under anesthesia, with or without arthroscopic lysis of adhesions, should be considered.

Posttraumatic arthritis, when it occurs, can cause significant disability. Conservative measures should be employed as with primary osteoarthritis. However, if exhausted, total shoulder arthroplasty can offer decreased pain and improved function.

66.10 Postoperative Care

One of the goals of operative fixation of glenoid fractures is to allow for early mobilization. Multiple studies have shown that passive and active-assisted range of motion can be safely initiated as early as the first day after operation.[15,16] If an anterior approach is used, and subscapularis taken down, passive external rotation and active internal rotation should be avoided for 4 to 6 weeks. Similarly, if the infraspinatus is taken down during a posterior approach, passive internal rotation and active external rotation should be avoided in the early postoperative period. Bracing can also be considered during this phase. Active range of motion and light weights can be initiated at 4 to 6 weeks, with strengthening and full return to activities begun at 12 weeks.

References

1. Ada JR, Miller ME. Scapular fractures. Analysis of 113 cases. Clin Orthop Relat Res. 1991(269):174–180.
2. Zlowodzki M, Bhandari M, Zelle BA, Kregor PJ, Cole PA. Treatment of scapula fractures: systematic review of 520 fractures in 22 case series. J Orthop Trauma. 2006;20(3): 230–233.
3. Lewis S, Argintar E, Jahn R, Zusmanovich M, Itamura J, Rick Hatch GF. Intra-articular scapular fractures: Outcomes after internal fixation. J Orthop. 2013;10(4): 188–192.
4. Sen RK, Sud S, Saini G, Rangdal S, Sament R, Bachhal V. Glenoid fossa fractures: Outcome of operative and nonoperative treatment. Indian J Orthop. 2014;48(1):14–19.
5. Cole PA, Freeman G, Dubin JR. Scapula fractures. Curr Rev Musculoskelet Med. 2013;6(1):79–87.
6. Adam FF. Surgical treatment of displaced fractures of the glenoid cavity. Int Orthop. 2002;26(3):150–153.
7. Hardegger FH, Simpson LA, Weber BG. The operative treatment of scapular fractures. J Bone Joint Surg Br. 1984;66(5):725–731.
8. Armitage BM, Wijdicks CA, Tarkin IS, et al. Mapping of scapular fractures with three-dimensional computed tomography. J Bone Joint Surg Am. 2009;91(9):2222–2228.
9. Cole PA, Gauger EM, Herrera DA, Anavian J, Tarkin IS. Radiographic follow-up of 84 operatively treated scapula neck and body fractures. Injury. 2012;43(3):327–333.
10. Schroder LK, Gauger EM, Gilbertson JA, Cole PA. Functional Outcomes After Operative Management of Extra-Articular Glenoid Neck and Scapular Body Fractures. J Bone Joint Surg Am. 2016;98(19):1623–630.
11. Bozkurt M, Can F, Kirdemir V, Erden Z, Demirkale I, Başbozkurt M. Conservative treatment of scapular neck fracture: the effect of stability and glenopolar angle on clinical outcome. Injury. 2005;36(10):1176–1181.
12. Pace AM, Stuart R, Brownlow H. Outcome of glenoid neck fractures. J Shoulder Elbow Surg. 2005;14(6): 585–590.
13. Romero J, Schai P, Imhoff AB. Scapular neck fracture—the influence of permanent malalignment of the glenoid neck on clinical outcome. Arch Orthop Trauma Surg. 2001;121(6):313–316.

14. Leung KS, Lam TP, Poon KM. Operative treatment of displaced intra-articular glenoid fractures. Injury. 1993;24(5):324–328.
15. Cole PA, Dubin JR, Freeman G. Operative techniques in the management of scapular fractures. Orthop Clin North Am. 2013;44(3):331–343, viii.
16. Schandelmaier P, Blauth M, Schneider C, Krettek C. Fractures of the glenoid treated by operation. A 5- to 23-year follow-up of 22 cases. J Bone Joint Surg Br. 2002;84(2):173–177.

67 Arthroscopic Reduction and Internal Fixation of Glenoid Rim Fractures

Devin R. Mangold, Joshua S. Dines, Jonathan D. Barlow, and Christopher L. Camp

Abstract

The goal of this arthroscopic approach is to obtain anatomic reduction of intra-articular glenoid fractures with labral suture anchors and rigid fixation with an extra-articular screw. Arthroscopic treatment of glenoid fractures minimizes the morbidity associated with traditional open approaches including infection, neurovascular injury, subscapularis injury, decreased postoperative motion, and a prolonged recovery. This technique can be used for simple intra-articular fractures of the glenoid when the fracture fragment can be mobilized and reduced by arthroscopic means.

Keywords: *glenoid, fractures, instability, arthroscopic, Bankart, intra-articular*

67.1 Goals of Procedure

Although intra-articular glenoid fractures are an uncommon injury, they can have important implications for shoulder stability and chondral preservation. While surgical stabilization is typically recommended, fixation can be technically challenging. Traditional open exposures used to treat intra-articular glenoid fractures are associated with significant morbidity, and intra-articular reduction and is frequently compromised. Accordingly, the goal of this arthroscopic approach is to obtain anatomic reduction of intra-articular glenoid fractures while reducing the morbidity associated with an open approach.

67.2 Advantages

Arthroscopic treatment of glenoid fractures minimizes the morbidity associated with traditional open approaches including infection, neurovascular injury, subscapularis injury, decreased postoperative motion, and prolonged recovery. Additionally, through an indirect reduction technique by achieving labral fixation, there is less need for provisional fixation with K-wires and reduction clamps, thereby lowering the risk of damage to neurovascular structures. Additionally, rigid fixation with an extra-articular screw offers superior stability compared to techniques utilizing suture anchors alone. Finally, intra-articular visualization is enhanced via an arthroscopic approach.

67.3 Indications

This technique can be used for simple intra-articular fractures of the glenoid when the fracture fragment can be mobilized and reduced by arthroscopic means.

67.4 Contraindications

This technique is not suited for complex, comminuted fractures or when anatomic reduction cannot be achieved arthroscopically. Additionally, this method requires an intact labrum and soft-tissue connection between the labrum and the fracture fragment.

67.4.1 Preoperative Preparation/positioning

Standard radiographs and CT scans are essential to adequately understand the fracture morphology (**Fig. 67.1**). 3D reconstructions can be particularly helpful to appreciate the nature of the fracture. MRI may also be helpful in identifying concomitant pathology.

After anesthesia is administered, an examination of the shoulder under anesthesia should be performed in order to gain a better sense of the magnitude of instability associated with the injury. Afterward the patient is placed in the lateral decubitus position on a beanbag and 10 to 15 lb of traction is applied to the extremity during the operation. Alternatively, the procedure may be performed in the standard beach-chair position. Intraoperative fluoroscopy is required for confirmation of safe placement of the extra-articular screw.

67.5 Operative Technique

The operative procedure begins with a standard diagnostic arthroscopy of the shoulder joint with a 30-degree arthroscope introduced through the standard posterior portal. A slightly more superolateral posterior portal can enhance glenoid visualization. A diagnostic arthroscopy is performed. Thorough evaluation of the integrity of the labrum is critical as an intact labrum is the basis for this treatment strategy. Two anterior portals are established with needle localization. The primary working portal is generally placed medially, just above the subscapularis. A 7.5-mm cannula is inserted in this location. In the far lateral aspect of the rotator interval, just anterior to the leading edge of the supraspinatus, a 5.5-mm cannula is placed.

While viewing from the posterior portal and working through one of the anterior portals, the fracture fragment is mobilized. This ensures that an anatomic reduction can be obtained. The fracture site is gently debrided with an arthroscopic elevator, shaver, or curette, removing any residual fracture hematoma between fragments (**Fig. 67.2**). An arthroscopic grasper can be useful to manipulate the fracture fragment as needed. A 70-degree arthroscope can help optimize visualization of the fracture line and the fragment itself. It is imperative to avoid significant displacement of the fracture fragment as this could disrupt any attached labral tissue, thereby impairing the ability to achieve indirect reduction through labral fixation. The labrum is carefully probed adjacent to the fracture line.

The next goal is to provisionally reduce and fix the fragment through repair of the adjacent labrum and capsule. A 3.0-mm (or similar-sized) suture anchor is placed in the rim of the intact glenoid immediately adjacent to the fracture

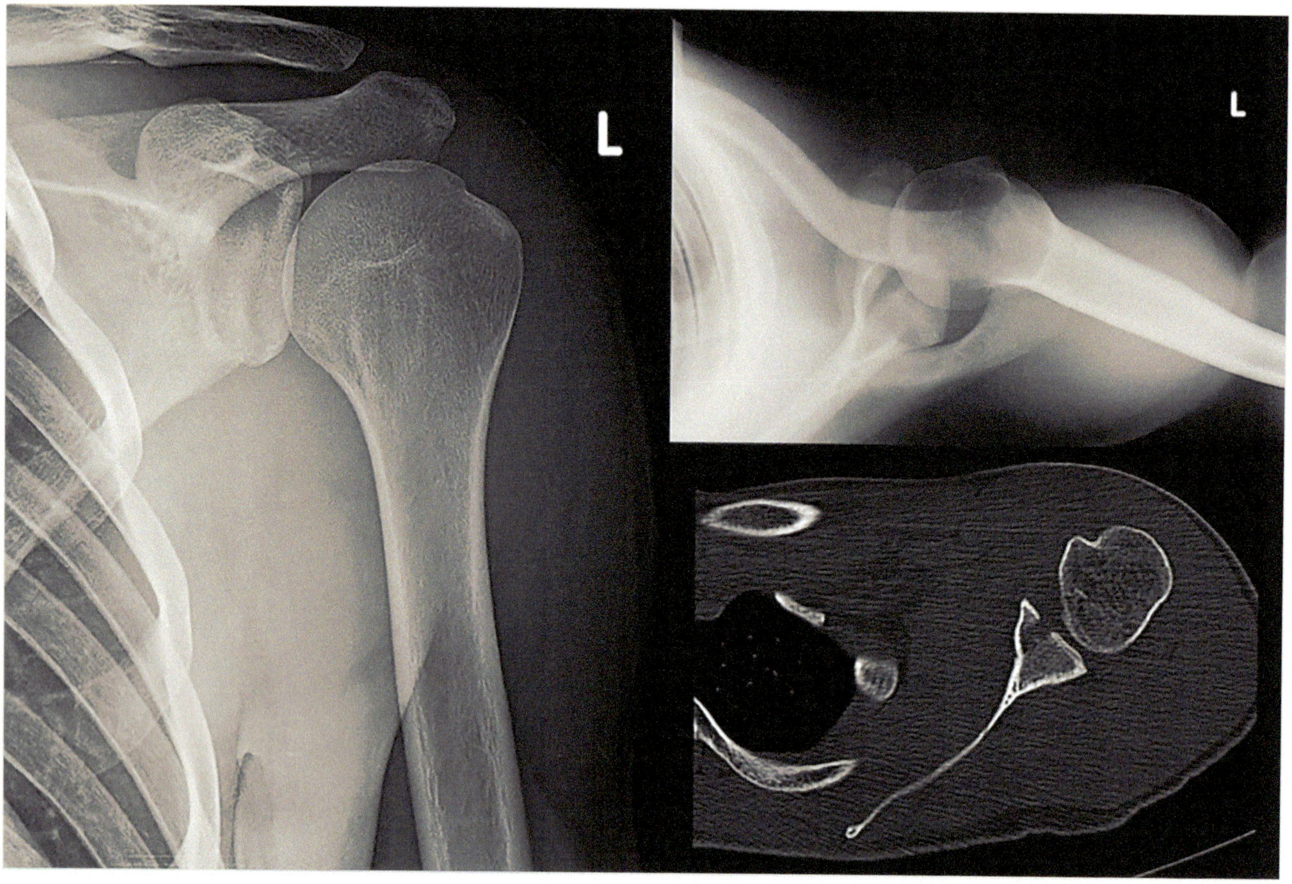

Fig. 67.1 Anteroposterior (*left*) X-ray, axillary X-ray (*top right*), and axial CT (*bottom right*) demonstrating intra-articular glenoid fracture involving the anterior glenoid.

fragment. One limb of the suture is passed around the labrum and the two limbs are tied arthroscopically, thereby creating a simple stitch around the labrum. In complete fractures, this step is repeated at the other junction between the intact glenoid and the fracture fragment. It is critical to ensure the suture anchors are placed in the intact portion of the glenoid to avoid malreduction of the glenoid. After labral fixation is completed, the fracture is thoroughly inspected to verify adequate reduction.

After confirming satisfactory reduction, bony fixation is obtained with an extra-articular screw. While viewing through the posterior portal, preliminary fixation is achieved with use of a K-wire through the anterior portal that gives the best angle to cross the fracture site orthogonally. If needed, a separate, percutaneous portal can be created. The trajectory and starting point of the K-wire are confirmed using intraoperative fluoroscopy to ensure safe placement and that there will not be intra-articular screw penetration. Once the K-wire is advanced to the desired depth, the appropriate screw length is determined. A cannulated 3.2-mm drill bit is passed over the K-wire, the path is drilled, and a fully threaded 3.5-mm screw is advanced through the drilled path. Final reduction is confirmed both by direct visualization through the arthroscope and via intraoperative fluoroscopy (**Figs. 67.3, 67.4**). Although these fragments are generally not large enough for multiple screws, an additional point of fixation could be considered for larger fractures.

67.6 Tips and Pearls/Expert Suggestions

Proper patient positioning is critical and the sterile field should be sufficient should open surgery be deemed necessary intraoperatively. Our preferred position is lateral decubitus as traction helps facilitate humeral head retraction. Given the infrequent use of fluoroscopy with arthroscopic shoulder surgery, fluoroscopic images should be obtained before prepping and draping to ensure adequate visualization. As in any arthroscopic procedure, portal placement is critical to ensure appropriate trajectory to accomplish the objectives of the procedure. The fracture fragment must be adequately mobilized to allow reduction; however, care must be taken to preserve soft-tissue attachments and not sacrifice the integrity of the bone. During fracture fragment drilling, there is risk that the fragment could spin with the drill bit. To prevent fracture fragment spinning, a grasper can be used to stabilize the fragment if needed. Finally, during placement of the screw, overtightening should be avoided to prevent further fragmentation of the bone.

67.7 What to Avoid

It is critical to ensure that adequate visualization of the fracture can be achieved arthroscopically. Furthermore, the fracture fragment must be able to be mobilized arthroscopically. During

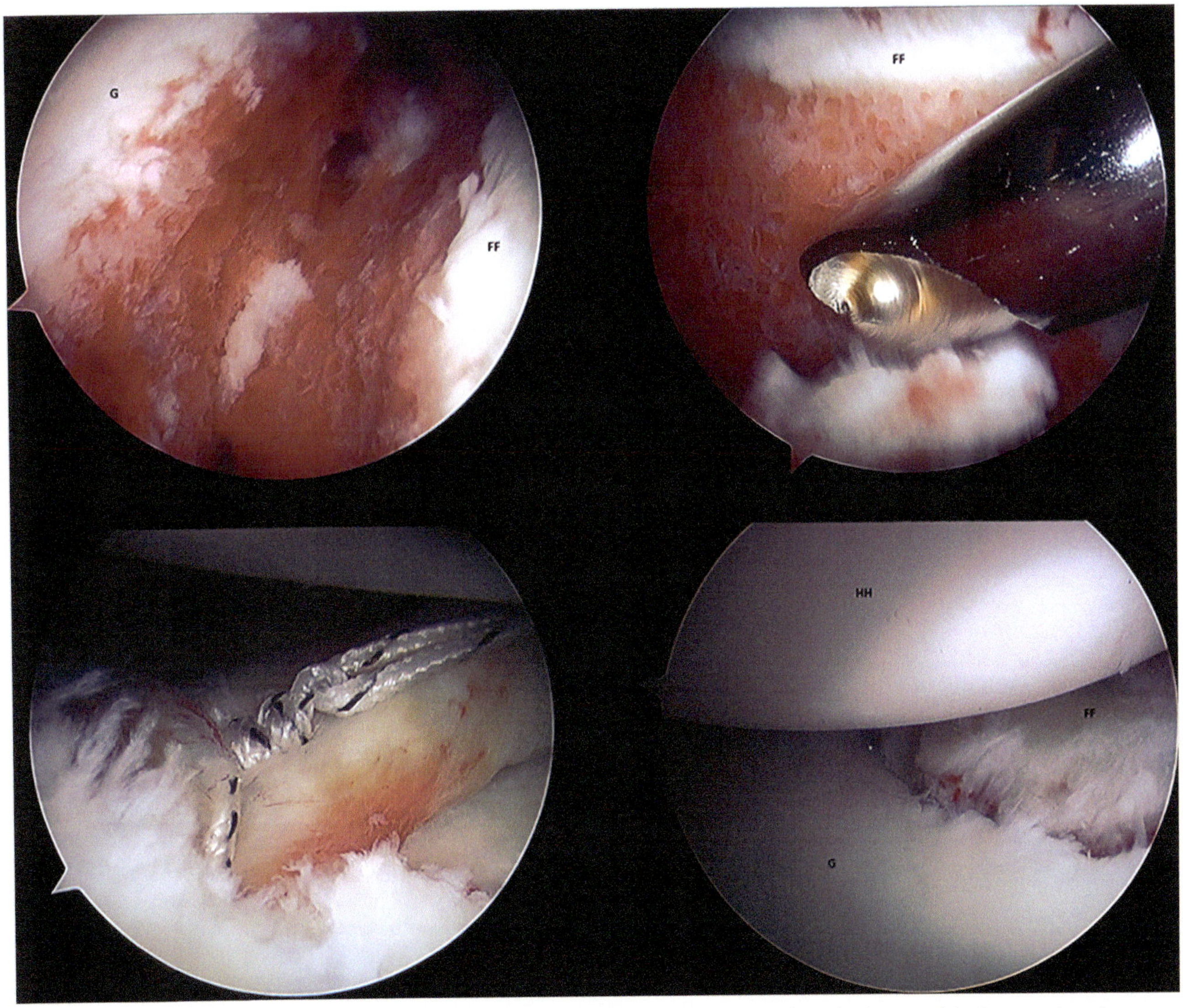

Fig. 67.2 *Top left*: Visualization of the fracture fragment through the posterior portal. *Top right*: Debridement of the fracture site using an arthroscopic shaver. *Bottom left*: Labral fixation with suture anchors. *Bottom right*: Preliminary reduction after labral repair. FF, fracture fragment; G, glenoid; HH, humeral head.

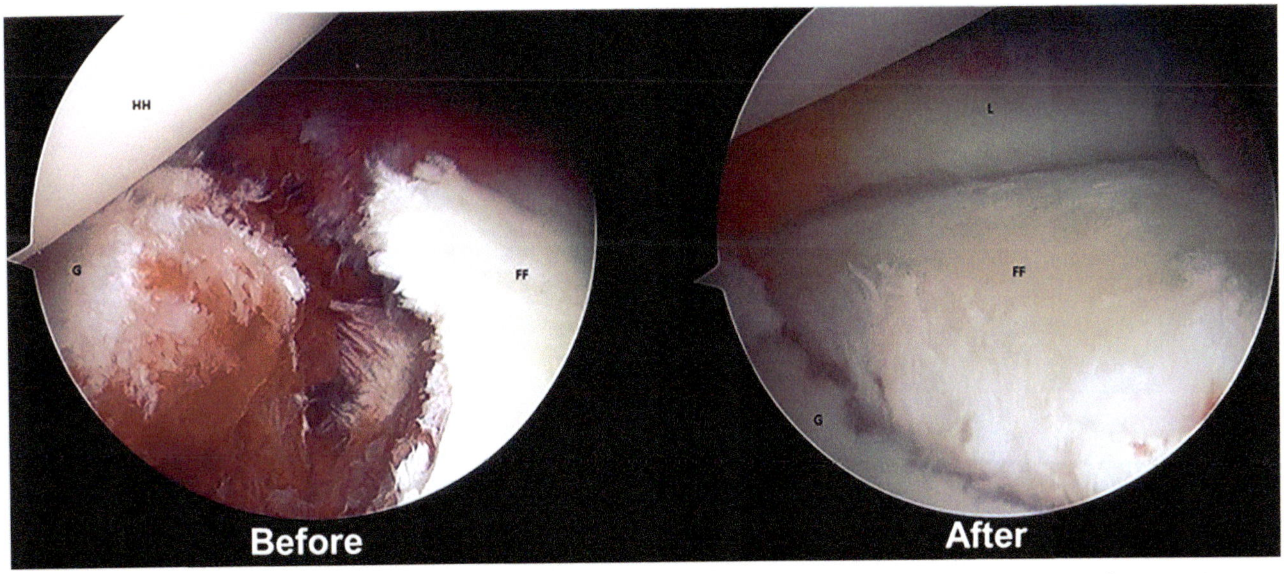

Fig. 67.3 Before and after pictures demonstrating anatomic reduction of the intra-articular glenoid fracture. FF, fracture fragment; G, glenoid; HH, humeral head; L, labrum.

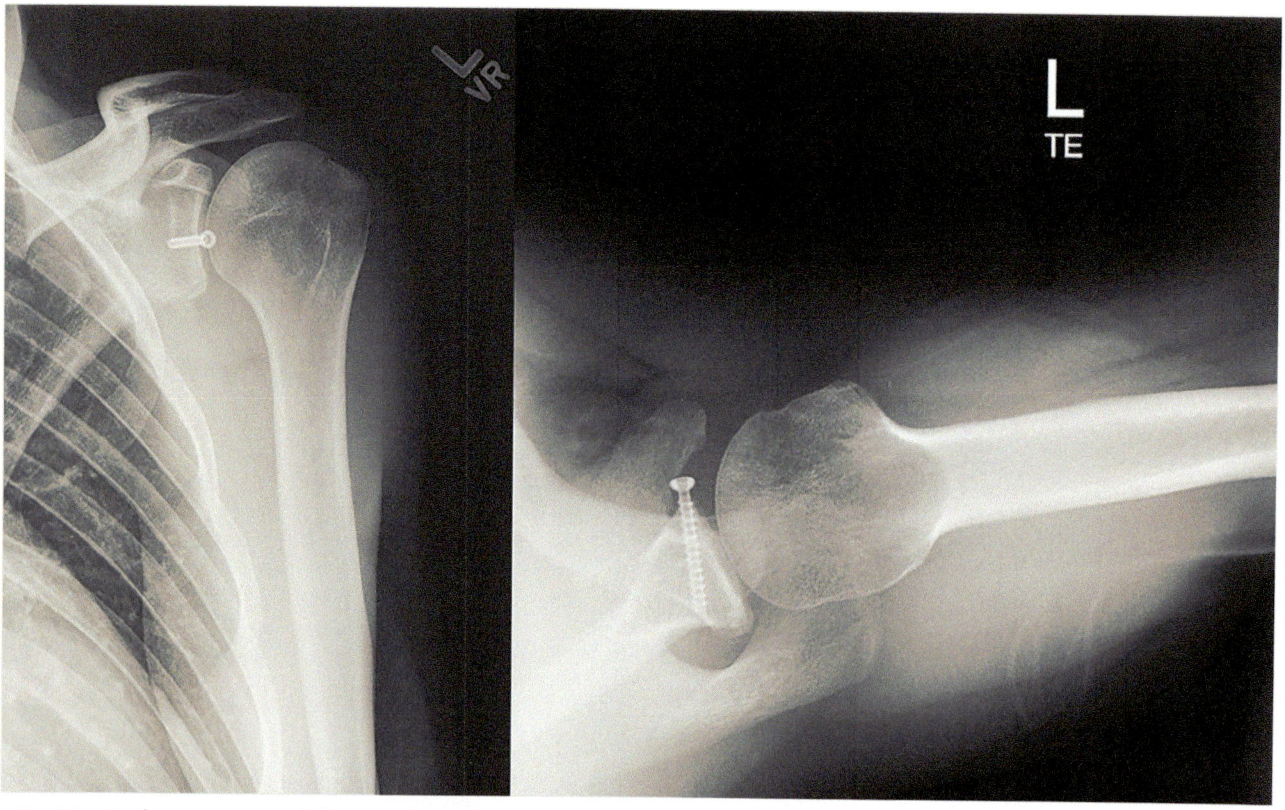

Fig. 67.4 Final anteroposterior (*left*) and axillary (*right*) X-rays.

mobilization and debridement of the fracture site, it is vital to maintain the labral soft-tissue connection to the fracture fragment. During placement of suture anchors, the surgeon must take care to ensure that the anchors pass through intact glenoid only and not through the fracture site. During drilling and placement of the extra-articular screw, care must be taken to ensure that there is no intra-articular violation by the drill bit or screw.

67.8 Complications/Bailout/Salvage

If the fracture cannot be adequately mobilized or reduced via arthroscopic means, conversion to open surgery should be considered and access to the glenoid can be achieved by a subscapularis split or tenotomy. If further fragmentation of the fracture occurs during screw placement making it impossible to reduce and there is concern for potential instability, consideration can be given to bone grafting with autograft (i.e., Latarjet) or allograft.

67.9 Postoperative Care

Patients remain non-weight-bearing on the operative extremity postoperatively and are placed in a sling for 6 weeks, coming out only to perform gentle range-of-motion exercises to help maintain joint mobility and prevent arthrofibrosis. Radiographs are typically obtained at 3- to 6-week intervals to ensure maintenance of fracture reduction until complete healing is observed. Strengthening is often delayed until approximately 6 weeks postoperatively. Patients return to normal activities typically around 16 weeks postoperatively.

Suggested Readings

Ideberg R, Grevsten S, Larsson S. Epidemiology of scapular fractures. Incidence and classification of 338 fractures. Acta Orthop Scand 1995;66(5):395–397

Sugaya H, Kon Y, Tsuchiya A. Arthroscopic repair of glenoid fractures using suture anchors. Arthroscopy 2005;21(5):635

Voleti PB, Camp CL, Sinatro AL, Dines JS. Arthroscopic fixation of glenoid rim fractures after reduction by labral repair. Arthrosc Tech 2016;5(2):e379–e383

68 Open Reduction and Internal Fixation of Midshaft Clavicle Fracture

Camden Tissue and David L. Helfet

Abstract

Historically, midshaft clavicle fractures have been treated conservatively. Recent clinical trials have demonstrated improved clinical outcomes with operative fixation of these displaced fractures and functional deficits in those treated conservatively. With operative care, open reduction and internal fixation with plates and screws is most commonly used. Multiple plate locations are possible. We believe that dual, orthogonal, mini-fragment plate fixation combines the advantages biomechanically of the different plate locations as well as allows use of low-profile plates that minimize the risk of hardware irritation. This technique reliably leads to anatomic union and decreases the number of secondary operations.

Keywords: *clavicle, midshaft, fracture, displaced, operative, plate, orthogonal, dual*

68.1 Goals of Procedure

Fractures of the clavicle are common with an incidence of 30 to 60 per 100,000 population per year.[1,2] Clavicle fractures comprise 35 to 44% of fractures about the shoulder and 2.6 to 4% of all fractures in the adult population.[2,3] Among those, fractures of the middle one-third of the clavicle account for the majority (69–81%).[1–3] The clavicle functions as a strut for the upper extremity. It is the only osseous attachment for the upper extremity to the axial skeleton and an important site for muscle insertion. Forces applied to the upper extremity are transmitted to the trunk via the clavicle and its articulation with the acromion process of the scapula and the manubrium of the sternum. The goal of surgery on the clavicle is to anatomically reconstruct the clavicular length, alignment, and rotation with stable, balanced internal fixation while preserving blood supply and allowing for early range of motion of the shoulder and rehabilitation. Further goals of the operation include recovery of muscle strength and endurance, patient satisfaction with shoulder function and appearance, and avoidance of nonunion or symptomatic malunion.

68.2 Advantages

Historically, fractures of the midshaft clavicle were treated conservatively in either a sling or a figure-of-8 brace. This treatment was driven by early studies reporting that the nonunion rate with conservative treatment of clavicle fractures is exceedingly rare (<1%).[4,5] Outcomes in these studies were often surgeon reported or radiographic. Any residual shoulder deformity was thought to be a cosmetic concern and shoulder function was unaffected. However, over the past 15 to 20 years, multiple prospective studies have shown less favorable outcomes. Conservatively treated displaced midshaft clavicle fractures have significantly decreased strength and endurance compared to the uninjured side.[6] Nonunion rates from 7 to 24% have been reported.[7–10] It is common (42%) to have pain or paresthesias 6 months after injury with conservative management.[7] Patients are dissatisfied with the cosmetic result of their shoulder and function overall.[6–8] Changes in the bony morphology can lead to altered scapular kinematics and changes in maximal muscle moments about the shoulder.[11–13] A recent study of cadavers found that the presence of an ipsilateral clavicle fracture was correlated with development of glenohumeral arthritis.[14]

Because of these numerous undesirable consequences uncovered in the literature, operative treatment has gained traction. High-level evidence comparing operative versus conservative treatment for displaced midshaft clavicle fractures found that operative treatment leads to faster time to union, better patient-reported outcomes, less nonunions, no symptomatic malunions, faster return to function, and better patient satisfaction with the shoulder.[15,16] Operative treatment has shown to be financially beneficial as well, with faster return to work, less pain medication requirement, and less need for physical therapy.[17]

68.3 Indications

The indications for surgical treatment of acute, midshaft clavicle fractures are shortening, displacement, or translation. The degree needed to indicate a patient for surgical treatment remains a topic of debate. Complete displacement, presence of comminution, advancing age, female gender, and initial shortening of 2 cm have all been associated with risk of nonunion and the risk of long-term sequelae.[6,8,9,18] Symptomatic malunions with shortening of the clavicle will have worse clinical outcomes. In our practice, we indicate patients with complete displacement or shortening of the clavicle for surgical management. Other indications for surgical treatment of midshaft clavicle fractures include open or impending open fracture with skin at risk, multiply traumatized patients in need of mobilization, concomitant neurovascular injuries, and fracture of glenoid neck of the scapula resulting in a "floating shoulder." Relative indications for surgery include patients in whom rapid return to work is desirable such as professional athletes or surgeons and patients in whom the cosmetic appearance of the shoulder is important such as professional models.

68.4 Contraindications

True contraindications to this procedure are rare. Relative contraindications include pediatric patients because of their inherent healing and remodeling abilities, nondisplaced and minimally displaced fractures, and patients with medical comorbidities that preclude surgery.

68.5 Preoperative Preparation/ Positioning

68.5.1 Physical Examination

As with any patient, a thorough history and physical examination is the important first step in management. Examination of the skin over the fracture site is mandatory as skin tenting and impending open fracture will alter the timing of treatment. The neurovascular examination is important to rule out injuries to the subclavian artery or vein or the brachial plexus as these may alter the surgical management. It is also prudent to examine the breath sounds and radiographs to rule out hemothorax or pneumothorax as these injuries have been reported in conjuncture with clavicle fractures.[19,20]

68.5.2 Imaging

Standard radiographs of the clavicle include anteroposterior view and a 45-degree cephalad view, also known as a "serendipity" view (**Fig. 68.1**). The "serendipity" view is useful in that the underlying thoracic structures no longer obscure the view of the clavicle. These two views will commonly provide adequate information about fracture pattern, displacement, and shortening to make surgical plans. If there is a borderline case, one can obtain upright views to allow gravity to gently stress the fracture site and show the true amount of displacement and shortening. Forty-one percent of patients who do not have complete displacement on supine films will have complete displacement on upright films.[21] If on physical examination, there is evidence of a neurovascular injury, one must rule out scapulothoracic dissociation. This can be done on chest radiographs by comparing the distance of the scapula from midline bilaterally. CT scans, though not usually necessary for treatment, can show evidence of scapulothoracic dissociation, intrathoracic injury, and details of the clavicle fracture fragments.

68.5.3 Positioning

The patient is placed supine on a standard radiolucent table (**Fig. 68.2**). A rolled towel is placed beneath the scapula to elevate the clavicle and allow for draping of the posterior shoulder. The patient's head is tilted away from the surgical field and secured. If the procedure is to be done under general endotracheal anesthesia, the endotracheal tube is secured on the opposite corner of the mouth to keep the tube out of the surgical field. Most commonly, we perform this procedure under regional (interscalene) block and sedation. The surgical field is isolated with adhesive drapes and surgical sterilization is performed. Stockinette is used to cover the hand and forearm and Ioban (3M, St. Paul, MN) is used to seal the surgical field from the surrounding areas including the axilla.

68.6 Operative Technique

The skin incision runs 7 to 8 cm just inferior to the anterior border of the clavicle and centered over the fracture site. Sharp dissection is carried down through the subcutaneous tissue. The supraclavicular nerves are identified and protected whenever possible. Next, the fracture is identified and any early fracture callus or soft tissue is removed using a scalpel, elevators, and curettes. Care must be taken to preserve soft-tissue attachment to the bone as much as possible, especially in the case of butterfly fragments.

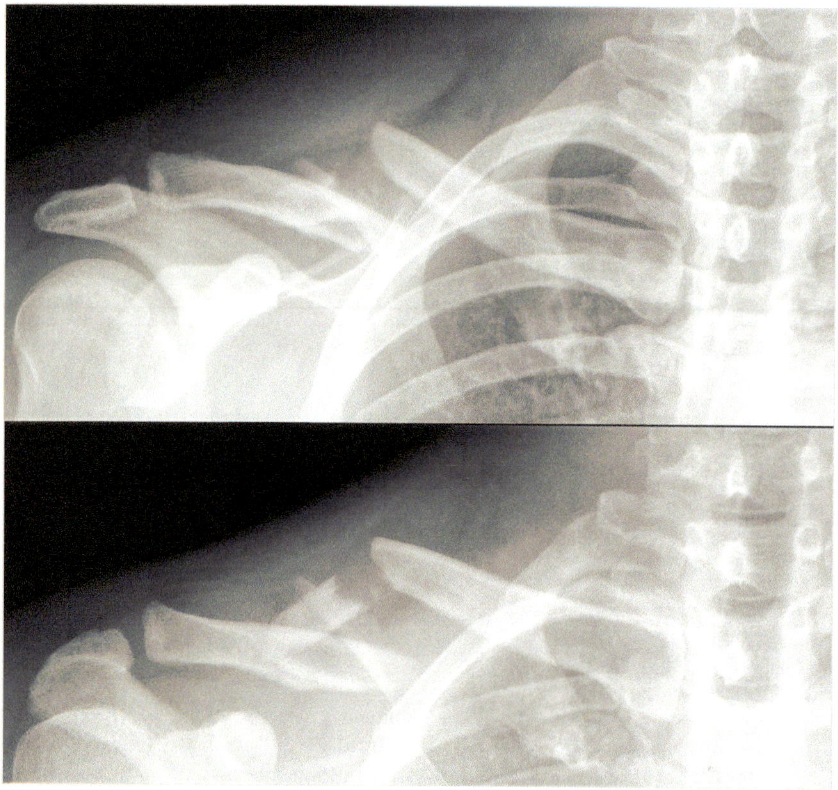

Fig. 68.1 Plain radiographs of a displaced midshaft clavicle fracture with multiple butterfly fragments including anteroposterior and "serendipity" views.

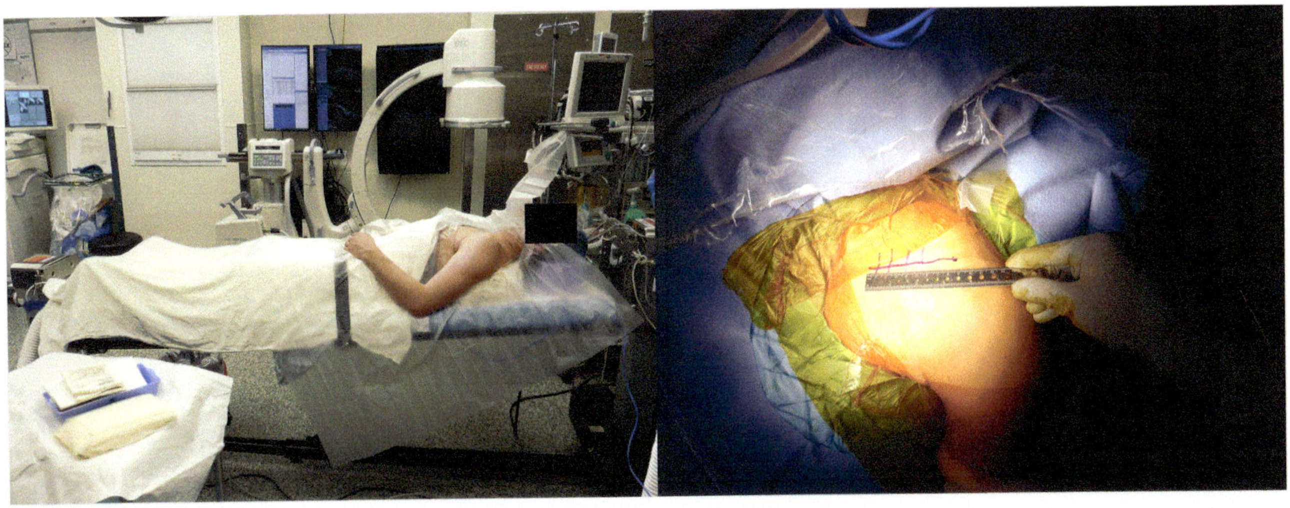

Fig. 68.2 Photograph of operative setup on a regular radiolucent table with a rolled towel placed under the scapula on the ipsilateral shoulder. On the right side, the planned incision is drawn just inferior to the anterior border of the clavicle and centered over the fracture.

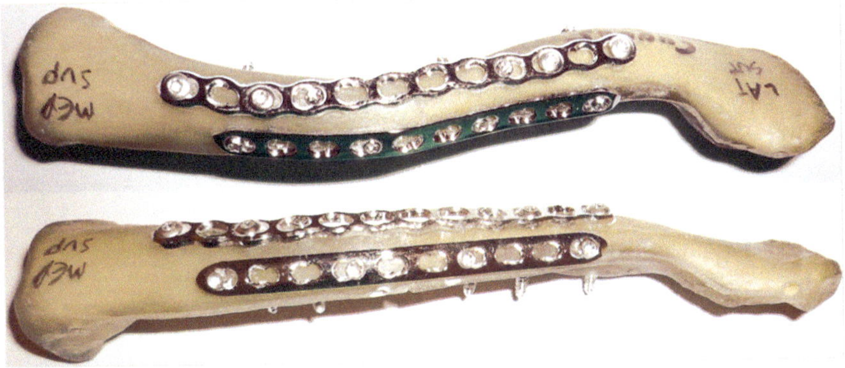

Fig. 68.3 Superior and anterior views of a saw bones model demonstrating the mini-fragment plates in orthogonal position to each other on the superior and anterior surfaces of the clavicle.

A variety of instruments are available to help achieve reduction. In the case of a simple fracture pattern, we find pointed reduction clamps to be most appropriate. Once the reduction has been exacted, provisional fixation is achieved using small (1.25-mm), smooth-tipped Kirschner wires. With comminuted fractures or complicated butterfly fragments, the reduction will be achieved using the plate as discussed below.

We find the best construct for displaced, midshaft clavicle fractures to be orthogonal dual mini-fragment plating. A Synthes (West Chester, PA) 2.4-mm limited contact plate is applied to the anterior surface of the clavicle and a Synthes 2.7-mm reconstruction plate is applied to the super surface (**Fig. 68.3**). The fracture pattern determines which plate will be placed first. For example, an oblique fracture running anterior to posterior is best served biomechanically by initial application of the anterior plate. The plate is anatomically contoured to the anterior surface of the clavicle. A forward-facing concave bend will be applied laterally for more laterally based fractures. A forward-facing convex bend will be placed medially for medial-based fractures. Minor incongruities between the plate and the bone are usually corrected during application of cortical screws or can be corrected with a standard reduction clamp. The 2.4-mm limited contact plate is then applied in such a fashion that it buttresses any anterior butterfly fragments and offers the opportunity for anterior to posterior lag screws using the plate as a washer (**Fig. 68.4**). At least three cortical screws will be applied to the anterior plate on the proximal and distal sides of the fracture to allow for maintenance of the reduction. The superior plate is similarly contoured with side benders to fit the superior surface of the clavicle and secured in place with cortical screws (**Fig. 68.5**). After the first plate is in place, application of the second plate is simple as the construct already has stability. The second plate functions to increase the strength of the construct. In cases with comminution or difficult reduction, one of the plates can be secured to the proximal aspect of the fracture and the main distal fragment can be reduced to the plate with a clamp and secured with cortical screws or vice versa.

After placement of all hardware, fluoroscopic imaging is obtained to confirm anatomic realignment of the clavicle and safe positioning of all screws. The wound is copiously irrigated with low-pressure normal saline. A deep drain is left in place and removed on postoperative day 1. Deep layers including the deltotrapezial fascia are closed using absorbable suture (**Fig. 68.6**). The skin is closed using a running, absorbable subcuticular suture and sealed with a layer of Dermabond (Ethicon, Somerville, NJ).

68.7 Tips and Pearls/Expert Suggestions

Multiple plating techniques are available for fixation of midshaft clavicle fractures. Traditionally, superior plating has been performed. The advantages of superior plating are ease of appli-

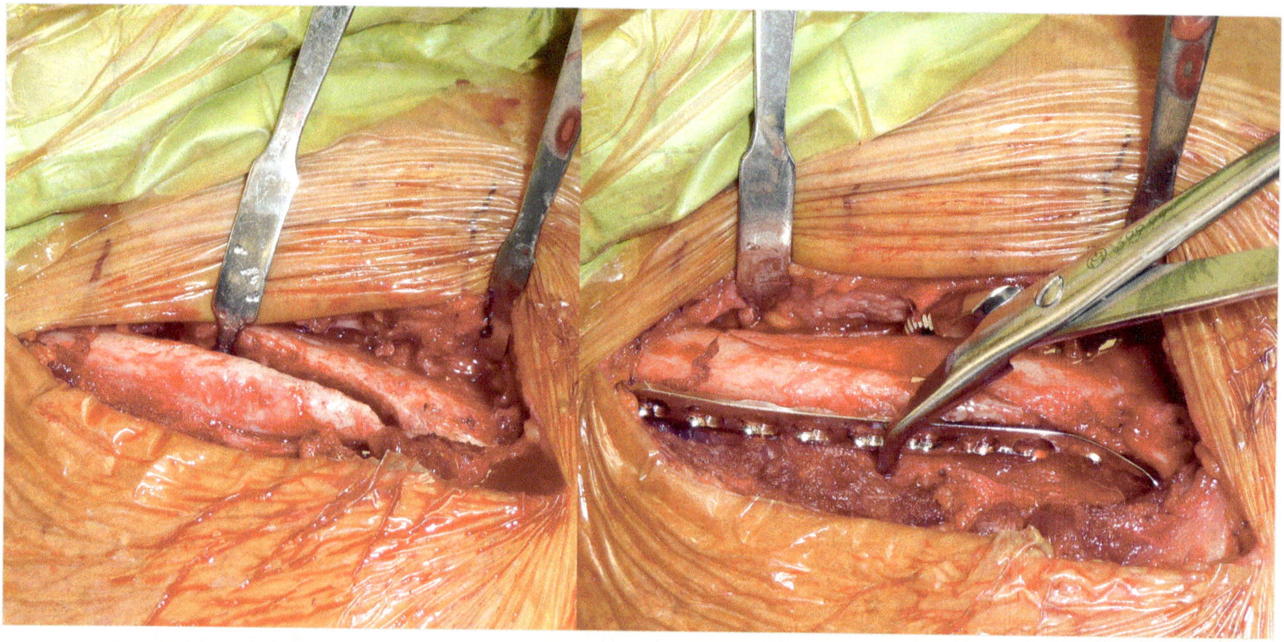

Fig. 68.4 Photograph of the fracture site after being cleared of intervening soft tissue and early fracture callus. On the right side, a 2.4-mm limited contact plate has been contoured and placed onto the anterior clavicle and fixed in place with a cortical screw laterally. A standard reduction clamp has been used to exact a reduction.

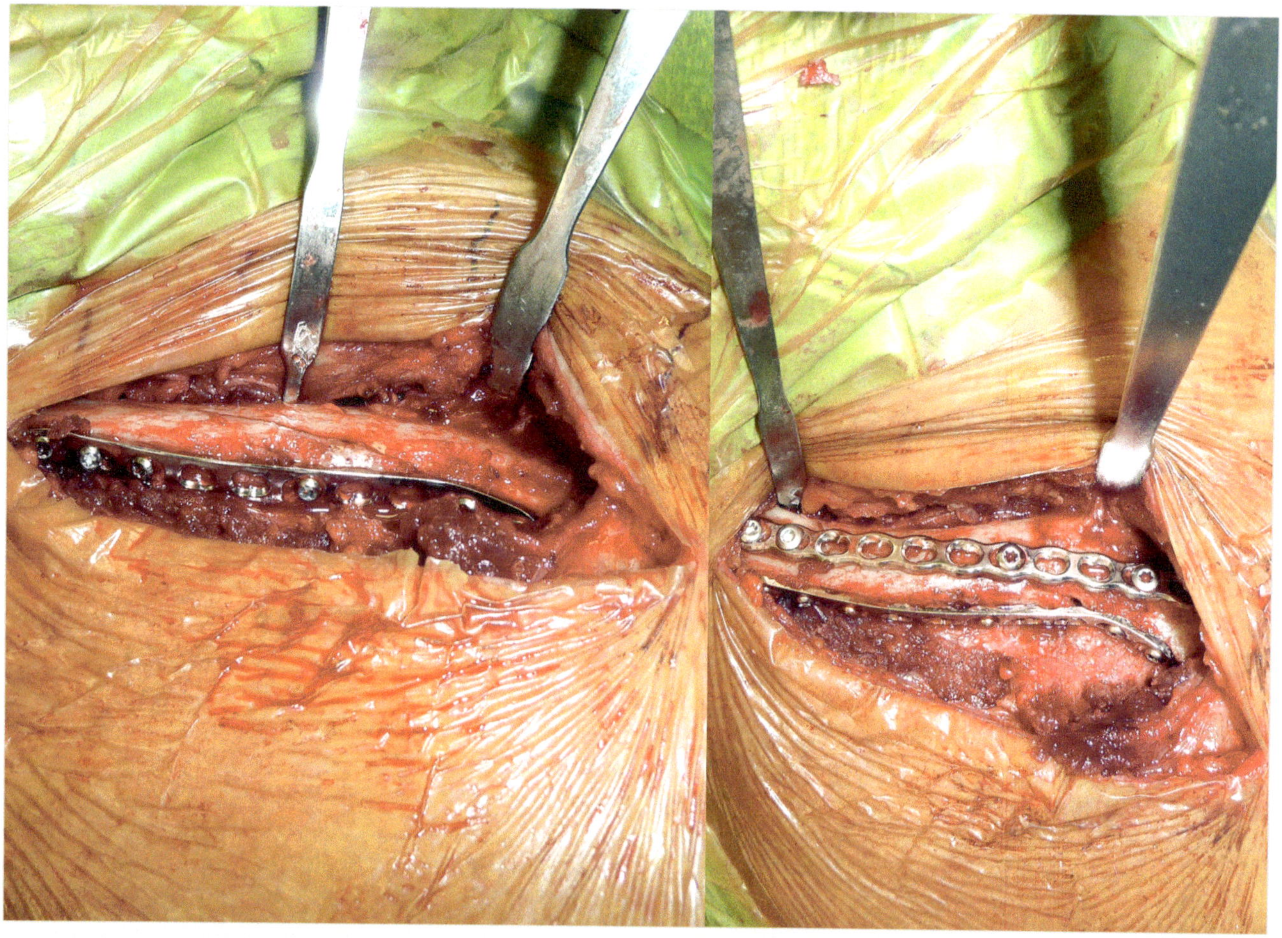

Fig. 68.5 Intraoperative photographs demonstrating placement of the superior 2.7-mm reconstruction plate. Lag screws have been placed perpendicular through the fracture line using the anterior plate as a washer. Notice the contour of the plates to fit the osteology of the clavicle.

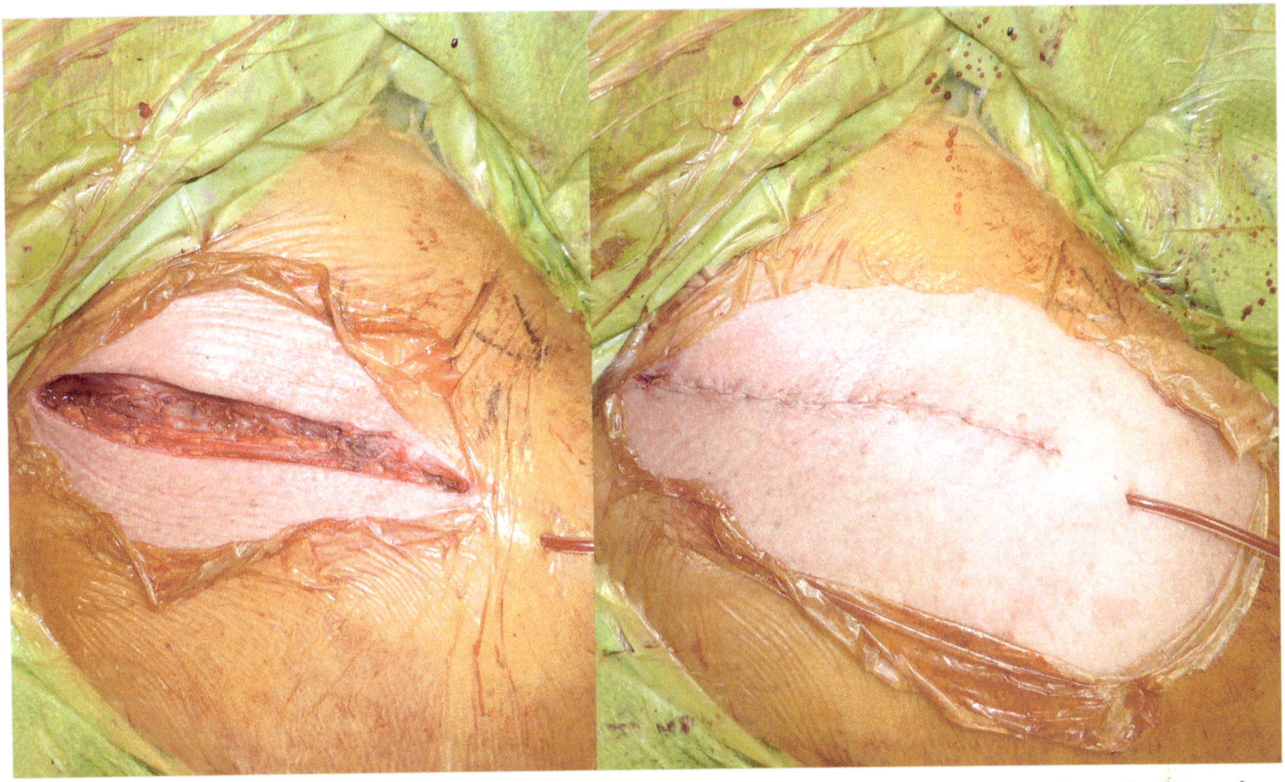

Fig. 68.6 Intraoperative photograph of closure. *Left:* After closure of the deltotrapezial fascia. *Right:* After running subcuticular closure of the skin. Notice the drain exiting laterally that will be removed on postoperative day 1.

cation and increased bending rigidity with an anterior bending load. Plating can also be performed on the anteroinferior surface of the clavicle. Advantages of anteroinferior plating include increased bending rigidity with a superior load, the ability to place longer screws laterally as the anterior to posterior width of the clavicle increases laterally, and the ability to place fixation perpendicular to the typical displacement pattern, thus affording increased stability. In the literature, biomechanical data comparing the two plating locations are conflicting.[22–26] The most common reason for repeat intervention in operatively treated clavicle fractures is hardware removal.[15] We utilize the dual-plating technique to combine the benefit of both plating locations, as well as allowing use of smaller, less prominent plates to decrease the potential for plate irritation. In a biomechanical study, dual mini-fragment plating was found to be no different than standard locking plate constructs in axial or torsional rigidity, and found to be more suitable for resisting the multiplanar bending forces experienced by the clavicle during shoulder motion.[27] The use of orthogonal plates also allows for buttressing of butterfly fragments and placement of lag screws through the plate regardless of fracture location.

68.8 What to Avoid

If operative fixation of a midshaft clavicle fracture is chosen, there are several techniques we believe advisable to avoid. Precontoured plates are available and have been used in several case series. These plates are designed to anatomically fit the clavicle, but a plate to fit all clavicles is not possible. Precontoured plates fit about 30% of clavicles anatomically and require further contouring in 73% of cases.[28] We believe that mini-fragment plates facilitate anatomic contouring to the clavicle and are less prominent than these precontoured plates. Also, many studies in the literature report on the use of intramedullary devices. While some authors have reported good results,[29–32] other studies comparing the technique to plate fixation have found less rotational stability,[33,34] high rates of implant-related pain,[35–37] higher rates of nonunion,[38] and higher overall complication rates.[39] There are case reports of intrathoracic pin migration.[40,41] With orthogonal plating, most of these complications are avoided.

68.9 Complications/Bailout/Salvage

As with any operation, multiple complications are possible. Infections, both deep and superficial, have been reported in a majority of studies at less than 10%.[42] Nonunion rates associated with plate fixation of clavicles is low.[9,10,15,31] Symptomatic malunions are reduced by operative fixation versus nonoperative management of the midshaft clavicle fracture, but they can still occur with poor technique. Implant-related complications are the most commonly reported with operative fixation including plate breakage, fixation failure, and hardware irritation. We believe the use of orthogonal plating with low-profile mini-fragment plates helps minimize these complications. Other rare complications include neurovascular injury (either from trauma or from iatrogenic injury by drill bits or clamps), painful neuromas of the supraclavicular nerves, refracture after hardware removal, and regional pain syndromes.[43]

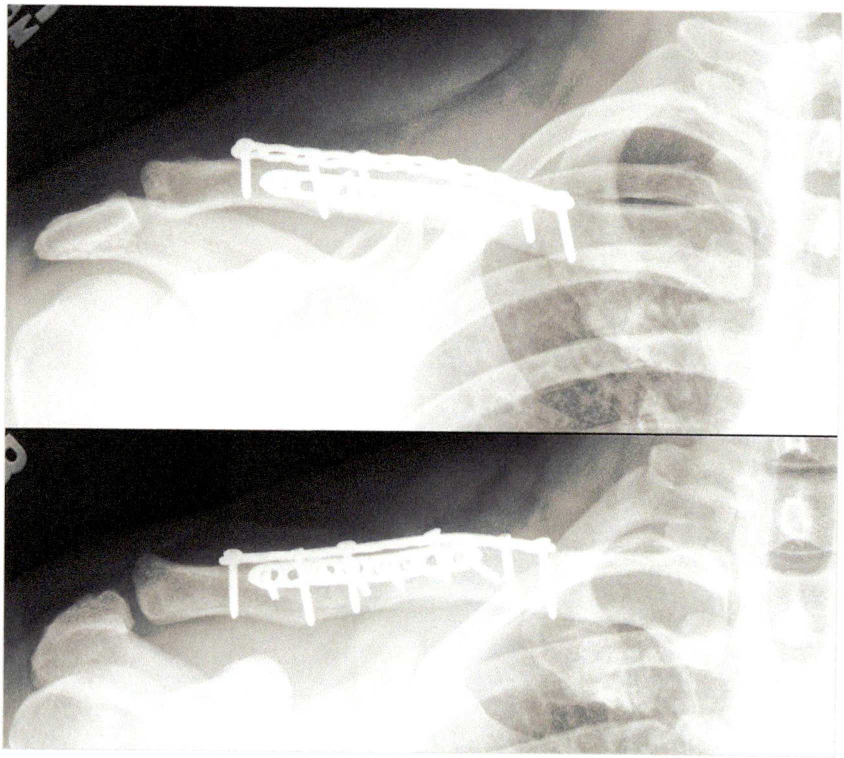

Fig. 68.7 Final radiographs 6 weeks postoperative showing complete healing in anatomic alignment and maintenance of hardware.

In case of any healing complication, the only salvage that will restore shoulder function is treatment of the nonunion or malunion. Nonunions can be treated with workup for the cause of the nonunion and revision fixation and bone grafting. Malunions can be treated with osteotomy and restoration of the native anatomy of the clavicle. Other options, including resection or leaving the patient with a nonunited or malunited clavicle, will negatively affect the patient's function.

68.10 Postoperative Care

The patients are admitted for pain control and discharged on postoperative day 1. Starting on postoperative day 1, the patient is instructed to perform pendulum exercises. The patient returns to clinic in 10 to 14 days and therapy is advanced to include wall walks, pulleys for stretching, and elastic band rotator cuff stretches. Partial weight bearing up to 10 kg is allowed at 3 weeks postoperatively and progressive weight bearing is allowed at 6 weeks postoperatively if pain has resided and radiographs show evidence of healing (**Fig. 68.7**).

References

1. Robinson CM, Ed F. Fractures of the clavicle in the adult. Epidemiology and classification. J Bone Joint Surg Br 1998;80(3):476–484
2. Nordqvist A, Petersson C. The incidence of fractures of the clavicle. Clin Orthop Relat Res 1994;300(300):127–132
3. Postacchini F, Gumina S, De Santis P, Albo F. Epidemiology of clavicle fractures. J Shoulder Elbow Surg 2002;11(5):452–456
4. Neer CS II. Nonunion of the clavicle. JAMA 1960;172(10):1006–1011
5. Rowe CR. An atlas of anatomy and treatment of midclavicular fractures. Clin Orthop Relat Res 1968;58(58):29–42
6. McKee MD, Pedersen EM, Jones C, et al. Deficits following nonoperative treatment of displaced midshaft clavicular fractures. J Bone Joint Surg Am 2006;88(1):35–40
7. Nowak J, Holgersson M, Larsson S. Sequelae from clavicular fractures are common: a prospective study of 222 patients. Acta Orthop 2005;76(4):496–502
8. Hill JM, McGuire MH, Crosby LA. Closed treatment of displaced middle-third fractures of the clavicle gives poor results. J Bone Joint Surg Br 1997;79(4):537–539
9. Zlowodzki M, Zelle BA, Cole PA, Jeray K, McKee MD; Evidence-Based Orthopaedic Trauma Working Group. Treatment of acute midshaft clavicle fractures: systematic review of 2144 fractures: on behalf of the Evidence-Based Orthopaedic Trauma Working Group. J Orthop Trauma 2005;19(7):504–507
10. Virtanen KJ, Remes V, Pajarinen J, Savolainen V, Björkenheim J-M, Paavola M. Sling compared with plate osteosynthesis for treatment of displaced midshaft clavicular fractures: a randomized clinical trial. J Bone Joint Surg Am 2012;94(17):1546–1553
11. Su W-R, Chen W-L, Chen R-H, Hong C-K, Jou I-M, Lin C-L. Evaluation of three-dimensional scapular kinematics and shoulder function in patients with short malunion of clavicle fractures. J Orthop Sci 2016;21(6):739–744
12. Shields E, Behrend C, Beiswenger T, et al. Scapular dyskinesis following displaced fractures of the middle clavicle. J Shoulder Elbow Surg 2015;24(12):e331–e336
13. Hillen RJ, Bolsterlee B, Veeger DHEJ. The biomechanical effect of clavicular shortening on shoulder muscle function, a simulation study. Clin Biomech (Bristol, Avon) 2016;37:141–146
14. Weinberg DS, Vallier HA, Gaumer GA, Cooperman DR, Liu RW. Clavicle fractures are associated with arthritis of the glenohumeral joint in a large osteological collection run-

ning title: clavicle fractures and glenohumeral joint arthritis. J Orthop Trauma 2016;30(11):605–611

15. Society COT; Canadian Orthopaedic Trauma Society. Nonoperative treatment compared with plate fixation of displaced midshaft clavicular fractures. A multicenter, randomized clinical trial. J Bone Joint Surg Am 2007;89(1):1–10
16. McKee RC, Whelan DB, Schemitsch EH, McKee MD. Operative versus nonoperative care of displaced midshaft clavicular fractures: a meta-analysis of randomized clinical trials. J Bone Joint Surg Am 2012;94(8):675–684
17. Althausen PL, Shannon S, Lu M, O'Mara TJ, Bray TJ. Clinical and financial comparison of operative and nonoperative treatment of displaced clavicle fractures. J Shoulder Elbow Surg 2013;22(5):608–611
18. Robinson CM, Court-Brown CM, McQueen MM, Wakefield AE. Estimating the risk of nonunion following nonoperative treatment of a clavicular fracture. J Bone Joint Surg Am 2004;86-A(7):1359–1365
19. Yates DW. Complications of fractures of the clavicle. Injury 1976;7(3):189–193
20. Taitsman LA, Nork SE, Coles CP, Barei DP, Agel J. Open clavicle fractures and associated injuries. J Orthop Trauma 2006;20(6):396–399
21. Backus JD, Merriman DJ, McAndrew CM, Gardner MJ, Ricci WM. Upright versus supine radiographs of clavicle fractures: does positioning matter? J Orthop Trauma 2014;28(11):636–641
22. annotti MR, Crosby LA, Stafford P, Grayson G, Goulet R. Effects of plate location and selection on the stability of midshaft clavicle osteotomies: a biomechanical study. J Shoulder Elbow Surg 2002;11(5):457–462
23. Prasarn ML, Ahn J, Paul O, et al. Dual plating for fractures of the distal third of the humeral shaft. J Orthop Trauma 2011;25(1):57–63
24. Favre P, Kloen P, Helfet DL, Werner CML. Superior versus anteroinferior plating of the clavicle: a finite element study. J Orthop Trauma 2011;25(11):661–665
25. Higgins TF, Klatt J, Bachus KN. Biomechanical analysis of bicondylar tibial plateau fixation: how does lateral locking plate fixation compare to dual plate fixation? J Orthop Trauma 2007;21(5):301–306
26. Celestre P, Roberston C, Mahar A, Oka R, Meunier M, Schwartz A. Biomechanical evaluation of clavicle fracture plating techniques: does a locking plate provide improved stability? J Orthop Trauma 2008;22(4):241–247
27. Prasarn ML, Meyers KN, Wilkin G, et al. Dual mini-fragment plating for midshaft clavicle fractures: a clinical and biomechanical investigation. Arch Orthop Trauma Surg 2015;135(12):1655–1662
28. Malhas AM, Skarparis YG, Sripada S, Soames RW, Jariwala AC. How well do contoured superior midshaft clavicle plates fit the clavicle? A cadaveric study. J Shoulder Elbow Surg 2016;25(6):954–959
29. Smekal V, Irenberger A, Struve P, Wambacher M, Krappinger D, Kralinger FS. Elastic stable intramedullary nailing versus nonoperative treatment of displaced midshaft clavicular fractures-a randomized, controlled, clinical trial. J Orthop Trauma 2009;23(2):106–112
30. Ngarmukos C, Parkpian V, Patradul A. Fixation of fractures of the midshaft of the clavicle with Kirschner wires. Results in 108 patients. J Bone Joint Surg Br 1998;80(1):106–108
31. Ferran NA, Hodgson P, Vannet N, Williams R, Evans RO. Locked intramedullary fixation vs plating for displaced and shortened mid-shaft clavicle fractures: a randomized clinical trial. J Shoulder Elbow Surg 2010;19(6):783–789
32. Assobhi JEH. Reconstruction plate versus minimal invasive retrograde titanium elastic nail fixation for displaced midclavicular fractures. J Orthop Traumatol 2011;12(4):185–192
33. Wilson DJ, Scully WF, Min KS, Harmon TA, Eichinger JK, Arrington ED. Biomechanical analysis of intramedullary vs. superior plate fixation of transverse midshaft clavicle fractures. J Shoulder Elbow Surg 2016;25(6):949–953
34. Renfree T, Conrad B, Wright T. Biomechanical comparison of contemporary clavicle fixation devices. J Hand Surg Am 2010;35(4):639–644
35. Andrade-Silva FB, Kojima KE, Joeris A, Santos Silva J, Mattar R. Clavicle fractures: pins, plates, and drilling down: commentary on an article by Fernando Brandao Andrade-Silva, MD, PhD, et al.: "single, superiorly placed reconstruction plate compared with flexible intramedullary nailing for midshaft clavicular fractures. A prospective, randomized controlled trial.". J Bone Joint Surg Am 2015;97(8):620–626
36. Frigg A, Rillmann P, Perren T, Gerber M, Ryf C. Intramedullary nailing of clavicular midshaft fractures with the titanium elastic nail: problems and complications. Am J Sports Med 2009;37(2):352–359
37. van der Meijden OA, Houwert RM, Hulsmans M, et al. Operative treatment of dislocated midshaft clavicular fractures: plate or intramedullary nail fixation? A randomized controlled trial. J Bone Joint Surg Am 2015;97(8):613–619
38. Millett PJ, Hurst JM, Horan MP, Hawkins RJ. Complications of clavicle fractures treated with intramedullary fixation. J Shoulder Elbow Surg 2011;20(1):86–91
39. Asadollahi S, Hau RC, Page RS, Richardson M, Edwards ER. Complications associated with operative fixation of acute midshaft clavicle fractures. Injury 2016;47(6):1248–1252
40. 40 Leppilahti J, Jalovaara P. Migration of Kirschner wires following fixation of the clavicle: a report of 2 cases. Acta Orthop Scand 1999;70(5):517–519
41. Tan L, Sun D-H, Yu T, Wang L, Zhu D, Li Y-H. death due to intra-aortic migration of Kirschner wire from the clavicle: a case report and review of the literature. Medicine (Baltimore) 2016;95(21):e3741
42. Wijdicks FJG, Van der Meijden OA, Millett PJ, Verleisdonk EJ, Houwert RM. Systematic review of the complications of plate fixation of clavicle fractures. Arch Orthop Trauma Surg 2012;132(5):617–625
43. Althausen PL, Shannon S, Lu M, O'Mara TJ, Bray TJ. Clinical and financial comparison of operative and nonoperative treatment of displaced clavicle fractures. J Shoulder Elbow Surg 2013;22(5):608–611

69 Open Reduction and Internal Fixation of Distal Clavicle Fractures

Sean McIntire, Bradley K. Deafenbaugh, and Lucas S. McDonald

Abstract

Clavicle fractures account for approximately 4% of all fractures, with distal clavicle fractures comprising 15 to 20% of all clavicle fractures. Treatment of distal clavicle fractures is more complex than midshaft clavicle fractures due to the potential involvement of the coracoclavicular ligaments, the acromioclavicular ligament, and the close proximity to the acromioclavicular joint. Although most distal clavicle fractures can be treated nonoperatively, surgical management is indicated for widely displaced fracture fragments, as these are associated with increased risk of nonunion. During surgical treatment, hardware purchase in the distal fracture segment may prove challenging due to a limited area for fixation. This chapter reviews two preferred operative techniques for open reduction and internal fixation of distal clavicle fractures: anatomic distal plate fixation (with or without coracoid augmentation) and hook plate fixation. We review indications for operative intervention, technique for fixation, postoperative care, and pearls/potential pitfalls in practice.

Keywords: *distal clavicle fracture, open reduction and internal fixation, anatomic distal plate, hook plate*

69.1 Goals of Procedure

The goals of distal clavicle surgical fixation are to provide anatomic reduction and stable fixation, resulting in fracture union and return to function for the patient.

69.2 Advantages

69.2.1 Advantages: Anatomic Distal Clavicle Plate

Advantages of fixation of distal clavicle fractures using a distal clavicle plate include the anatomic contour of the plate and the ability to augment the construct with coracoclavicular fixation. No scheduled hardware removal is required with this technique, potentially limiting the number of surgical interventions required.

69.2.2 Advantages: Hook Plate

Advantages of using a hook plate include the ability to address fracture patterns in which the distal fragment is too small to provide adequate screw purchase. The stout fixation provided by the hook plate also allows for earlier initiation of shoulder motion.

69.3 Indications

Absolute indications for distal clavicle fracture fixation include open fractures, traumatic acromioclavicular (AC) joint arthrotomy, neurovascular injury, and impending skin compromise. Relative indications for surgical management include displaced distal clavicle fractures.

69.4 Contraindications

Contraindications for distal clavicle fracture fixation include fractures in patients not healthy enough to undergo operative intervention and minimally displaced fractures. Hardware implantation is also contraindicated in the presence of active infection.

69.5 Preoperative Preparation/Positioning

Open reduction and internal fixation (ORIF) of distal clavicle fractures is accomplished in either the supine or the beach-chair position and is based on surgeon preference. Supine positioning is a simple setup with easier fluoroscopic imaging, while the beach-chair position is more familiar to many surgeons. For supine positioning, the patient is placed on a reversed cantilever radiolucent table (**Fig. 69.1a, b**). "Flat-top" radiolucent tables with support at the head and the feet make it difficult to obtain inlet and outlet images of the clavicle. If a flat-top table is used, the patient should be positioned as far distal on the table as possible, permitting maximum c-arm tilt. In the supine position, the patient's operative shoulder is positioned on the edge of the bed and the patient's nonoperative arm is tucked to the side of the body. The c arm is placed on the opposite side, perpendicular to the table. A radiolucent arm board can be attached to the table on the operative side and positioned against the side of the bed for operative extremity support. A small towel bump is positioned beneath the patient's ipsilateral scapula and the patient's head and neck are gently rotated away from the operative clavicle, improving access. The endotracheal tube should be secured on the opposite side of the involved clavicle and the sternal notch should be included in the prep and drape. The entire operative arm is prepped and draped free, permitting easy manipulation of the extremity during reduction and fixation. In the beach-chair position, the bed is elevated 30 to 45 degrees and the patient's hips and knees are positioned in a gently flexed position and supported by a foam wedge or pillows (**Fig. 69.2**). The bed is rotated 90 degrees so the c arm can be brought in either parallel to the table from above the patient or perpendicular from the side of the table to obtain adequate fluoroscopic views. With either position, the surgeon should confirm that adequate fluoroscopic views can be obtained before proceeding with sterile preparation and draping.

69.6 Operative Technique

69.6.1 Surgical Approach

The clavicle and AC joint are marked and an incision is made along the inferior border of the clavicle. The incision should extend laterally past the AC joint for adequate exposure. Before

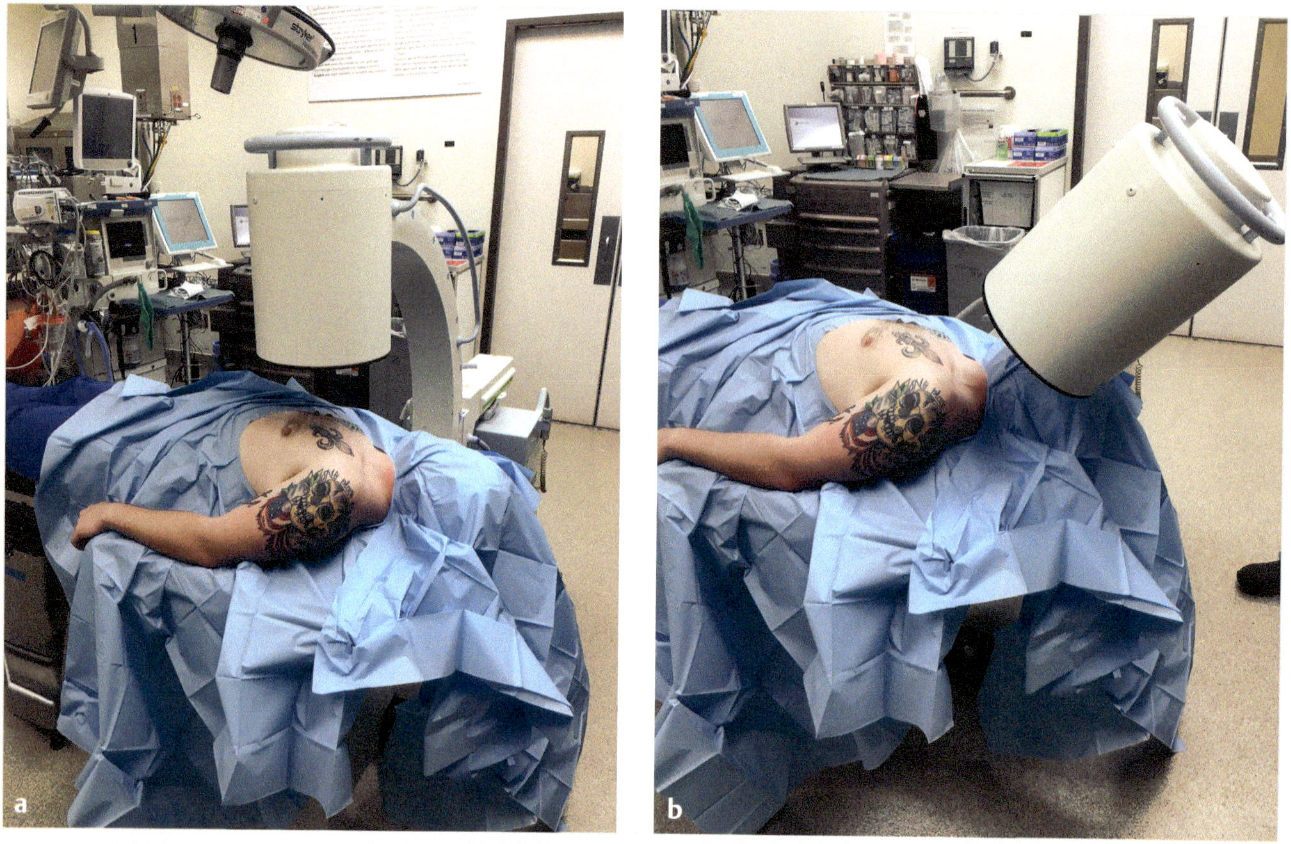

Fig. 69.1 (a,b) Flat top with reversed cantilever radiolucent table. The C arm is positioned on the nonoperative side permitting orthogonal radiographs of the distal clavicle.

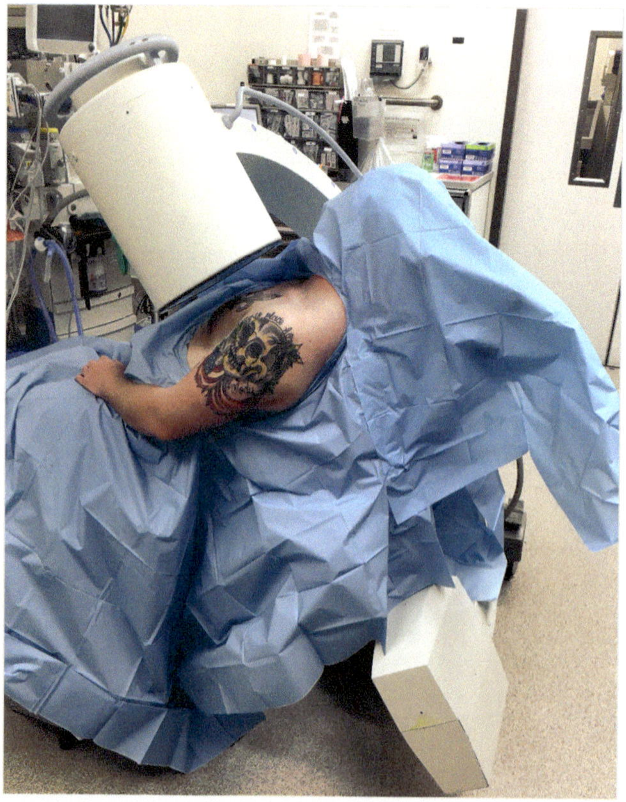

Fig. 69.2 The beach-chair position with the patient situated laterally and the arm free. The C arm is positioned on the nonoperative side (as shown) or brought in from the head permitting orthogonal radiographs of the distal clavicle.

making the incision, preinjecting the incision line with a local anesthetic with epinephrine solution aids hemostasis. As the dissection proceeds through the subcutaneous tissues, sensory branches of the supraclavicular nerve are encountered crossing perpendicular to the surgical field. When possible, these branches are identified and preserved. In most cases, however, one or more of these branches must be sacrificed to obtain exposure, and patients must be counseled on the risk of postoperative anterior chest wall numbness. The fracture site is exposed by sharply elevating muscle fibers of the trapezius posteriorly and the deltoid anteriorly. Care should be taken to preserve soft-tissue attachments, when possible, to preserve osseous blood supply. The fracture hematoma is evacuated and the fracture edges are meticulously cleaned to obtain adequate visualization for reduction.

69.6.2 Fixation with Anatomic Distal Clavicle Plate

We recommend the beach-chair position when using this implant due to the ease of placing supplemental coracoid fixation if needed, and the ability to use a commercially available arm holder. Reduction of distal clavicle fractures can be challenging due to the firm coracoclavicular ligaments that are often attached to the distal fragment. This makes manipulation of lateral fragments difficult because they are less mobile than the fragments in a middle third pattern. Trying to reduce the lateral fragment, with the attached conoid and trapezoid ligaments, to the more superior medial fragment can result in comminution

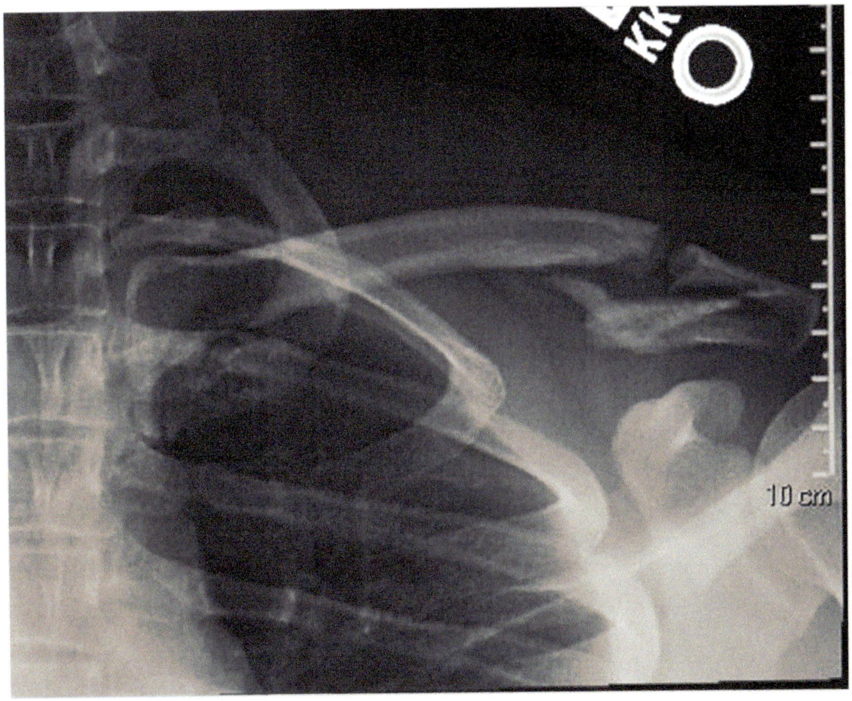

Fig. 69.3 Anteroposterior radiograph of a left distal clavicle fracture with superior displacement. There is no widening of the coracoclavicular distance when considering the inferior/distal fracture fragment.

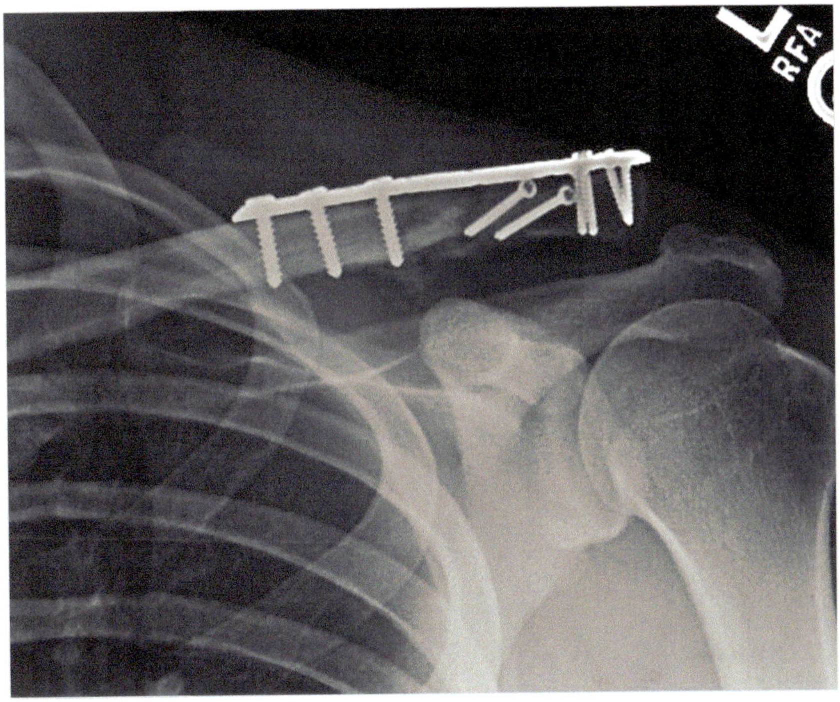

Fig. 69.4 Postoperative radiograph of the left distal clavicle fracture demonstrating anatomic distal clavicle fracture fixation including lag screw fixation, bicortical screws medially and locking screws distally. Due to robust fixation in lateral fragment and no injury to the coracoclavicular ligaments, no supplemental fixation was performed.

of the lateral fragment. The majority of the reduction force is therefore concentrated on reducing the more mobile medial fragment to the less mobile lateral fragment. Once the fragments are reduced and held with reduction forceps, lag screw fixation is performed if possible. The size of the fragments often requires smaller screw sizes, generally 2.4 or 2.7 mm in diameter. After provisional fixation, an anatomically contoured distal clavicle plate (Arthrex, Naples, FL) is placed superiorly in neutralization mode. These precontoured plates have a wide distal flare, permitting a cluster of smaller diameter screws to be placed into the distal fragment. Bicortical screw fixation is performed medially with nonlocking cortical screws, with at least six cortices (three screws) utilized. Distally in the smaller fragment locking screws are typically employed and a locking screw guide is used to drill before screw placement. If there is considerable comminution at the fracture site, but the distal fragment is large enough to accommodate appropriate screw fixation, the comminuted fragments are bypassed and the distal clavicle plate is used in a bridging fashion (**Figs. 69.3, 69.4**).

69.6.3 Coracoclavicular Ligament Repair/Reinforcement

If the lateral fixation is tenuous, or the injury pattern involves the coracoclavicular ligaments, additional fixation to the coracoid process is recommended. This can be performed in an open or arthroscopic method. We prefer open treatment, as exposure of the coracoid is straightforward when combined with ORIF of the fracture. The coracoid process is identified and a deltoid split is performed to the base of the coracoid, clearing both medially and laterally to ensure a central location for the drill hole and permitting retrieval of a shuttling suture from beneath the coracoid. A guide pin is drilled bicortically, confirming a central location at the base of the coracoid with direct palpation. A right-angle retractor is placed under the coracoid to prevent inadvertent advancement of the guide pin and the coracoid is drilled bicortically with a 3-mm cannulated drill. A nitinol wire is passed through the drill and retrieved laterally with a hemostat or 90-degree clamp. A preloaded button from the acute AC repair kit (Arthrex) is shuttled retrograde through the coracoid. Fluoroscopy is then used to confirm placement under the coracoid. A second bicortical drill hole through the clavicle is created traversing to an appropriate hole in the plate and the sutures again shuttled. The sutures are passed through the distal clavicle plate button (Arthrex) that fills an appropriate hole in the plate, and tightened. Suture limbs are then tied and cut short.

69.6.4 Fixation with a Hook Plate

When the lateral fracture segment is small or comminuted and cannot accept screw fixation, or reduction cannot be obtained as previously described, a hook plate (DePuy Synthes, Westchester, PA) can be used. Patient positioning can be in either the beach-chair or the supine position and is the surgeon's preference. With a hook plate, the lateral flare or hook of the plate is positioned underneath the acromion, posterior to the AC joint. A small rent in the trapezial fascia is made just posterior to the distal clavicle and the hook is slid along the undersurface of the acromion. The hook plate flare comes in different hook depths and may require trialing to match the patient's anatomy. Once the hook is appropriately positioned, the medial shaft of the plate is levered down onto the superior aspect of the medial fracture fragment, effecting a reduction. A clamp is then used to hold the reduction in place. The plate is subsequently secured to the medial fragment with 3.5-mm bicortical screws. Although a hook plate provides robust fixation and is an excellent option for these fracture patterns, its positioning underneath the acromion necessitates a second surgery for removal once healing occurs. The plate is removed 3 to 4 months postoperatively to avoid further impingement and possible erosion of the acromion at the bone–hook interface (**Figs. 69.5–69.7**).

69.7 Tips and Pearls/Expert Suggestions

69.7.1 Pearls/Pitfalls: Anatomic Distal Clavicle Plate

Distal clavicle plates should only be used when the surgeon feels there is adequate bone stock in the distal fragment to accommodate multiple screws. Techniques to reduce axial pullout include gaining bicortical fixation with standard screws in the distal fragment, or placing screws with divergent paths.[1] If the screw holes are large enough, screws with a larger thread may also be used to gain increased purchase in the distal bone, although the screw head may sit more prominently over the screw hole of the plate. Additionally, if injury to the coracoclavicular or AC ligaments has occurred, or if backup fixation for the construct is needed, supplemental fixation to the coracoid process may decrease stress on the fracture construct during the healing phase. Adherence to postoperative activity restrictions is imperative to decrease stresses placed on the fracture repair. We utilize a specific distal clavicle system (Arthrex) due

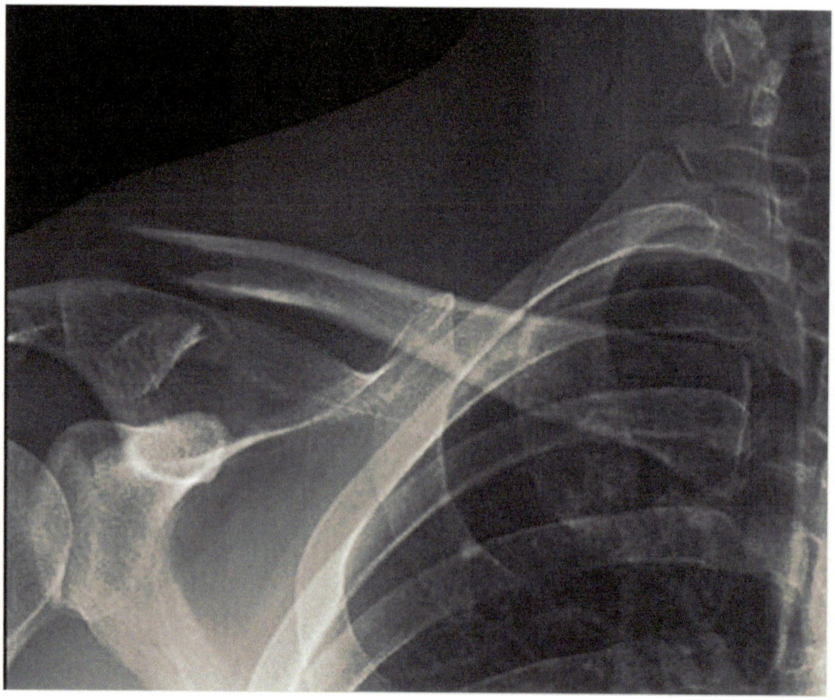

Fig. 69.5 Anteroposterior radiograph of the right distal clavicle fracture with small distal fragment. With this small fracture fragment, insufficient fixation is possible with anatomic plating. Coracoclavicular widening is present.

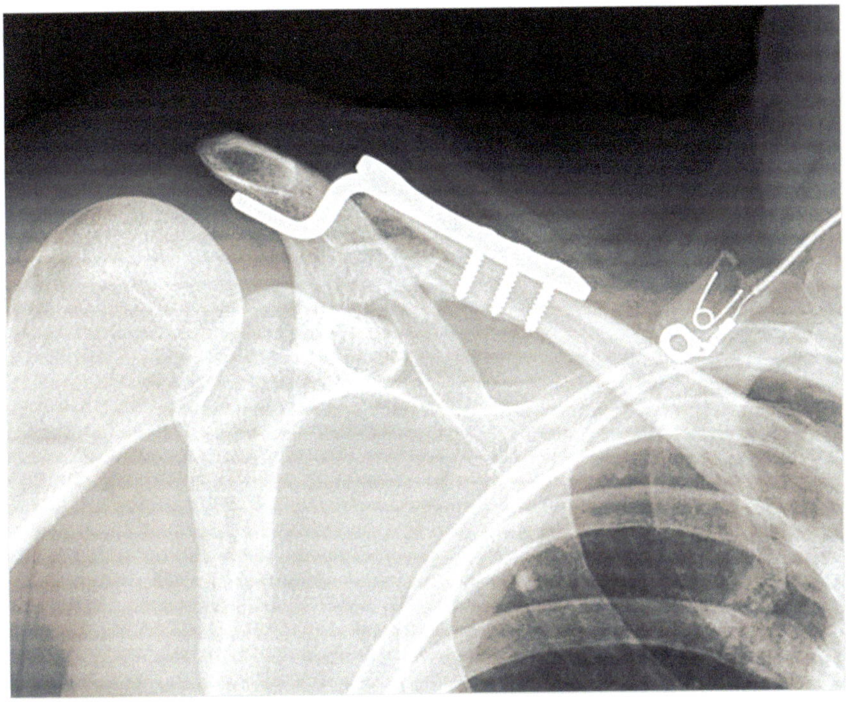

Fig. 69.6 Anteroposterior radiograph of the right distal clavicle fracture demonstrating hook plate fixation with bicortical screw fixation medially and reduction of the fragment with reduction of the coracoclavicular widening.

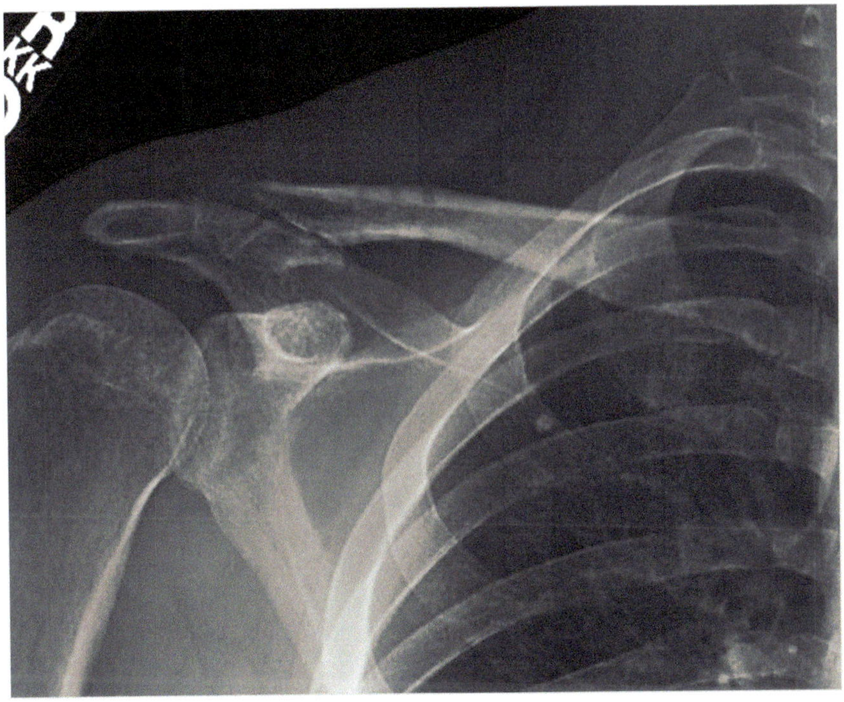

Fig. 69.7 Anteroposterior radiograph of the right distal clavicle fracture after healing and removal of the hook plate.

to its ability to augment the fixation through the plate, and the available guides that make the procedure smoother from a technical standpoint.

69.7.2 Pearls/Pitfalls: Hook Plate

When a hook plate is chosen, it is often due to small lateral fragments preventing adequate distal fixation with an anatomic distal clavicle plate. In these patterns, the medial fragment may be difficult to reduce inferiorly and hold in place with clamps or k-wires. The hook plate is helpful in this situation, as once the hook of the plate is positioned under the acromion, the plate itself can be used to lever down the medial segment, reducing the fracture. Due to the soft tissue and osseous concerns surrounding the AC joint, hook plate removal is recommended after bony union occurs. This is typically performed approximately 3 to 4 months after initial fixation. The need for a second procedure is the primary drawback of hook plate fixation, balanced by the advantage of being a more rigid initial fixation construct. If present, impingement symptoms and radiographic findings of osteolysis usually resolve after hook plate removal.

69.8 What to Avoid

Key points to avoid with this procedure include incomplete closure of soft-tissue structures, inadequate fragment fixation, and prolonged retained hook plate hardware. After fixation, appropriate soft-tissue closure starting with the deltotrapezial fascia must be performed to provide coverage to the plate and prevent fluid or hematoma accumulation, which may lead to deep infection. With hook plate fixation, patients should begin early range-of-motion therapy to prevent stiffness due to the stout nature of the construct. The hook plate also should not be left in longer than is necessary to achieve union, due to the irritating effect the plate has on the rotator cuff and the AC joint.

69.9 Complications/Bailout/Salvage

69.9.1 Complications: Anatomic Distal Clavicle Plate

Soft-tissue complications including infection or hardware irritation are a concern. Though not required, patients may request hardware removal due to prominence leading to discomfort, or for cosmetic reasons.[2] Documented nonunion rates range from 0 to 5%.[2,3] Peri-implant fractures have also been described, requiring further surgical treatment.[3] The most concerning complication is the potential for construct failure, especially considering the small area for screw fixation distal to the fracture. Axial screw pullout can occur, even with the use of locking screw technology.[1] This is best prevented with supplemental coracoid fixation reinforcing the construct when necessary and a slow postoperative rehabilitation protocol until fracture union. If revision surgery is necessary, this can be accomplished by either adding coracoid fixation if not used initially or revising to a hook plate and using the distal acromion as the supplemental fixation.

69.9.2 Complications: Hook Plate

Soft-tissue complications of infection and hardware irritation are a primary concern. Additionally, if significant comminution exists in the distal fragment, nonunion may occur. Peri implant fractures have been documented with minimal trauma.[4,5] Complications specific to the hook plate include rotator cuff impingement, subacromial bursitis, and inferior acromial osteolysis, along with AC joint arthrosis.[4,6,7] Rotator cuff impingement and subacromial bursitis are treated with hook plate removal. AC joint arthrosis is addressed with distal clavicle resection if symptoms persist after hook plate removal. Described methods of hardware failure include hook displacement from under the acromion as well as proximal screw pull.[8]

69.10 Postoperative Care

69.10.1 Postoperative Care: Anatomic Distal Clavicle Plate

The patient is non-weight-bearing on the operative extremity in a sling for a minimum of 6 weeks. This reduces the inferior traction placed on the construct by the weight of the operative extremity and may help prevent fixation failure. To avoid stiffness, wrist and elbow range-of-motion exercises in the sling are encouraged beginning postoperative day 1. Postoperative visits are scheduled for 2 weeks, 6 weeks, 3 months and 6 months with radiographic and clinical evaluation. Physical therapy is initiated at 6 weeks with full active and passive range of motion, followed by gradual strengthening and an expected return to activities as tolerated by 3 months postoperatively.

69.10.2 Postoperative Care: Hook Plate

Due to the robust fixation provided by the hook plate, physical therapy with gentle active range-of-motion exercises can be initiated immediately following surgery. The positioning of the hook underneath the acromion often keeps patients from tolerating shoulder abduction or forward flexion past 90 degrees. A sling is used for comfort and may be discontinued when tolerated. The patient is scheduled for plate removal at 3 to 4 months following the index procedure.

References

1. Brouwer KM, Wright TC, Ring DC. Failure of superior locking clavicle plate by axial pull-out of the lateral screws: a report of four cases. J Shoulder Elbow Surg 2009;18(1):e22–e25
2. Shin SJ, Ko YW, Lee J, Park MG. Use of plate fixation without coracoclavicular ligament augmentation for unstable distal clavicle fractures. J Shoulder Elbow Surg 2016;25(6):942–948
3. Andersen JR, Willis MP, Nelson R, Mighell MA. Precontoured superior locked plating of distal clavicle fractures: a new strategy. Clin Orthop Relat Res 2011;469(12):3344–3350
4. Tiren D, van Bemmel AJM, Swank DJ, van der Linden FM. Hook plate fixation of acute displaced lateral clavicle fractures: mid-term results and a brief literature overview. J Orthop Surg 2012;7:2
5. Klein SM, Badman BL, Keating CJ, Devinney DS, Frankle MA, Mighell MA. Results of surgical treatment for unstable distal clavicular fractures. J Shoulder Elbow Surg 2010;19(7):1049–1055
6. Renger RJ, Roukema GR, Reurings JC, Raams PM, Font J, Verleisdonk EJMM. The clavicle hook plate for Neer type II lateral clavicle fractures. J Orthop Trauma 2009;23(8):570–574
7. Meda PVK, Machani B, Sinopidis C, Braithwaite I, Brownson P, Frostick SP. Clavicular hook plate for lateral end fractures: a prospective study. Injury 2006;37(3):277–283
8. Haidar SG, Krishnan KMK, Deshmukh SC. Hook plate fixation for type II fractures of the lateral end of the clavicle. J Shoulder Elbow Surg 2006;15(4):419–423

70 All-Arthroscopic Coracoclavicular Ligament Reconstruction for Type V Acromioclavicular Separation

Xinning Li and Nicholas R. Pagani

Abstract

In this chapter, we discuss the operative indications, advantages, contraindications, operative technique, pearls, and pitfalls of the arthroscopic coracoclavicular (CC) ligament reconstruction for acromioclavicular (AC) separations. Utilizing the all-arthroscopic technique described is advantageous due to decreased risk of patient morbidity through smaller surgical incisions and possible accelerated recovery time compared to open techniques. Additionally, using the arthroscopic technique allows the surgeon to address the concomitant shoulder pathology. The senior author (X.L.) recommends the use of arthroscopic CC ligament reconstruction for type V AC separations in the setting of both acute and chronic injuries.

Keywords: *arthroscopic CC ligament reconstruction, AC joint injury, acromioclavicular, coracoclavicular*

70.1 Goals of Procedure

Acromioclavicular (AC) joint injuries are found in approximately 9% of all shoulder girdle injuries and are associated with injuries occurring from a direct collision or axially directed force on the affected shoulder. Among AC joint injuries that are managed surgically, a number of key elements are essential to a successful postoperative outcome depending upon surgical technique utilized. These include anatomic reduction of the AC joint, direct repair or reconstruction of the coracoclavicular (CC) ligaments, protection of the CC ligament repair, or reconstruction with synthetic material to maintain AC joint stability during the acute phases of healing, repair of the deltoid and trapezial fascia, and distal clavicular resection in patients with evidence of AC osteoarthritis.[1] Many open surgical techniques are currently employed to achieve these goals. Recent surgical advancements have led to the development of an arthroscopically assisted CC ligament reconstruction with free tendon grafts or synthetic material.[2] Here we describe a technique for an all-arthroscopic CC ligament reconstruction utilizing a semitendinosus allograft and biocomposite tenodesis screws without disruption of the deltoid attachment onto the distal clavicle as seen with the open technique.

70.2 Advantages

This all-arthroscopic surgical technique minimizes soft-tissue dissection and reduces skin and wound complications in comparison to open CC ligament reconstruction. As a result, this technique leads to decreased patient morbidity and facilitates faster postoperative recovery with earlier return to work or sport. Additionally, the surgeon is able to address intra-articular shoulder pathology at the same time of the arthroscopic CC ligament reconstruction surgery. The portal location described and utilized with this technique, as well as its use of 30- and 70-degree arthroscopes, allows for proper visualization of all relevant anatomy and appropriate debridement of the coracoid base and distal clavicle. The use of tendon grafts (autograft or allograft) in CC ligament reconstruction is associated with lower rates of failure and early complications as compared to cortical fixation button (a commonly employed technique in modern arthroscopically assisted AC stabilization procedures for acute AC separations).[3] Moreover, AC joint reconstruction using a semitendinosus graft has been shown to achieve better Oxford Shoulder Score and Nottingham Score than the classic modified Weaver–Dunn procedure.[2]

70.3 Indications

AC joint injuries are classified as types I to VI using the Rockwood system. This classification system is based on the extent of damage to the AC and CC ligaments as well as the displacement of the distal clavicle.[4] Type I and II injuries of the AC joint involve either sprain or tear of the AC ligament without tear of the CC ligaments and are managed nonsurgically with sling immobilization, early shoulder range of motion, and physical therapy. Type III, IV, V, and VI injuries all involve tears of both the AC and CC ligaments with varying displacements of the distal clavicle. Surgical management is indicated for patients with type IV, V, and VI AC joint injuries. The management of type III AC joint injury remains controversial; however, surgical intervention is typically considered in active patients with high functional demand on the shoulder.[5] It should be noted that the all-arthroscopic CC ligament reconstruction technique described here is significantly easier to perform on type V AC joint separation compared to type III due to the portal positions and the amount of the displacement of the distal clavicle.

70.4 Contraindications

All-arthroscopic CC ligament reconstruction is contraindicated if the distal clavicle is not reducible under general anesthesia. Advanced age is a relative contraindication to arthroscopic AC joint reconstruction due to poorer overall bone quality. This all-arthroscopic technique is very difficult to perform in patients with chronic type V AC joint separations who have calcification of the CC ligaments or heterotopic bone formation in the CC interval. The senior author (XL) recommends a mini-open approach for these cases.

70.5 Preoperative Preparation/Positioning

The patient is placed in the beach-chair position. The author prefers a semitendinosus allograft for this procedure; however, a semitendinosus autograft is also applicable for this technique. A no. 2 braided suture is used to prepare the graft via whip stitch across the entire length of the graft for augmentation. Additional no. 2 braided suture is passed on either end of the graft in a Krakow fashion in order to facilitate passage of the graft (**Fig. 70.1a**). Graft thickness is measured to guide the size of the tunnel drilled on the distal clavicle.

70.6 Operative Technique

This all-arthroscopic technique utilizes four portals (**Fig. 70.1b**): a medial portal (portal M—located just medial to the coracoid process), an anterolateral primary viewing portal (portal V), an accessory anterolateral portal (portal A—located 1 cm lateral to the anterolateral corner of the acromion), and an AC joint portal (portal B—located just lateral to the AC joint). A standard 30-degree arthroscope is utilized for the majority of the procedure. A 70-degree arthroscope is utilized for visualization of the coracoid and clavicular undersurfaces during the debridement and drilling of the distal clavicle.

Starting with the 30-degree arthroscope located in the standard posterior portal, a spinal needle is used to locate the rotator interval anteriorly. A radiofrequency (RF) device is then introduced through the rotator interval, and debridement of the rotator interval and coracoid base is subsequently performed. Adequate debridement of the coracoid base is essential for the success of this all-arthroscopic procedure. One trick is to establish the anterior portal slightly lateral in the rotator interval to be able to debride the top and bottom of the coracoid base. Alternatively, a 70-degree arthroscope can be used in the posterior viewing portal to facilitate this step if visualization of the coracoid base is difficult.

Following debridement of the rotator interval and coracoid base, the 30-degree arthroscope is moved to portal V. This is performed with the assistance of a switching stick. Portal V serves as the primary viewing portal for this technique and provides an excellent view of the subscapularis tendon and coracoid base (**Fig. 70.2**). The RF device is inserted through accessory portal A to perform further debridement of the superior and inferior aspects of the coracoid base (**Fig. 70.2**). In order to locate

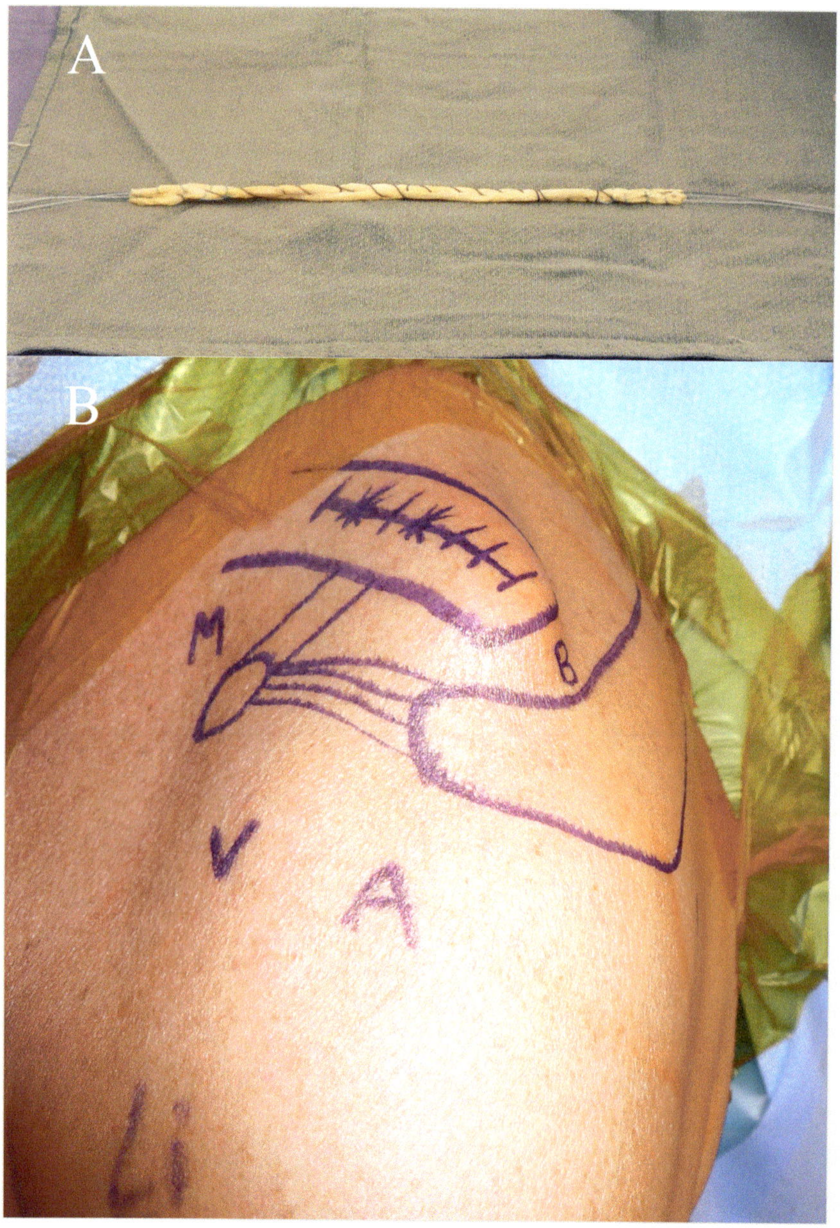

Fig. 70.1 (a) Semitendinosus allograft preparation used for the coracoclavicular ligament reconstruction. A no. 2 braided suture (Arthrex FiberWire) is used to whip stitch the entire allograft to reinforce the biomechanical strength of the reconstruction. **(b)** The four portals utilized in the all-arthroscopic technique (portal M: medial portal; portal V: anterolateral viewing portal; portal A: accessory anterolateral portal; portal B: acromioclavicular joint portal).

a working portal medial to the coracoid base, a spinal needle is inserted to assist in establishing portal M (**Fig. 70.3a**). Once direct visualization of the spinal needle is achieved, a trocar is placed to widen the tunnel and also to further debride the soft tissue on the medial side of the coracoid base. The RF device is then inserted through the M portal for thorough debridement of the medial aspect of the coracoid base and release of the pectoralis minor tendon (**Fig. 70.3b**) to help facilitate with the graft passage. Debridement is complete once the RF can be passed from the medial to inferior aspect of the coracoid base.

A 90-degree suture passer is introduced into the M portal such that the tip of the passer can be visualized on the medial and inferior side of the coracoid base. The suture shuttle device is passed medially around the undersurface of the coracoid base and the suture passer is then deployed. Using a grasper inserted through portal A, the deployed suture is grasped (**Fig. 70.4a**) and a no. 2 braided suture is subsequently shuttled around the base of the coracoid. The limbs of this suture are used in a future step to facilitate passage of the semitendinosus graft around the coracoid base.

Next, debridement of the inferior aspect of the clavicle is performed. The anterior and posterior borders of the clavicle are delineated using three spinal needles, which serve as reference guides for the anterior and posterior extents of the clavicle during subsequent debridement (**Fig. 70.4b**). The undersurface of the distal clavicle is visualized via a 70-degree arthroscope inserted in portal V. The clavicle undersurface is debrided using the RF wand inserted through the accessory portal B. Thorough soft-tissue debridement past 4.5 cm from the distal clavicle is critical for accurate drill tunnel positioning for the conoid and

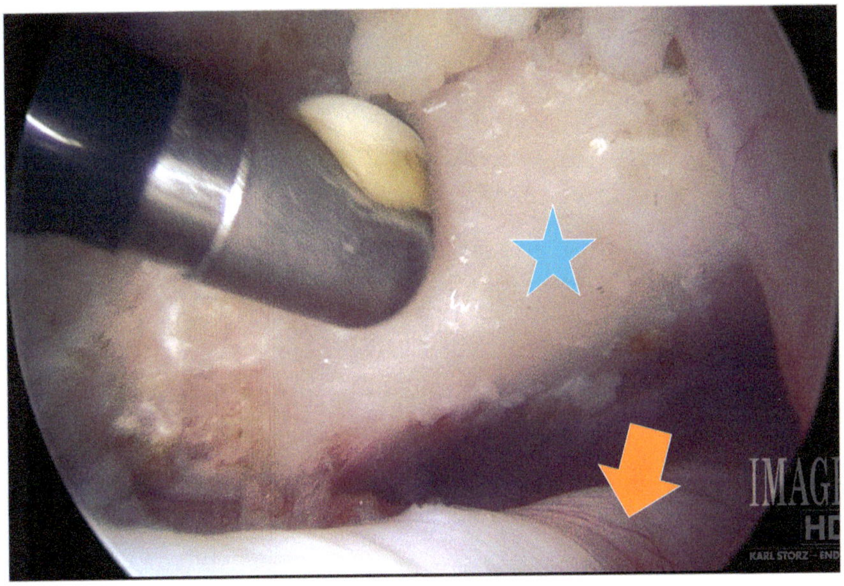

Fig. 70.2 Arthroscopic viewing with a 30-degree arthroscope using portal V. A radiofrequency wand is inserted into the anterior glenohumeral joint via the accessory portal A to further debride the base of the coracoid (*blue star*) and the subscapularis tendon (*orange arrow*).

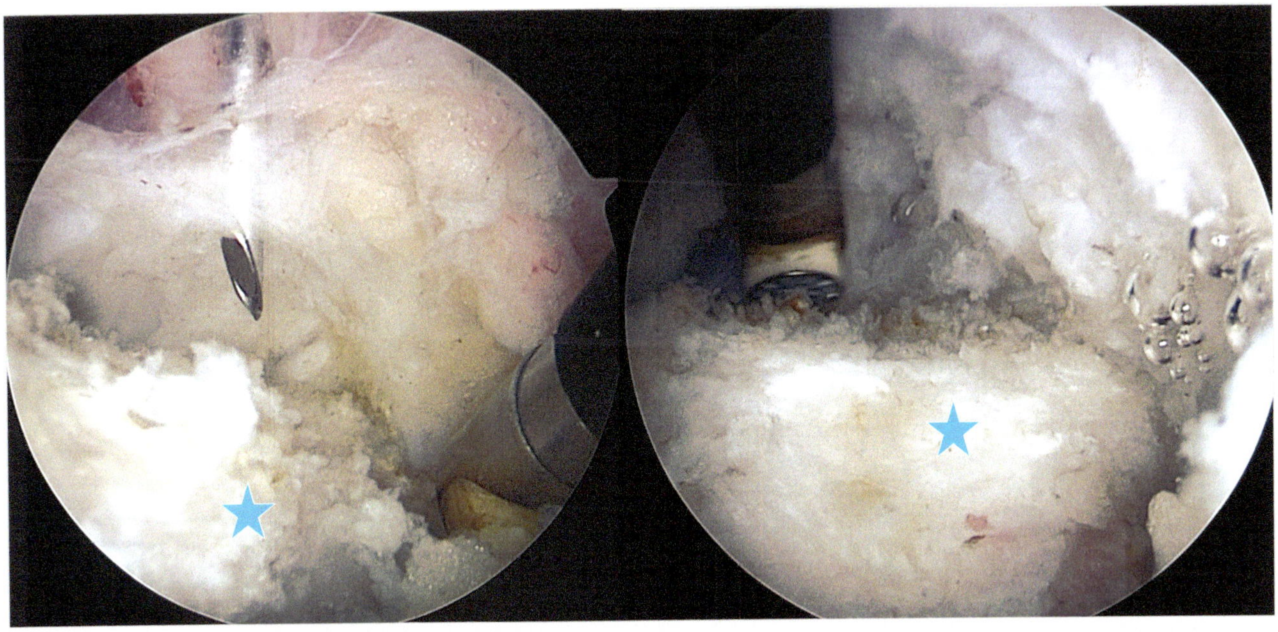

Fig. 70.3 **(a)** Viewing from portal V using a 30-degree arthroscope. A spinal needle is used to help locate the medial aspect of the coracoid base (*blue star*) via portal M. **(b)** A radiofrequency wand is used via portal M to help debride the pectoralis minor off the medial aspect of the coracoid (*blue star*) to help facilitate graft passage around the base.

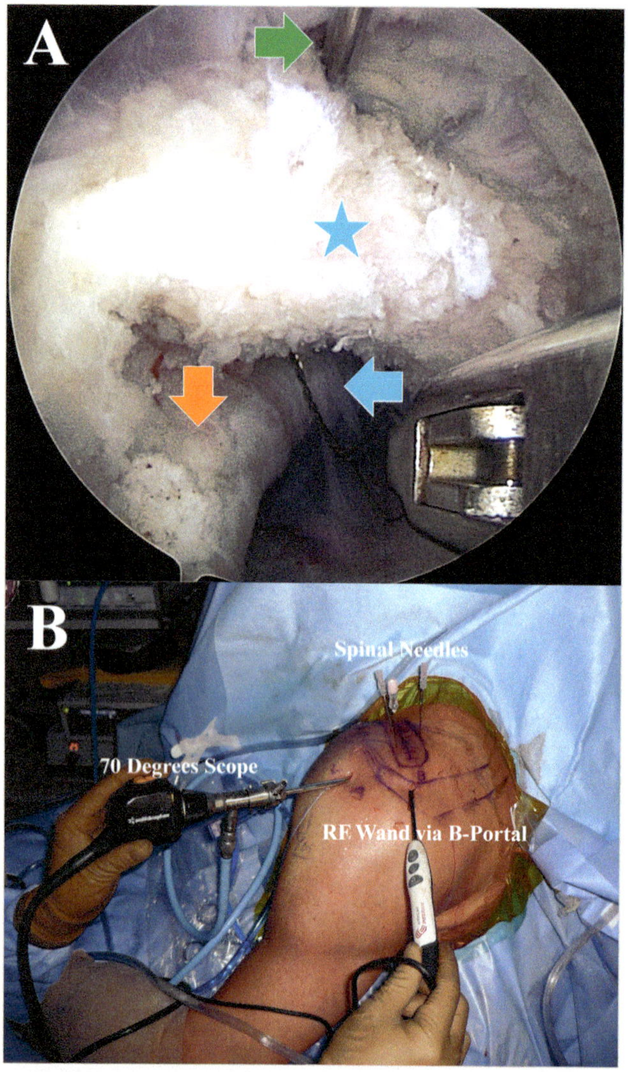

Fig. 70.4 (a) This shows the grasper inserted through portal A that is used to grasp the deployed chia (DePuy-Mitek Ideal Passer, 90-degree suture passer) and shuttle it around the coracoid base. A no. 2 suture is shuttled around the coracoid base with this chia passer, where the suture is ultimately to be used in aiding passage of the semitendinosus graft around the coracoid base. (b) Three spinal needles anterior and posterior to the distal clavicle serve as reference guides for the anterior and posterior margins of the clavicle, so the clavicle can be appropriately debrided with the radiofrequency wand from accessory portal B.

the trapezoid tunnel position.

Following thorough debridement and complete visualization of the inferior clavicle, a 3-cm incision is made in line with and superior to the distal clavicle at the location of the conoid (4.5 cm from the distal clavicle) and trapezoid tunnels (3.0 cm from the distal clavicle). Two clavicular drill tunnels (for the conoid and trapezoid) are now prepared. The senior author (XL) prefers to use either a 5.0- or a 5.5-mm cannulated headed reamer over a drill bit for the two tunnels and 5.5 × 8 mm polyetheretherketone (PEEK) tenodesis screws for the fixation (Arthrex, Naples, FL). The senior author (X.L.) finds that semitendinosus grafts will fit perfectly into a 5.0- or 5.5-mm tunnel. The tunnel position for the conoid medially is located approximately 4.5 cm from the distal clavicle and slightly in the posterior aspect of the clavicle. The tunnel position for the trapezoid laterally is located around 3.0 cm from the distal clavicle (1.5 cm lateral to the conoid drill tunnel) and slightly anterior on the distal clavicle. The conoid and trapezoid drill tunnels are created over guide pins from the superior to the inferior direction. The two drill guide pins are visualized arthroscopically on the inferior aspect of the distal clavicle using the 70-degree arthroscope via portal V during this process. Once the guide pin is drilled, either a curette or an arthroscopic grasper can be used to hold the pins and protect the soft tissue from injury. Once the two tunnels are made, the RF wand is used to debride the tunnels superiorly and inferiorly.

Following preparation of the two clavicular drill tunnels, the 90-degree suture passer (Ideal Passer with Chia; DePuy-Mitek Sports Medicine, Raynham, MA) is introduced through the medial (conoid) drill tunnel. The lateral limb of the no. 2 braided suture that was previously looped around the coracoid base is now shuttled through the medial (conoid) drill tunnel using a grasper and the deployed suture passer via portal A (**Fig. 70.5a**). This step results in the medial limb of the suture still exiting through portal M and the lateral limb of the suture now exiting through the medial (conoid) drill tunnel. In similar fashion to the previous step, the suture shuttle is next introduced through the lateral (trapezoid) drill tunnel and the suture passer is deployed. The medial limb of the suture is then shuttled through the lateral (trapezoid) drill tunnel with the use of a grasper inserted through portal A. The result of these steps is a crisscross pattern of the no. 2 braided suture around the coracoid base with the medial limb exiting through the lateral (trapezoid) drill tunnel and the lateral limb exiting through the medial (conoid) drill tunnel (**Fig. 70.5b**).

Attention is now turned to preparation of the semitendinosus allograft for passage. Mineral oil is applied along the surface of the graft to facilitate passage through the drill tunnels. Using the no. 2 suture, the graft is passed through one drill tunnel, around the coracoid base, and out the opposite drill tunnel. Following this maneuver, the two ends of the graft will be visualized through the 3-cm superior incision at the distal end of the clavicle. A biocomposite screw is now inserted into the medial (conoid) drill tunnel to secure this limb of the graft. The AC joint is then reduced using a superiorly directed force on the ipsilateral upper extremity and an inferiorly directed force on the clavicle. While holding this reduction, a second biocomposite screw is inserted into the lateral (trapezoid) drill tunnel.

The residual two ends of the tendon graft are sutured upon themselves with a no. 2 braided suture (**Fig. 70.6a**) and the final reconstruction is seen arthroscopically (**Fig. 70.6b**). Currently, the senior author (X.L.) also prefers to augment the reconstruction with a FiberTape (2.0-mm thickness, Arthrex) hand tied over the top of the clavicle that is passed around the coracoid base. This is passed at the same time as the semitendinosus allograft.

70.7 Tips and Pearls/Expert Suggestions

- The all-arthroscopic CC ligament reconstruction technique described here is significantly easier to perform on Rockwood type V AC joint separation compared to type III. This is due to the increased displacement of the distal clavicle seen with the type V injuries, which allows the RF device to

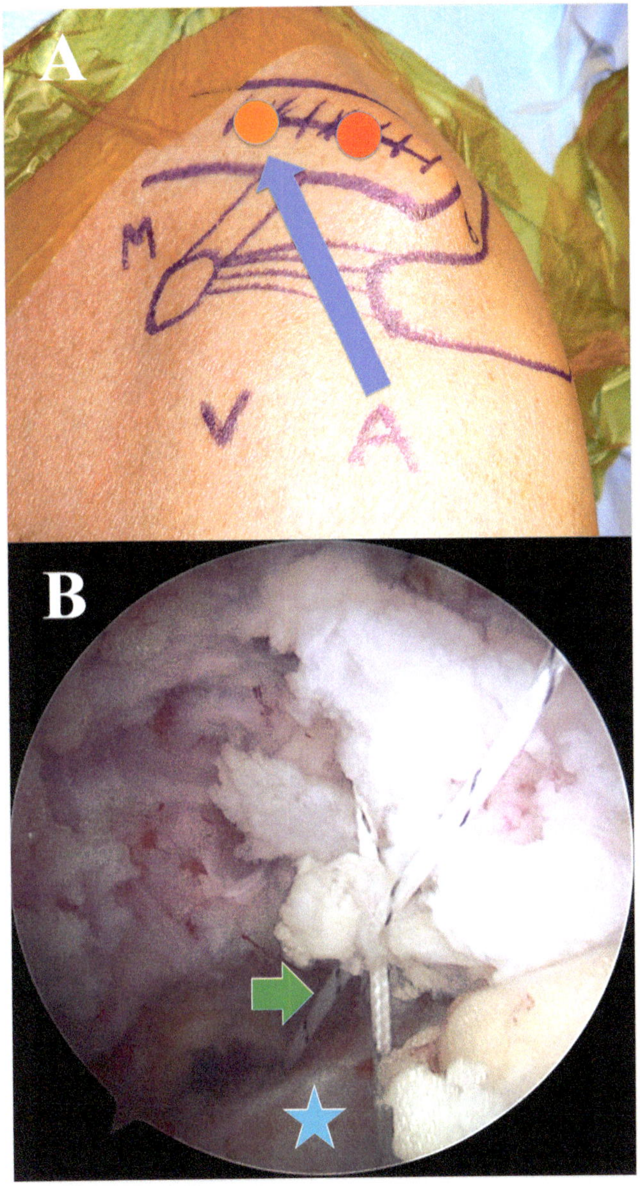

Fig. 70.5 (a) The *arrow* points to the two clavicular drill tunnels as represented by the two *circles*. A no. 2 suture is passed from portal A to the medial drill tunnel in preparation for graft passage. (b) An arthroscopic image showing the crisscross pattern of the no. 2 suture around the coracoid base.

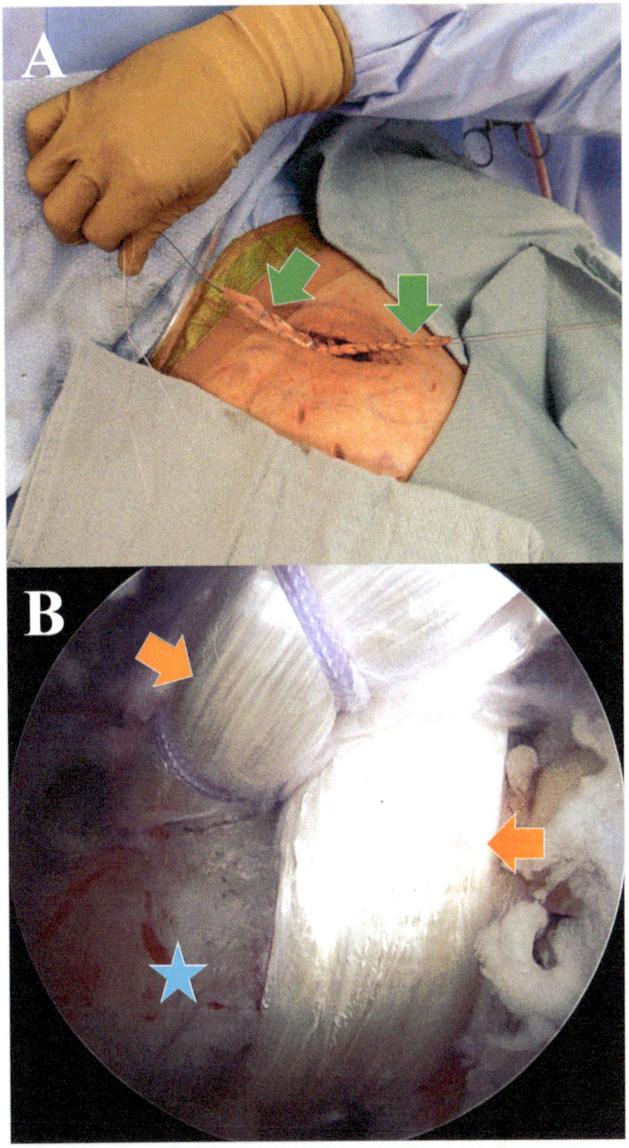

Fig. 70.6 (a) The residual two ends of the allograft graft are sutured upon themselves with no. 2 sutures after placement of the 5.5 × 8 mm tenodesis screws (Arthrex). (b) The final coracoclavicular ligament reconstruction using semitendinosus allograft is visualized arthroscopically via portal V using a 30-degree arthroscope.

debride the undersurface via assessor portal B.

- Always suture the residual graft over the distal clavicle after fixation with no. 2 braided sutures using a figure of 8 technique to help reinforce the reconstruction.
- Use a tape-like material around the coracoid base and tie over the top of the clavicle to further help augment the repair that will decrease stretching of the graft.
- Using a tenodesis screw that is a line-to-line fit to the size of the tunnel will give you the best fixation and screw purchase. If you drill a 5.0- or 5.5-mm tunnel, use the 5.0-mm screw.
- Perform a minimal (5–8 mm) distal clavicle resection at the time of CC ligament reconstruction to help prevent future AC joint arthrosis and pain.
- In revision setting, the senior author prefers to use semitendinosus autograft.

70.8 What to Avoid

Any patient with calcification of the CC ligament or heterotopic bone formation in the CC ligament interval is not a candidate for this arthroscopic CC ligament reconstruction procedure. Arthroscopic dissection of this region in the setting of extra bone formation is dangerous and should be avoided. The senior author prefers a mini-open technique in these patients.

70.9 Complications/Bailout/Salvage

If the surgeon encounters difficulties with passage of the graft, the anterior deltoid can be taken down to help facilitate a mini-open approach to help with graft passage. Bailout to open CC ligament reconstruction is needed if further difficulties are encountered with graft passage. In cases of revision AC separation, mini-open CC ligament reconstruction with semitendinosus autograft is preferred.

If the distal clavicle is fractured during the procedure, a plate fixation should be performed and the graft can be passed around the clavicle and underneath the plate to help secure the fixation and reduction of the CC ligament space and AC joint.

70.10 Postoperative Care

This all-arthroscopic technique offers the added advantage of expedient postoperative recovery. Sling immobilization is required for 4 weeks following AC joint and CC ligament reconstruction with semitendinosus allograft tendon. Physical therapy is then initiated at week 2 with focus on upper extremity range of motion and strength. Patients will start with passive range of motion in the supine position with forward flexion, abduction, and external rotation at week 2. When the range of motion is started in the supine position, this will help alleviate stress from the AC joint and the CC reconstruction. Transition from passive ROM to active ROM is done between weeks 6 and 10 depending on the patient. Strengthening is started in weeks 8 to 10 when the patient retains at least 80% of his or her passive ROM compared to the contralateral side. Overhead athletes may begin a throwing program at 18 weeks postoperatively. Return to heavy labor work is allowed when the patient is within 90% of the motion and strength of the contralateral normal side. This is usually around 4 to 6 months after surgery.

References

1. Li X, Ma R, Bedi A, Dines DM, Altchek DW, Dines JS. Management of acromioclavicular joint injuries. J Bone Joint Surg Am 2014;96(1):73–84
2. Hegazy G, Safwat H, Seddik M, Al-Shal EA, Al-Sebai I, Negm M. Modified Weaver-Dunn procedure versus the use of semitendinosus autogenous tendon graft for acromio-clavicular joint reconstruction. Open Orthop J 2016;10: 166–178
3. Rush LN, Lake N, Stiefel EC, et al. Comparison of short-term complications between 2 methods of coracoclavicular ligament reconstruction: a multicenter study. Orthop J Sports Med 2016;4(7):2325967116658419
4. Rockwood C, Williams G, Young DDisorders of the acromio-clavicular joint. In: Rockwood CJ, Matsen F, eds. The Shoulder. 3rd ed. Philadelphia, PA: WB Saunders Co; 2004:521–586
5. Smith TO, Chester R, Pearse EO, Hing CB. Operative versus non-operative management following Rockwood grade III acromioclavicular separation: a meta-analysis of the current evidence base. J Orthop Traumatol 2011;12(1):19–27

71 Open Acromioclavicular Joint Reconstruction

Neil S. Kumar and Augustus D. Mazzocca

Abstract

This chapter reviews the operative technique for open anatomic coracoclavicular ligament reconstruction (ACCR). The procedure aims to reestablish the natural biomechanics of the shoulder and alleviate pain. Indications for reconstruction following acromioclavicular (AC) joint disruption include persistent pain or distal clavicle instability after 3 to 4 weeks of nonoperative treatment. Preoperative bilateral Zanca views and axillary lateral radiographs identify injury pattern and concomitant pathology. Reconstruction focuses on restoring natural anatomical relationships. Trapezoid and conoid tunnels are placed 25 and 45 mm medial to the AC joint, respectively, to re-create the native anatomy and avoid the inferior bone density of the lateral clavicle. A third tunnel is placed 10 mm medial to the joint and paired with an acromial tunnel for a figure-of-8 suture fixation. Peroneus longus allograft is combined with a high-strength nonabsorbable suture for biologic and nonbiologic fixation. Reduction is achieved with scapular elevation and an anteriorly directed force on the distal clavicle. Tenodesis screws and suture technique create internal biologic and nonbiologic braces. The deltotrapezial fascia is critical to sagittal stability of the distal clavicle and must be repaired anatomically. Strengthening is started at 12 weeks postoperatively with return to collision sports at 6 months.

Keywords: *acromioclavicular joint, coracoclavicular ligament, distal clavicle instability, ligament reconstruction*

71.1 Goals of Procedure

Open anatomic coracoclavicular ligament reconstruction (ACCR) aims to reestablish the natural biomechanics of the shoulder and alleviate pain. The goals of surgery are to restore shoulder range of motion (ROM) and strength, allowing the patient to return to full activities.

71.2 Advantages

Restoration of normal acromioclavicular (AC) joint anatomy plays a vital role in achieving stability of the distal clavicle. Open surgery provides direct visualization of the AC joint and distal clavicle, helping the surgeon achieve the goal of anatomic reconstruction. Acromial and clavicular tunnel locations can be directly measured from the AC joint and related to key bony landmarks, allowing for accurate tunnel placement. High-grade dislocations may disrupt the fascia and cause the distal clavicle to "buttonhole" through the tissue, preventing reduction. Open visualization allows the surgeon to release the clavicle and repair traumatic fascial tears, which is essential to maintain anteroposterior stability of the distal clavicle.

71.3 Indications

In the treatment algorithm of the senior author, the major indication for open ACCR is increasing or persistent shoulder pain, particularly with subjective distal clavicle instability, which limits the patient from participation in activities after 3 to 4 weeks of nonoperative treatment. Tented skin "at risk" secondary to significant distal clavicle deformity also warrants surgical intervention.

Type I and II injuries are typically lower energy[1] and are treated nonoperatively with pain relief modalities, early shoulder motion, and periscapular and shoulder strengthening for 6 to 12 weeks. These injuries inherently maintain some degree of ligamentous stability of the distal clavicle and, therefore, are surgically treated with distal clavicle excision. However, surgery is indicated only if chronic pain and dysfunction develop, which in our clinical experience is rare.

The evidence regarding treatment for type III injuries is still inconclusive.[2] In the practice of the senior author, these patients complete 3 to 4 weeks of nonoperative treatment to reduce pain, improve ROM, and increase use of the injured upper extremity. If significant improvements are made, rehabilitation is completed; patients who do not show marked progress undergo surgical reconstruction. It is important to note that many variables are examined when choosing the length of nonsurgical treatment, particularly for athletes or heavy laborers. Type of labor or sport, especially those involving contact or overhead activity, must be considered. Other factors such as competition level, years of eligibility remaining, and whether injury occurred in- or offseason are also reviewed.

High-energy type IV, V, and VI dislocations are treated operatively. Such injuries frequently involve trauma to the deltotrapezial fascia and may lead to "buttonholing" of the distal clavicle, requiring surgical reduction.[1] Nonsurgical treatment risks the morbidity of persistent pain, restricted ROM, and shoulder girdle weakness.[3]

71.4 Contraindications

Contraindications to ACCR include nerve injury to the ipsilateral upper extremity limiting shoulder function or ongoing chronic infection. Relative contraindications include significant distal clavicle bone loss, displaced coracoid fracture, and poor skin quality overlying the AC joint.

71.5 Preoperative Preparation/ Positioning

71.5.1 Imaging

A standing bilateral Zanca view radiograph with the arms by the side is performed to allow side-to-side comparison of the coracoclavicular (CC) distance. A cross-body adduction view may show the distal clavicle overriding the acromion, indicating AC joint instability. An axillary lateral X-ray determines distal clavicle sagittal position. Shoulder radiographs can reveal additional trauma, such as coracoid or glenoid fractures.

MRI can be obtained if concerns exist for concomitant soft-tissue injuries. In younger patients, biceps or superior labral anterior and posterior (SLAP) tears should be suspected; rotator cuff tears occur more often in older patients. CT scan can confirm suspected coracoid fracture.

71.5.2 Positioning

Following intubation, the patient is placed in the beach-chair position. The head is slightly rotated away from the surgical site to allow for conoid tunnel drilling. The hips are flexed to 60 to 70 degrees and a pillow is placed under the knees. Sequential compression devices are used on both lower extremities. The patient is positioned as far laterally on the table as possible and the torso is elevated with a bump placed under the medial border of the scapula. The patient is secured to the table with tape across the torso and with a safety belt across the thighs. The scapular bump is also secured with tape to prevent loss of positioning when manipulating the upper extremity.

The mini C arm is used to obtain a Zanca view of the operative shoulder and a reduction maneuver, typically scapular elevation with anterior translation of the clavicle, is fluoroscopically reviewed to visualize joint reduction. The operative field is prepped to include the sternoclavicular joint medially and the scapular spine posteriorly.

71.6 Operative Technique

71.6.1 Surgical Approach

The coracoid, acromion, AC joint, and lateral one-half of the clavicle are marked (**Fig. 71.1**). We utilize a curved incision along Langer lines approximately 30 mm medial to the AC joint. The incision extends 20 mm posterior to the posterior border of the clavicle and to the anterior tip of the coracoid process. This incision allows access anteriorly to the coracoid, medially to the conoid tubercle, and laterally to the lateral border of the acromion. Extending the incision posteriorly toward the scapular spine can improve exposure of the distal clavicle and AC joint.

The skin is sharply incised and needle-tip electrocautery is used to complete the dissection to the level of the deltotrapezial fascia. Self-retaining retractors aid dissection and maintain strict hemostasis. Skin flaps superficial to the fascial layer are raised medially and laterally to improve exposure. Flaps should be kept as thick as possible to avoid postoperative wound complications. A full-thickness fascial incision in line with the clavicle is made on the superior clavicular surface between the trapezius insertion posteriorly and deltoid origin anteriorly (**Video 71.1**). The fascial incision continues over the acromion posterior to the posterior border of the clavicle. It is critical to extend the fascial cut a few millimeters lateral to the AC joint and to the conoid tubercle medially in order to place anatomic drill holes; we typically ensure access up to 5 cm medial to the AC joint. The anterior clavicle is skeletonized to create a full-thickness periosteal flap including the deltoid origin. Of note, the deltoid has a second origin that lies on the deep and inferior surface of the clavicle, which must be dissected subperiosteally as well. Once both deltoid layers are dissected, a tagging suture is placed. The trapezius insertion is skeletonized with subperiosteal dissection off the posterior clavicular border and a tagging suture is placed. At this time, a provisional reduction maneuver is performed with an anteriorly directed force on the distal clavicle with scapular elevation. Direct and fluoroscopic visualization can verify anatomic joint reduction and identify interfering soft tissue.

Blunt dissection is used at this point to determine the medial and lateral borders of the coracoid process. Needle-tip electrocautery is used to peel the soft tissues off of the superior surface (**Fig. 71.2**). Here, extreme care must be taken to keep the dissection on the bony coracoid surface to avoid injuring surrounding neurovascular structures, such as the lateral cord, musculocutaneous nerve, and axillary artery. Once the coracoid can be visualized to the anterior tip, blunt dissection of the medial and lateral borders creates a plane for the curved suture passer. A high-strength nonabsorbable shuttling suture is passed from medial to lateral around the anterior coracoid process. The suture typically "settles" posteriorly at the base of the coracoid; the surgeon should ensure the suture rests anteriorly toward the tip of the coracoid process to avoid injuring the suprascapular nerve during graft passage.

71.6.2 Tunnel Preparation

The conoid tunnel is marked approximately 45 mm medial to the AC joint posterior to the midline of the clavicle (**Video 71.2**). Placing this tunnel slightly medial captures the better bone quality of the medial clavicle compared to lateral bone.[4] The trapezoid

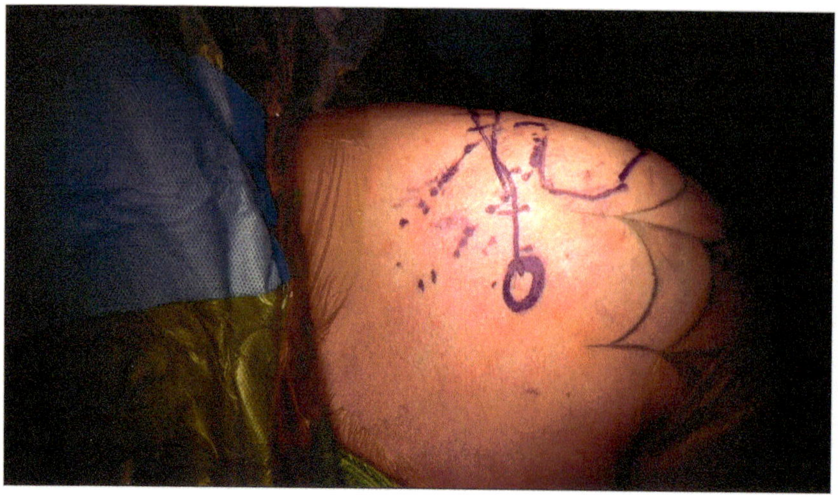

Fig. 71.1 The incision extends 20 mm posterior to the posterior border of the clavicle and to the anterior tip of the coracoid process.

tunnel is marked approximately 25 mm medial to the AC joint just anterior to the midline. A third mark, 10 mm medial to the AC joint, is made for AC joint suture fixation. A guide wire is placed bicortically from superior to inferior at the conoid tunnel, angling the wire slightly anteriorly. A Cobb elevator is used at the inferior clavicle to prevent lung injury. A second guide wire is introduced at the trapezoid tunnel perpendicular to the clavicle (**Fig. 71.3**). A cannulated 5.0-mm reamer is passed over the guide wires bicortically. In order to prevent eccentric tunnels, the drill is disconnected from the reamer after broaching the far cortex and removed manually. A 5.5-mm tap is used for both tunnels and interference screw lengths are measured and recorded.

Smaller tunnels are used for supplemental suture fixation of the AC joint (**Video 71.3**). At the most lateral clavicle marking, a 2.4-mm drill is used from the anterior border of the clavicle to the posterior border with a Cobb elevator placed posteriorly to protect the soft tissues. A suture is passed through the tunnel with a loop exiting posteriorly. The complementary acromial tunnel begins at the anterolateral angle and exists posteriorly in line with the posterior border of the clavicle. The 2.4-mm drill is introduced and a suture is passed through the tunnel with a loop exiting posteriorly. A high-strength, nonabsorbable suture is passed through the clavicle from posterior to anterior. The anterior limb should be extended as this is passed through the acromion from posterior to anterior. This technique allows for figure-of-8 suture fixation of the AC joint (**Fig. 71.4**).

71.6.3 Coracoclavicular Fixation

The allograft ends are tubularized into a "bullet tip" with high-strength nonabsorbable suture to ease graft passage through the tunnels. A standard whip stitch is completed on both ends and tied over the graft end. Frayed edges are debrided sharply. The graft plus a no. 2 high-strength nonabsorbable suture are passed from medial to lateral using the shuttle suture; the additional suture serves as nonbiologic fixation. The graft should be passed around the coracoid in such a manner that the conoid tunnel will accept the thinner end of the graft (**Video 71.4**). The graft and suture are cyclically tensioned around the coracoid to ensure they lie anteriorly. The straight suture passer shuttles the graft and one free suture limb through the conoid tunnel from inferior to superior. Approximately 20 mm of allograft should exit the tunnel superiorly. The remaining graft and free suture limb are shuttled through the trapezoid tunnel. The thicker graft end should pass through the trapezoid tunnel because the lateral clavicle typically has poorer bone quality.

Anatomic reduction of the AC joint is visualized directly and fluoroscopically. A pointed bone reduction clamp maintains

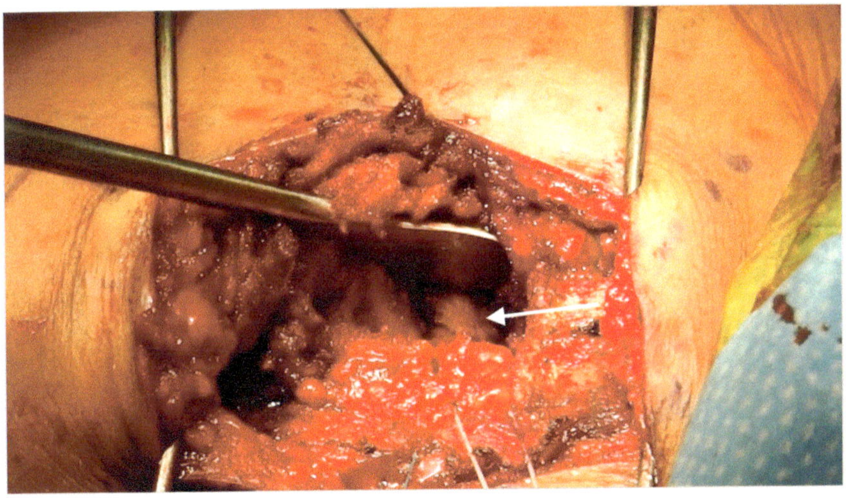

Fig. 71.2 The coracoid (*arrow*) is fully visualized to ease suture hook passage.

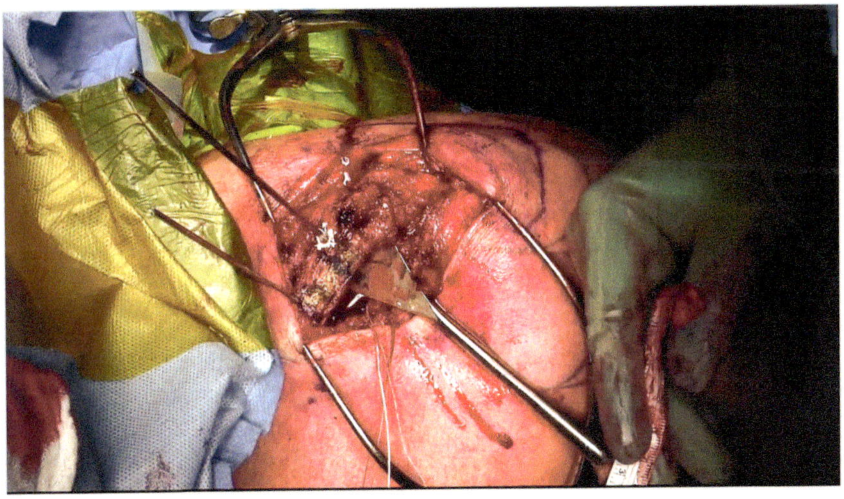

Fig. 71.3 Guide wires are placed 25 and 45 mm medial to the acromioclavicular joint to mark the trapezoid and conoid tunnels, respectively.

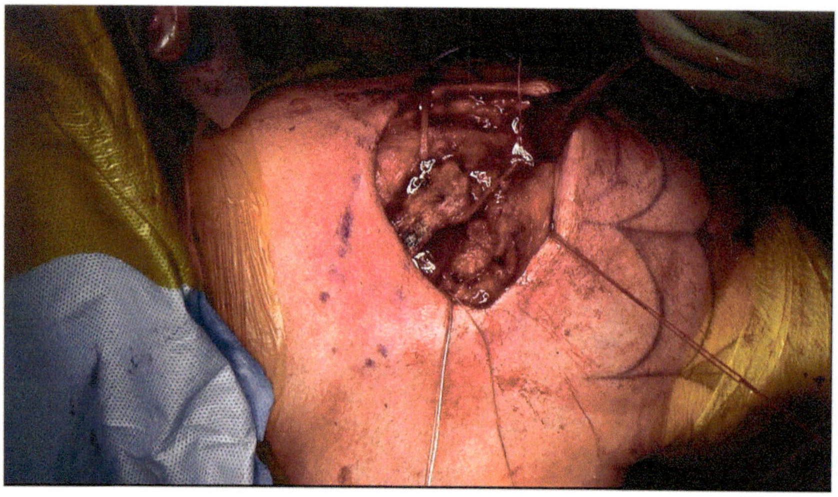

Fig. 71.4 The anterior clavicular suture limb is passed through the acromion from posterior to anterior.

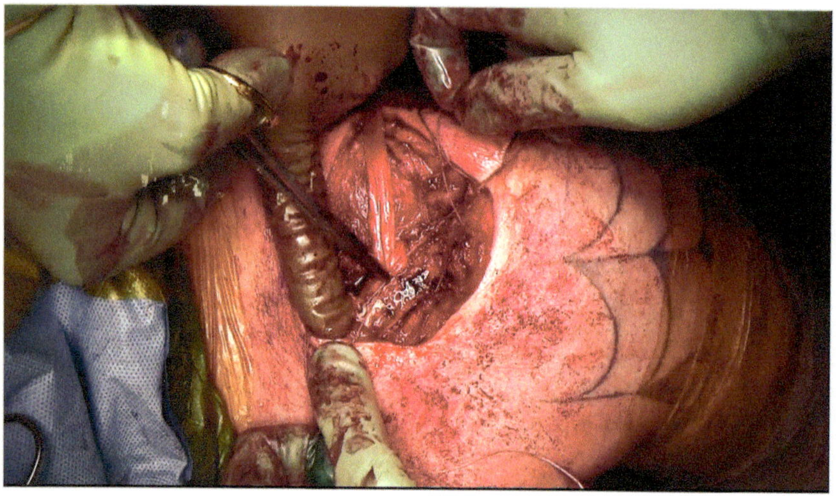

Fig. 71.5 Following allograft tenodesis, the nonbiologic fixation suture is used to form an internal brace.

reduction. At this point, the graft is tensioned to remove slack. With the joint reduced and tension on the graft maintained, a 5.5-mm tenodesis interference screw is placed in the anterior aspect of the conoid tunnel utilizing the nonbiologic fixation suture. The graft is retensioned and the second interference screw is placed in the anterior aspect of the trapezoid tunnel. The two limbs of the free suture are tied over the superior clavicle to form an internal brace (**Fig. 71.5**). Finally, the excess conoid graft is tied to the base of the excess trapezoid graft to create a biologic brace.

71.6.4 Acromioclavicular Fixation

The remaining capsuloligamentous structures of the AC joint are primarily repaired with interrupted sutures. Nonbiologic augmentation via high-strength, nonabsorbable, figure-of-8 suture is tensioned and tied with the joint anatomically reduced (**Fig. 71.6**). Biologic augmentation of the AC joint capsule reconstructs the anterior and posterior AC ligaments (**Video 71.5**). The excess graft from the trapezoid tunnel is laid over the posterior aspect of the joint and sutured to periosteum and the posterior ligaments. The graft is then laid superiorly and anteriorly over the AC joint and sutured to the anterior periosteum and remaining ligaments (**Fig. 71.7**). If graft length is sufficient, the remainder is sutured medially "onto itself" at the trapezoid tunnel, completing the biologic brace of the AC joint.

71.6.5 Wound Closure

Anatomic repair of the deltotrapezial fascia is critical to maintain coronal and sagittal plane stability of the distal clavicle. We utilize an interrupted inverted modified Donati technique, which invests the fascia over the superior surface of the clavicle and prevents skin irritation from bulky knots (**Fig. 71.8**, **Video 71.6**). The suture is initially passed superficial to deep through the deltoid fascia and similarly taken superficial to deep through the trapezial flap. The suture is then passed deep to superficial through the trapezial fascia and finished with a deep-to-superficial throw through the deltoid flap. All fascial sutures are sewn and clamped with hemostats prior to knot tying. The surgical assistant holds tension on the repair by pulling the hemostats, and the surgeon ties the sutures medially to laterally. Fascial closure is done with a nonabsorbable polyester suture. The deep dermal layer is closed with interrupted inverted 2–0 Vicryl sutures, and the skin is closed with a running 3–0 monofilament suture.

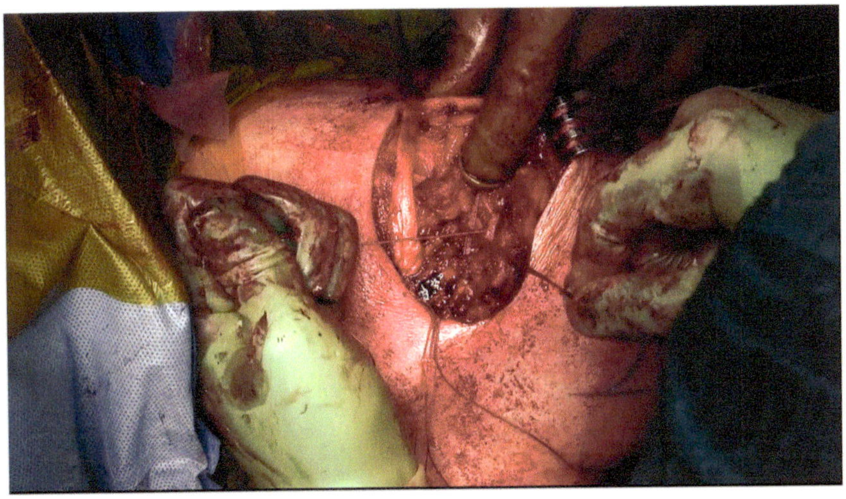

Fig. 71.6 While maintaining joint reduction, the high-strength nonabsorbable figure-of-8 acromioclavicular joint suture is tensioned and tied.

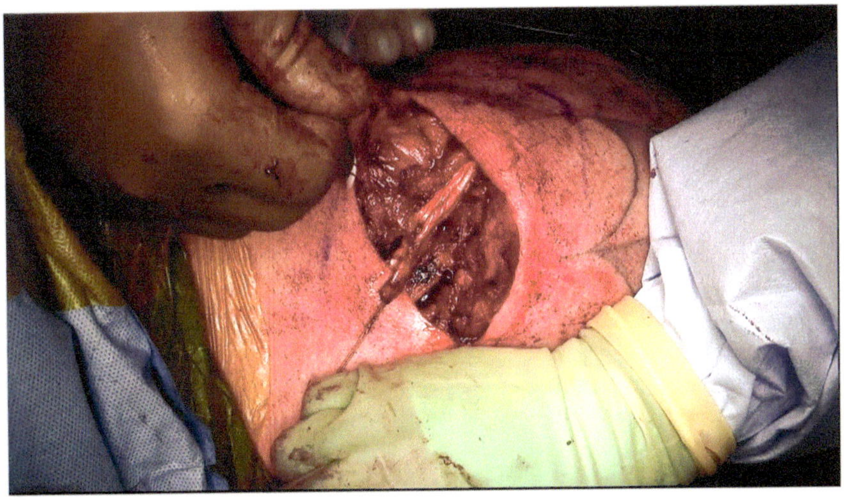

Fig. 71.7 The graft is secured first to the periosteum over the posterior acromioclavicular joint, then to the anterior periosteum, and then to itself at the trapezoid tunnel.

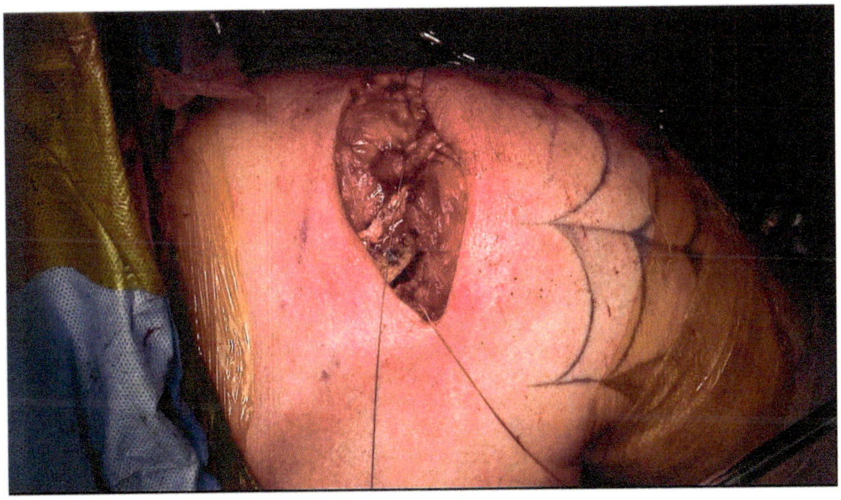

Fig. 71.8 An interrupted inverted modified Donati technique is used to close the deltotrapezial fascia over the acromioclavicular joint and clavicle.

71.7 Tips and Pearls/Expert Suggestions

- Positioning the patient as laterally as possible on the table allows the arm to move easily throughout the entire ROM, frees the scapula for reduction, and increases surgical field visualization.
- Reduction is achieved typically with support of the elbow and anterior translation of the clavicle. The mini C arm is utilized to check joint reduction intraoperatively.
- We prefer peroneus longus allograft for biologic reconstruction because it is easily attainable, has the required length of 110 mm, and does not require significant trimming to allow passage through the clavicular tunnels.
- The length of the tenodesis screws should not exceed 12 mm, no matter the measured length of the tunnels. Most procedures are performed with either 8- or 10-mm screws.
- The surgeon should maintain at least 20 mm of distance between the tunnels to prevent fracture and keep the tunnels greater than 3 mm from the anterior or posterior clavicular borders to prevent blowout during interference screw placement.

- It is important to note that the coracoid shuttling suture should be placed toward the anterior coracoid process, not at the base where the suture typically settles, to protect the suprascapular nerve during graft passage.

71.8 What to Avoid

- Ensure deltotrapezial fascial dissection utilizes full-thickness flaps and avoids violation of the musculature.
- Clavicular tunnels accepting allograft should not be less than 5 mm to prevent fracture during graft passage. Tunnels should be re-reamed in 0.5-mm increments if increased size is needed.
- Avoid placing the trapezoid tunnel less than 25 mm medial to the end of the clavicle in order to avoid the poorer bone quality of the distal clavicle.
- The senior author no longer performs concomitant distal clavicle excision to avoid postoperative anteroposterior instability of the distal clavicle.
- Fascial knots should be buried and placed as posteriorly as possible to avoid skin irritation.

71.9 Complications/Bailout/ Salvage

At times, the central aspect of the allograft can be bulbous and very difficult to pass. Significant tension on an impassable graft can lead to tendon bunching or shredding at the inferior tunnel aperture. If the tunnel is widened and the central graft still does not pass, the interfering tissue can be sharply debrided. Should the graft bunch and lose integrity, a limited debridement is performed to remove only the deformed aspect and a tenodesis screw is placed in one tunnel to "lock" the graft. The figure-of-8 AC suture is tied with the distal clavicle reduced. The remaining allograft is then maximally tensioned and fixed with a tenodesis screw.

In the presence of a coracoid fracture, a tunnel is created in the supraspinatus fossa to obtain inferior fixation. Dissection is used directly posterior to the coracoid base to visualize the fossa. Ideally, the location of the tunnel should be at the supraspinatus myotendinous junction. The supraspinatus is dissected off of the scapula bluntly and a 5-mm tunnel is created to allow graft passage. A curved suture passer is used inferior to superior to pass a suture shuttle. The surgeon should prevent iatrogenic injury to the suprascapular nerve.

71.10 Postoperative Care

Patients are initially immobilized for 6 to 8 weeks using a Lerman Shoulder Brace (DJO Inc., Vista, CA) or Gunslinger Shoulder Orthosis (Hangar Prosthetics and Orthotics, Inc., Bethesda, MA). A home exercise program emphasizes elbow, wrist, and hand ROM. Sling removal is allowed for grooming and hygiene as well as supervised supine gentle passive motion. After 8 weeks, active assist ROM is begun and progressed to upright active motion as pain allows. Closed chain exercises focus on scapular control. Motions that stress the AC joint, such as cross-body adduction, end-range forward flexion, and internal rotation, are avoided. At 12 weeks, full active ROM is allowed and resistance training is started. Strengthening exercises initially focus on scapular stabilization and retraction to prevent asymmetry during shoulder flexion and abduction. Weight training is progressed as tolerated once obtaining adequate scapular control. After 6 months, patients are cleared to return to contact sports and heavy lifting including overhead weightlifting, bench press, and shoulder press. Full strength typically returns at 9 to 12 months postoperatively.

References

1. Galatz LM, Williams GRAcromioclavicular joint injuries. In: Bucholz RW, Heckman JD, Court-Brown C, eds. Rockwood and Green's Fractures in Adults. Vol. 2. 6th ed. Philadelphia, PA: Lippincott Williams & Wilkins; 2006:1331–1364
2. Virk MS, Apostolakos J, Cote MP, Baker B, Beitzel K, Mazzocca AD. Operative and nonoperative treatment of acromioclavicular dislocation: a critical analysis review. JBJS Rev 2015;3(10):1–12
3. Dunphy TR, Damodar D, Heckmann ND, Sivasundaram L, Omid R, Hatch GF III. Functional outcomes of type V acromioclavicular injuries with nonsurgical treatment. J Am Acad Orthop Surg 2016;24(10):728–734
4. Mazzocca AD, Edgar CM, Beitzel K, Imhoff AB, DeBerardino TM, Arciero RAOpen surgical reconstruction of acute and chronic acromioclavicular joint instability. In: Craig EV, ed. The Shoulder. Philadelphia, PA: Lippincott Williams & Wilkins; 2013:231–242

72 Sternoclavicular Joint Reconstruction

Joseph M. Gentile and Russell Warren

Abstract
Sternoclavicular joint reconstruction with a biologic graft is a reliable surgical treatment for sternoclavicular joint dislocations and/or instability. We present our technique with surgical pearls and tips for optimal success.

Keywords: *sternoclavicular joint, instability, dislocations, graft reconstruction*

72.1 Goals of Procedure

- Improve pain and functional limitations.
- Ideally, restore full range of motion as well as return to preinjury sporting and daily activities.

72.2 Advantages

This technique is a biologic reconstruction, allowing avoidance of complications associated with hardware such as prominence and potential need for removal or possibly lethal migration as has been reported. This type of construct utilizing graft material, and its variations, has been shown to be superior to other techniques (i.e., subclavius tendon reconstruction and intramedullary ligament reconstruction) by biomechanical studies[1] and to have satisfactory clinical outcomes via various case reports.[2–5]

72.3 Indications

- Posterior dislocations as they are potentially life threatening due to the proximity of the medial clavicle to adjacent vital anatomic structures.
- Severely displaced or irreducible anterior dislocations.
- Recurrent symptomatic anterior instability or subluxations that have failed nonoperative treatment.

72.4 Contraindications

- No previous trial of closed reduction and/or sling immobilization.

72.5 Preoperative Preparation/ Positioning

Proper imaging is important prior to surgical intervention. Diagnosis is frequently missed; in one series, over 70% were undiagnosed in the primary care or emergency setting.[6] Standard X-rays will miss displacement of the medial clavicle. The "serendipity view" can be performed with the X-ray beam tilted 40 degrees cephalad in order to better assess anterior or posterior translation of the clavicle at the sternoclavicular joint (SCJ). CT scans are most reliable to assess both direction and magnitude of displacement. Alternatively, MRA can help assess the proximity of the mediastinal vessels.

The patient may be positioned supine, or in a modified beach-chair position with chest elevated approximately 30 to 60 degrees and a rolled towel or gel pad between the scapulae. The entire operative extremity including the anterior chest is prepped and draped (**Fig. 72.1**). The arm may be placed in an arm holder or left free supported on an arm board or a Mayo stand.

72.6 Operative Technique

An incision is made over the proximal clavicle and is carried to the mid-sternum. After dissecting through the subcutaneous tissue, the platysma is incised and raised as a separate layer in line with the incision. Periosteum is reflected off the clavicle superiorly and inferiorly. The capsule of the SCJ is also reflected superiorly and inferiorly, thus exposing the intra-articular disc, which is removed to allow for passage of our graft through the SCJ. In some patients, this disc has been torn, causing pain. Arthroscopic instruments are useful to complete the resection. Periosteum is then elevated off the sternum as well as the insertion of the ipsilateral sternocleidomastoid superiorly in order to visualize the sulcus of the superior sternum (**Fig. 72.2**). In dissecting the soft tissues off the clavicle and sternum, try to create a layer that can be reapproximated to the SCJ. Dissection of both the sternum and the clavicle should be sufficient to allow for passage of your soft-tissue graft. Our graft of choice is allograft semitendinosus; alternatively, gracilis or palmaris longus can be used, either auto- or allograft. The graft is prepared at either end with a no. 2 braided suture in a whip stitch fashion and each end is sized. Guide pins and cannulated drills can be used to make uni- or bicortical drill holes for graft passage, but we prefer to use a pneumatic burr in a unicortical fashion for both increased control and safety. Holes are made approximately 10 mm lateral to the SCJ on the clavicle and 10 mm medial to the SCJ on the sternum (**Fig. 72.3**). They are typically

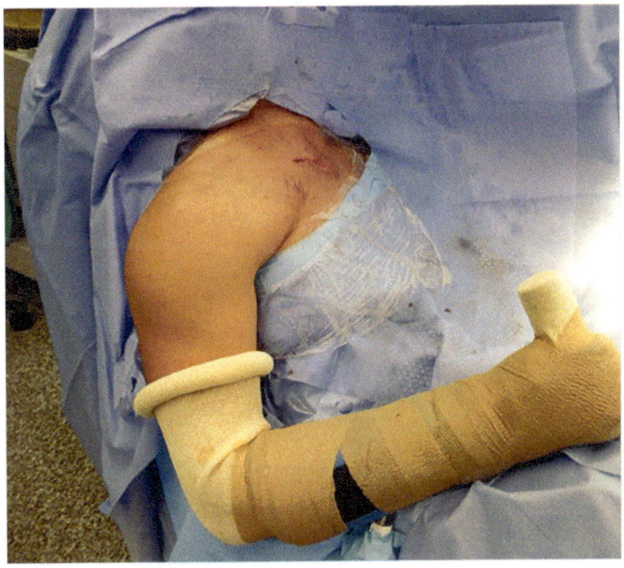

Fig. 72.1 Patient positioning.

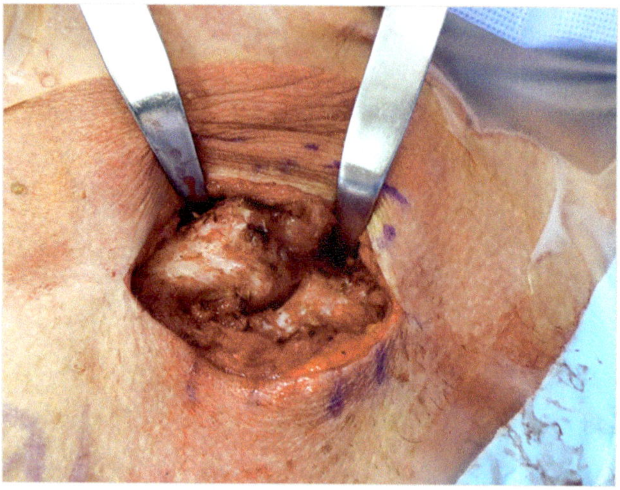

Fig. 72.2 Dissection of the sternoclavicular joint.

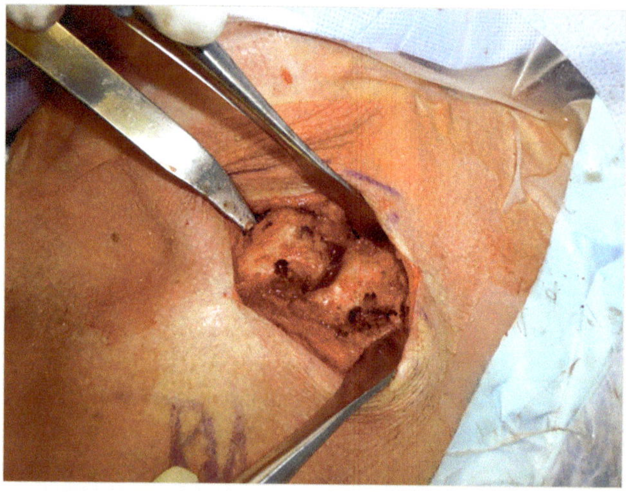

Fig. 72.3 Burr holes for passage of the graft.

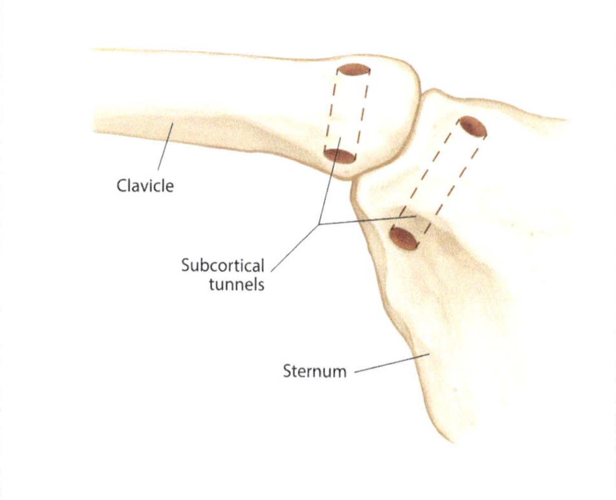

Fig. 72.4 Schematic of burr holes and subcortical tunnels.

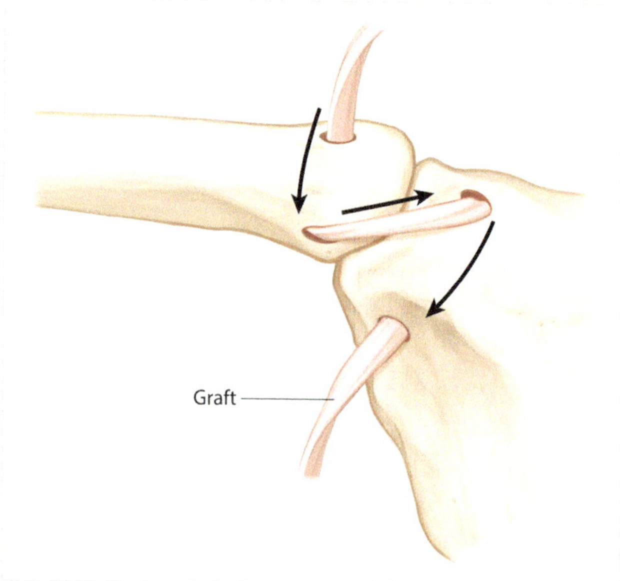

Fig. 72.5 Graft is passed from superior to inferior through the clavicular tunnel, then taken diagonally across the sternoclavicular joint and passed from superior to inferior through the sternum.

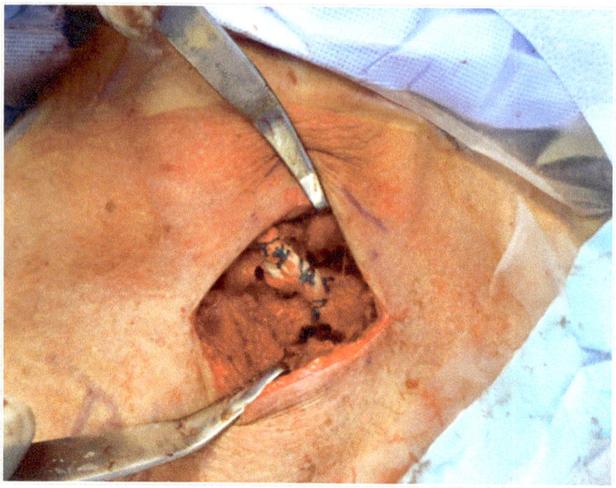

Fig. 72.6 Completed construct.

3 to 4.5 mm in size, depending on the size of the graft. These holes are connected with a sharp curette to form subcortical tunnels (**Fig. 72.4**). No posterior dissection is required unless significant scarring is present. Shuttling sutures or devices can be used to assist in graft passage. The graft is passed in a simple figure-of-8 fashion passing anteriorly or if desired passing through the SCJ (**Fig. 72.5**).

If subluxed or dislocated, the SCJ should be reduced, taking care not to over-reduce and posteriorly displace the clavicle. The articular surfaces of the SCJ should be aligned. If reduction is not possible, the clavicle can be shortened to allow reduction. Fixation is achieved when sutures are placed between the free ends of the graft as well as at any points the graft crosses itself (**Fig. 72.6**). Augmentation of fixation is an option with the addition of tenodesis screws, analogous to CC joint reconstruction, which may minimize the amount of potentially prominent suture material anteriorly.[7] Periosteum and joint capsule are then repaired using a no. 0 nonabsorbable suture, followed by the platysma, subcutaneous tissue, and skin in layers.

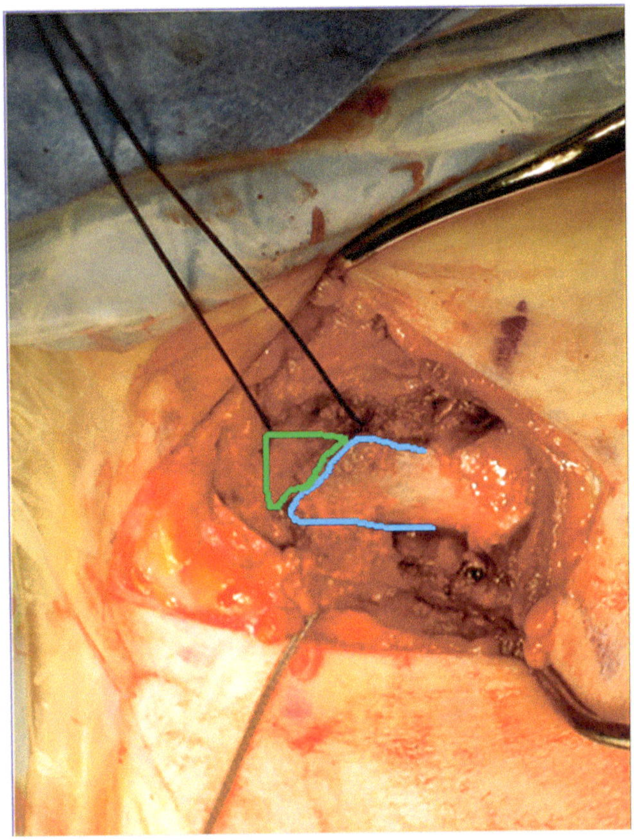

Fig. 72.7 Left sternoclavicular joint fracture-dislocation, reduced. Medial epiphyseal fragment is outlined in *green* and lateral clavicular fragment in *blue*. Heavy sutures are placed in the periosteal sleeve, superior and inferior.

72.7 Tips and Pearls/Expert Suggestions

If acute, posterior dislocations are relatively easy to reduce. In particular, in patients younger than 25 years, manipulation of the clavicle from underneath the manubrium is easily done in the first few days after injury, but generally beyond this time period an open procedure is necessary. If chronic, the clavicle can scar onto the vessels, making dissection difficult and warranting a pre-op MRA and surgery performed in an OR with vascular capability and a thoracic surgeon. Once the clavicle is pulled laterally, using the arm to manipulate, it should reduce to the medial component. Acute cases can be sutured to the medial component to create stability. As the medial clavicular epiphysis begins to ossify at the age of 18 to 20 years, and does not fully ossify until the age of 22 to 26 years, individuals in this age range can sustain a fracture dislocation through the medial clavicular epiphysis as the sternoclavicular ligaments primarily insert on the epiphysis (**Fig. 72.7**). This leaves the physis unprotected outside the capsule. There is generally a robust periosteal sleeve, connected to the sternoclavicular ligaments, which can be repaired once the clavicle is reduced to the manubrium and epiphyseal fragment and creates a stable construct (**Fig. 72.8**). Chronic (posterior) cases may need a graft procedure, similar to those with anterior instability, using a semitendinosus tendon.

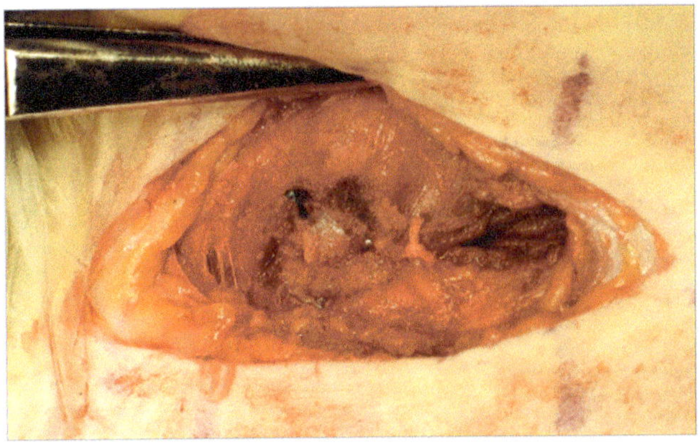

Fig. 72.8 Completed repair of surrounding periosteum and ligamentous sleeve.

72.8 What to Avoid

Posterior displacement of the clavicle should be avoided during reduction in order to prevent injury to the adjacent vital structures as well as over-reduction, which can compromise outcomes. Techniques have been described which utilize bicortical holes through the sternum and/or the clavicle; this requires not only exposure posteriorly of these structures but also the risk of drill passage posteriorly into vital structures in near proximity if not properly prevented.

72.9 Complications/Bailout/ Salvage

For chronic posterior dislocations, it is prudent to have vascular or thoracic surgeon assistance or backup available as well as be in the correct surgical setting (potentially even a vascular suite) in case damage to the posterior vital structures occurs or has occurred due to the initial injury. Persistent instability and pain are the common reasons for failure after initial reconstruction surgery.[8] Revision procedures can be performed including medial clavicular resection, especially if degeneration in the joint is seen.

72.10 Postoperative Care

Sling immobilization is required for 6 weeks. Shoulder pendulums three times a day are allowed. At 6 weeks, shoulder range of motion is initiated below 90 degrees and the sling is weaned. Range of motion is advanced to full at 12 weeks and strengthening is initiated. Return to sports activities or manual work activities are allowed by 5 to 6 months after surgery.

References

1. Spencer EE Jr., Kuhn JE. Biomechanical analysis of reconstructions for sternoclavicular joint instability. J Bone Joint Surg Am 2004;86-A(1):98–105
2. Petri M, Greenspoon JA, Horan MP, Martetschläger F, Warth RJ, Millett PJ. Clinical outcomes after autograft reconstruction for sternoclavicular joint instability. J Shoulder Elbow Surg 2016;25(3):435–441

3. Kusnezov N, Dunn JC, DeLong JM, Waterman BR. Sternoclavicular reconstruction in the young active patient: risk factor analysis and clinical outcomes at short-term follow-up. J Orthop Trauma 2016;30(4):e111–e117
4. Sabatini JB, Shung JR, Clay TB, Oladeji LO, Minnich DJ, Ponce BA. Outcomes of augmented allograft figure-of-eight sternoclavicular joint reconstruction. J Shoulder Elbow Surg 2015;24(6):902–907
5. Sewell MD, Al-Hadithy N, Le Leu A, Lambert SM. Instability of the sternoclavicular joint: current concepts in classification, treatment and outcomes. Bone Joint J 2013;95-B(6):721–731
6. Terra BB, Rodrigues LM, Pádua DV, Martins MG, Teixeira JC, De Nadai A. Sternoclavicular dislocation: case report and surgical technique. Rev Bras Ortop 2015;50(4):472–477
7. Sabatini JB, Shung JR, Clay TB, Oladeji LO, Minnich DJ, Ponce BA. Outcomes of augmented allograft figure-of-eight sternoclavicular joint reconstruction. J Shoulder Elbow Surg 2015;24(6):902–907
8. Sewell MD, Al-Hadithy N, Le Leu A, Lambert SM. Instability of the sternoclavicular joint: current concepts in classification, treatment and outcomes. Bone Joint J 2013;95-B(6):721–731

73 Pectoralis Major Repair

Lionel E. Lazaro and Frank A. Cordasco

Abstract
This chapter will provide the reader with an overview of the indications, contraindications, preoperative preparation, operative technique, and the authors' tips, pearls, key points, and postoperative rehabilitation.

Keywords: *pectoralis tendon tear, pectoralis tendon repair, sternocostal head tear, bench pressing, NFL injuries*

73.1 Goals of Procedure

Rupture of the pectoralis major (PM) can lead to significant functional deficits, especially during labor-intensive actions and athletic activities.[1–5] The objective of the anatomical repair is to restore the function of the PM as a potent adductor, internal rotator, and dynamic stabilizer of the glenohumeral joint.[6–8]

73.2 Advantages

In the elderly and the low-demand patient, nonoperative treatment can result in good functional outcomes during activities of daily living.[1,2,9–12] However, athletes and laborers treated nonoperatively are unable to return to their preinjury level of activity.[1,2,4,5] Several studies have demonstrated surgical treatment provides the ability to return to a preinjury level of activity with great patient satisfaction and enhanced cosmesis.[2–5,7–10,13–21]

73.3 Indications

Injuries proximal to the muscle–tendon junction, muscle contusions and strains, partial tears, and complete tears (Tietjen's classification[22] types I, II, IIIA, and IIIB) in the low-demand patient are treated without surgery.[2] Tendon ruptures at the insertion site or intrasubstance in the athletes (Tietjen's classification types IIIC and IIID, and Bak et al's modification types IIIE and IIIF), workers, and patients with cosmetic deformity of axillary fold are indicated for surgical repair.[13,22] Surgical treatment of chronic injuries can lead to satisfactory outcomes, and should not prohibit surgical treatment.[5,7,16]

73.4 Contraindications

Complete tears in patients with multiple comorbidities and low-demand (elderly, nonworker, and sedentary) patients are contraindicated for surgical repair.

73.5 Preoperative Preparation

A detailed history and focused physical examination is of paramount importance. Patients usually recall the injury and are able to describe the mechanism of injury. They complain of weakness, swelling, ecchymosis, asymmetry, and pain in the axilla and chest wall. In acute injuries, the amount of swelling, pain, and ecchymosis may confound the clinical scenario particularly if presented in the emergency department or primary care setting.[2,20,23–27] Advanced imaging is extremely helpful, especially during the acute presentation, to provide for further clarity of the clinical picture and facilitate an accurate and timely diagnosis.[2,20,23–27]

MRI is the favored imaging technique. Imaging can differentiate between partial and complete tears, whether the tear involves both the clavicular head (CH) and sternocostal heads (SH) or often in the context of weight training, an isolated SH tear.[20,27–29] MRI can also facilitate the distinction between acute and chronic PM tendon injuries.[26] At our institution, an axial fast-spin echo (FSE) MRI is obtained first, then the oblique coronal images are determined and acquired based upon the orientation of the axial images in parallel to the long axis of the PM tendon complex. Additionally, a coronal inversion recovery sequence is acquired in a comparable mode.

73.5.1 Positioning

Following combined regional and general anesthesia, the patient is placed in the beach-chair position with the operative arm in a positioner (**Fig. 73.1**). The operative area is covered and sealed using an Ioban drape (3M, St. Paul, MN).

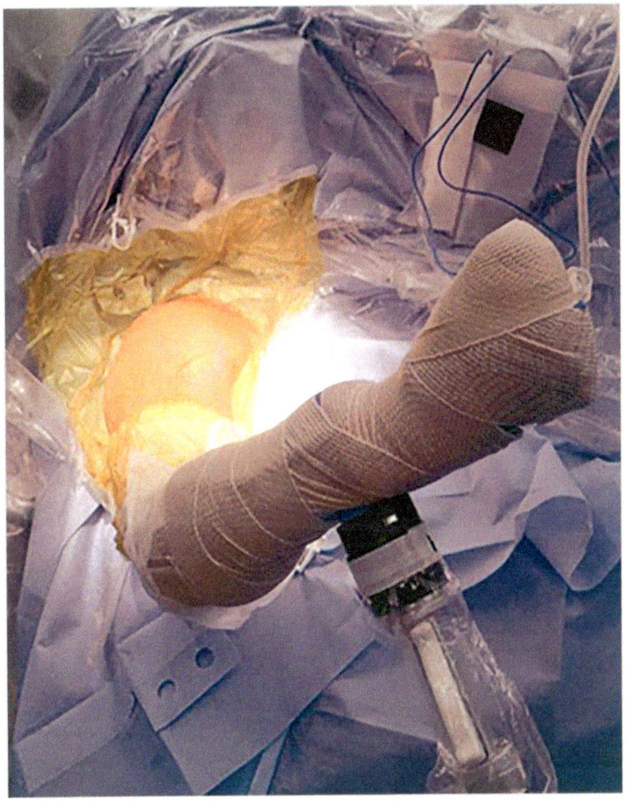

Fig. 73.1 Photograph depicting the patient in the beach-chair position with the operative arm in a mechanical arm holder. The surgical area is covered and sealed using an Ioban drape.

73.6 Operative Technique

The distal part of the deltopectoral approach is used for surgical exposure (**Fig. 73.2**). In cases of CH and SH tears, the torn and retracted tendon is identified on the deep, posterior aspect of the muscle, released from adhesions, and mobilized. When an isolated SH tear is present, the deltopectoral interval will be intact. Cordasco et al have reported that isolated SH tears occur in the majority of weight training injuries (described as indirect injuries) compared to injuries that involve both the CH and SH, which have occurred with trauma, so-called direct injuries.[20] The approach will not, in general, require a deltopectoral interval takedown, as it is important to leave the CH insertion intact. By developing a plane inferior to the CH, the SH stump can be identified and repaired without compromising the CH insertion. The tendon edges are then debrided of mechanically incompetent tissue. In general, two sets of locking no. 2 FiberWire sutures (Arthrex, Naples, FL) are applied to each torn head, using a modified Krackow suture arrangement with four suture limbs for each head (**Figs. 73.3, 73.4**). These stiches are deployed to the superior and inferior areas of each ruptured tendon.

To identify the PM footprint, lateral to the bicipital groove, a retractor is placed along the lateral side of the humerus to retract the anterior deltoid. The humeral insertion site is debrided, while protecting the long head of the biceps. Electrocautery is utilized to mark the site of implant placement. A 3.2-mm guide pin (Arthrex) is utilized to establish four unicortical drill holes. These are placed in a staggered fashion, leaving a sufficient bone bridge to avoid increasing the risk of fracture. To gain intramedullary (IM) length to flip the cortical buttons, the drill holes are angled. The titanium buttons are preloaded with two no. 2 FiberWire (high-

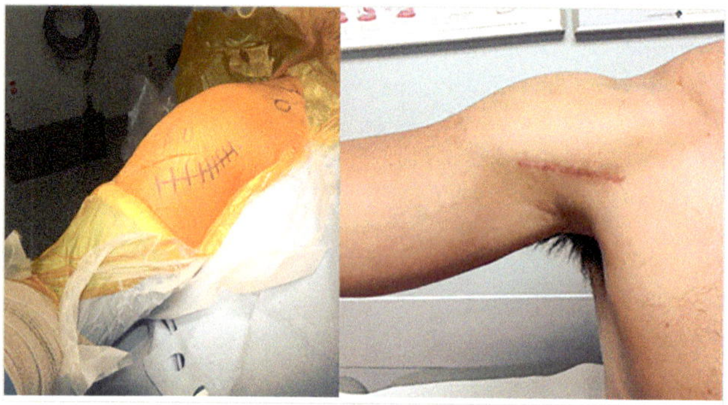

Fig. 73.2 The left photograph depicts the marking of the planned incision utilizing the distal aspect of the deltopectoral approach. The right photograph demonstrates healed incision utilizing the distal aspect of the deltopectoral approach. (Adapted from Lazaro L and Cordasco FA: Pectoralis Major Injury. In: Arciero RA, Cordasco FA, Provencher MT eds: Shoulder and Elbow Injuries in Athletes. Elsevier, Philadelphia. 2018, p. 387–401.)

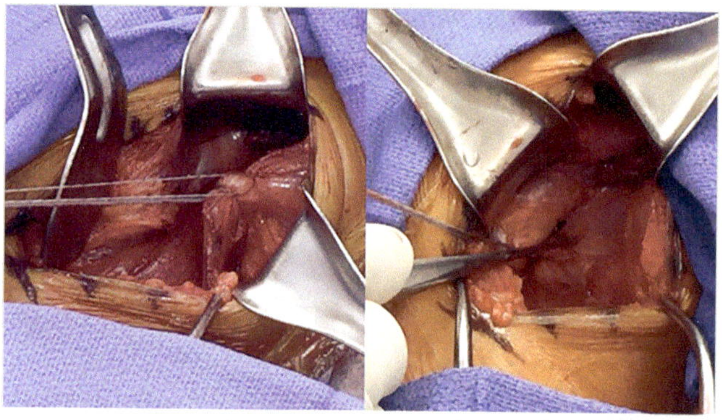

Fig. 73.4 The left photograph demonstrates the high-strength nonabsorbable sutures applied to the sternocostal head. The right photograph demonstrates tendon reduced and secured to the footprint. (Adapted from Lazaro L and Cordasco FA: Pectoralis Major Injury. In: Arciero RA, Cordasco FA, Provencher MT eds: Shoulder and Elbow Injuries in Athletes. Elsevier, Philadelphia. 2018, p. 387–401.) Prevention, Treatment and Return to Sport. In press.)

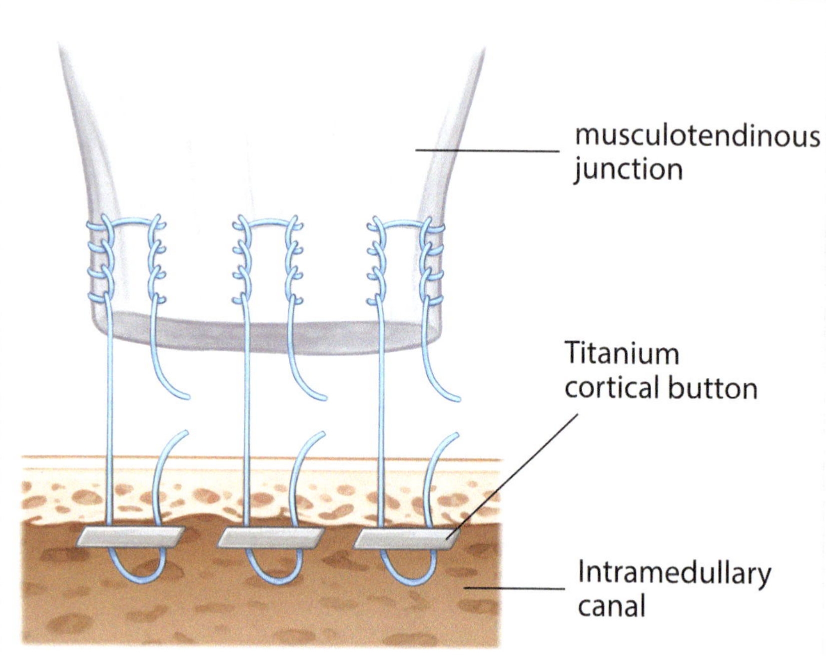

Fig. 73.3 Depiction of the fixation construct with the intramedullary unicortical implant and the high-strength nonabsorbable sutures applied to one of the tendon heads.

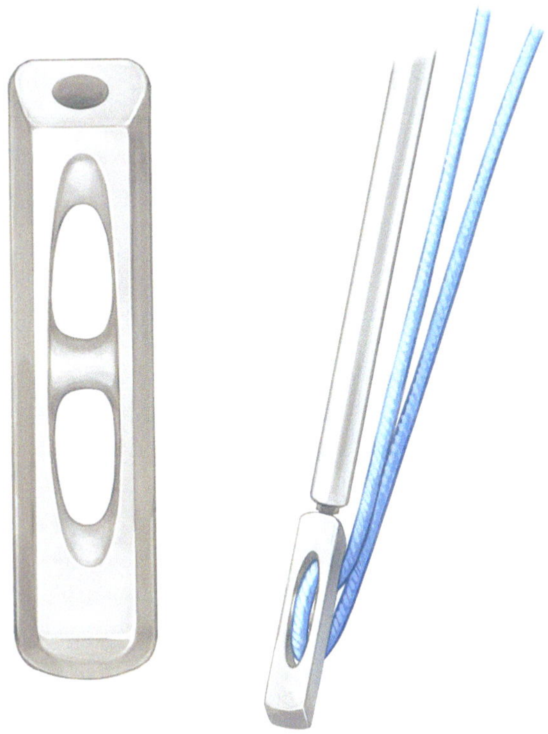

Fig. 73.5 The implant (titanium cortical button) utilized for the repair.

strength nonabsorbable) sutures (**Fig. 73.5**). The button is deployed into the IM canal and the tendon reduction is performed by tensioning the suture limbs to the footprint.[1,30] The anatomic reduction and fixation are performed with the arm in adduction and neutral position. The SH is reduced first, given that the footprint is more posterior and more proximal than the CH (**Fig. 73.6**). Sutures in the SH are tensioned first, then the CH, and then secured by standard knots.

Generally, a total of four buttons (two per head) are used for complete ruptures. Fluoroscopy is then used to confirm correct button position (**Fig. 73.7**). Following wound irrigation, a layered closure is performed and the arm is then placed in a sling in an adducted position.

73.7 Tips and Pearls/Expert Suggestions

73.7.1 Pearls

- In cases of isolated SH tears, the surgical approach is best performed by elevating the CH superiorly to access the retracted stump of the SH. It is not generally necessary to compromise the deltopectoral interval.
- The drill should be angled slightly when drilling the unicortical drill hole, to facilitate deployment of the button in narrower IM canals.
- Prior to reduction and fixation, the arm is placed into an adducted and neutral position to reduce tension forces on the surgical repair.
- To maintain direct visualization of each head during reduction and fixation, the SH is reduced and fixed first. The insertion site is more posterior and proximal relative to the CH insertion.
- To confirm adequate deployment of the implants, intraoperative fluoroscopy is obtained at the end of the procedure.

73.7.2 Pitfalls and Risks

- To decrease risk of fracture, adequate bone bridges between drill holes should be maintained.
- Given the metallic composition of the implants, a metal-suppressive MRI sequence may be needed to minimize metal artifact in the unusual event that postoperative imaging is necessary.

73.7.3 Key Points

- Surgical repair of PM rupture in active adults, athletes, and laborers achieves better functional outcomes than nonoperative treatment.
- The unicortical buttons are associated with a lower risk of fracture, compared with bicortical fixation.
- Tensioning button fixation has the advantage of reducing the tendon to the footprint by pulling it to the footprint as opposed to suture anchor or transosseous techniques that push the knot to the footprint.
- When athletes achieve their sport- and position-specific rehabilitation criterion, they can return to contact sports between 5 and 6 months.

73.8 What the Authors Personally Have Found Is Important to Make the Case Go Smoothly

- PM tears should be repaired surgically as soon as possible after the injury, preferably within a week to 10 days. This will facilitate the approach and dissection and minimize surgical time.
- Appropriate preoperative advanced imaging and planning is vital.
- Correct positioning and draping is essential to allow for complete access to the planned surgical area.
- Maintaining hemostasis is important to sustain direct visualization.
- Adequate release of scar tissue and mobilization of the ruptured tendon is paramount.
- Altering the surgical approach depending upon whether the repair involves a complete CH and SH tear or an isolated SH tear.

73.9 What to Avoid

- Precise dissection and careful retraction is essential to avoid injury to the pectoralis nerve, especially inferior and medial to the coracoid.[31]
- Excellent exposure and direct visualization of the lateral lip of the bicipital grove (footprint region) while prepping the bone, drilling, and placing the implants is essential to avoid

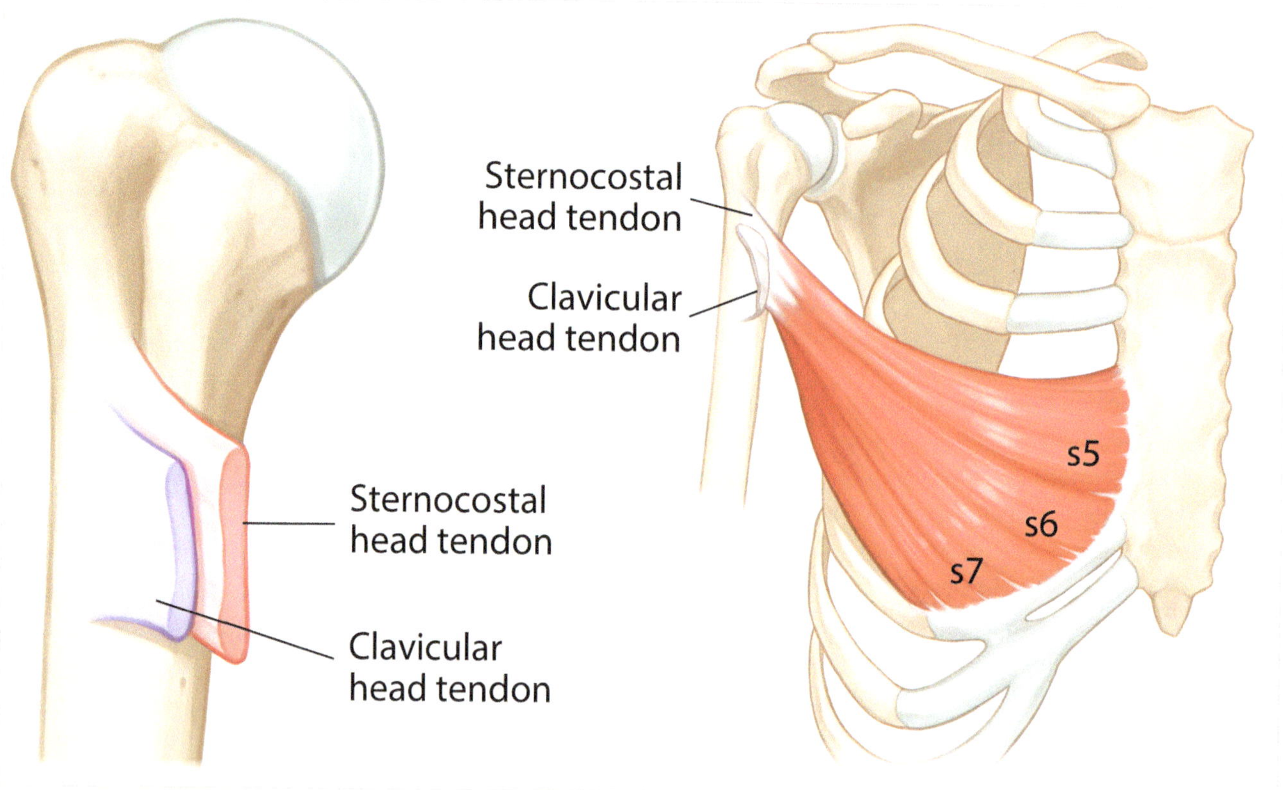

Fig. 73.6 The bilaminar conjoined tendon along the lateral lip of the bicipital grove. The clavicular head and the superior segments of the sternocostal head constitute the anterior and inferior tendon laminar fibers. The middle portion of the sternocostal head constitutes the inferior **U**-shaped insertion to the anterior and posterior laminar fibers. The lower portion of the sternocostal head constitutes the more proximal segment of the posterior laminar fibers, inserting more proximal in the humerus than the anterior layer.

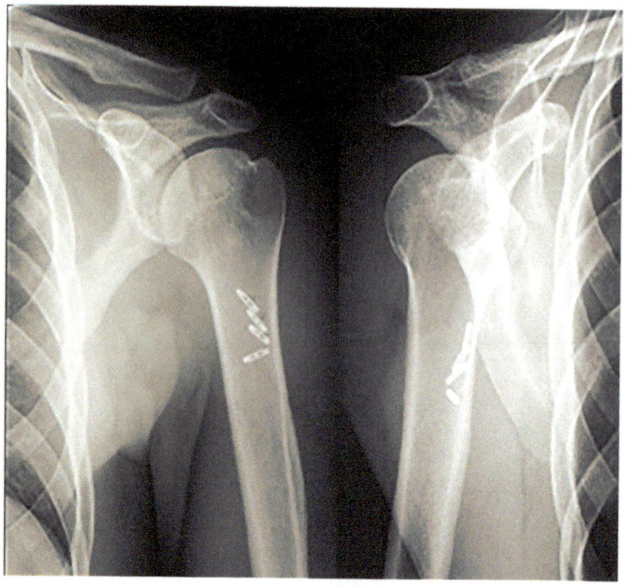

Fig. 73.7 Radiographs demonstrate the intramedullary implants applied in a staggered fashion lateral to the bicipital grove.

injury or subsequent compression to the long head of the biceps.

- Drill holes are placed in staggered fashion to maintain adequate bony bridge and avoiding a stress riser and humeral fracture.
- To minimize the risk of failure, avoid performing a tendon to bone repair under increased tension. If the released tendon cannot be reapproximated to the footprint without tension, then an allograft should be considered to perform the repair. This is not usually necessary except in the most chronic injuries.
- Avoid compromising the deltopectoral interval in isolated SH repairs.

73.10 What Can Go Wrong and How to Manage

A chronic PM rupture can be challenging because of the increase scarring and poor quality of the remnant tissue. After meticulous dissection, extensive release and debridement of the available tissue may not be sufficient to reapproximate the native tendon to the footprint. In those cases, a primary repair of tendon to bone cannot be performed, and an Achilles tendon allograft can be used for the surgical repair. The proximal edge of the allograft is fixed to the musculotendinous junction with a modified Krackow suture technique.[32,33]

In the rare case that the cortical button failed to deploy or flip in the medullary canal and you are able to remove the implant, attempts can be made to revise the unicortical drill hole in a greater angle to facilitate deployment. If that maneuver fails, another fixation method will need to be utilized, such as suture anchors or transosseous suture techniques.[2,5]

73.11 Postoperative Care

Depending on the quality of the repaired tissue and the chronicity of the injury, the patients are instructed to use a sling for 4 to 6 weeks. Progressive range-of-motion exercises are implemented from 6 to 12 weeks. At 3 months following surgery, additional strengthening and sport-specific rehabilitation begins. In the senior author's experience, the patients can return to full activities at 5 to 6 months postoperatively.[20]

References

1. Kang RW, Mahony GT, Cordasco FA. Pectoralis major repair with cortical button technique. Arthrosc Tech 2014;3(1):e73–e77
2. Haley CA, Zacchilli MA. Pectoralis major injuries: evaluation and treatment. Clin Sports Med 2014;33(4):739–756
3. de Castro Pochini A, Ejnisman B, Andreoli CV, et al. Pectoralis major muscle rupture in athletes: a prospective study. Am J Sports Med 2010;38(1):92–98
4. Zeman SC, Rosenfeld RT, Lipscomb PR. Tears of the pectoralis major muscle. Am J Sports Med 1979;7(6):343–347
5. Schepsis AA, Grafe MW, Jones HP, Lemos MJ. Rupture of the pectoralis major muscle. Outcome after repair of acute and chronic injuries. Am J Sports Med 2000;28(1):9–15
6. Petilon J, Carr DR, Sekiya JK, Unger DV. Pectoralis major muscle injuries: evaluation and management. J Am Acad Orthop Surg 2005;13(1):59–68
7. Quinlan JF, Molloy M, Hurson BJ. Pectoralis major tendon ruptures: when to operate. Br J Sports Med 2002;36(3):226–228
8. Cordasco FA and Delos, D: Pectoralis Major Rupture: Diagnosis and Treatment. In: Iannotti, Miniaci, Williams and Zuckerman eds: Disorders of the Shoulder: Diagnosis and Management, 3rd Edition Vol II: Shoulder Sports Injuries. Philadelphia, Lippincott Williams & Wilkins, 2013, p. 371-380.
9. Wolfe SW, Wickiewicz TL, Cavanaugh JT. Ruptures of the pectoralis major muscle. An anatomic and clinical analysis. Am J Sports Med 1992;20(5):587–593
10. McEntire JE, Hess WE, Coleman SS. Rupture of the pectoralis major muscle. A report of eleven injuries and review of fifty-six. J Bone Joint Surg Am 1972;54(5):1040–1046
11. Scott BW, Wallace WA, Barton MA. Diagnosis and assessment of pectoralis major rupture by dynamometry. J Bone Joint Surg Br 1992;74(1):111–113
12. Beloosesky Y, Grinblat J, Weiss A, Rosenberg PH, Weisbort M, Hendel D. Pectoralis major rupture in elderly patients: a clinical study of 13 patients. Clin Orthop Relat Res 2003(413):164–169
13. Bak K, Cameron EA, Henderson IJ. Rupture of the pectoralis major: a meta-analysis of 112 cases. Knee Surg Sports Traumatol Arthrosc 2000;8(2):113–119
14. de Castro Pochini A, Andreoli CV, Belangero PS, et al. Clinical considerations for the surgical treatment of pectoralis major muscle ruptures based on 60 cases: a prospective study and literature review. Am J Sports Med 2014;42(1):95–102
15. Pavlik A, Csépai D, Berkes I. Surgical treatment of pectoralis major rupture in athletes. Knee Surg Sports Traumatol Arthrosc 1998;6(2):129–133
16. Hanna CM, Glenny AB, Stanley SN, Caughey MA. Pectoralis major tears: comparison of surgical and conservative treatment. Br J Sports Med 2001;35(3):202–206
17. Park JY, Espiniella JL. Rupture of pectoralis major muscle. A case report and review of literature. J Bone Joint Surg Am 1970;52(3):577–581
18. Kretzler HH Jr, Richardson AB. Rupture of the pectoralis major muscle. Am J Sports Med 1989;17(4):453–458
19. Antosh IJ, Grassbaugh JA, Parada SA, Arrington ED. Pectoralis major tendon repairs in the active-duty population. Am J Orthop 2009;38(1):26–30
20. Cordasco FA, Mahony GT, Tsouris N, Degen RM. Pectoralis major tendon tears: functional outcomes and return to sport in a consecutive series of 40 athletes. J Shoulder Elbow Surg 2016
21. Cordasco FA. Outcome of Pectoralis Major Tendon Repair : Does Study Design Matter?: Commentary on an article by Drew W. Nute, MD, et al: "Return to Function, Complication, and Reoperation Rates Following Primary Pectoralis Major Tendon Repair in Military Service Members." J Bone Joint Surg Am. 2017 Jan 4;99(1):e4. doi: 10.2106/JBJS.16.00786
22. Tietjen R. Closed injuries of the pectoralis major muscle. J Trauma 1980;20(3):262–264
23. Lee J, Brookenthal KR, Ramsey ML, Kneeland JB, Herzog R. MR imaging assessment of the pectoralis major myotendinous unit: an MR imaging-anatomic correlative study with surgical correlation. AJR Am J Roentgenol 2000;174(5):1371–1375
24. Weaver JS, Jacobson JA, Jamadar DA, Theisen SE, Ebrahim F, Kalume-Brigido M. Sonographic findings of pectoralis major tears with surgical, clinical, and magnetic resonance imaging correlation in 6 patients. J Ultrasound Med 2005;24(1):25–31
25. Miller MD, Johnson DL, Fu FH, Thaete FL, Blanc RO. Rupture of the pectoralis major muscle in a collegiate football player. Use of magnetic resonance imaging in early diagnosis. Am J Sports Med 1993;21(3):475–477
26. Connell DA, Potter HG, Sherman MF, Wickiewicz TL. Injuries of the pectoralis major muscle: evaluation with MR imaging. Radiology 1999;210(3):785–791
27. Carrino JA, Chandnanni VP, Mitchell DB, Choi-Chinn K, DeBerardino TM, Miller MD. Pectoralis major muscle and tendon tears: diagnosis and grading using magnetic resonance imaging. Skeletal Radiol 2000;29(6):305–313
28. Egan TM, Hall H. Avulsion of the pectoralis major tendon in a weight lifter: repair using a barbed staple. Can J Surg 1987;30(6):434–435
29. Ohashi K, El-Khoury GY, Albright JP, Tearse DS. MRI of complete rupture of the pectoralis major muscle. Skeletal Radiol 1996;25(7):625–628
30. Sherman SL, Lin EC, Verma NN, et al. Biomechanical analysis of the pectoralis major tendon and comparison of techniques for tendo-osseous repair. Am J Sports Med 2012;40(8):1887–1894
31. Provencher MT, Handfield K, Boniquit NT, Reiff SN, Sekiya JK, Romeo AA. Injuries to the pectoralis major muscle: diagnosis and management. Am J Sports Med 2010;38(8):1693–1705
32. Zacchilli MA, Fowler JT, Owens BD. Allograft reconstruction of chronic pectoralis major tendon ruptures. J Surg Orthop Adv 2013;22(1):95–102
33. Joseph TA, Defranco MJ, Weiker GG. Delayed repair of a pectoralis major tendon rupture with allograft: a case report. J Shoulder Elbow Surg 2003;12(1):101–104

Index

Note: The notations *f* or *t* indicate figures or tables, respectively.

S

T

U

V

W

Z